PULMONARY
VASCULAR DISEASES

LUNG BIOLOGY IN HEALTH AND DISEASE

Executive Editor: **Claude Lenfant**
Director, Division of Lung Diseases
National Institutes of Health
Bethesda, Maryland

PULMONARY VASCULAR DISEASES

Edited by

Kenneth M. Moser

University of California, San Diego
School of Medicine
San Diego, California

MARCEL DEKKER, INC.   New York · Basel

Library of Congress Cataloging in Publication Data

Main entry under title:

Pulmonary vascular diseases.

(Lung biology in health and disease ; v. 14)
Includes bibliographical references and indexes.
1. Lungs–Blood-vessels–Diseases. I. Moser,
Kenneth M. II. Series.
RC756.L83 vol. 14 [RC776.V37] 616.2'4'008s
ISBN 0-8247-6609-1 [616.2'4] 79-22995

MARCEL DEKKER, INC.
270 Madison Avenue, New York, New York 10016

Current printing (last digit):
10 9 8 7 6 5 4 3 2 1

PRINTED IN THE UNITED STATES OF AMERICA

CONTRIBUTORS

Edward H. Bergofsky, B.S., M.D.   Professor of Medicine and Head, Pulmonary Disease Division, Department of Medicine, State University of New York at Stony Brook, Stony Brook, Long Island, New York

Leon Cudkowicz, F.R.C.P., M.D.   Professor, Department of Medicine, Wright State University School of Medicine, Dayton, Ohio

Lewis Dexter, A.B., M.D.   Professor Emeritus, Department of Medicine, Peter Bent Brigham Hospital, Harvard Medical School, Boston, Massachusetts

Jesse E. Edwards, B.S., M.D.   Senior Consultant in Anatomic Pathology, Department of Pathology, United Hospitals, St. Paul, Minnesota; Professor of Pathology, Department of Pathology, University of Minnesota, Minneapolis, Minnesota

Gabriel Gregoratos, A.B., M.D.   Associate Clinical Professor, Division of Cardiology, Department of Medicine, University of California San Diego School of Medicine, San Diego, California

Donald Heath, M.D., Ph.D., F.R.C.P., F.R.C.Path.   George Holt Professor of Pathology, Department of Pathology, University of Liverpool, Liverpool, England

Joel S. Karliner, M.D., F.A.C.P., F.A.C.C.   Associate Professor, Department of Medicine; Director of Clinical Cardiology, Division of Cardiology, University of California, San Diego, School of Medicine, San Diego, California

Kenneth M. Moser, M.D.   Director, Pulmonary Division; Professor, Department of Medicine, University of California, San Diego, School of Medicine, San Diego, California

Joseph K. Perloff, B.A., M.A., M.D.   Professor, Departments of Medicine and Pediatrics, University of California, Los Angeles, School of Medicine, Los Angeles, California

John T. Reeves, M.D., B.S.   Professor, Department of Medicine, University of Colorado Medical Center, Denver, Colorado

Paul Smith, B.Sc., Ph.D.   Senior Lecturer, Department of Pathology, University of Liverpool, Liverpool, England

William M. Thurlbeck, M.B., Ch. B., F.R.C.P.(C), F.R.C.Path., F.C.C.P.
Professor and Head, Department of Pathology, University of Manitoba; Director, Department of Pathology, Health Sciences Center, Winnipeg, Manitoba, Canada

Norbert F. Voelkel, M.D.   Research Fellow, Cardiovascular Pulmonary Research Laboratory, University of Colorado Medical Center, Denver, Colorado

C.A. Wagenvoort, M.D., F.R.C.Path.   Professor and Chairman, Department of Pathological Anatomy, University of Amsterdam, Amsterdam, The Netherlands

Noeke Wagenvoort   Department of Pathological Anatomy, University of Amsterdam, Amsterdam, The Netherlands

FOREWORD

Most of us who are asked to name how the great advances in modern medicine and surgery have come about, would probably respond by listing some Nobel laureates and the discoveries closely linked with their names: for example, Roentgen and X-rays; Koch and the tubercle bacillus; Fleming and penicillin; Enders and culture of polio virus; Banting and insulin. Yet, once in awhile, an event that is ineligible for a Nobel Prize has had just as important an impact on medical advance as one that was eligible and won an award. One such event was Abraham Flexner's 1910 report "Medical Education in the United States and Canada" that resulted in a considerable decrease in the number of American medical schools and a considerable increase in their quality and in the scientific content of their curricula. Another was the opening of the Johns Hopkins Medical School in 1893, staffed by four professors, each outstanding as a scientist in his specialty and each believing in joining scientific research, medical education, and patient care.

Sometimes a book or a series of books has had a strong influence on the advance of medical science. One such book was the first edition of Osler's *Medicine* (1892) because Osler's emphasis on how little physicians knew for sure led John Rockefeller's adviser on philanthropy to recommend the building of the great Institute for Medical Research, which opened in 1904 and for decades was the foremost institution for research in basic medical sciences in the United States. Another was the first (1941) edition of Goodman and Gilman's *Pharmacological Basis for Medical Practice* that revolutionized teaching and research on the action and use of drugs; as one professor of pharmacology stated in 1941, no professional pharmacologist could from then on teach at a lower level than that of the superb text used by his students!

In the field of respiration and the lungs, there are some classic monographs and a comprehensive *Handbook of Physiology* that have heightened the interest of scientists, students, and physicians in this subject and stimulated them to enter pulmonary research. One can safely predict that this new series of monographs, "Lung Biology in Health and Disease," will have an even greater impact on young (and older) researchers because it is the first truly comprehensive, monumental work in this field. It does not deal just with cellular processes or just with clinical problems but with the entire spectrum of basic sciences and of lung function, metabolic functions, and respiratory defense mechanisms. The series will also include volumes that apply to modern biological knowledge to elucidate mechanisms of pulmonary and respiratory disorders (immunologic, infectious, and genetic disorders, physiology and pharmacology of airways, genesis and resolution of pulmonary edema, and abnormalities of respiratory regulation). Other volumes will deal with the biology of specific pulmonary diseases (e.g., cancer, chronic obstructive pulmonary disease, disorders of the pulmonary circulation, and abnormalities associated with occupational and environmental factors) and with early detection and specific diagnosis.

This series shows the lung as a challenging organ, with many problems calling for innovative research. If it attracts some imaginative, creative, and perceptive young scientists to attack these difficult problems, the tremendous effort in writing, editing, and publishing these volumes will be well worthwhile. The volumes cannot win the Nobel Prize, but someone may who was challenged by them.

Julius H. Comroe, Jr.
San Francisco, California

PREFACE

This volume was designed to provide a comprehensive review of what is known and what is not known about the pulmonary vascular bed. While the reader must judge whether that objective was achieved, publication of this book is, in a sense, a symbol of triumph over adversity. The nature of this adversity is the fact that certain historical and political factors have operated in the past to place the pulmonary vascular bed at a disadvantage as an object of investigative and clinical concern.

The key historical event was the labeling of this vascular bed as the "lesser circulation." Presumably, this description was not used in the pejorative sense; but it seems to have operated in that way, intentional or not. Who would deign to study the lesser circulation when one could attack questions about the "greater circulation"? Furthermore, was not the lesser circulation simply a passive system of tubes leading from right ventricle to left atrium, where the really important events would occur? Of course, along the way, the blood perfusing these passive conduits did participate in gas exchange, but that was a "pulmonary" not a "hemodynamic" or circulatory event. Which brings us to the political problems experienced by the pulmonary vascular bed; namely, under whose aegis does concern with this bed properly fall?

It turns out that such concern does not fall exclusively within one domain; it cuts across many. That fact is in one way positive, because this bed should be (and is) an interdisciplinary "meeting ground." Those concerned with this bed are a conglomerate of individuals who are "card carriers" in various disciplines. Some cardiologists, despite the temptation to be associated with the "greater circulation," have focused their work on this circulation; some pulmonologists, despite the lures of lung mechanics, gas exchange, and other overtly "pulmonary" concerns, have labored in this field; and these two groups have been joined by hematologist-coagulationists (mainly under the impetus of embolic disease); by some pathologists; and, lately, by investigators with biochemical, pharmacologic, and other concerns.

This volume stands as a testimonial to the fact that the lesser circulation has grown up as an object of research interest over the years; and has done this despite the threat that it tends to fall between the cracks of strictly disciplinary blocks from which the structure of science is built. The contents of this book clearly reflect the interdisciplinary composition of those workers who form the ranks of the pulmonary vascular cadre.

The first two chapters both deal with the normal anatomy of the two circulations which supply the lungs—the pulmonary and bronchial—and the responses of these vascular beds to disease. Yet, neither is written by an "anatomist." Rather, Drs. C.A. and Noelke Wagenvoort, who carry the label pathologists, and Dr. Leon Cudkowicz, a department chairman in medicine, share with us their substantial knowledge.

The third chapter, by Dr. Edward Bergofsky, deals with the multiplicity of factors which serves to control the behavior of the pulmonary vascular, a field which involves consideration of anatomy, histology, pulmonary physiology, gas exchange, and pharmacology.

Against the background provided by the first three chapters, Chapter 4, by Drs. Karliner, Gregoratus, and myself, provides a conceptual framework for the diagnosis of pulmonary vascular disease in humans and examines in detail the current status of those techniques which are available to detect the causes and degree of such disease.

Chapters 5 through 11 address the individual types of pulmonary vascular disorders which occur in humans. Chapter 5, which I contributed, details the types of agents and conditions which may obstruct the lumens of pulmonary arteries and veins by embolism, thrombosis, or inflammation. In Chapter 6, Drs. Heath and Smith describe the mechanisms by which primary lung diseases impact on the pulmonary vascular bed and the consequences of such impact. Dr. Dexter, in Chapter 7, reviews the ways in which acquired heart diseases, particularly mitral stenosis, alter pulmonary vascular anatomy and performance.

In Chapter 8, Dr. Perloff examines how congenital heart disease influences the pulmonary vascular bed and explores certain bedside and laboratory techniques of special value in this context. Dr. Edwards, in Chapter 9, provides a lucid and comprehensive review of the many congenital abnormalities which may involve in the pulmonary vessels themselves.

Drs. Reeves and Voelkel, in Chapter 10, bring us up to date about what is known about the cause(s) and course of that still-mysterious entity which serves as a prototype of intrinsic pulmonary arterial disease: primary pulmonary hypertension. Chapter 11, by Dr. Thurlbeck, describes in depth the several neoplastic conditions that can involve the pulmonary vascular bed and compromise its function.

This comprehensive treatment of the pulmonary vascular bed will indicate, at the least, that its diminutive appellation "lesser" does not apply to the rate at which we are gaining knowledge about it. Hopefully, it will also serve as a roadmap to guide those who, in the future, will be exploring the many fascinating unknowns which exist at this time.

This comment would not be complete without my thanking all the contributors to this volume. They tolerated with laudatory grace and good humor the lash, scissors, and blue pencil of an obsessive editor whose concern for the English language and love of the simple sentence are only a micrometer less than his devotion to medical science. I thank them for their forebearance. They have been excellent and supportive companions on the long road we have travelled from proposal to print.

Kenneth M. Moser

INTRODUCTION

There is no doubt that the blood when thinned, passes in the vena arteriosa to
the lung to permeate its substance and mingle with air, its thinned part purified;
and then passes in the arteria venosa to reach the left cavity of the two cavities
of the heart, having mixed with air and become fit for the creation of the
spirit.

Ibn Nafis, Cairo, thirteenth century

Nafis' description, followed by Harvey's observations and Malpighi's discovery of
the pulmonary capillaries, both in the seventeenth century, established the anatomical foundations of our present knowledge of the pulmonary circulation. But
we had to wait for the advent of cardiac catheterization in the first half of the
twentieth century (Forssman 1929 and Cournand and Richards 1941) before
entering the domain of the quantitative study of cardiovascular function in health
and disease. Though tremendous progress has been made in our knowledge of
the heart and the systemic circulation functions, the pulmonary circulation, however, still presents us with many mysteries. Yet by its very nature, the circulatory
system, for which there is no conceivable substitute, is intriguing and fascinating.
It is affected by alterations in the performance of the heart and of the systemic
circulation. In turn, any alteration of the pulmonary circulation reflects on
heart function and on the integrity of the respiratory and nonrespiratory functions of the lung. Indeed, the pulmonary circulation has a pivotal role in the
study of "Lung Biology in Health and Disease." For this reason, this series of
monographs would be lacking if one of the volumes was not devoted to the pulmonary circulation.

Although simply titled *Pulmonary Vascular Diseases*, this volume discusses
the "small circulation" in health and in disease. It is an asset to the series that
Dr. Kenneth M. Moser accepted to edit it and was successful in assembling a
roster of pioneers in this field from both this country and from abroad. It is a
privilege to acknowledge the efforts of Dr. Moser and of the authors, and to
express my own appreciation on behalf of the series.

Claude Lenfant
Bethesda, Maryland

CONTENTS

PULMONARY
VASCULAR DISEASES

1

Pulmonary Vascular Bed
Normal Anatomy and Responses to Disease

C. A. WAGENVOORT and NOEKE WAGENVOORT

University of Amsterdam
Amsterdam, The Netherlands

I.   Introduction

In several respects the lungs are unique with regard to their blood supply.
Like all other organs in the body they have their share of the systemic
circulation, since they receive arterialized blood by way of the bronchial
arteries. The bronchial circulation, however, is a modest one in terms of
contributing to the blood supply of the lungs. The lungs are the only organs
having a double circulation since blood is also, and mainly, provided by the
pulmonary vasculature. The pulmonary circulation carries the entire output
of the right ventricle, thus causing the lungs to be the most richly supplied
organs in the body in terms of total blood flow received.

Since the pulmonary circulation is subservient to the essential function
of the lungs, respiration, lung vessels, and lung tissue are closely interwoven.
Generally, neither respiration nor circulation can be studied successfully without consideration of the other. Also, with regard to secondary lung functions
such as metabolic processes and the interception of blood-borne particulate
matter, the lung vessels play an important role.

Morphologically, there are great differences between virtually all parts of the pulmonary vasculature on the one hand and their counterparts in the systemic vasculature on the other. Vascular structure, to a large extent, depends on the demands posed by the hemodynamic situation. Therefore, the pulmonary vessels that in a normal individual are faced with pressures much lower and a blood flow much higher than in the systemic circulation, tend to be more thin walled and wider than the comparable segments of the systemic vasculature.

The structure of the lung vessels also depends on the age of the individual. This is most striking when the lungs of newborn infants are compared to those of young adults, but there are also characteristic age changes in old individuals which may be considered normal for that age group. Therefore, in our description of the normal anatomy of the pulmonary vasculature, these age-related aspects will be included.

II. Normal Anatomy

The pulmonary arterial tree may be divided into an extrapulmonary and an intrapulmonary part. The latter consists of elastic and muscular arteries and arterioles. The arterioles supply the alveolar capillaries. From there the blood is carried away by the pulmonary venules and veins. Additional attention will be given to anastomotic connections between various vessels and to the pulmonary lymphatics.

A. Extrapulmonary Arteries

Course and Structure

The extrapulmonary part of the arterial vasculature of the lung is formed by pulmonary trunk and main pulmonary arteries. The origin of the pulmonary trunk from the right ventricle is in front of the aortic orifice but somewhat more cranial and to the left. The pulmonary trunk runs in an obliquely upward course to the left and dorsally over a distance of approximately 4.5 cm before it divides in a left and a right main pulmonary artery. This bifurcation is located just under the aortic arch (Fig. 1).

The left main pulmonary artery is almost a continuation of the pulmonary trunk as it veers to the hilus of the left lung while curving over the left upper lobe bronchus at the site of its origin from the main bronchus. The right main pulmonary artery arises at a right angle from the pulmonary trunk and follows a horizontal course to the right, behind the ascending aorta, to reach the hilus of the right lung in front of the right main bronchus. The

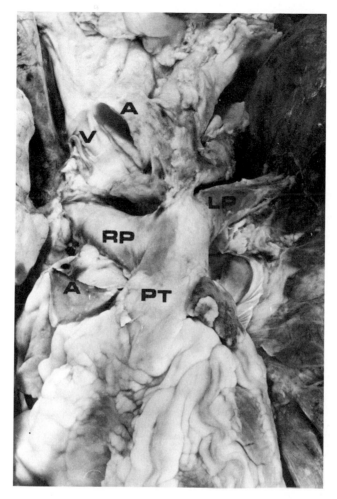

FIGURE 1 Base of heart and lung hili in a woman aged 59 years. The pulmonary trunk (PT) continues to the left as the left main pulmonary artery (LP). Parts of aorta (A) and superior vena cava (V) are removed to show the course of the right main pulmonary artery (RP).

ligament of the ductus arteriosus connects the beginning of the left main pulmonary artery with the wall of the aorta. Its original orifice from the left main pulmonary artery usually can be recognized inside as a small dimple or scar.

The posterior wall of the pulmonary trunk is the site of a glomus, lying in its adventitia. It has been suggested [1] that this glomus receives its blood

supply from the pulmonary trunk and that, therefore, it could act as a chemoreceptor for pulmonary arterial blood. Later studies have shown that this so-
called glomus pulmonale is supplied by systemic branches [2], even though in
fetal life a small arterial branch from the pulmonary trunk is sometimes observed [3]. Thus, it has a function not different from that of the aortic and
carotid glomera.

The caliber of the pulmonary trunk in normal individuals is in the same
range as that of the ascending aorta. Its wall thickness, however, is much less
and usually no more than 60 to 75% of that of the aortic wall (Fig. 2).

The histologic structure of the pulmonary trunk and that of the main
pulmonary arteries are similar. Essentially, these arteries are of the elastic type,
but in contrast to what is found in the aortic media with its continuous, parallel, and regularly arranged elastic laminae, in the pulmonary trunk these
laminae tend to be interrupted and fragmented (Fig. 3). Moreover, between
the elastic membranes there is a greater amount of mucopolysaccharides and
collagen in addition to the smooth muscle cells connecting the laminae (Fig. 4).

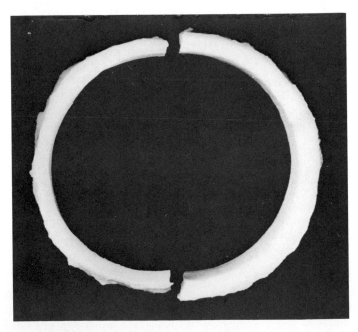

FIGURE 2   Pulmonary trunk (left) as compared to aorta (right), in a man aged
27 years. Two halves of cross-sectional slices, fixed in expanded state, are compared. The vessels have similar caliber, but the wall of the pulmonary trunk is
much thinner than that of the aorta (×1.7).

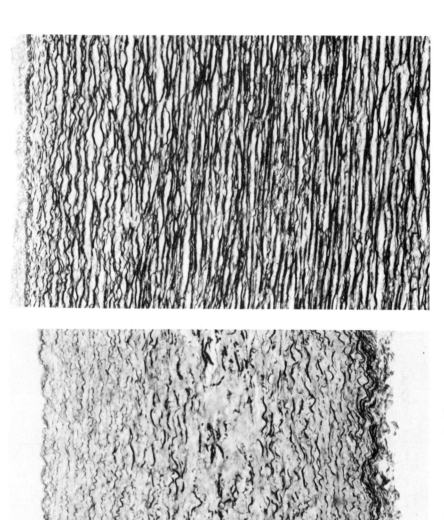

FIGURE 3 Pulmonary trunk (left) as compared to aorta (right) in a man aged 27 years. Interrupted and fragmented elastic laminae in the pulmonary trunk contrast with the intact and regular ones in aorta (Both: Elastic van Gieson's, X90).

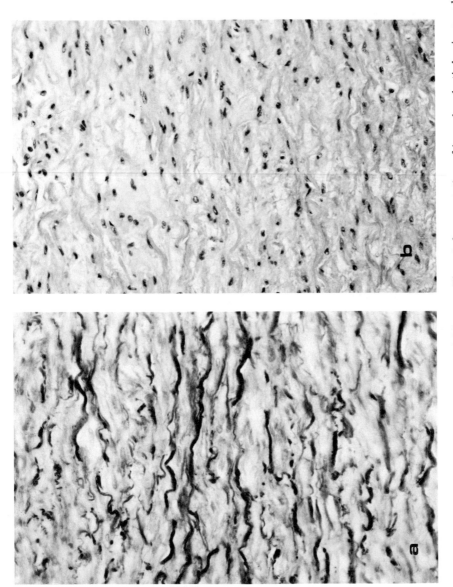

FIGURE 4 Pulmonary trunk, in a man aged 29 years. There is fragmentation of irregular elastic laminae and deposition of mucopolysaccharides and collagen in between [(a) Elastic van Gieson's; (b) H & E, X300].

There is, however, great variation in the elastic configuration of the pulmonary trunk so that in some normal individuals the elastic pattern is rather dense, somewhat resembling that of the aorta (Fig. 5), while there are other extremes in which the elastic fibers are very fragmented and scanty.

The intima of pulmonary trunk and main arteries is thin in young individuals, where it consists of a single endothelial layer overlying a basement membrane. The adventitia, composed of fibrous tissue, contains vasa vasorum,

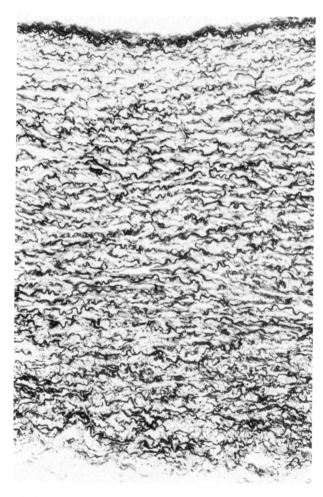

FIGURE 5 Pulmonary trunk, in a woman aged 58 years. Although the pulmonary arterial pressure was normal, the elastic configuration resembles that of the aorta (Elastic van Gieson's, ×90).

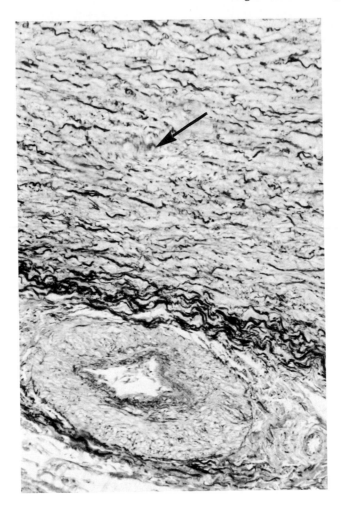

FIGURE 6   Pulmonary trunk, in a woman aged 41 years. A large vas vasorum lies in the adventitia; a small one (arrow), well within the media (Elastic van Gieson's, ×140).

which may penetrate the outer third of the media (Fig. 6) and, occasionally, the middle of the media [4,5]. The number of vasa vasorum is greater than in the aorta [6].

Age Changes

As in systemic vessels, age has its imprint on the structure of the pulmonary arteries, and the pulmonary trunk and main arteries are not exceptions to this rule. It may be difficult to decide whether such an alteration in the wall of these arteries should be labeled normal or pathologic. Atherosclerosis, for instance, is a pathologic process, but since, as we will see, there are few individuals over the age of 40 to 50 years who have not at least some traces of atheroma in their large pulmonary arteries [7], one is inclined to designate these minimal or mild lesions as normal age changes. On the other hand, we should realize that most of these observations apply to the Western world. While in this locale some degree of atherosclerosis also is rarely absent from elastic systemic arteries, its incidence in native Africans is very low [8]. Similar data, to our knowledge, are not available for the pulmonary trunk and main arteries. However, it is very likely that, as in systemic arteries, even this mild form of atheroma is a pathologic process that, though increasing with age, is related to a cultural pattern and thus should not be regarded as normal.

These considerations may apply equally to some other structural vascular changes which are commonly observed in old individuals. When they are discussed under the main heading of normal anatomy, it is because they tend to occur in the vast majority of the cases in our material, without being distinctly related to disease.

In the media of the pulmonary trunk, the amount of elastic tissue tends to diminish with age, being replaced by collagen. Often this coincides with an increased capacity and a decreased extensibility of the pulmonary trunk [9, 10]; dilatation of the trunk and main arteries also may be conspicuous. The calcium content of the arterial wall, though generally much lower than that of the aorta, increases gradually with age [11].

A mild degree of diffuse intimal fibrosis (Fig. 7) is commonly observed in the elderly and may affect both the pulmonary trunk and the main arteries. There is usually no apparent relation to cardiac or pulmonary disease. This lesion may be completely absent even in very old individuals.

Small patches of atheroma, easily overlooked when the intimal surface is not wiped clean after the vessels are cut open, are observed particularly near the ramifications of secondary and tertiary pulmonary arterial branches (Fig. 8) and to a lesser extent at the bifurcation of the pulmonary trunk. These patches are usually small and hardly raised but stand out by their yellow color due to their content of lipid-laden macrophages (Fig. 9). More severe degrees of atherosclerosis are generally related to elevation of pulmonary arterial pressure or to hypercholesterolemia.

Structure in Fetal and Perinatal Life

During fetal and immediate postnatal life, the pulmonary trunk has a structure identical to that of the aorta. This applies both to the wall thickness, which is approximately equal in the two vessels (Fig. 10), and to their elastic configuration. The fetal and neonatal pulmonary trunk and main pulmonary

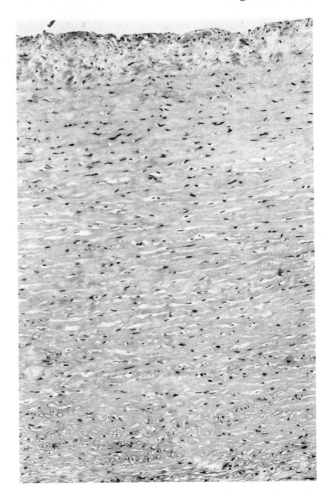

FIGURE 7   Pulmonary trunk, in a woman aged 58 years. There is mild intimal fibrosis (H & E, ×90).

arteries are typical elastic arteries with a dense and regular arrangement of parallel elastic membranes, separated by scarce smooth muscle cells and collagenous fibers (Fig. 11).

     After birth, the elastic tissue gradually diminishes and is replaced by collagen. From the fourth month onward, and particularly after the first year of life, the elastic laminae are noticeably swollen and disrupted and become gradually more and more fragmented [12,13]. This is accompanied by a relative decrease in thickness of the media as compared to that of the aorta.

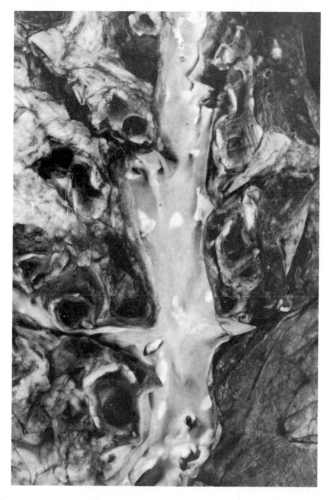

FIGURE 8 Primary branch of main pulmonary artery cut open lengthwise, in a man aged 69 years. Multiple small plaques of atherosclerosis, representing age changes, are particularly located near ramifications.

B. Intrapulmonary Elastic Arteries

From the hilus the secondary and subsequent branches of the pulmonary artery retain an elastic structure. In the adult, however, they differ from the main pulmonary arteries in keeping a regular elastic configuration with parallel and intact laminae (Fig. 12), without the disruption and fragmentation of these laminae to be found in the extrapulmonary vessels. This elastic structure is

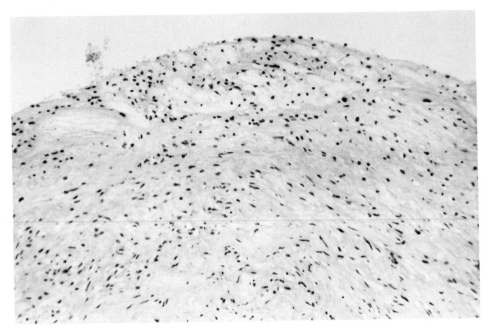

FIGURE 9   Histological section of one of the atherosclerotic patches depicted in Figure 8. The patch is slightly raised and contains lipid-laden macrophages (H & E, ×140).

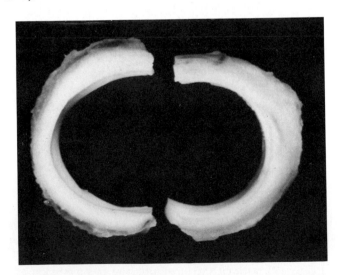

FIGURE 10   Pulmonary trunk (left) as compared to aorta (right), in a stillborn female infant. Two halves of cross-sectional slices, fixed in expanded state, are shown. Both the caliber and wall thickness are approximately equal (×7).

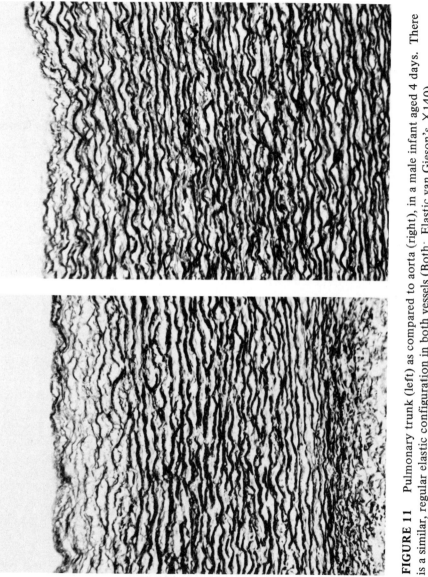

FIGURE 11 Pulmonary trunk (left) as compared to aorta (right), in a male infant aged 4 days. There is a similar, regular elastic configuration in both vessels (Both: Elastic van Gieson's, ×140).

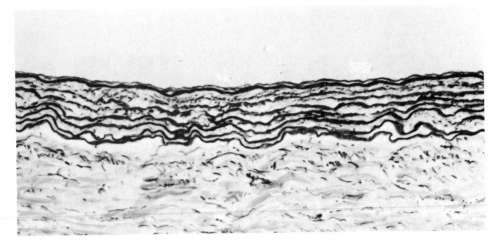

FIGURE 12   Elastic pulmonary artery with regular, parallel elastic laminae, in a girl aged 4 years (Elastic van Gieson's, ×230).

maintained down to branches of a caliber in the range of 1 mm. Between 1000 and 500 μm external diameter, a transition from the elastic to the muscular type takes place. Smaller branches are entirely muscular.

As in the main arteries, the largest elastic intrapulmonary arteries often show small patches of atheroma, particularly at the sites of branching. These patches are common in individuals over the age of 40 or 50 years, in the absence of any apparent underlying cardiac or pulmonary condition, so that they may be regarded as a normal age change.

In the fetus and newborn infant, the elastic intrapulmonary arteries are scarce and gradually increase in number [14]. They have a regular elastic configuration. Rather commonly, the largest elastic arteries exhibit a layer of intimal cellular proliferation over considerable distances (Fig. 13). This layer usually does not attain a thickness of more than half of the arterial media. In the course of the first postnatal year it tends to disappear without leaving traces. Its significance is not understood.

C.   Muscular Pulmonary Arteries and Arterioles

Course and Structure

Within the lung the branches of the pulmonary arterial tree, as shown in a postmortem arteriogram (Fig. 14), tend to follow a dichotomous system. This applies to the elastic as well as to the muscular arteries (Fig. 15). They fol-

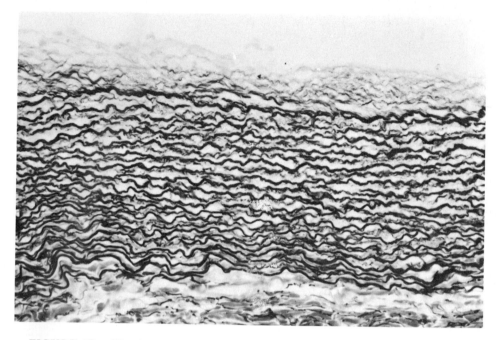

FIGURE 13   Elastic pulmonary artery with a layer of cellular intimal proliferation, in a stillborn male infant (Elastic van Gieson's, X230).

low the ramifications of the bronchial tree, and in histologic sections they are in close proximity to the bronchi and bronchioles down to a level where the respiratory bronchioles break up into the alveolar sacs.

It has been shown, however [15–17], that in addition to these dichotomous divisions there are numerous, usually small, muscular branches, arising perpendicularly from both elastic and larger muscular pulmonary arteries.

These so-called supernumerary branches, which do not accompany the bronchi and bronchioles, supply adjacent pulmonary lobules and generally are difficult to identify in a pulmonary arteriogram. Even so, when studied in histologic serial sections, they appear to be numerous and according to Elliott and Reid [15], may, at least in the periphery of the lungs, even outnumber the dichotomous branches. In structure they do not differ from the latter.

As we have seen, the gradual transition of the elastic to the muscular type of pulmonary artery in the adult lies between 1000 and 500 μm, and arteries of smaller caliber are generally completely muscular. The muscular coat of these vessels is continuous down to an external vascular diameter of approximately 70 μm. Smaller branches are generally amuscular.

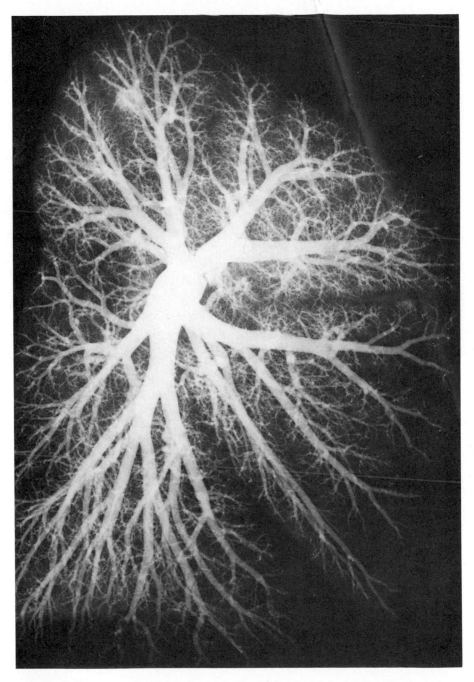

FIGURE 14 Normal right pulmonary arteriogram showing dichotomous ramifications, in a man aged 46 years.

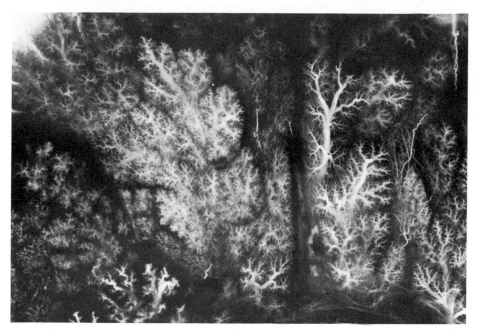

FIGURE 15   Pulmonary arterial tree after injection with barium sulfate, in a 4-month-old boy. The lung tissue has been cleared with benzene to show the mode of ramification of large and small pulmonary arterial branches.

The adventitia of the larger muscular pulmonary arteries, consisting of dense fibrous tissue, is rather thick, often 2 or 3 times as thick as the media. In smaller arteries its thickness decreases rapidly, also in comparison to the medial thickness.

The media differs from that of systemic muscular arteries in two major respects. It is relatively thin, and it is bounded on either side by an elastic lamina (Fig. 16). In systemic arteries there is always an internal elastic lamina but the external one is usually incomplete or absent, although sometimes a condensation of adventitial elastic fibers may mimic a single lamina.

The media of muscular pulmonary arteries is composed of smooth muscle cells that are circularly or nearly circularly arranged (Fig. 17). Between these muscle cells there are scanty reticulin and collagen fibers, often not recognizable with the light microscope, but easily seen with the electron microscope. In the larger muscular arteries occasional thin elastic fibers may occur.

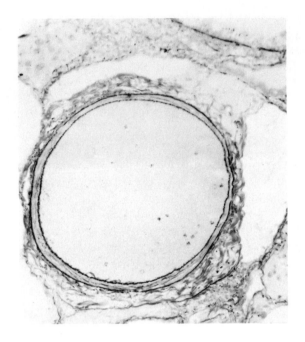

FIGURE 16   Normal
muscular pulmonary artery
with wide lumen and thin
media bounded by elastic
laminae, in a youth aged
18 years (Elastic van
Gieson's, ×140).

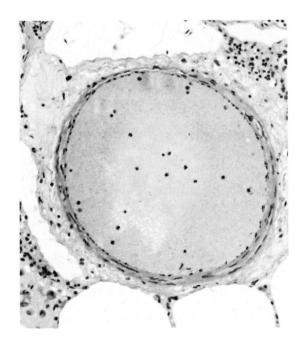

FIGURE 17   Normal
muscular pulmonary artery
with wide lumen and cir-
cularly arranged smooth
muscle cells in thin media.
Same case as Figure 16
(H & E, ×160).

The thickness of the media may best be expressed as a percentage of the external vascular diameter. On the average, this thickness in normal, uninjected lungs is in the range of 5%, against 15 to 20% in systemic arteries [18–20]. Injection of the pulmonary arteries with fixative or contrast medium yields lower values [21]. Individual arteries usually vary from 2 to 8%, although occasional vessels are much more thick walled, up to 15 or 20% of the external diameter. This seems to indicate that some vessels may be constricted while others in the same lung are not.

Generally, the muscular pulmonary arteries are thus thin walled, with a wide lumen which is in keeping with the low resistance and pressures prevailing in the pulmonary circulation. In spite of the pulmonary blood flow being much greater in the lower lobes than in the upper lobes [22], there are no recognizable qualitative or quantitative differences in pulmonary arterial structure in the various lobes of the normal lungs [20,23], nor is there any difference according to the sex of the individual.

The transition of a muscular to a nonmuscular part of the pulmonary arterial tree lies, as we have seen, at a caliber of approximately 70 μm. This transition is not sharp, first because occasional vessels of 80 or even 90 μm may be nonmuscular while sometimes an artery in the range of 60-μm external diameter has a complete muscular coat. But second—and this is a more important reason—the media changes gradually from a complete layer to a discontinuous one (Fig. 18). The circularly arranged smooth muscle cells in this intermediate segment follow a more and more widening spiral course, so that muscular and nonmuscular portions alternate (Fig. 19). The term "pulmonary arteriole," which has often been used in a rather loose and varying way, is best applied to branches with such a transition [24]. The distal parts of these arterioles, which are nonmuscular, have a wall consisting of a single elastic lamina as a continuation of the external elastic lamina, lined on the inner side by the intima.

The intima of normal muscular pulmonary arteries is thin, consisting of an endothelial layer resting upon a basement membrane and overlying few reticulin and collagen fibers.

Age Changes

Although often the media of muscular pulmonary arteries is somewhat irregular and fibrotic in old age and unequal in thickness even in the same vascular cross section, the average medial thickness is in the same range as that of younger adults [20]. Subsequent reports [23,25] indicated that in old individuals the media is increased in thickness, but in these studies the arteries were injected. It has since been pointed out that decreased vascular extensibility, at least partly due to increased intimal fibrosis, will resist dilatation by

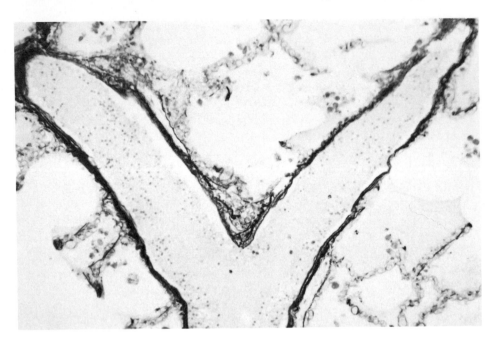

FIGURE 18   Normal pulmonary arteriole longitudinally cut from same case as Figure 16. Thin muscular segments bounded by two elastic laminae alternate with amuscular segments (Elastic van Gieson's, ×140).

injection pressure, so that the arteries of the aged tend to be less wide and thus somewhat more thick walled than those of the young [5,26].

Intimal fibrosis is a very common age change (Fig. 20). An occasional patch of intimal fibrosis may be found even in children. In young adults, minimal to mild intimal fibrosis becomes gradually more common. In the older age groups there is generally a sharp increase in the incidence and extent of intimal fibrosis, even though it varies greatly in various individuals [7,20]. The intimal fibrosis is patchy with an irregular distribution, so that it may be absent in many cross sections. Warnock and Kunzmann [26] observed it in just under 50% of the cross-sectioned arteries they measured.

In smokers, the thickness of the intima of pulmonary arteries tends to be greater than in nonsmokers [27]. Naeye and Dellinger [28] found bundles of longitudinal smooth muscle cells in the intima of normal pulmonary arteries in smokers and even in nonsmokers. The occurrence of such muscle bundles is well known in patients with chronic bronchitis (p. 96) and therefore may well be observed in smokers, but we could find no evidence of it in nonsmoking, old individuals. On the other hand, it must be realized that at an

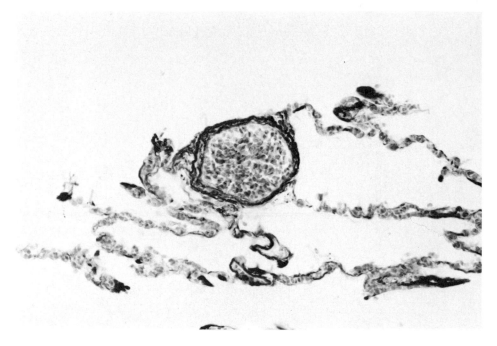

FIGURE 19   Normal pulmonary arteriole in cross section, in a woman aged 47 years. On one side there is a muscular, and on the other side, an amuscular wall (Elastic van Gieson's, ×230).

ultrastructural level, most if not all cells constituting the patches of intimal fibrosis do have the characteristics of smooth muscle cells (Fig. 21) but they are arranged in a haphazard way and cannot be recognized as such with light microscopy [29].

These age changes are generally more common in the upper parts of the lungs than in the lower parts. In view of their appearance it is suggestive that reparative processes, including thrombosis with subsequent organization, are basic to the formation of the intimal plaques. This could well be a response to various injuries to the lung, occurring in the course of time.

Structure in Fetal and Perinatal Life

Pulmonary hemodynamics differ substantially in the prenatal as compared to the postnatal period. In fetal life the lungs have no function with regard to blood oxygenation. The fetus derives its oxygen from the placenta. Oxygenated blood reaches the right atrium by way of the ductus venosus and the inferior vena cava. From here, the greater part flows through the patent

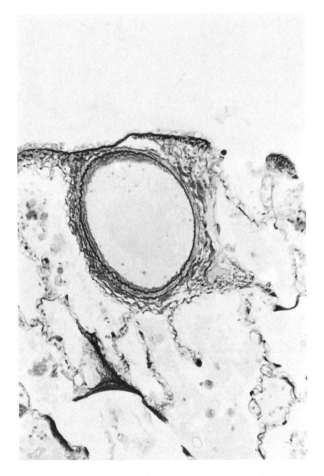

FIGURE 20   Muscular pulmonary artery, in a woman aged 28 years. There is a crescent-shaped layer of mild intimal fibrosis as an age change (Elastic van Gieson's, ×150).

foramen ovale to the left side of the heart and to the systemic circulation. The remaining part of the blood, together with the blood from the superior vena cava, flows to the right ventricle and the pulmonary trunk, but again, the largest proportion is diverted by way of the ductus arteriosus to the systemic circulation, so that only 10 to 15% of the right ventricular stroke volume reaches the lungs [30].

This arrangement guarantees that the ascending aorta and the aortic arch, with their coronary and cerebral arterial branches, contain well-oxygenated blood, while more distally after the entrance of the ductus arteriosus into the aorta there is a mixture of well-oxygenated and poorly oxygenated blood supplying the lower parts of the body.

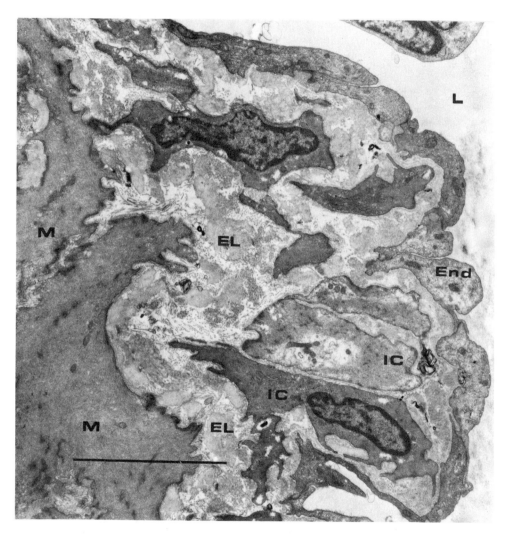

FIGURE-21 Electronmicrograph of detail of muscular pulmonary artery, in a man aged 56 years. There is intimal fibrosis as an age change. The circularly arranged smooth muscle cells of the media (M) are separated from the thickened intima by the internal elastic lamina (EL). The intimal cells (IC) have the characteristics of smooth muscle cells; End, endothelial layer; L, lumen. Bar indicates 5 μm.

The high pulmonary resistance and low flow in the fetus find their reflection in the muscular pulmonary arteries more than in any other part of
the pulmonary circulation, so that the differences between these vessels and
their postnatal counterparts are particularly striking.

Fetal muscular pulmonary arteries and arterioles have thick walls, while
their lumina are narrow (Fig. 22). This applies to fetuses of 20-weeks gesta-
tion as well as to newborn infants. The thickness of the media in this period
is in the range of 15 to 25% of the external arterial diameter [31]. The
arteries have essentially the same structure as in later life; that is, the media is
bounded by an internal and an external elastic lamina, but these laminae are
very thin and in fetuses sometimes hardly stain with various methods for the
demonstration of elastin.

When the total amount of arterial smooth muscle tissue is calculated,
either by comparing the surface area of the media to the area of lung tissue
[31] or to the intimal area [32], it appears that this increases during gesta-
tion. Since, during fetal life, the medial smooth muscle cells do not change in
size [33], this means that there must be a gradual growth and multiplication

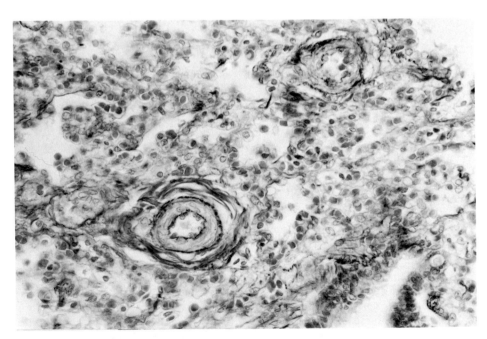

FIGURE 22 Muscular pulmonary arteries with narrow lumina and thick media,
in a stillborn male infant (Elastic van Gieson's, ×350).

of the branches of the pulmonary arteries. This has also been shown in fetal lambs [34]. This increase in number continues during the first postnatal months, or even longer [35,36].

At the time of birth, the hemodynamic situation changes instantly. With pulmonary respiration the oxygenation of the blood is now localized in the lungs. The resistance in the pulmonary circulation decreases, the ductus arteriosus becomes functionally closed, and the whole right cardiac output now flows through the lungs. The increased pulmonary venous return with a concomitant rise in left atrial pressure causes closure of the foramen ovale.

This sudden change finds its expression in a transition of the fetal to the postnatal type of muscular pulmonary artery. Within the first 2 to 3 weeks they become considerably wider, first particularly the smallest arteries and arterioles, which were almost closed during fetal life (Fig. 23). The largest arteries open up somewhat more slowly [31]. This conspicuous early dilatation of the pulmonary arteries is followed by a more gradual widening of the lumen and decrease of medial thickness, so that at an age variably given as 6

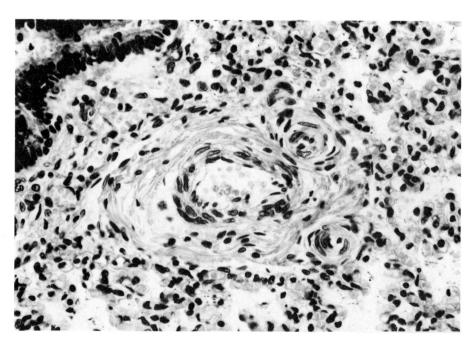

FIGURE 23 Muscular pulmonary artery with two small arterioles, from the same case as Figure 22. While the lumen of the artery is narrow, those of the arterioles are virtually closed (H & E, ×350).

months to 1½ years the media/diameter ratio has attained the same values existing in adult life [37–39].

The intima of the fetal pulmonary arteries and arterioles consists essentially of a single layer of endothelial cells. Due to the contracted state of the vessels, these cells tend to bulge into the lumen, thus contributing to the obstruction of the vessels. During postnatal arterial dilatation they become flatter.

Bundles of longitudinal smooth muscle cells (Fig. 24) can often be observed in the intima of small pulmonary arteries and arterioles [40]. They probably contribute to the narrowing of these vessels and to their high resistance in fetal life. We did not find them in newborn infants after the age of 10 days [41].

D. Alveolar Capillaries

The main constituents of the alveolar walls are the dense networks of alveolar capillaries. These networks are supplied by amuscular terminal branches of the arterioles and drained by small venules (Fig. 25). The meshes within these

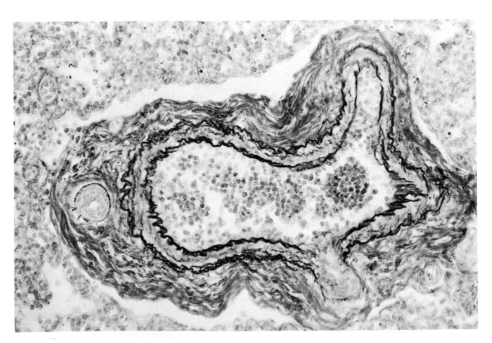

FIGURE 24   Muscular pulmonary artery with two arterioles, from the same case as Figure 22. The arterioles are narrowed by bundles of longitudinally arranged intimal smooth muscle cells (Elastic van Gieson's, ×230).

networks are roughly hexagonal (Fig. 26), bordered by capillary segments which have a length in the range of 10 to 15 μm and an average diameter of 8.3 μm [42,43]. These capillaries are generally wider than systemic capillaries, but their caliber depends on the degree of filling. In congested lungs they are distinctly dilated. The capillary networks of adjacent alveoli communicate [44,45], so that the pulmonary blood generally perfuses several alveoli before it is carried off to the venous system. In fact, in a single alveolar wall there is only one alveolar meshwork intertwined with a flat interstitial meshwork [46].

The wall of the alveolar capillary, constituting the air-blood barrier, is very thin at an ultrastructural level and has a thickness in the range of 1.6 to 1.8 μm [47]. It consists essentially of five layers. An attenuated cytoplasmic layer of epithelial cells lines the wall at the site of the alveolar space. It rests on a thin and sometimes indistinct basement membrane. On the opposite site, a similar thin layer of cytoplasm formed by the endothelial cells borders on the capillary lumen. This layer also overlies a similar basement membrane. Between the two basement membranes there is generally a thin interstitial space containing a few reticulin and collagen fibers [48], although both membranes may sometimes fuse. Locally, the interstitial space may be consider-

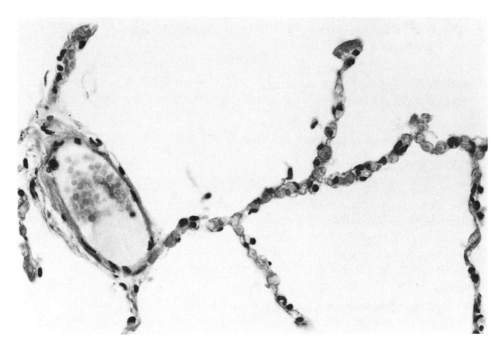

FIGURE 25   Normal alveolar walls with alveolar capillaries, in a woman aged 49 years. To the left a pulmonary venule (H & E, ×350).

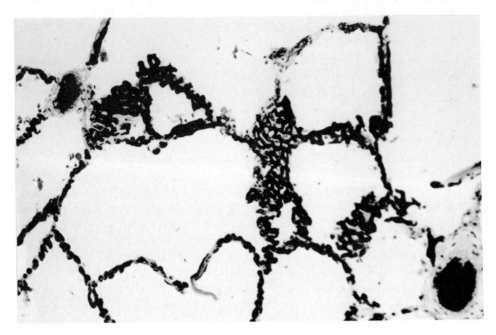

FIGURE 26   Alveolar capillaries after injection with India ink, in a man aged
57 years. The capillaries form dense hexagonal meshes. To the right a pulmonary arteriole (H & E, ×140).

ably thicker and fairly rich in collagen. Pericytes are observed in pulmonary
capillaries but are much smaller in number than in systemic capillaries [49].

E.   Pulmonary Venules and Veins

Course and Structure

From the capillary networks the blood is drained by small amuscular branches,
the collecting venules, to somewhat wider pulmonary venules (Fig. 27). These
pulmonary venules are also essentially amuscular, although with increasing
caliber they may gradually contain occasional smooth muscle cells. For the
greater part, however, the wall of the venule consists solely of an endothelial
layer, resting upon a thin basement membrane and overlying a single elastic
lamina [45].

Distinction between a pulmonary venule and a pulmonary arteriole is
generally not possible in histologic sections since both are amuscular and
situated in the lung parenchyma without the localization in interlobular fibrous
septa or near bronchioles, characteristic of larger venous and arterial branches,

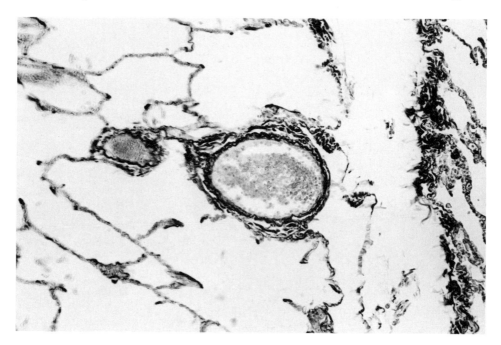

FIGURE 27   Pulmonary venules just before entering an interlobular septum, in a woman aged 47 years. The venules are amuscular (Elastic van Gieson's, ×140).

respectively. The only safe method of distinction may be their tracing in histologic serial sections to prove that they connect with larger vessels clearly recognizable as veins or as arteries. The venules merge into larger pulmonary veins which, at a caliber of 60 to 100 μm, are generally to be found within the interlobular fibrous septa. At this point the structure of the venous wall (Fig. 28) is also distinctly different from that of an artery. It is thinner and composed of irregularly arranged elastic fibers, interspersed with smooth muscle cells and collagen [50]. An internal elastic lamina is usually recognizable. Generally, the endothelial layer is separated from this lamina only by its basement membrane. In contrast to the systemic veins, the pulmonary veins contain no valves. The adventitia is thin and composed of collagenous and elastic fibers. In the absence of an external elastic lamina, the demarcation between media and adventitia is indistinct.

In the larger pulmonary venous trunks the structure of the wall is essentially similar. Occasionally, small clumps of fairly large cells rich in cytoplasm have been observed in the venous adventitia or sometimes outside the vascular wall though in close proximity to the adventitia. These groups of

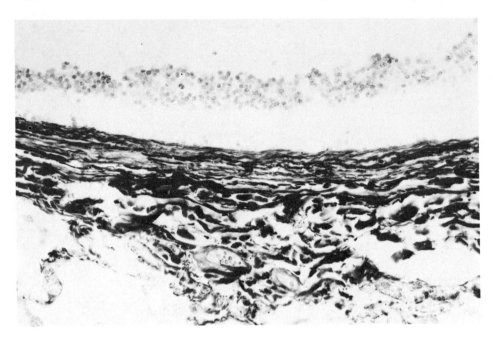

FIGURE 28   Pulmonary vein, in a man aged 52 years. The venous wall is relatively thin and contains irregularly arranged elastic fibers (Elastic van Gieson's, X230).

cells have been interpreted as local hyperplasia of chemoreceptor cells [51] or as chemodectomas [52], suggesting that normally cells sensitive to oxygen or carbon dioxide may be present in these locations. More recently, electron microscopic studies [53,54] have thrown doubt upon the concept of pulmonary venous chemoreception, since the ultrastructure of the cells does not resemble that of chemoreceptor cells elsewhere in the body.

The extrapulmonary part of the venous trunks is surrounded by a coat of cardiac muscle as an extension from the left atrial wall. In small rodents, such as rats and mice, this coat of striated muscle tissue may extend within the lung far into the periphery [55]. In human lungs the cardiac muscle usually stops abruptly at the hilus, although occasionally it can be observed just within the lung tissue [56].

Age Changes

The pulmonary veins may show changes with age, although these are usually less striking than those in arteries. In old individuals there is fragmentation and loss of elastic membranes and an increase of collagen, resulting in a decreased elasticity of the vessels.

The intima is usually thickened. Sometimes this happens in the form of a hyaline intimal fibrosis, almost completely devoid of cells (Fig. 29). Smaller veins and venules may become distinctly narrowed by this process, without resulting in obliteration.

Structure in Fetal and Perinatal Life

The walls of pulmonary veins and venules in perinatal life tend to be extremely thin. In spite of this they are usually not so collapsed as those in adults, allowing morphometric assessment of their wall thickness. Throughout the perinatal period the medial thickness of the uninjected veins is in the range of 3 to 4% of their external diameter [57]. Their wall composition resembles that of adult pulmonary veins.

F.   Anastomoses

It is generally agreed that in the normal lung there are no connections between different precapillary branches of the pulmonary artery, or between pulmonary

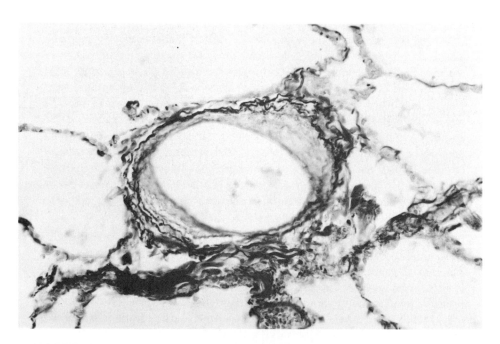

FIGURE 29   Small pulmonary vein with hyaline intimal fibrosis as an age change, in a woman aged 57 years (Elastic van Gieson's, ×230).

veins. Other forms of anastomoses do occur, although for most forms it may be said that their functional significance is either limited or controversial.

Controversy is particularly great with regard to arteriovenous anastomoses. Their occurrence is denied by some authors, while others claim that they are not only present in the normal lung but that they are even of large caliber. The confusion, to a great extent, appears to have been brought about by the nature of the methods applied in the study of these anastomoses.

Prinzmetal et al. [58] injected glass spherules into the arteries of various organs, and notably into the pulmonary artery. They recovered spherules as large as 300 μm in diameter from the pulmonary venous blood and concluded that these could only have arrived there by way of arteriovenous anastomoses of an adequate caliber. Similar studies by Tobin and Zariquiev [59], Rahn et al. [60], and Niden and Aviado [61] confirmed these results for glass spherules from up to 200 to 500 μm in diameter.

Morphologic methods, particularly tracing of pulmonary arteries and veins, although successful in the demonstration of other types of anastomoses, even of small connecting channels, were hardly successful with regard to pulmonary arteriovenous anastomoses. Some authors found them in small numbers and of small caliber [40,62], while many others, in spite of extensive studies, were unable to demonstrate any at all [63-66]. They were also absent in corrosion casts of the pulmonary vasculature [67].

The discrepancy in the results of the various methods may in part be due to overdistention of capillaries under pressure. In lungs of animals, particles of 75 μm could be forced through the capillary bed [68,69]. Moreover, the risk of spilling spherules during injection so that they entered samples of pulmonary venous blood was recognized. However this may be, it seems very unlikely that arteriovenous anastomoses of an appreciable caliber and in any significant number could occur in the normal lung without being demonstrable by the study of histologic serial sections. Admittedly, in most of these studies, the pulmonary arteries were traced down to a caliber where they lost their media. This leaves open the possibility of anastomoses between the nonmuscular portions of distal arterioles and venules, although in that case their caliber would necessarily be very small.

Bronchopulmonary arterial anastomoses, connections between bronchial and pulmonary arteries, do occur in normal lungs (Fig. 30). They are of rather small caliber, as their external diameter rarely exceeds 250 μm. Usually it is in the range of 100 μm or less [64,70]. They have been demonstrated by using serial sections. Some authors reported they were fairly common [63,71-73], while others believe they are generally scarce [64,65,74], or even absent [75,76]. In part, these varying results depend on the age of the individual. In newborn infants, and particularly in early childhood, broncho-

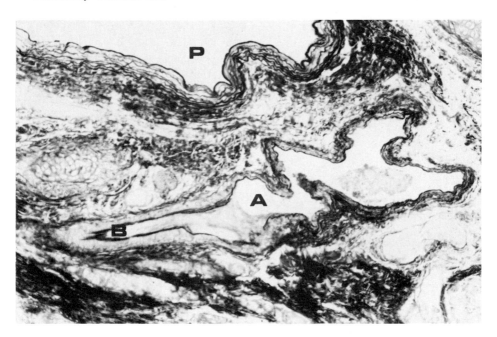

FIGURE 30   Bronchopulmonary arterial anastomosis (A) connecting a bronchial artery (B) to an elastic pulmonary artery (P), in a girl aged 1 year. There is obstructing intimal fibrosis at the bronchial arterial end (Elastic van Gieson's, ×90).

pulmonary arterial anastomoses are much more common and of relatively wider caliber than in adults, but they tend to disappear or to be obliterated in later life so that they are very uncommon in normal adults [64-66,70]. Here, their functional significance is no doubt negligible. In infants we do not know their function or the direction of the blood flow within these anastomoses.

Bronchopulmonary arteries, representing branches of bronchial arteries but supplying the lung tissue (Fig. 31), as well as pulmobronchial arteries that, although derived from pulmonary arteries, supply the bronchial walls and interstitium, are particularly observed in the perinatal period [64].

In the normal lung the most common type of vascular anastomosis is that between bronchial and pulmonary veins (Fig. 32). The peripheral part of the bronchial venous system depends for its drainage on adjacent pulmonary veins. There are thus numerous and often wide connections between the bronchial venous plexus around the bronchi and bronchioli and the pulmonary veins [77].

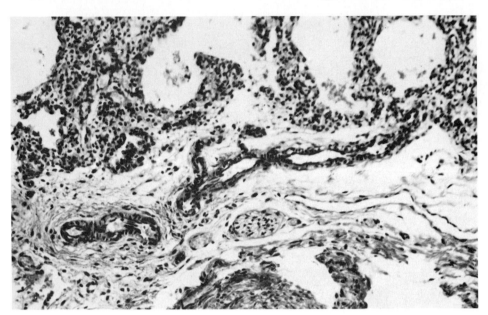

FIGURE 31   Bronchopulmonary artery in a stillborn female infant. A bronchial artery (left) supplies the lung tissue (top) with multiple small branches (H & E, ×140).

G.   Lymphatics

It has been shown by injection studies that there is a very extensive and dense network of lymph vessels in the lungs. These pulmonary lymphatics are particularly numerous around bronchi and bronchioli and around pulmonary arterial branches (Fig. 33). They begin as blind sacs at the level of respiratory bronchioles and their accompanying pulmonary arteries, so that the alveolar walls do not possess lymphatics [72,78,79]. Moreover, there are numerous lymphatics in the interlobular fibrous septa connected to extensive networks in the pleura. Within the interlobular septa there is no clear association with the pulmonary veins.

The structure of pulmonary lymphatics resembles that of lymph vessels elsewhere. The wall is very thin, consisting of an endothelial layer overlying a thin basement membrane. Occasional reticulin and elastic fibers reinforce the wall. The endothelial cells contain within their cytoplasm some thin and thick filaments, suggesting that their permeability can be regulated at the sites of intercellular junctions [80]. The larger lymphatics within the pleura, interlobular septa, and also along the larger bronchi may be provided with a distinct muscular coat (Fig. 34). Valves are numerous within their course.

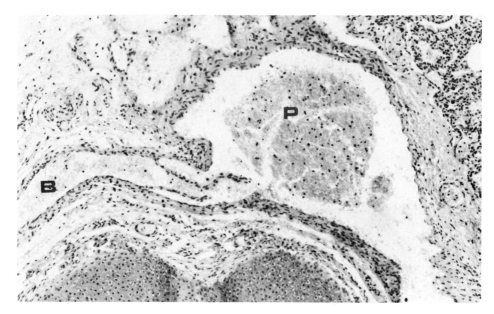

FIGURE 32   Bronchopulmonary venous anastomosis connecting a bronchial vein (B) with a pulmonary vein (P), from the same case as Figure 31. A valve protrudes into the pulmonary vein (H & E, ×140).

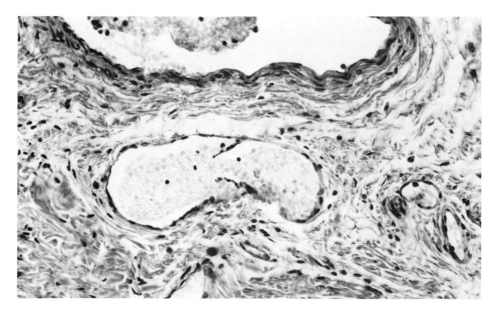

FIGURE 33   Pulmonary lymphatic with wall consisting of endothelial layer, in a girl aged 1 year. It contains a bicuspid valve (H & E, ×230).

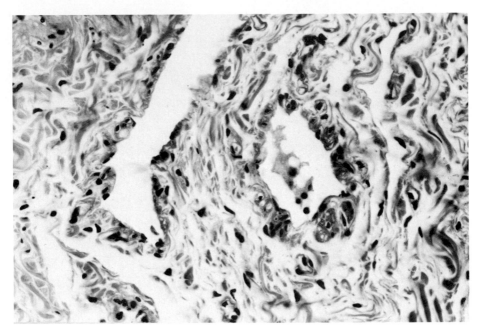

FIGURE 34   Pulmonary lymphatics with layers of smooth muscle in their walls, in a woman aged 20 years (H & E, ×350).

III.   Responses to Disease

A.   Introduction

The vessels of the lung may react to abnormal stimuli in many ways. In fact, the variety of alterations that may be found in response to disease or to disturbed hemodynamics is much greater in the pulmonary than in the systemic vasculature. This is related to the central position the lungs occupy in the circulation, not only receiving the whole right cardiac output but also sieving out all the particulate matter entering or being formed in the systemic veins. Moreover, in no other organ is the vasculature so intimately interwoven with both organ structure and function as in the lungs.

Lung diseases, particularly if diffuse, as well as changes in composition of alveolar air, such as hypoxia, will elicit marked alterations in the vessels of the lung. Particularly common, and also of great practical importance, are those vascular lesions that are formed in response to an increased pressure in the pulmonary circulation and that in turn may elevate this pressure. There are many forms of pulmonary hypertension and also many forms of hypertensive pulmonary vascular disease. In principle, it is possible from the morphologic picture of the lung vessels to decide upon the type of pulmonary hypertension and thus to make a classification on the basis of biopsy or autopsy material [81,82].

Vascular alterations may also result from decreased pulmonary flow, various types of lung diseases, vascular tumors, and congenital malformations of lung vessels. Most of these latter conditions are dealt with in other chapters.

Within the pulmonary arterial system, lesions may be found in the pulmonary trunk and main arteries as well as in the elastic intrapulmonary arteries. These changes are never so conspicuous and so varied as in the muscular pulmonary arteries and arterioles which constitute the most reactive part of the pulmonary vasculature. But also in capillaries, venules, and veins, and even in anastomoses and pulmonary lymphatics, pronounced alterations, often characteristic for the type of underlying condition, do occur.

B. Extrapulmonary Arteries

Lesions of Adventitia

Pulmonary hypertension has little or no effect on the adventitia of the pulmonary trunk and main arteries [6]. The vasa vasorum are often enlarged if there is thrombosis of main arteries, because they play a part in recanalization of the thrombosed areas.

Lesions of Media

In disease, the media of the pulmonary trunk and main pulmonary arteries may show alterations both in its thickness and in its configuration with regard to smooth muscle cells, elastic fibers, collagen fibers, and ground substance.

In the presence of pulmonary hypertension, the medial thickness is usually increased and may equal that of the aorta. This is independent of the type of pulmonary hypertension.

Structural changes of the media are more conspicuous in patients who have had pulmonary hypertension from birth than in those who acquired it in later life. In children with congenital cardiac shunts, such as a ventricular septal defect or a patent ductus arteriosus, the "aortic" configuration normally present in newborn infants usually fails to change into the "adult" configuration. In other words, the media of the pulmonary trunk continues to exhibit a dense arrangement of regular intact elastic membranes (Fig. 35) not unlike that in the aorta [12]. Exceptions to the rule are not uncommon since disruption and fragmentation of elastic membranes may sometimes be found in patients with congenital cardiac shunts.

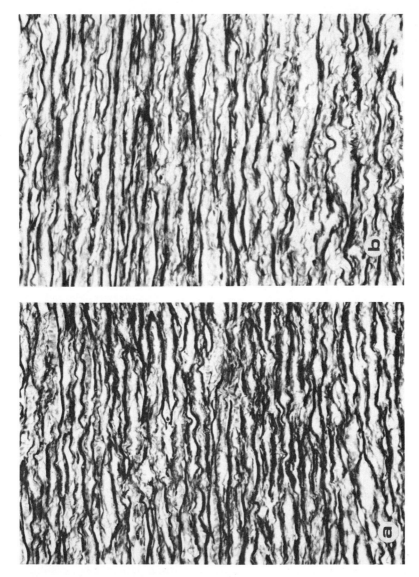

FIGURE 35   Pulmonary trunk (a) as compared to aorta (b), in a man aged 31 years with a ventricular septal defect of the endocardial cushion type and pulmonary hypertension. There is an "aortic" configuration of the elastic tissue in the pulmonary trunk (Both: Elastic van Gieson's, X90).

If pulmonary hypertension is acquired, as in rheumatic mitral stenosis or chronic bronchitis, the adult configuration of the media, already present when the pressure became elevated, is retained. Therefore, in these cases, the elastic tissue in the wall of the pulmonary trunk and main arteries is generally scarce, while the elastic membranes are disrupted and fragmented. Usually there is a marked increase both in collagen and ground substance in the media in these cases. Sometimes there is an excess amount of acid mucopolysaccharides, and, for instance in patients with mitral valve disease, the pulmonary trunk may be friable in spite of an increased wall thickness. Excessive fragmentation and deposition of acid mucopolysaccharides have also been described in the absence of pulmonary hypertension in cases of Marfan's syndrome and idiopathic dilatation of the pulmonary trunk [83].

The structure of the pulmonary trunk has been used to decide whether, in patients with primary pulmonary hypertension, the condition was acquired or present from birth. In this way, it has been shown that occasionally, usually in very young patients with this disease, the pulmonary arterial pressure was likely to have been increased from birth or from a time soon after birth. In the majority of the patients, however, the adult configuration was found at the time of death, so that it seemed likely that they had an acquired form of primary pulmonary hypertension [84–86].

If the pulmonary flow is decreased, as in patients with tetralogy of Fallot, the media of the pulmonary trunk and main arteries may be much thinner than normal (Fig. 36). This atrophic media may contain very little elastic tissue [12], but this is not necessarily so.

Calcification of the media, usually in a mild form, is seen in some patients with pulmonary hypertension. Severe calcification is found in infants suffering from infantile calcifying arteriopathy, a rare disorder of obscure etiology in which multiple systemic arteries are involved but sometimes also the large elastic pulmonary arteries.

Lesions of Intima

As we have seen, both diffuse fibrosis of the intima and atherosclerosis occur regularly in the absence of disease in adult, particularly old, individuals. Both types of alteration are more extensive and more pronounced if the pulmonary arterial pressure is elevated. In pulmonary hypertension, marked intimal fibrosis may be found in young individuals (Fig. 37), even in young children [87]. Also, marked atherosclerosis of the large pulmonary arteries is common in all types of pulmonary hypertension (Fig. 38).

Even so, the very severe degrees of atherosclerosis with ulceration of atheromatous plaques and subsequent thrombosis, so commonly found in the

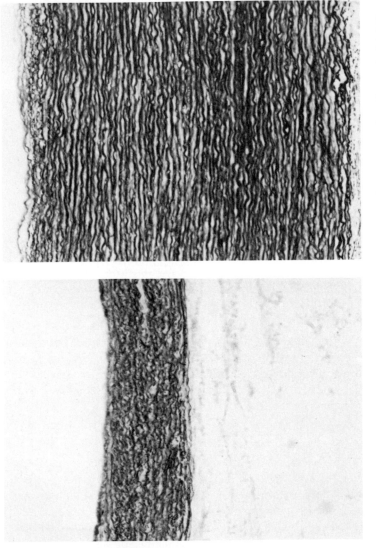

FIGURE 36 Pulmonary trunk (left) with severe medial atrophy, compared to the aorta (right), in a girl aged 12 years with tetralogy of Fallot (Both: Elastic van Gieson's, ×90).

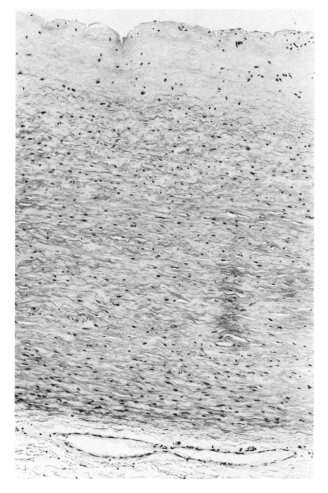

FIGURE 37   Pulmonary trunk with marked diffuse intimal fibrosis, in a boy aged 15 years with a ventricular septal defect and pulmonary hypertension (H & E, ×90).

aorta, are rare in the large pulmonary arteries. Calcification of the plaques is sometimes prominent but generally much less marked than in aortic atherosclerosis.

If a thrombus, virtually always of embolic origin, is incorporated into the wall of the pulmonary trunk or one of the main arteries, the lumen may become considerably narrowed or even almost obstructed by the organized

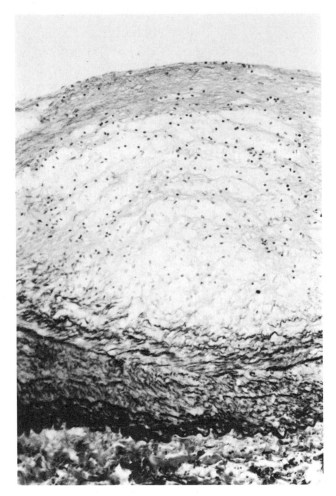

FIGURE 38   Main pulmonary artery with extensive patch of atherosclerosis, in a woman aged 23 years with patent ductus arteriosus and pulmonary hypertension (Elastic van Gieson's, ×140).

mass which forms a large, fibrotic intimal plaque (Fig. 39). By progressive recanalization and shrinkage of these thrombotic masses, fibrotic bands and web-like structures may be spread out in the arterial lumen (Fig. 40).

Lesions of Whole Wall

Among the conditions affecting the whole wall of the large extrapulmonary arteries, vasculitis is rare and much more uncommon than in systemic arteries

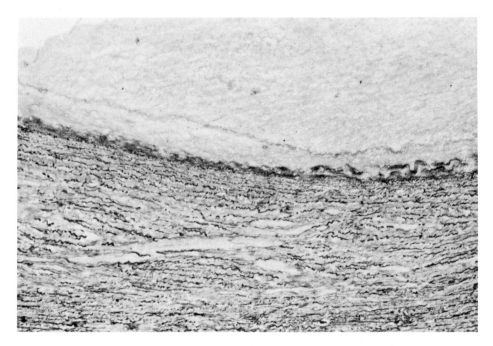

FIGURE 39   Main pulmonary artery with intimal fibrosis due to organization of a thromboembolus, in a woman aged 37 years with chronic thromboembolism (Elastic van Gieson's, ×50).

of comparable caliber. Arteritis of the pulmonary trunk has been described as being due to syphilis [88], to Takayashu's disease [89-91], and to the condition known as giant cell arteritis [92,93].

Saccular aneurysms affect mainly the pulmonary trunk, less often its main branches. They may be multiple (Fig. 41). These aneurysms are uncommon. Pulmonary hypertension in the presence of acquired valvular disease, ventricular septal defect, or, particularly, patent ductus arteriosus, is the most common causative factor [88]. Other causes are syphilis [94], trauma [95, 96], bacterial infections [97,98] and Marfan's syndrome [99,100]. In the latter condition the wall of the pulmonary trunk exhibits changes similar to those usually seen in the aorta, that is, excessive fragmentation and loss of elastic tissue and marked deposition of acid mucopolysaccharides [83].

Dissecting aneurysms of the pulmonary trunk are even more rare [101-103]. Also, in these cases there is usually pulmonary hypertension. They may cause death by cardiac tamponade when they rupture into the pericardial cavity.

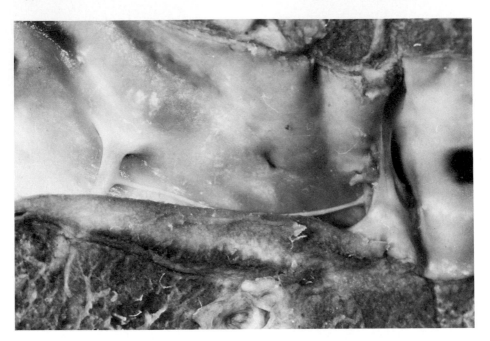

FIGURE 40   Bands and weblike structures in main pulmonary artery near the hilus, in a man aged 71 years with embolic pulmonary hypertension.

Diffuse dilatation of the pulmonary trunk and of both main pulmonary arteries is commonly associated with pulmonary hypertension irrespective of its cause (Fig. 42). This form of dilatation is sometimes very pronounced. Local aneurysm formation within a dilated vessel has been described [104].

In the presence of pulmonic stenosis a poststenotic dilatation affecting the pulmonary arteries sometimes over a considerable distance, may occur [105,106]. Idiopathic dilatation of the pulmonary arteries is an uncommon condition. It usually does not give rise to severe symptoms, although incompetence of the pulmonary valve has been reported [107-109]. Even without the development of an aneurysm the wall of the pulmonary artery may rupture with fatal hemorrhage. Partial rupture has also been described. Often in these instances there is so-called cystic medionecrosis of the arterial wall. Rupture is almost always due to pulmonary hypertension, notably in patients with mitral stenosis [110-113], patent ductus arteriosus [114,115], ventricular septal defect [116], primary pulmonary hypertension [117], chronic pulmonary embolism [118], or lung diseases [119]. The tear may start in a patch of atherosclerosis [120].

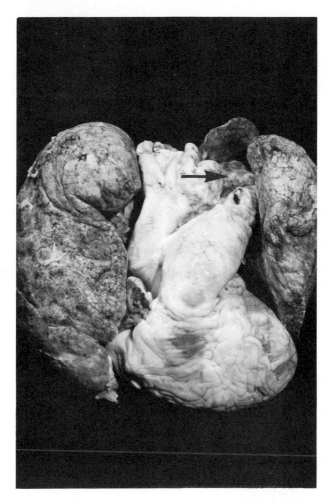

FIGURE 41 Heart-lung specimen with a large aneurysm of the pulmonary trunk and a second aneurysm (arrow) of the left main pulmonary artery, in a woman aged 76 years with primary pulmonary hypertension.

C. Elastic Pulmonary Arteries

Lesions of Media

Generally, the changes that occur in response to abnormal hemodynamic situations in the media of elastic pulmonary arteries are not very conspicuous. In pulmonary hypertension there is some increase in thickness of the media as well as in the amount of elastic tissue. Atrophy of the media may be seen in patients with pulmonic stenosis or tetralogy of Fallot.

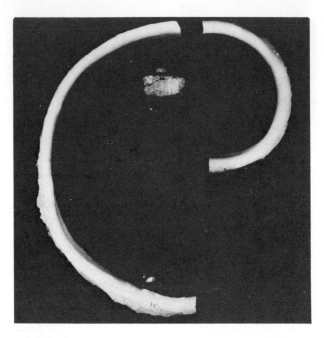

FIGURE 42   Pulmonary trunk (left) as compared to aorta (right), in a man aged 31 years with a ventricular septal defect of the endocardial cushion type and pulmonary hypertension. Two halves of cross-sectional slices, fixed in expanded state, are contrasted. There is extreme diffuse dilatation of the pulmonary trunk (×1.7).

Lesions of Intima

As in the pulmonary trunk and main arteries, atherosclerosis of elastic pulmonary arteries is common in all forms of pulmonary hypertension (Fig. 43). It also occurs in young children with congenital heart disease. Since within the lungs the pulmonary arteries retain an elastic structure down to a caliber of approximately 1-mm external diameter, these arteries are the smallest in the body in which true atheroma can be observed. In young children with pulmonary hypertension, atherosclerotic patches may be found in arteries of a caliber between 500 and 300 μm.

Thromboemboli, by a process of organization, ultimately produce eccentric patches of intimal fibrosis in elastic pulmonary arteries. Subsequent recanalization may result in the formation of band-like and web-like structures, that may be numerous in patients with chronic thromboembolism (Fig. 44).

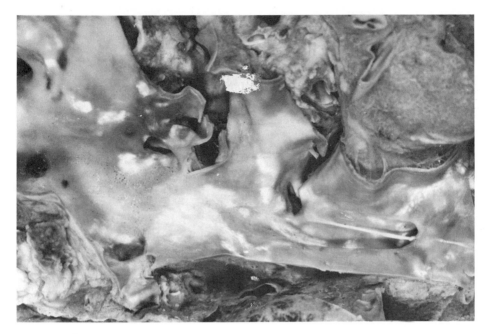

FIGURE 43   Large, elastic pulmonary arteries, cut open lengthwise, with pronounced atherosclerosis, in a woman aged 84 years with embolic pulmonary hypertension. There is also a band resulting from recanalization of an embolus.

Lesions of Whole Wall

The elastic pulmonary arteries are not often the site of arteritis. Occasionally they are involved in inflammatory processes of the lungs, for instance, tuberculosis.

Saccular aneurysms of the intrapulmonary elastic arteries are often mycotic, sometimes following endocarditis [121-124]. They are mostly multiple. Saccular aneurysms also occur in pulmonary hypertension, for instance due to patent ductus arteriosus [125] or primary pulmonary hypertension [126]. Moreover, thromboemboli in some instances, by their impact on the arterial wall, are supposed to cause damage to the wall resulting in aneurysms [127], while occasionally a congenital origin (Fig. 45) has been accepted [128].

Dissecting aneurysms of elastic pulmonary arteries have been described, usually in patients with pulmonary hypertension [129-131].

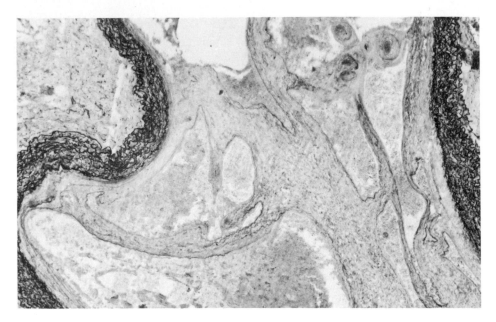

FIGURE 44   Elastic pulmonary artery with multiple band-like and web-like structures due to organization and recanalization of thromboemboli, in a man aged 54 years with embolic pulmonary hypertension (Elastic van Gieson's, ×50).

D.   Muscular Pulmonary Arteries and Arterioles

As the muscular pulmonary arteries, including the muscularized portions of the arterioles, form by far the most reactive part of the pulmonary vasculature, the changes in these arteries, observed in response to hemodynamic alterations, usually tend to be both more early and more pronounced than in other pulmonary vessels. This applies particularly to the media, which may change its thickness very rapidly according to functional requirements. Although intimal reactions generally take more time, they may become also very prominent, with severe and lasting consequences for the pulmonary circulation. In contrast, lesions of the adventitia are usually less spectacular. In pulmonary hypertension the muscular pulmonary arteries are often coiled (Fig. 46).

Lesions of Adventitia

Lung processes may involve the adventitia of muscular pulmonary arteries, and commonly it is the only part of the vascular wall thus affected. Such changes will be considered together with alterations of the whole wall. Specific adventitial lesions are uncommon, but adventitial thickening with

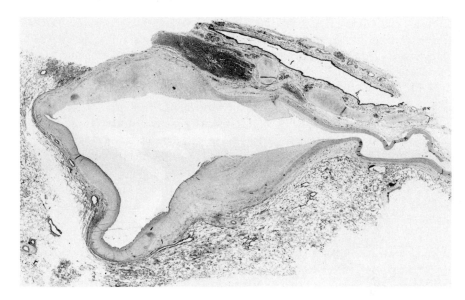

FIGURE 45   Aneurysm of elastic pulmonary artery, in a woman aged 26 years with a small ventricular septal defect but without pulmonary hypertension. The aneurysm is supposedly of congenital origin. There are patches of intimal fibrosis (H & E, ×8).

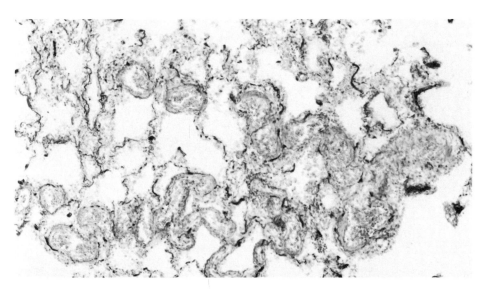

FIGURE 46   Markedly coiled muscular pulmonary arteries, in a woman aged 23 years with patent ductus arteriosus and pulmonary hypertension (Elastic van Gieson's, ×90).

fibrosis (Fig. 47) is characteristic of pulmonary venous hypertension. This fibrosis, which may be due to perivascular edema, may cause the adventitial thickness to increase from a normal average of 4.6% to 10.5% in patients with mitral stenosis [133].

Bundles of longitudinal smooth muscle cells may occur in the adventitia, often in a reduplication of the external elastic lamina (Fig. 48). These are particularly common in patients with pulmonary venous hypertension, as in mitral valve disease, but are also observed in chronic lung disease and other conditions. Their function is probably related to that of intimal smooth muscle bundles (p. 72).

Lesions of Media

Vasoconstriction

In most instances, thickening of the muscular coat of the pulmonary arteries is due either to their constriction or to hypertrophy of their media. The two

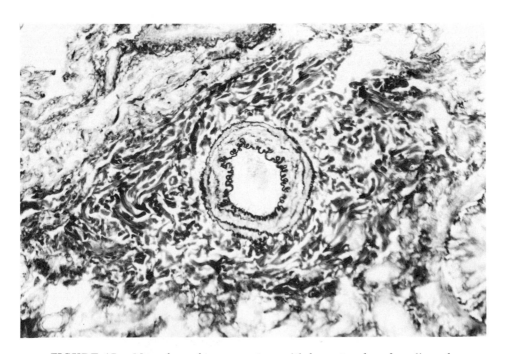

FIGURE 47   Muscular pulmonary artery with hypertrophy of media and severe fibrotic thickening of adventitia, in a girl aged 14 years with mitral stenosis (Elastic van Gieson's, ×140).

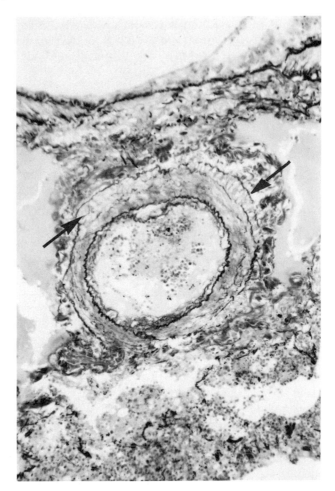

FIGURE 48   Muscular pulmonary artery with bundles of longitudinal smooth muscle cells in a reduplication of the external elastic lamina, in a woman aged 27 years with mitral stenosis (Elastic van Gieson's, ×140).

processes may cause this thickening independently or in combination with each other, and it is often difficult to decide to what extent each has contributed.

Vasoconstriction of muscular pulmonary arteries causes narrowing of the lumen, crenation of the internal and sometimes also of the external elastic lamina, and an increased thickness of the media. All these features may be present, however, in the absence of active arterial contraction, when the vessels are studied in collapsed, formalin-fixed lung tissue. This implies that vasoconstriction cannot be judged reliably in such material. Neither is it advisable to inject the pulmonary arteries with fixative or contrast material, because by this procedure the vessels dilate, often unpredictably and excessively, so that vasoconstriction can no longer be assessed.

However, if the lungs are inflated in situ by instillation with fixative through the trachea, the blood vessels in the lung are generally distended. In normal rat lungs it could be shown that in this way the elastic laminae of virtually all muscular pulmonary arteries were smooth, while the media was much thinner than that in collapsed lungs. On the other hand, when pulmonary arterial vasoconstriction is induced in rats, either by application of fulvine or by hypoxia, inflation of lung tissue does not abolish the crenation of the elastic laminae or the increase in medial thickness [134,135], so that an impression of the degree of arterial contraction may be gained.

A more reliable characteristic of vasoconstriction can be demonstrated at an ultrastructural level. Electron microscopic studies of constricted pulmonary arteries and veins of the rat have shown that the medial smooth muscle cells form cytoplasmic excrescences of their surface (Fig. 49), particularly adjacent to the internal, to a lesser extent also to the external elastic lamina [134]. In this way it could be shown that if vasoconstriction is abolished, for instance by discontinuation of hypoxia, the excrescences disappear while medial hypertrophy may persist [135].

In normal adult human lungs with their thin-walled muscular pulmonary arteries, as in the lungs of animals that normally have a thin pulmonary arterial media, such as the dog and the rat, vasoconstriction is usually not noticeable in histologic sections. Even so, it is striking that sometimes occasional pulmonary arteries are much more thick walled than the great majority while having a markedly crenated internal elastic lamina. This suggests that arterial constriction may occur in some arteries in an otherwise normal lung [136].

In some animals like the rabbit, which normally have a thick pulmonary arterial muscular coat, constriction may be very conspicuous [137]. The arteries may even become completely occluded as the intima is rumpled up and blocks what remains of the lumen (Fig. 50). Such an excessive vasoconstriction has been observed in the rabbit after isolated lung perfusion or after intravenous injection of packed cells. We found that if only one lung is perfused the phenomenon is unilateral. It may occur in less than 30 min, indicating that medial hypertrophy does not contribute to the pronounced thickening of the media.

Pronounced vasoconstriction is also readily observed in the smallest pulmonary arteries and arterioles of the normal fetal and neonatal lung, both in the human (p. 24) and in various animals, but in these instances the arterial media also is thick, as compared to that of the adult arteries.

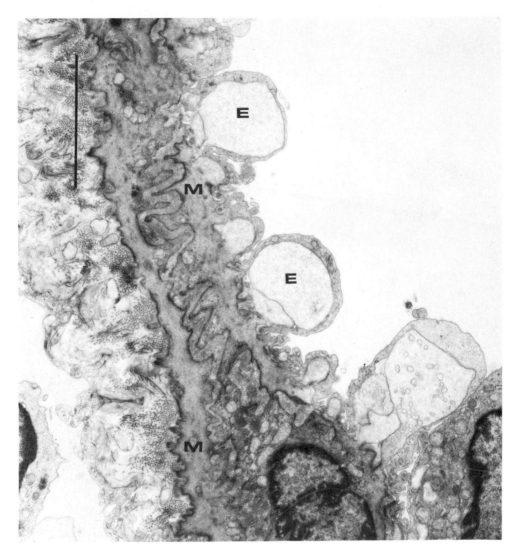

FIGURE 49 Electron micrograph of detail of pulmonary venous wall in a rat, 3 weeks after intraperitoneal application of fulvine. As an expression of vaso-constriction, cytoplasmic excrescences (E) from medial smooth muscle cells (M) protrude into the lumen. These excrescences are poor in organelles and covered by endothelium. Bar indicates 5 μm.

Medial Hypertrophy

Increased tone and contraction of arterial smooth muscle eventually leads to an actual increase of medial smooth muscle tissue. In part this is due to hy-

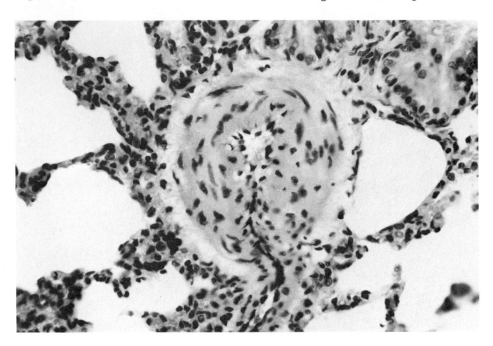

FIGURE 50   Severe vasoconstriction of muscular pulmonary artery in a rabbit after a 60-min perfusion of whole blood. The lumen is subtotally occluded, a branch completely obstructed (H & E, ×350).

pertrophy, as individual muscle cells increase in size; for the greater part it is due to hyperplasia, that is, an increase in number of muscle cells. The term medial hypertrophy has always conveniently been applied to the increase of medial smooth muscle produced in either way. If medial hypertrophy has developed, the capacity of the artery for vasoconstriction is augmented.

Medial hypertrophy of muscular pulmonary arteries is generally judged from the increase in medial thickness (Fig. 51). Although vasoconstriction, as we have seen, contributes to this thickness, a marked increase always connotes hypertrophy of the media. Generally, in normal adult human lungs, an average thickness of the media of over 7% of the external diameter indicates hypertrophy; this ratio may increase to 15% and sometimes to over 20% (Fig. 52).

In newborn infants that normally have a thick media, and the same applies to some animals, an increased thickness may be difficult to judge without morphometric evaluation. On the other hand, particularly in infants with obstruction of pulmonary venous flow, as in congenital mitral stenosis, medial

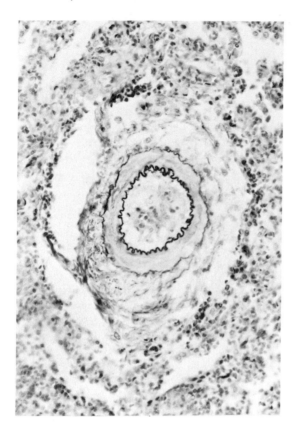

FIGURE 51 Muscular pulmonary artery with medial hypertrophy, in a boy aged 5 years with persistent truncus arteriosus and pulmonary hypertension (Elastic van Gieson's, ×230).

hypertrophy may be excessive, with individual arteries showing a medial thickness of over 30% of the external diameter.

Sometimes, medial hypertrophy may be masked by vascular dilatation which reduces the thickness of the media. In these instances it may be necessary to assess the amount of arterial smooth muscle by calculating the cross-sectional medial surface area per unit of lung surface area [21] or by comparing it to the intimal surface area, when intimal lesions are absent [32]. Although this method permits the assessment of hypertrophy only, thus eliminating the effect of contraction or dilatation, it is very time consuming and not easily applicable to routine examination.

Medial hypertrophy is the most common alteration in muscular pulmonary arteries. It is found in any form of pulmonary hypertension, whether due to congenital or acquired heart disease, to lung diseases or hypoxia, to embolism, or to the idiopathic form of pulmonary hypertension. It is unlikely

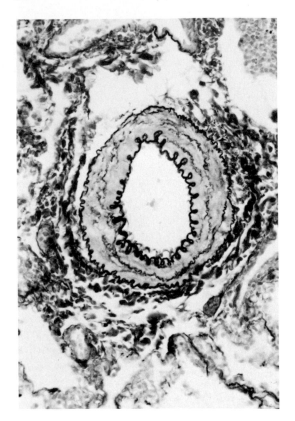

FIGURE 52 Muscular
pulmonary artery with
severe medial hypertrophy,
in a girl aged 12 years with
patent ductus arteriosus
and total anomalous pul-
monary venous connection
(Elastic van Gieson's,
×230).

that it is ever absent when the pulmonary arterial pressure is significantly
elevated. Reports to the contrary are probably caused either by misjudgment
in the absence of morphometric studies or by the secondary effect of dilatation.

Even in patients in whom a pulmonary arterial pressure within normal
limits had been established by cardiac catheterization, the muscular pulmonary
arteries may sometimes exhibit medial hypertrophy. We observed this, for instance, in a number of patients with mild mitral stenosis or with aortic
stenosis. It is likely that intermittent elevation of pressure during exercise is
responsible for the medial hypertrophy in these cases.

Not distinctly related to elevation of pressure is medial hypertrophy in
pulmonary arteries, in or adjacent to areas of lung fibrosis, or near a bronchial
carcinoma. Sometimes all arteries in the affected lobe are involved, while
those in other parts or in the contralateral lungs have a normal media. Possibly, the development of bronchopulmonary anastomoses in the diseased lung
tissue is basic to the development of medial hypertrophy in these pulmonary
arteries [138].

Muscularization of Arterioles

Since normal arterioles, according to the definition we gave earlier (p. 19), are arterial branches with a transition of a muscular to a nonmuscular wall, it follows that, particularly at a small caliber, they have only a discontinuous muscular coat or none at all. In pulmonary hypertension, these small branches develop circular smooth muscle cells in their walls, so that in the adult human lung, branches of an external diameter of 30 to 40 μm sometimes, and in children, of 20 μm or less, exhibit a continuous muscular media (Fig. 53). In effect, this muscularization of arterioles is a form of medial hypertrophy.

Although it is possible that this muscularization in some instances is brought about by proliferation of smooth muscle cells in a distal direction, it is more likely that muscle cells have developed from endothelial cells or multifunctional mesenchymal cells [139]. Mitotic figures in pulmonary vascular

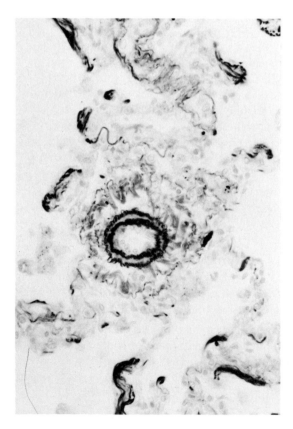

FIGURE 53 Pulmonary arteriole with muscularization, in a man aged 18 years with mitral stenosis (Elastic van Gieson's, X350).

walls are observed occasionally but are generally rare even in cases of pulmonary hypertension.

Muscularization of arterioles is usually not conspicuous in embolic pulmonary hypertension but is common in patients with congenital heart disease with a left-to-right shunt, in those with pulmonary venous hypertension, and particularly in those with pulmonary hypertension due to hypoxia. In the latter condition the increase in arterial smooth muscle may well be largely restricted to this form of medial hypertrophy, as the media of the larger muscular arteries may be normal or only mildly hypertrophied [140,141].

Longitudinal Muscle Bundles in Media

Small bundles, more uncommonly crescent-shaped or circumferential layers, of longitudinally arranged smooth muscle bundles may be found within the media [5]. They usually occur in association with intimal and/or adventitial longitudinal smooth muscle bundles and probably have a similar function. We have observed them in patients with rheumatic mitral stenosis (Fig. 54), as well as in those with congenital heart disease with a left-to-right shunt.

Dilatation and Atrophy

Dilatation and medial atrophy of muscular pulmonary arteries cause thinning of the muscular layer, alone or in combination. It is even more difficult than in the case of vasoconstriction versus medial hypertrophy to decide which of the two factors is responsible or predominates, since the assessment of medial cross-sectional surface area is of little help in these instances. Although theoretically this surface area is decreased in medial atrophy and unchanged in dilatation, the small variations with regard to normally thin-walled arteries rarely permit a conclusion. When pulmonary arteries associated with bronchioles have lost virtually, sometimes even completely, their medial smooth muscle tissue, it is safe to assume that atrophy is involved. In these instances the vessels are usually dilated as well.

Dilatation is sometimes focal, as in the small telangiectases of the lung, occasionally observed in patients with cirrhosis of the liver; more often it is a diffuse process. As such, it may be found in patients with acute pulmonary congestion. In the presence of a very large pulmonary blood flow, as in some patients with an atrial septal defect, it may mask medial hypertrophy [142].

Medial atrophy, generally in combination with dilatation, is observed in patients with isolated congenital pulmonic stenosis and particularly with tetralogy of Fallot [143]. In these patients a poststenotic dilatation could be assumed, but this does not seem probable since not only the most peripheral pulmonary arteries but also the pulmonary veins are usually wider than normal. It is

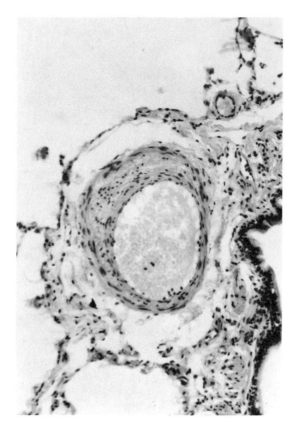

FIGURE 54 Muscular pulmonary artery with a crescent-shaped layer of longitudinally arranged smooth muscle cells within the media, in a man aged 57 years with mitral stenosis (H & E, ×140).

more likely that an increased blood volume is basic to the general vascular dilatation, but also in that case the atrophy of the muscular coat, which is sometimes very striking (Fig. 55), remains unexplained. In the presence of a pulmonic stenosis the pulmonary arterial pressure curve is flattened, and it seems likely that this, through the absence of high systolic pressure peaks, is basic to a dysfunction atrophy of the arterial muscular media in these instances. In patients with complete transposition of the large arteries, medial atrophy may be present as well [144].

In the presence of severe intimal fibrosis the media often becomes atrophic in these areas, probably since the smooth muscle cells are inhibited in their function by the rigid core of the thickened intima. This secondary medial atrophy is much more common in plexogenic pulmonary arteriopathy than in other forms of pulmonary hypertension. Dilatation of muscular arteries may also be part of the so-called dilatation lesions, discussed later (p. 80).

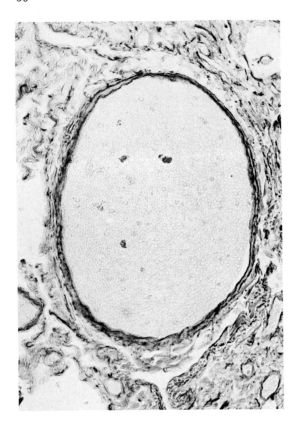

FIGURE 55   Severe
medial atrophy of a mus-
cular pulmonary artery, in
a woman aged 19 years
with tetralogy of Fallot.
The muscular coat is either
thin or completely absent
(Elastic van Gieson's,
×140).

Medial Fibrosis and Calcification

In some conditions, more often in pulmonary venous hypertension and in lung
diseases than in other forms of pulmonary hypertension, the muscular pulmonary arteries exhibit not only hypertrophy but also fibrosis of their media.
There is a marked increase of collagen and sometimes of elastic fibers which
are interspersed between the circular smooth muscle fibers. This fibrosis and
elastosis may contribute considerably to the thickness of the media. In
patients with mitral stenosis the number of smooth muscle cells per medial
surface area is distinctly lower than the relative numbers in comparable arteries from patients with, for instance, a ventricular septal defect.

The deposition of calcium in the walls of muscular pulmonary arteries
and arterioles is usually limited to the intima (Fig. 56), particularly to the internal elastic lamina. Sometimes, also, the external elastic lamina is involved,
as in primary pulmonary hemosiderosis. Uncommonly there is more extensive
medial calcification and very rarely bone formation in the arterial wall.

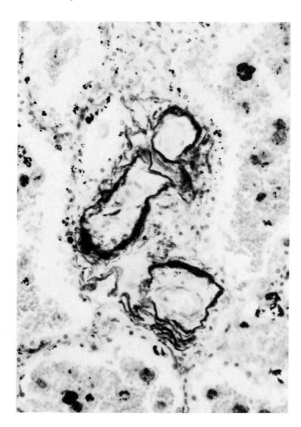

FIGURE 56 Pulmonary arterioles with calcification of elastic laminae, in a girl aged 11 years with primary pulmonary hemosiderosis (von Kossa stain, ×230).

Lesions of Intima

Cellular Proliferation

The earliest intimal changes in response to an elevated pulmonary arterial pressure tend to escape our observation unless electron microscopic studies are done. In histologic sections there may be some swelling of the endothelial cells, that may protrude into the lumen, particularly in the presence of arterial contraction.

At an ultrastructural level the subendothelial space is widened and the cytoplasm of the endothelial cells shows an increase of organelles, indicating an active cellular metabolism. Moreover, vacuoles, sometimes of considerable size, are formed [145,146].

The role of the endothelial cells in intimal cellular proliferation is probably very limited, although in experimental pulmonary hypertension we observed an occasional mitotic figure within the endothelium. The layers of proliferating cells in the intima are entirely or almost entirely composed of cells with all the characteristics of smooth muscle cells [29]. They have abundant myofilaments and electron-dense bodies, while their nuclei also resemble closely those of smooth muscle cells, and in our experience the only difference with medial smooth muscle cells is that they are often not spindle shaped.

There is much evidence to indicate that most cells in cellular intimal proliferation are derived from the media. In histologic sections it can be observed that usually in the early lesions the proliferating cells are arranged perpendicularly to the media (Fig. 57), and in electron microscopic preparations there are often indications that they penetrate the internal elastic lamina. How these cells migrate and whether they are derived from mature medial smooth muscle cells, from multipotential cells [147,148] or from vasoformative reserve cells [149] is still undecided.

Cellular intimal proliferation is particularly frequent in small arteries and arterioles in patients with congenital heart disease with a left-to-right

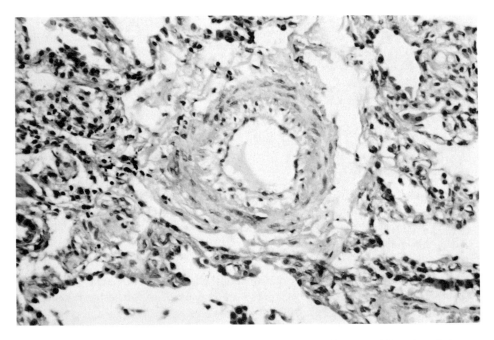

FIGURE 57   Muscular pulmonary artery with early cellular proliferation, in a boy aged 6 years with a ventricular septal defect. The intimal cells are perpendicular to the media (H & E, ×230).

shunt. In mitral valve disease larger muscular pulmonary arteries are more often involved (Fig. 58). The lesions are reversible in the sense that, when the cause of the pulmonary hypertension is removed, a thick cellular layer may regress to a thin layer of compact intimal fibrosis (p. 92).

Generally, this intimal change is absent or uncommon in infants younger than 1 or 2 years of age. If pulmonary hypertension develops in a patient in whom the muscular pulmonary arteries are not adapted to a high pressure, it may develop within a few weeks. Such an event occurred in a boy aged 15 years with tetralogy of Fallot in whom corrective surgery was performed but who developed acute pulmonary hypertension because the patch over his ventricular septal defect loosened [136].

Concentric Laminar Intimal Fibrosis

Among the various forms of intimal fibrosis in muscular pulmonary arteries, concentric-laminar intimal fibrosis is characteristic for the pattern of pulmonary vascular lesions that has been termed "plexogenic pulmonary arteriopathy" [150]. This pattern is characteristic for pulmonary hypertension due

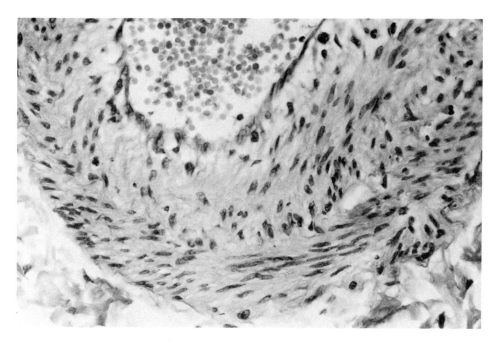

FIGURE 58   Detail of large, muscular pulmonary artery with cellular intimal proliferation, in a woman aged 40 years with mitral stenosis. The intimal cells are perpendicular to the media (H & E, ×350).

to congenital heart disease with a shunt, as well as for primary pulmonary hypertension.

It develops on the basis of cellular intimal proliferation. Gradually in these cellular layers, collagen fibers, and sometimes also elastic fibers, are deposited in such a way that a concentric onionskin-like arrangement is formed, with narrowing and often obstruction of the lumen (Fig. 59). This arrangement is also recognizable in a hematoxylin stain (Fig. 60). The cells within these layers retain their smooth muscle-like appearance at an ultrastructural level and therefore do not differ from those in other forms of intimal fibrosis [29]. Even so, the peculiar concentric-laminar structure has certain implications, as these intimal alterations tend to be progressive, and either do not regress or regress minimally after closure of a ventricular septal defect or of a patent ductus arteriosus.

There is a rough but distinct correlation between the degree of concentric-laminar intimal fibrosis on the one hand and the elevation of pulmonary arterial pressure and resistance on the other [142]. If intimal fibrosis is

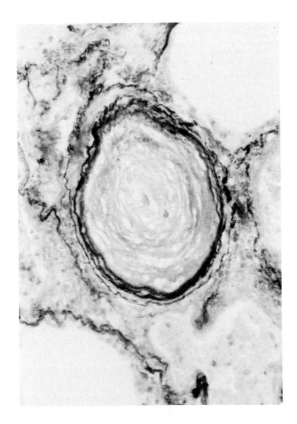

FIGURE 59   Muscular pulmonary artery with concentric-laminar intimal fibrosis, in a woman aged 19 years with primary pulmonary hypertension (Elastic van Gieson's, ×140).

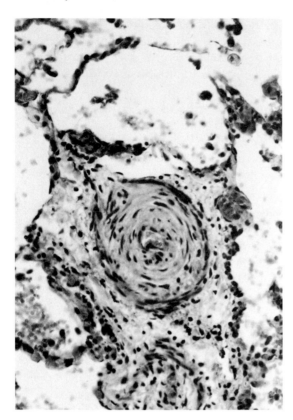

FIGURE 60 Muscular pulmonary artery with concentric-laminar intimal fibrosis, in a girl aged 6 years with primary pulmonary hypertension (H & E, ×230).

mild in a lung biopsy taken during surgical closure of a defect, it does not stand in the way of a favorable postoperative course. Severe and widespread intimal lesions of this type usually indicate a poor prognosis.

In some instances this type of intimal fibrosis is crescent shaped rather than concentric. If there is severe intimal fibrosis in an arterial branch, this may protrude at the site of its orifice from a larger artery into the parent vessel so that it forms an eccentric patch. As always in the evaluation of pulmonary vascular lesions, the presence of concentric-laminar intimal fibrosis should not be judged from an occasional artery, but the total picture of the lung vessels should be taken into account. Uncommonly, an onionskin type of intimal lesion is observed in young patients with mitral stenosis, but then usually in very few arteries.

Postthrombotic Intimal Fibrosis

It has long been known from experiments in animals that thrombi injected intravenously, after being trapped in the pulmonary arteries, produce, by subsequent organization, eccentric patches of intimal fibrosis [151-153]. Similar lesions are extraordinarily common in the human. Occasional small patches of eccentric intimal fibrosis in muscular pulmonary arteries may be found regularly at autopsy in adult individuals. Obviously, these have no clinical significance.

In chronic embolic pulmonary hypertension, however, these changes are usually very numerous and contribute to the mechanical obstruction of the pulmonary arterial bed (Fig. 61), even though the obliteration is generally over only a short distance. Therefore, in a histologic section, pulmonary arteries with an obstructed lumen are seen next to many arterial cross sections with a normal patent lumen.

From the morphologic point of view it is not possible to tell whether this intimal fibrosis results from organization of thromboemboli or of locally formed thrombi. In tetralogy of Fallot, for instance, there is often a marked tendency to thrombosis in the pulmonary arteries, and in these patients this

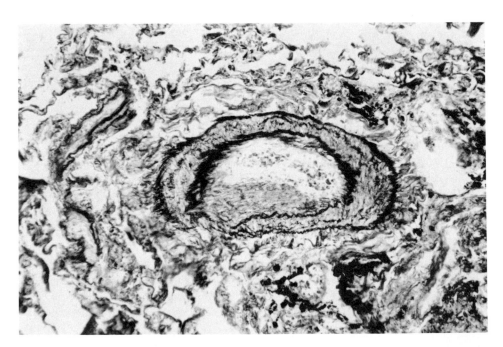

FIGURE 61   Muscular pulmonary artery with patch of eccentric intimal fibrosis due to organization of thromboembolus, in a woman aged 35 years with embolic pulmonary hypertension (Elastic van Gieson's, ×140).

form of eccentric intimal fibrosis is sometimes just as common as in patients with chronic pulmonary embolism.

Also in this type of intimal fibrosis, the organizing cells are ultrastructurally identical to muscle cells, and this remains so after the whole thrombus is incorporated into the vascular wall. Iron pigment may be present in the intimal patch, but this is not common.

Recanalization first produces small capillary-like channels. These may widen to large spaces, so that ultimately broad (or less often thin) intravascular fibrous septa stand out in the lumen as remnants of the original organized clot (Fig. 62). These fibrous septa are often particularly widespread and delicate (Fig. 63) in tetralogy of Fallot [143,154]. They are comparable to the bands and webs in the larger elastic arteries.

Diffuse Eccentric Intimal Fibrosis

Particularly in patients with pulmonary venous hypertension, but also in some patients with fibrosis of the lungs, the muscular pulmonary arteries may be

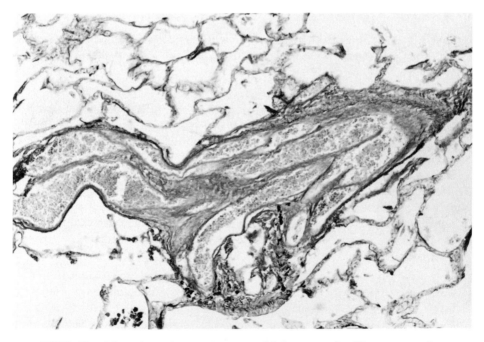

FIGURE 62 Muscular pulmonary artery with intravascular fibrous septa due to organization and recanalization of thromboemboli, in a woman aged 39 years with embolic pulmonary hypertension (Elastic van Gieson's, ×90).

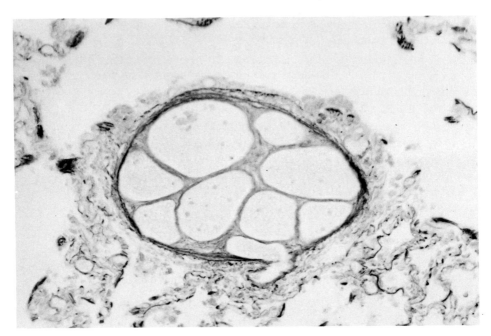

FIGURE 63   Muscular pulmonary artery with very delicate intravascular fibrous septa, in a woman aged 19 years with tetralogy of Fallot (Elastic van Gieson's, ×140).

the site of severe intimal fibrosis. In contrast to the intimal changes observed in cases of thromboembolism or tetralogy of Fallot, these alterations are diffuse in the sense that they are present over long distances in the arteries. Although often pronounced and causing considerable narrowing of the lumen, obliteration of the arteries is uncommon (Fig. 64). In mitral valve disease all arteries of both lungs are essentially involved, although the intimal fibrosis is usually more severe in the upper parts of the lungs [155]. Few, if any, arterial crosssections exhibit a normal intima. In various lung diseases this type of intimal fibrosis is limited to the fibrotic areas or their immediate environment.

Even though the intimal fibrosis may happen to be circumferential in some arteries, it is not concentric-laminar as in plexogenic pulmonary arteriopathy. The cellular components again resemble smooth muscle cells in every aspect. The fibrotic layer is more loosely constructed than that in patients with ventricular septal defect or primary pulmonary hypertension. This may explain the fact that, even in the presence of severe intimal fibrosis, the pulmonary arterial pressure in patients with mitral stenosis is often not markedly

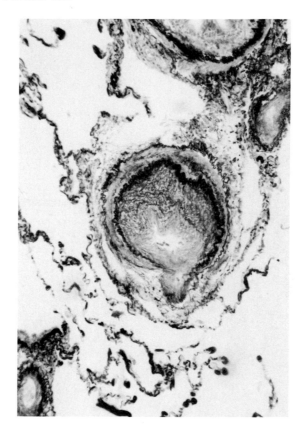

FIGURE 64 Muscular pulmonary artery with pronounced diffuse eccentric intimal fibrosis, in a man aged 64 years with mitral stenosis (Elastic van Gieson's, ×140).

elevated. Generally, there is a poor correlation between intimal changes and pulmonary arterial pressure in these cases. Consequently, severe intimal changes in a lung biopsy do not indicate an unfavorable outcome of an operation, as they do in patients with congenital heart disease.

Intimal Elastosis

Collagen is the predominant fiber component in most forms of intimal fibrosis, though occasional elastic fibers are not uncommon in the thickened intimal layer. In some instances the intimal elastic tissue is very pronounced (Fig. 65). This elastosis is particularly observed in patients with congenital heart disease with left-to-right shunts, sometimes in young children. It is also regularly to

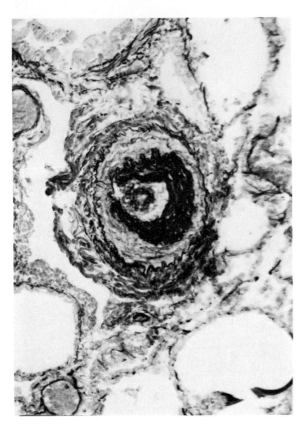

FIGURE 65 Muscular
pulmonary artery with in-
timal elastosis, in a boy
aged 10 years with a
ventricular septal defect
(Elastic van Gieson's,
×140).

be found in mitral valve disease. It does not distinctly correlate with hemodynamic data.

Longitudinal Muscle Bundles in the Intima

As we have seen, the cells present in the various forms of intimal fibrosis are
all or mostly smooth muscle cells on ultrastructural analysis. Generally, however, these cells have an haphazard arrangement, and in histologic sections they
are not recognizable as such.

Often, bundles of longitudinally arranged muscle cells, clearly recognizable as such under the light microscope, develop within the thickened intima
(Fig. 66). These bundles may be isolated, crescent shaped, or circumferential.
Intimal muscle bundles occur characteristically in small, muscularized arterioles
in hypoxic pulmonary hypertension, whether due to living at high altitudes,
to chronic bronchitis, or to other hypoxic states [156–158].

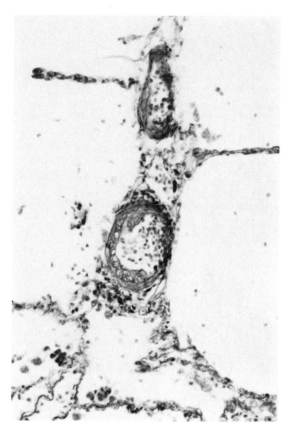

FIGURE 66   Pulmonary arteriole with distinct muscular media and a layer of longitudinal smooth muscle cells in the intima, in a man aged 37 years with Pickwickian syndrome (Elastic van Gieson's, ×225).

These bundles are also common in pulmonary venous hypertension but then usually in larger muscular pulmonary arteries (Fig. 67). Less regularly they are observed in patients with congenital heart disease. In uncommon cases, patients with a ventricular septal defect may have considerable thickening of the intimal layer, even to the point of complete obstruction of the pulmonary arterial lumen, which is composed entirely or predominantly of longitudinal smooth muscle cells. There are indications that these patients, in spite of the severe intimal thickening, do very well after corrective surgery, so that apparently these vessels to some extent become patent again after closure of a defect.

The smooth muscle cells that occur normally in the intima of small arterioles of newborn infants (p. 26) tend to persist in the presence of pulmonary hypertension, while normally they disappear within days after birth. In infants with an elevated pulmonary arterial pressure some arterioles

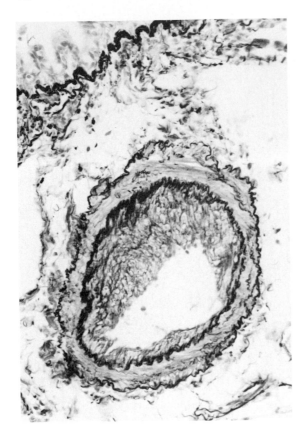

FIGURE 67 Muscular pulmonary artery with longitudinal smooth muscle bundles in the thickened intima, in a woman aged 44 years with mitral stenosis (Elastic van Gieson's, ×230).

at the site of branching have a ring-like structure consisting of smooth muscle cells and protruding into the lumen of the parent artery (Fig. 68). These sphincter-like structures are sometimes seen in normal neonatal arteries but more often in systemic than in pulmonary vessels [159].

The effect of the longitudinal intimal muscle cells, and probably the same applies to medial (p. 58) and adventitial (p. 50) smooth muscle bundles, is apparently that they enhance the action of the circular muscle cells of the media by preventing overdistention of the vessel [160].

Uncommonly, circular smooth muscle bundles develop in the thickened and fibrotic intima, thus forming a second muscular coat (Fig. 69), usually immediately beneath the endothelial layer [136].

Calcification and Iron Incrustation

Deposits of calcium and iron salts are found mainly in the internal elastic lamina, but also in the media and sometimes in a thickened intima. It is ob-

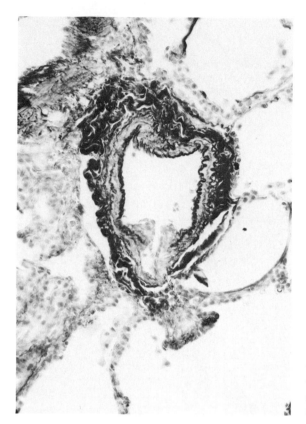

FIGURE 68 Muscular pulmonary artery with ring-like structure consisting of smooth muscle cells, protruding from the orifice of a branch, in a boy aged 6 months with complete transposition of the large vessels and ventricular septal defect (Elastic van Gieson's, ×230).

served in patients with a disturbed calcium metabolism, with primary pulmonary hemosiderosis, and less often in patients with secondary hemosiderosis [161]. In some instances there is no distinct reason why this incrustation occurs.

Lesions of Whole Wall

Arteritis and Fibrinoid Necrosis

Pulmonary arteritis implies an inflammatory process involving the walls of the arteries of the lungs. The term fibrinoid necrosis is used when—generally in a short vascular segment, sometimes only in a part of its circumference—the arterial wall becomes necrotic with imbibition of fibrin. This process usually is first visible in the media, but both the intima and the adventitia may become involved as well. Pulmonary arteritis may occur in the absence of recognizable necrosis, while fibrinoid necrosis is regularly observed without an inflammatory cellular exudate in the vascular wall. The combination of both

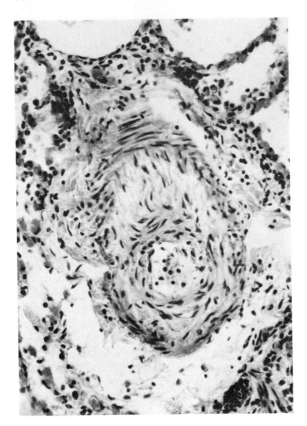

FIGURE 69   Muscular pulmonary artery with marked intimal fibrosis, in which a second circular smooth muscular layer has developed, in a girl aged 6 years with primary pulmonary hypertension (H & E, X230).

processes, however, is very common, and in many instances arteritis and fibrinoid necrosis are difficult to separate.

There are many clinicopathologic entities associated with pulmonary arteritis and fibrinoid necrosis, in which the cause and pathogenesis are unknown [162]. Known causes include infectious arteritis. The muscular pulmonary arteries may become involved in a wide variety of infectious processes, generally more readily spreading from the luminal side when the vessel is blocked by an infected embolus than from the surrounding lung tissue (Fig. 70). If the artery is lying in an area of pneumonia, as long as the blood flow through the pulmonary arteries is undisturbed, the vascular wall appears to be very resistant to the infectious process and arteritis does not appear until in a late stage [136].

Granulomatous arteritis is uncommonly observed in patients with pulmonary tuberculosis. When it does occur, the granuloma usually affects all layers of the arterial wall, although sometimes a small granuloma that appar-

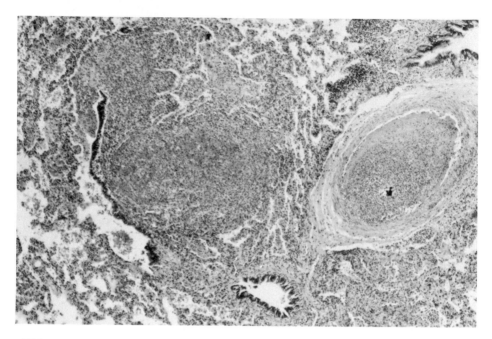

FIGURE 70 Two muscular pulmonary arteries, each containing an infected embolus, in a boy aged 9 years with sepsis. In the artery to the right there is beginning inflammatory involvement of its wall; in that to the left, the wall is largely destroyed (H & E, ×55).

ently is limited to the intima may protrude into the lumen. Also, in sarcoidosis, the granulomas may sometimes involve vascular walls.

Pulmonary arteritis may occur as a manifestation of a generalized systemic disease, such as polyarteritis nodosa, systemic lupus erythematosus, scleroderma, dermatomyositis, and rheumatic-rheumatoid disorders. Generally, the lung vessels are less often involved than the systemic vessels in these conditions, and in polyarteritis nodosa, for instance, the lung vessels are often spared [163]. There is regularly a combination of arteritis and fibrinoid necrosis in these disorders, and the inflammatory exudate, consisting of polymorphonuclear leukocytes or of mononuclear cells, may extend well into the surrounding parenchyma of the lung.

In patients with generalized vasculitis resulting from drug allergy, the pulmonary arteries are commonly involved with a morphologic picture resembling that in polyarteritis nodosa [164].

An ill-defined group of disorders of unknown cause is that of the granulomatous vasculitides which often involve or are even limited to the muscular pulmonary arteries. This group has been designated as "pathergic granulomatoses" on the basis that the cause in any of these disorders should be attributed to a disturbance of the immune reaction in these patients [165]. Liebow [166] listed the following conditions as "pulmonary angiitis and granulomatosis": (1) classic Wegener's granulomatosis, (2) limited form of Wegener's granulomatosis, (3) lymphomatoid granulomatosis, (4) necrotizing sarcoid granulomatosis, and (5) bronchocentric granulomatosis. Lie [162] added (6) Churg-Strauss allergic granulomatosis. The histopathologic characteristics of these various conditions, inasmuch as the pulmonary arteries are concerned, tend to overlap. In the Churg-Strauss granulomatosis, eosinophils predominate in the cellular infiltrate [167].

Another form of pulmonary arteritis and fibrinoid necrosis, of particular interest with regard to the pulmonary circulation, is that occurring in severe pulmonary hypertension. In these cases there is always fibrinoid necrosis (Fig. 71), but inflammatory exudate involving the surrounding lung tissue may be absent, present, or even extensive (Fig. 72). Fibrinoid necrosis has a characteristic localization, namely, in a small branch, shortly after its ramification from a larger artery. The lesion may be circumferential or may involve only part of the circumference. The affected part of the arterial wall is swollen, has lost its nuclei, and has a pink color in routine histologic sections. Usually the lumen in this area is the site of a fibrin clot.

It is likely that spastic bouts of arterial constriction are responsible for the vascular necrosis with subsequent imbibition of the wall by fibrin [168], and that the inflammation is a later reaction secondary to the necrosis. If Crotalaria alkaloids such as fulvine are administered to rats, an identical form of fibrinoid necrosis (Fig. 73) is produced in the pulmonary arterial walls [169,170], and this is preceded by intense arterial vasoconstriction [134].

Fibrinoid necrosis of muscular pulmonary arteries with or without arteritis is particularly common in patients with primary pulmonary hypertension and, to a lesser extent, in those with congenital cardiac disease with a left-to-right shunt. In these forms of pulmonary hypertension vasoconstriction is supposed to play a predominant part [171]. It is uncommon in patients with mitral stenosis and rare in other conditions associated with pulmonary hypertension.

These vascular alterations are generally observed in the more severe cases of pulmonary hypertension. Their presence in a lung biopsy taken when a cardiac malformation is corrected usually indicates a doubtful prognosis for the patient.

Plexiform Lesions

In the more severe cases of vasoconstrictive pulmonary hypertension, the complicated and striking changes known as plexiform lesions can often be de-

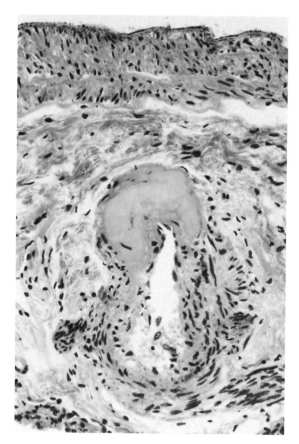

FIGURE 71 Muscular pulmonary artery with fibrinoid necrosis, in a boy aged 2 years with primary pulmonary hypertension. The affected area (top) is localized shortly after branching from a parent artery (H & E, ✕230).

tected. Their frequency in the lung vessels varies greatly. In some cases they are fairly numerous; in others, it may be necessary to study multiple lung sections to find a single example. Apart from the very early stages, plexiform lesions are so easily recognizable, particularly in a hematoxylin stain, and so characteristic that they gave rise to the term plexogenic pulmonary arteriopathy to indicate the morphologic vascular pattern of which they form one of the latest stages [150].

In its full-blown form, a plexiform lesion consists of a localized dilatation in a muscular pulmonary artery or arteriole shortly after its ramification from a larger vessel. The wall of this aneurysm-like dilatation is thin and shows signs of destruction, usually with interruption of elastic laminae. The former lumen of this dilated area is filled up with proliferating cells, often with dark nuclei that form strands and septa with capillary-like channels in between (Fig. 74). In this way a plexus is formed that looks like, and has even been misinterpreted as, a small angioma.

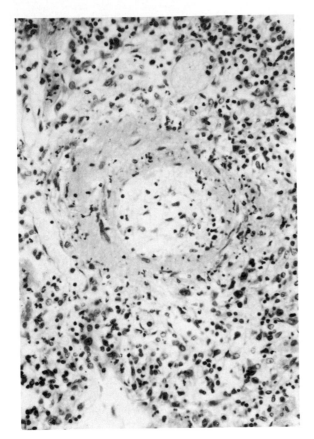

FIGURE 72   Muscular
pulmonary artery with
fibrinoid necrosis and
arteritis, in a girl aged 13
years with primary pulmo-
nary hypertension (H & E,
×230).

The proximal part of the branch shows usually medial hypertrophy and
sometimes but not always concentric-laminar intimal fibrosis. Distal to the
plexus the artery and its branches are wide and thin walled (Fig. 75).

There is much morphologic and experimental evidence that plexiform
lesions develop in areas previously affected by fibrinoid necrosis. Fibrinoid
necrosis and sometimes arteritis are often recognizable in the initial part of the
branch containing the plexiform lesion. In either alteration, the localization is
in the same area shortly after the branching point. Transitional stages between
fibrinoid necrosis with early cellular proliferation to the mature plexiform
lesions can often be observed (Fig. 76).

In experimental animals in which a shunt between systemic and pulmonary circulations has been created so that they developed pulmonary hypertension, the sequence of the lesions can be determined. In this way it could
be shown that fibrinoid necrosis and arteritis preceded the plexiform lesions
[172–174].

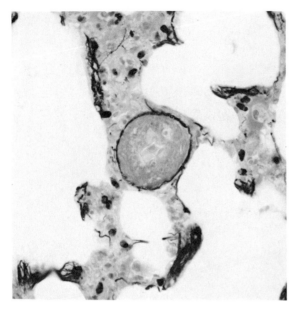

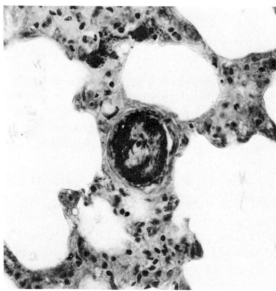

FIGURE 73 Muscular pulmonary artery with fibrinoid necrosis in a rat, 4 weeks after intraperitoneal application of fulvine. [(top) Elastic van Gieson's, (bottom) Phosphotungstic acid hematoxylin; both: ×350.]

Plexiform lesions are present in patients with primary pulmonary hypertension, with pulmonary hypertension due to congenital cardiac disease with a shunt, or in association with hepatic injury. Also, in patients with tetralogy of Fallot in whom pulmonary hypertension has occurred as a result of the

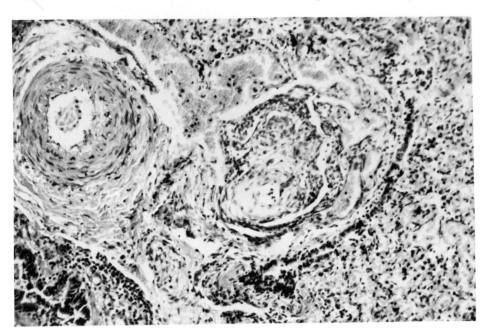

FIGURE 74   Plexiform lesion (right) in a branch of a muscular pulmonary artery (left), in a boy aged 5 years with a ventricular septal defect (H & E, ×140).

surgical creation of a shunt, plexiform lesions have been observed occasionally [175,176]. The only other condition in which plexiform lesions may occur is pulmonary schistosomiasis. If this is associated with severe pulmonary hypertension, fibrinoid necrosis and arteritis as well as plexiform lesions may be found, in addition to the granulomas around the ova of the Schistosoma parasite.

   If a lung biopsy reveals plexiform lesions when a patient is operated upon for a cardiac defect, this generally must be taken as an ominous sign.

Dilatation Lesions

Plexiform lesions are sometimes included within the group of so-called dilatation lesions, and, as we have seen, dilatation is one of their features. As we have pointed out before [81], we prefer to treat them as an alteration separate from the other dilatation lesions because they represent one of the most characteristic lesions of hypertensive pulmonary vascular disease, while this certainly does not apply to the group of dilatation lesions as a whole.

   We will therefore use the term *dilatation lesions* for those alterations based on arterial distention but lacking an intraluminal plexus. Such changes

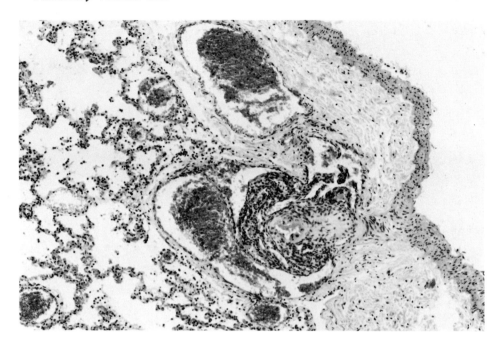

FIGURE 75 Plexiform lesion in a branch shortly after ramification from a parent artery (right), in a girl aged 5 years with a ventricular septal defect. The distal branches are dilated (H & E, X90).

may occur in the form of "vein-like branches" or as clusters of markedly dilated arteries [177]. These vessels, by the secondary thinning of the originally hypertrophied media, may sometimes mimic normal pulmonary arteries but often have almost entirely lost their muscular coat by excessive distention. Large clusters of this type are known as angiomatoid lesions.

Lungs that contain dilatation lesions may or may not simultaneously contain fibrinoid necrosis and plexiform lesions. All these alterations have the same significance with regard to the severity of the pulmonary hypertension. In some cases they are exceedingly numerous. The clusters are usually situated in branches shortly after ramifications (Fig. 77), a localization similar to that of the plexiform lesions. Whether fibrinoid necrosis plays a part in their pathogenesis is not clear.

E.   Alveolar Capillaries

In congestion of the lungs, the alveolar capillaries are dilated and engorged with blood. Leakage of fluid through the capillary walls causes pulmonary

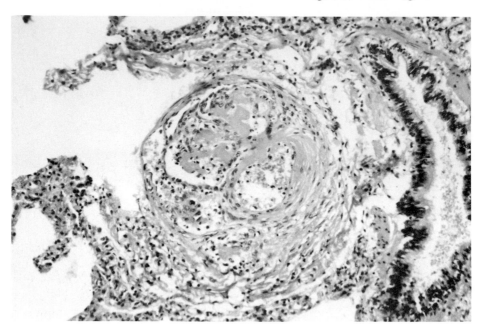

FIGURE 76   Early plexiform lesion with beginning recanalization of fibrin
clot, in a girl aged 9 years with a patent ductus arteriosus. There is destruction
of the wall of the arterial branch (H & E, ×140).

edema, and the transudate may become hemorrhagic through diapedesis of
erythrocytes. The capillaries may also rupture.

By their intimate connection with the lung tissue, the alveolar capillaries
rarely escape damage in the presence of lung disease. In atelectasis of the
lungs the alveolar walls become collapsed, and to a certain extent this also
applies to the capillaries. Even so, there is no immediate decrease of pulmonary blood flow in the nonventilated parts of the lungs [178,179]. A subsequent gradual decrease in flow is probably in part the result of narrowing of
pulmonary arteries and arterioles and in part of collapse and kinking of the
capillaries.

In pulmonary emphysema the alveolar walls are stretched or even
destroyed and this leads to narrowing and disappearance of large numbers of
alveolar capillaries. In view of the very large reserve of the pulmonary capillary bed, it is unlikely that this contributes significantly to the elevation of
pulmonary arterial pressure observed in many patients, particularly with centrilobular emphysema or with a combination of emphysema and chronic

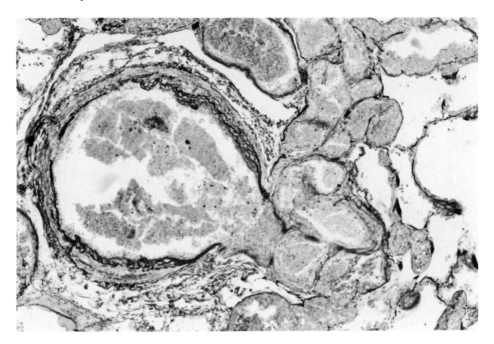

FIGURE 77   Muscular pulmonary artery with a dilatation lesion in a branch, in a woman aged 36 years with primary pulmonary hypertension (Elastic van Gieson's, X90).

bronchitis [180]. It is far more likely that hypoxic vasoconstriction of muscular pulmonary arteries is responsible for the pulmonary hypertension in these instances. In pulmonary emphysema, some of the capillaries that remain intact increase considerably in width [181]. These have been termed flow capillaries.

In all forms of interstitial fibrosis, the alveolar walls become thickened by the deposition of collagen fibers. If the fibrosis is severe the capillaries become compressed and distorted. Eventually, obliteration of alveolar capillaries results. However, the development of severe pulmonary hypertension on the basis of capillary destruction is uncommon.

In the presence of pulmonary hypertension, irrespective of its cause, the basal membranes of the alveolar capillaries are thickened. This has been shown in acquired as well as in congenital heart disease and also in primary pulmonary hypertension [182-185]. Moreover, the endothelial cells are swollen and edematous and the cytoplasm may contain an increased amount of lamellar structures and organelles.

F.   Pulmonary Venules and Veins

Lesions of Adventitia

As in the pulmonary arteries, the pulmonary venous adventitia tends to become markedly thickened and fibrotic in patients with mitral stenosis or other forms of pulmonary venous hypertension.

Lesions of Media

Although the pulmonary veins have a muscular coat thinner than that of pulmonary arteries containing relatively fewer muscle cells, there is increasing evidence that they are capable of constriction. This could already be assumed on the basis of the marked medial hypertrophy of pulmonary veins in cases of pulmonary venous hypertension, but active constriction of veins also has been demonstrated in response to pharmacologic agents and hypoxia [186–188].

This has now also been corroborated by morphologic evidence. When fulvine is administered to rats it appears that the veins of the lung constrict (Fig. 78) in the same way as the arteries [169]. Morphologically, the smooth muscle cells of the venules and veins exhibit all the features of contraction. Their nuclei show deep indentations, and their cytoplasm forms excrescences similar to those in the constricted pulmonary arteries. These excrescences are even more prominent than in the arteries as there is no internal elastic lamina to withstand them [134,170]. They often protrude deep into the endothelial cells and may even push the endothelial nuclei to the lumen.

Medial hypertrophy of pulmonary veins (Fig. 79) is usually present and often conspicuous in patients with pulmonary venous hypertension such as mitral stenosis [189]. It may be particularly severe in young, even newborn, infants with congenital mitral stenosis, aortic atresia, or other cardiac malformations with impaired pulmonary venous flow [57]. Both large and small pulmonary veins are usually affected.

A characteristic change, observed in the pulmonary veins under the same circumstances, is arterialization (Fig. 80). This implies that the elastic configuration of the venous wall, normally irregular and haphazard, is altered in such a way that elastic laminae are formed on either side of the thickened media [50]. Often there is no more than a rough indication of external and internal elastic laminae, but sometimes the arterial wall is mimicked so accurately that the arteries and veins become virtually indistinguishable and serial histologic sections may be necessary to identify the vessels. Medial hypertrophy and arterialization are as a rule present at the same time.

Medial atrophy of pulmonary veins is sometimes suggestive in patients with tetralogy of Fallot but is difficult to distinguish from venous dilatation, which is discussed in connection with lesions of the whole vascular wall (p. 86).

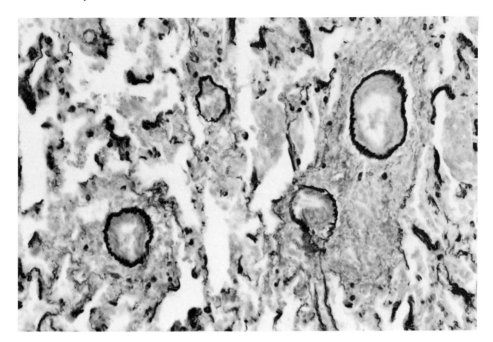

FIGURE 78 Pulmonary veins showing pronounced constriction of their walls, in a rat 3 weeks after intraperitoneal application of fulvine. The elastic laminae are markedly crenated. The muscular pads are accentuated (Elastic van Gieson's, ×230).

Lesions of Intima

While mild intimal fibrosis occurs regularly as an age change in the pulmonary veins of adults, it tends to be much more severe in most forms of pulmonary venous hypertension (Fig. 81). Usually it is patchy and eccentric. Complete obliteration is uncommon. In chronic hypoxia, intimal fibrosis of pulmonary veins may be present and more pronounced than is usually seen as an age change (Fig. 82).

In pulmonary veno-occlusive disease, a rare condition affecting mainly children and young adults, numerous pulmonary veins and venules are narrowed or even completely obliterated by sometimes loose, sometimes more dense and collagen-rich connective tissue (Fig. 83). There is much evidence that venous thrombosis is basic to this type of intimal fibrosis. It seems likely that at least in some cases the thrombosis is brought about by viral infection, although other etiologic factors may well be involved [190,191].

Pulmonary venous thrombosis is otherwise not very common, although it occurs sometimes in patients with tetralogy of Fallot or with infectious [192] or neoplastic processes in the lungs.

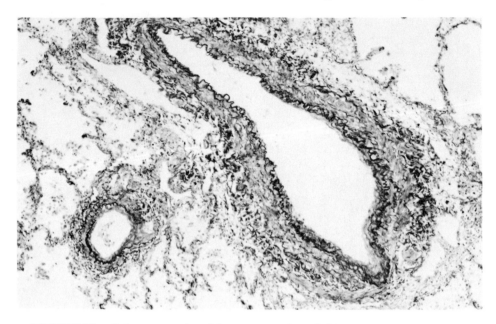

FIGURE 79   Pulmonary vein with pronounced medial hypertrophy, in a man aged 63 years with aortic stenosis and mitral incompetence (Elastic van Gieson's, ×90).

Lesions of Whole Wall

Dilatation of pulmonary venous and venular walls occurs in acute congestion of the lungs and is sometimes excessive. In mitral valve disease varices of pulmonary veins may develop [193]. These pulmonary varices are also known to occur in the absence of pulmonary hypertension and are then considered to be congenital malformations [194], but it is likely that in part they are the result of dilatation secondary to pulmonary venous hypertension, as they may regress after repair of the mitral valve disease [195].

Other alterations including the whole pulmonary venous wall include phlebitis in patients with infectious, allergic, or other conditions associated with pulmonary vasculitis, as discussed in connection with arteritis (p. 72). Fibrinoid necrosis is usually absent or inconspicuous, but in experiments with fulvine it could be shown that it may occur in the pulmonary veins of the rat [170].

G.   Anastomes

An increase in number and size of bronchopulmonary arterial anastomoses has been established in various forms of lung disease, notably in patients with

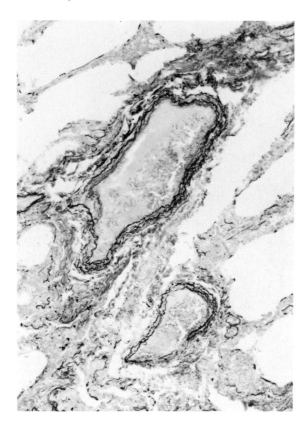

FIGURE 80   Pulmonary
veins with arterialization,
in a woman aged 27 years
with mitral stenosis. There
is a distinct internal and
external elastic lamina
(Elastic van Gieson's,
X90).

chronic bronchitis and emphysema and particularly in patients with bronchiectasis [77,196,197]. It is likely that, at least in part, these anastomoses
develop de novo in areas of granulation tissue [196]. Marked intimal fibrosis
(Fig. 84) may occur in these enlarged anastomoses. Also, in lung diseases associated with fibrosis, for instance in pulmonary tuberculosis, bronchopulmonary arterial anastomoses are often numerous and enlarged [198].

Anastomoses between bronchial arteries and pulmonary arteries obstructed by thromboemboli may develop with time [199]. In tetralogy of
Fallot, among numerous collateral arteries, many can be considered to represent bronchopulmonary arterial anastomoses. Like the pulmonary arteries,
these anastomoses are usually wide and thin walled, although eccentric intimal
thickening by postthrombotic intimal fibrosis is often present.

Bronchopulmonary venous anastomoses are dilated in pulmonary congestion. In pulmonary veno-occlusive disease they may become obstructed by
postthrombotic obliteration just like the small pulmonary veins [200].

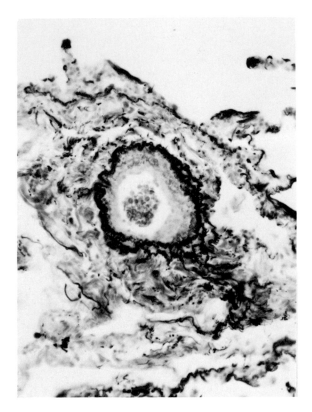

FIGURE 81 Pulmonary vein with marked intimal fibrosis, in a woman aged 29 years with mitral stenosis (Elastic van Gieson's, ×230).

H. Lymphatics

Dilatation of pulmonary lymphatics is a very common change and rarely absent in any form of congestive lung disease (Fig. 85). Sometimes this dilatation produces the picture of focal lymphangiectasis, circumscribed areas consisting of clusters of extremely dilated lymph vessels. Dilatation may also be observed when the lymphatics are blocked by infectious or neoplastic processes.

I. Regression of Vascular Lesions

Some pulmonary vascular lesions appear to be partly or completely reversible when the abnormal stimuli that caused them are removed. Complete regression is achieved with regard to medial alterations like medial hypertrophy and atrophy.

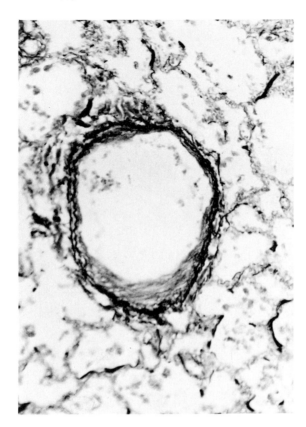

FIGURE 82   Pulmonary vein with mild intimal fibrosis, in a boy aged 16 years living at an altitude of 3500 m in the Andes (Elastic van Gieson's, X140).

When medial hypertrophy of the muscular pulmonary arteries was induced in dogs by the surgical creation of a shunt between systemic and pulmonary circulations, it could be shown that this regressed to normal or near normal after subsequent closure of the shunt [201-203]. In patients with a congenital cardiac defect, the reversibility of pulmonary vascular lesions could be studied when banding of the pulmonary artery was performed, thus providing an artificial stenosis that protected the pulmonary vascular bed from large flow and pressure. When this was later followed by a corrective operation of the defect, and when lung biopsies were taken on both occasions, the effect of the decreased pulmonary arterial pressure on the vascular lesions could be evaluated.

Dammann et al. [204] in this way found that medial hypertrophy regressed to normal or near normal in 8 of 10 patients; in our own material we established this in 11 of 20 patients, while some decrease in mean medial thickness was found in the other 9 as well.

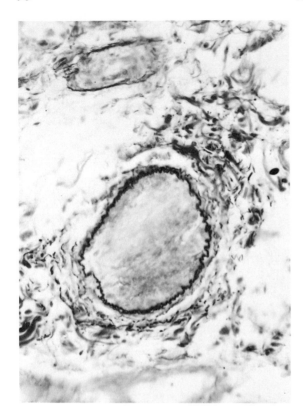

FIGURE 83   Pulmonary
vein with complete ob-
literation by intimal
fibrosis, in a girl aged 4
years with pulmonary
veno-occlusive disease
(Elastic van Gieson's,
X230).

It is more difficult to assess regression of medial atrophy, as similar
opportunities to compare sequential lung biopsies are rarely provided. Even
so, it is very likely that medial atrophy, which is an almost constant feature in
patients with tetralogy of Fallot [143], is reversible. It may even change to
medial hypertrophy if a palliative shunt created between systemic and pulmonary circulations was inadvertently so large that pulmonary hypertension
ensued.

In our material, the early intimal alterations of muscular pulmonary arteries, consisting of loose cellular proliferation, were reversible to a large extent. If cellular proliferation was present in the biopsy taken at a banding
operation, only mild sequelae were to be found in the later biopsy in the form
of a thin, compact layer of intimal fibrosis. The lumen in these instances was
largely restored. Dammann et al. [204], in three patients with mild intimal
thickening, saw no intimal lesions in the second biopsies.

If intimal *fibrosis* is present at the time of the banding operation, reversibility is usually minimal, particularly when much collagen is deposited in

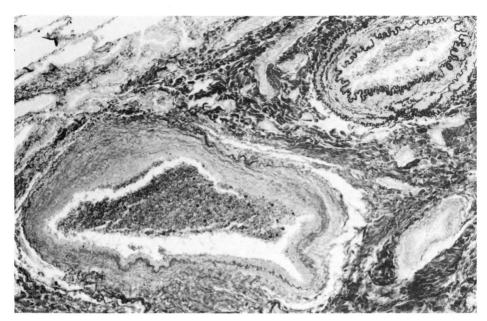

FIGURE 84   Large bronchopulmonary anastomosis with intimal fibrosis adjacent to a pulmonary artery of transitional type with medial hypertrophy, in a man aged 19 years with bronchiectasis (Elastic van Gieson's, X90).

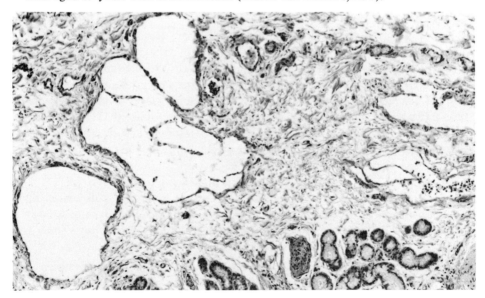

FIGURE 85   Pulmonary lymphangiectases, in a woman aged 31 years with mitral incompetence. The valves in the dilated lymphatics are recognizable (H & E, X90).

the lesions or when the lumen is obliterated. This may well be different in patients with mitral stenosis where the intimal fibrosis is of a more loose texture. In one patient in whom we could study the lungs 10 years after successful commissurotomy, the severe intimal fibrosis present in the lung biopsy had regressed to thin, compact, collagen-rich layers, while the lumen was largely restored.

To some extent, restoration of a vascular lumen is also observed after thrombotic or thromboembolic obstruction of a pulmonary artery. This is achieved by fibrinolysis, by retraction of the organized mass, and by recanalization.

IV. Classification of Pulmonary Vascular Disease

Some of the alterations occurring in the pulmonary vasculature are very common. Medial hypertrophy of muscular pulmonary arteries, for instance, may be found in a large variety of conditions, usually but not even always associated with pulmonary hypertension. Other changes, such as the plexiform lesions, are limited to certain forms of hypertensive pulmonary vascular disease. On the basis of the types and combinations of vascular lesions, therefore, the pathologist may decide when studying lung tissue from a biopsy or from autopsy material what the underlying condition or group of conditions is that caused the pulmonary vascular changes.

While in this way a classification of pulmonary vascular disease, based on these patterns of lesions, is possible [81,82], one should be aware of some hazards. The material studied must be representative for the lungs as a whole. Particularly, small lung biopsies are not always adequate in this respect. It should also be realized that, particularly in the earlier stages of the disease, the pattern may be incomplete, while in other patients more than one pattern may be present. Finally, in many instances it is often at best possible to indicate a group of diagnoses rather than a single diagnosis. The pattern that is now called plexogenic pulmonary arteriopathy occurs in congenital heart disease with a left-to-right shunt and also in the classic or vasoconstrictive form of primary pulmonary hypertension. Another pattern indicates chronic pulmonary venous hypertension, but it cannot be decided whether this is due to mitral valve disease, chronic left ventricular failure, or obstruction of pulmonary veins by mediastinal processes from the lung vessels alone.

Even so, in spite of these limitations, the study of the pulmonary vasculature may be profitable from the diagnostic point of view when a lung biopsy is available, or it may contribute to the postmortem evaluation of the case at autopsy. The following classification may be helpful for this purpose.

A. Plexogenic Pulmonary Arteriopathy

Medial hypertrophy, cellular intimal proliferation, concentric-laminar intimal fibrosis, fibrinoid necrosis of arteries, pulmonary arteritis, plexiform lesions, and dilatation lesions are the characteristic changes.

This pattern occurs, very often in its complete form, in "classical" vasoconstrictive primary pulmonary hypertension. Moreover, it is found in congenital cardiac disease with a left-ro-right shunt. This group includes ventricular septal defect, patent ductus arteriosus, truncus arteriosus persistens, single ventricle, aortico-pulmonary septal defect, and atrial septal defect. The changes are often particularly severe and occur at a very early stage in common atrioventricular canal and in complete transposition of the great vessels associated with a ventricular septal defect. In such instances plexiform lesions, which usually are uncommon below the age of 2 years, may be found in infants as young as 3 weeks [41,205-207], although always in their early stages.

There are also cases on record of plexogenic pulmonary arteriopathy in patients with complete transposition of the great vessels with an intact ventricular septum [208-210] and in patients with hepatic injury [211-214]. In these instances a causal relationship between the underlying condition and the elevated pulmonary arterial pressure seems likely. However, such a connection is not proven and the pulmonary hypertension could be considered as "primary."

Acquired cardiac shunts, such as perforation of the ventricular septum due to myocardial infarction or rupture of an aortic aneurysm into the pulmonary artery, in principle could produce plexogenic pulmonary arteriopathy. However, the serious underlying disease rarely will allow the patient to live beyond the stages of medial hypertrophy or cellular intimal proliferation. An acquired form of pulmonary hypertension producing this pattern of lesions is observed in patients with tetralogy of Fallot in whom the creation of too large a shunt between both circulations results in the equivalent of a wide patent ductus arteriosus [175,176].

Plexogenic pulmonary arteriopathy is always a severe type of hypertensive pulmonary vascular disease, tending to be progressive and reversible only in its earlier stages.

B. Thromboembolic Pulmonary Hypertension

Mild medial hypertrophy (sometimes absent), recognizable thrombi in arteries without or with organization, eccentric patches of intimal fibrosis, and intra-arterial fibrous septa are the characteristic changes.

Chronic, often "silent," pulmonary thromboembolism may have an insidious course, protracted over many years, often in the absence of any recognizable episodes of embolism. Recognizable thrombi, though more numerous than in most other conditions, may be absent, but their sequelae in the form of organized plaques incorporated into the arterial wall are always recognized. The most characteristic feature is formed by the intravascular fibrous septa based upon progressive recanalization of the thrombotic masses [5].

Although we have seen cases of chronic thromboembolism in which medial hypertrophy was an outstanding feature, the increase in medial thickness is usually mild and may be absent. This probably indicates that mechanical obstruction, rather than vasoconstriction, is basic to the elevation of pressure.

The obstructive lesions are focal and often far apart, so that sometimes, in a single histologic section, very few arteries exhibit intimal fibrosis or fibrous septa.

It must be emphasized that primary thrombosis of pulmonary arteries is likely to produce exactly the same pattern of lesions as thromboembolism. Such primary thrombosis is probably rare in comparison to an embolic process, but it is occasionally suggested by the presence of the vascular alterations not only in the arteries but also in the pulmonary veins.

C. Pulmonary Venous Hypertension

Severe arterial medial hypertrophy; muscularization of arterioles; severe intimal fibrosis, usually eccentric, sometimes circumferential but not laminar; uncommonly, pulmonary arteritis; pulmonary venous medial hypertrophy and arterialization with mild to moderate intimal fibrosis; dilatation of lymphatics; hemosiderosis; and interstitial fibrosis of lung tissue are the characteristic changes.

Pulmonary venous hypertension may be caused by a wide variety of conditions all having in common an obstruction to the outflow of the pulmonary venous blood. Acquired conditions like mitral stenosis or incompetence, aortic incompetence, or chronic left ventricular failure are the most common causes [5]. Sometimes, the pattern of pulmonary vascular lesions is produced by a left atrial myxoma or by stenosis of pulmonary veins as a result of mediastinal processes [215].

In principle, exactly the same alterations in the lung vessels can be produced by congenital cardiovascular malformations such as congenital mitral stenosis, aortic atresia, cor triatriatum, total anomalous pulmonary venous connection, or congenital stenosis of pulmonary veins. In some of the latter conditions, medial hypertrophy of both pulmonary arteries and pulmonary veins and venous arterialization tend to be very severe and may occur in young infants. In aortic atresia, for instance, we have found it present at birth [216].

In contrast to other forms of pulmonary hypertension, in pulmonary venous hypertension there is a regional distribution of the vascular lesions. Probably related to the hydrostatic pressure in the lower parts of the lungs, coming on top of the increased left atrial pressure [217], medial hypertrophy of pulmonary arteries and veins in cases of rheumatic mitral stenosis is more pronounced at the bases of the lungs than in the apices. On the other hand, intimal fibrosis is often more conspicuous in the upper parts of the lungs [155].

While in patients with congenital cardiac defects associated with a left-to-right shunt there is a rough correlation between the degree of arterial medial hypertrophy and intimal fibrosis on the one hand and the elevation of pulmonary vascular pressure and resistance on the other, such a correlation is absent or indistinct in pulmonary venous hypertension. This is probably based upon the relatively low number of smooth muscle cells in the arterial media of these patients and on the different structure of the intimal fibrotic plaques (p. 68).

D. Pulmonary Veno-Occlusive Disease

Varying but usually mild arterial medial hypertrophy; sometimes arterial thrombi; pronounced intimal fibrosis and obliteration of pulmonary veins and venules, sometimes with thrombi and intravascular fibrous septa; focal areas of hemosiderosis; and interstitial fibrosis of lung tissue are the characteristic changes.

Pulmonary veno-occlusive disease, a rare condition affecting mainly children and young adults, is distinctive from the previous group because the lesions of the pulmonary veins and venules are primary and not secondary to an increased pressure.

The lesions are almost certainly based upon local thrombosis of the vessels, with subsequent organization. The etiology, however, is not clear. In a considerable number of cases it appears likely that a respiratory, possibly viral, infection has initiated the changes [191,218], but probably other factors may be involved, so that the condition is possibly not an etiologic entity [191].

The clinical diagnosis of pulmonary veno-occlusive disease is difficult, and usually the condition is labeled as "unexplained pulmonary hypertension." The fact that the pulmonary arterial wedge pressure in these patients is only mildly elevated, or even normal, contributes to the problems. Carrington and Liebow [218] explained the low wedge pressure on the basis of obstruction of the small anastomosing veins and venules so that the capillary pressure falls following arterial blockage by the wedged catheter.

E.   Hypoxic Pulmonary Hypertension

Medial hypertrophy of small muscular pulmonary arteries and arterioles is
present; larger arteries are not or are less affected. Bundles or layers of
longitudinal smooth muscle fibers in arterioles and sometimes in venules are
the characteristic changes.

The characteristic features of hypoxic pulmonary hypertension are
particularly observed in the smallest pulmonary arteries that are in close contact with alveolar air spaces, suggesting that alveolar hypoxia may have a direct
effect on these vascular walls. The changes may be found in any form of
bronchial obstruction, such as chronic bronchitis and centrilobular emphysema
[141,219], impaired respiratory movements such as muscular disorders, kyphoscoliosis [220,221], and Pickwickian syndrome [156,222], and even in
chronic upper airway obstruction due to enlarged adenoids. Moreover, the
pattern is present in individuals who develop pulmonary hypertension in
response to hypoxia prevailing at high altitudes [158,223].

In addition to the pulmonary vascular changes, right ventricular hypertrophy and a distinct increase in size of the carotid bodies due to hypertrophy of the type-I glomus cells are seen [140,221,224].

F.   Pulmonary Vascular Changes in Lung Diseases

Marked medial hypertrophy and intimal fibrosis of both pulmonary arteries
and veins, particularly or exclusively in or around areas of diseased lung tissue,
are the characteristic changes.

This is not a distinct or well-defined pattern. On the other hand, it is
useful to recognize that there are often pronounced changes in both pulmonary arteries and veins in close association with areas of lung tissue that are
altered by fibrosis, granulomatosis, or tumor. As this frequently happens in
the absence of pulmonary hypertension, the lung vessels in other areas are
normal and a lung biopsy taken from an affected area may easily be
misinterpreted.

These vascular changes are nonspecific and independent of the underlying pulmonary process. They may be found in any form of fibrotic lung
disease, whether focal or interstitial, in infectious diseases, and in pneumoconioses and granulomatous disorders. Also, in lungs or lung lobes that are
the site of a bronchial carcinoma, these pulmonary vascular lesions are usually
present [138]. Often there are, in addition, vascular changes characteristic of
chronic hypoxia.

G. Pulmonary Vascular Changes
in Decreased Pulmonary Flow

Medial atrophy and wide lumen with thrombotic lesions and delicate intravascular fibrous septa in pulmonary arteries and, to lesser extent, in pulmonary veins; and marked development of collateral arteries, are the characteristic changes.

In patients with tetralogy of Fallot the lung vessels, particularly the pulmonary arteries, are wide and thin walled. The media may become so atrophic in some cases that all arterial smooth muscle disappears [143]. These features also may be recognized in pulmonic stenosis, tricuspid atresia, and in complete transposition of the great arteries with intact ventricular septum [144] but almost never to the same extent. The marked tendency to thrombosis of lung vessels in patients with tetralogy of Fallot results, particularly in older children and adults, in the development of organized masses incorporated into the vascular wall and of intravascular fibrous septa, first described by Rich [154].

Wide and thin-walled arteries, and even thrombi with early organization, may be observed in infants. In pulmonic atresia such alterations have been noticed very shortly after birth [216,225].

References

1. Krahl, V. E., The glomus pulmonale. A preliminary report, *Bull Sch. Med. Maryland,* **45**:36–38 (1960).
2. Becker, A. E., The glomera in the region of the heart and great vessels, *Pathol. Eur.,* 1:410–424 (1966).
3. Boyd, J. D., The inferior aortico-pulmonary glomus, *Br. Med. Bull.,* **17**: 127–131 (1961).
4. Tobin, C. E., Some observations concerning the pulmonic vasa vasorum, Surg. Gynecol. Obstet., **111**:297–303 (1960).
5. Wagenvoort, C. A., and N. Wagenvoort, *Pathology of Pulmonary Hypertension.* New York, London, Sydney and Toronto, Wiley & Sons, 1977.
6. Harris, P., and D. Heath, *The Human Pulmonary Circulation. Its Form and Function in Health and Disease,* 2nd ed. Edinburgh, London, and New York, Churchill Livingstone, 1977.
7. Brenner, O., Pathology of the vessels of the pulmonary circulation, *Arch. Intern. Med.,* **56**:211–237 (1935).
8. Drury, R. A. B., The mortality of elderly Ugandan Africans, *Trop. Geograph. Med.,* 24:385–392 (1972).

9. Meyer, W. W., H. Richter, P. Schollmeyer, and E. Simon, Das Fassungs-vermögen und die Volumendehnbarkeit des aortalen Windkessels und der Pulmonalis in Abhängigkeit von Alter, Arteriosklerose und Hochdruck, *Verh. Dtsch. Ges. Kreislaufforsch.,* 23:346–352 (1957).

10. Harris, P., D. Heath, and A. Apostopoulos, Extensibility of the human pulmonary trunk, *Br. Heart J.,* 27:651–659 (1965).

11. Gray, S. H., F. P. Handler, J. O. Blache, J. Zuckner, and H. T. Blumenthal, Aging processes of aorta and pulmonary artery in negro and white races, *Arch. Pathol.,* 56:238–253 (1953).

12. Heath, D., E. H. Wood, J. W. DuShane, and J. E. Edwards, The structure of the pulmonary trunk at different ages and in cases of pulmonary hypertension and pulmonary stenosis. *J. Pathol. Bacteriol.,* 77:443–456 (1959).

13. Farrar, J. F., J. Blomfield, and R. D. K. Reye, The structure and composition of the maturing pulmonary circulation, *J. Pathol. Bacteriol.,* 90:83–96 (1965).

14. Ferencz, C., M. Libi-Sylora, and J. Greco, Age-related characteristics of the human pulmonary arterial tree, *Circulation,* Suppl. II, 34:107 (1967).

15. Elliott, F. M., and L. Reid, Some new facts about the pulmonary artery and its branching patterns, *Clin. Radiol.,* 16:193–198 (1965).

16. Robertson, B., The normal intrapulmonary arterial pattern in infancy and early childhood; a micro-angiographic and histological study, *Acta Pathol. Microbiol. Scand.,* 71:481–501 (1967).

17. Cumming, G., R. Henderson, K. Horsfield, and S. S. Singhal, The functional morphology of the pulmonary circulation. In *The Pulmonary Circulation and Interstitial Space.* Edited by A. P. Fishman and H. H. Hecht. Chicago and London, University Press, 1969.

18. Granston, A. S., Morphologic alterations of the pulmonary arteries in congenital heart disease, *Proc. Inst. Med. Chicago,* 22:116–117 (1958).

19. Heath, D., and P. V. Best, The tunica media of the arteries of the lung in pulmonary hypertension, *J. Pathol. Bacteriol.,* 76:165–174 (1958).

20. Wagenvoorts, C. A., and N. Wagenvoort, Age changes in muscular pulmonary arteries, *Arch. Pathol.,* 79:524–528 (1965).

21. Wagenvoort, C. A., Vasoconstriction and medial hypertrophy in pulmonary hypertension, *Circulation,* 22:535–546 (1960).

22. West, J. B., and C. T. Dollery, Distribution of blood flow and ventilation-perfusion ratio in the lung, measured with radio active CO_2, *J. Appl. Physiol.,* 15:405–410 (1960).

23. Simons, P., and L. Reid, Muscularity of pulmonary artery branches in the upper and lower lobes of the normal young and aged lungs, *Br. J. Dis. Chest,* 63:38–44 (1969).

24. Edwards, J. E., Functional pathology of the pulmonary vascular tree in congenital cardiac disease, *Circulation,* 15:164–196 (1957).

25. Semmens, M., The pulmonary artery in the normal aged lung, *Br. J. Dis. Chest,* 64:65–72 (1970).

26. Warnock, M. L., and A. Kunzmann, Changes with age in muscular pulmonary arteries, *Arch. Pathol.,* 101:175–179 (1977).

27. Auerbach, O., A. P. Stout, E. C. Hammond, and L. Garfinkel, Smoking habits and age in relation to pulmonary changes. Rupture of alveolar septums, fibrosis and thickening of walls of small arteries and arterioles, *N. Engl. J. Med.*, **269**:1045–1054 (1963).

28. Naeye, R. L., and W. S. Dellinger, Pulmonary arterial changes with age and smoking, *Arch. Pathol.*, **92**:284–288 (1971).

29. Balk, A. G., K. P. Dingemans, and C. A. Wagenvoort, The ultrastructure of the various forms of pulmonary arterial intimal fibrosis, *Virchows Arch. [Pathol. Anat.]*, **382**:139–150 (1979).

30. Rudolph, A. M., The changes in the circulation after birth. Their importance in congenital heart disease, *Circulation*, **41**:343–359 (1970).

31. Wagenvoort, C. A., H. N. Neufeld, and J. E. Edwards, The structure of the pulmonary arterial tree in fetal and early postnatal life, *Lab. Invest.*, **10**: 751–762 (1961).

32. Naeye, R. L., Arterial changes during the perinatal period, *Arch. Pathol.*, **71**:121–128 (1961).

33. Naeye, R. L., Development of systemic and pulmonary arteries from birth through early childhood, *Biol. Neonate*, **10**:8–16 (1966).

34. Levin, D. L., A. M. Rudolph, M. A. Heymann, and R. H. Phibbs, Morphological development of the pulmonary vascular bed in fetal lambs, *Circulation*, **53**:144–157 (1976).

35. Reid, L., The embryology of the lung. In Ciba Foundation Symposium: *Development of the Lung.* Edited by A.V.S. de Reuck and R. Porter. London, Churchill, pp. 109–124, 1967.

36. Davies, G., and L. Reid, Growth of the alveoli and pulmonary arteries in childhood, *Thorax*, **25**:669–681 (1970).

37. Civin, W. H., and J. E. Edwards, The postnatal structural changes in the intrapulmonary arteries and arterioles, *Arch. Pathol.*, **51**:192–200 (1951).

38. Dammann, J. F., and C. Ferencz, The significance of the pulmonary vascular bed in congenital heart disease. I. Normal lungs. II. Malformations of the heart in which there is pulmonary stenosis, *Am. Heart J.*, **52**:7–17 (1956).

39. Lucas, R. V., J. W. St. Geme, R. C. Anderson, P. Adams, and D. J. Ferguson, Maturation of the pulmonary vascular bed: A physiologic and anatomic correlation in infants and children, *Am. J. Dis. Child.*, **101**:467–475 (1961).

40. Von Hayek, H., Über einen Kurzschluszkreislauf (arteriovenöse Anastomosen) in der menschlichen Lunge, *Z. Anat. Entwicklungsgesch.*, **110**: 412–422 (1940).

41. Wagenvoort, C. A., The pulmonary arteries in infants with ventricular septal defect, *Med. Thorac.*, **19**:354–361 (1962).

42. Weibel, E. R., and D. M. Gomez, A principle for counting tissue structures on random sections, *J. Appl. Physiol.*, **17**:343–348 (1962).

43. Weibel, E. R., Principles and methods for the morphometric study of the lung and other organs, *Lab. Invest.*, **12**:131–155 (1963).

44. Staub, N. C., The interdependence of pulmonary structure and function, *Anesthesiology*, **24**:831–854 (1963).

45. Reeves, J. T., J. E. Leathers, and M. B. Quigley, Microradiography of pulmonary arterioles, capillaries, and venules of the rabbit, *Anat. Rec.*, **151**: 531–546 (1965).
46. Weibel, E. R., Morphological basis of alveolar-capillary gas exchange, *Physiol. Rev.*, **53**:419–495 (1973).
47. Weibel, E. R., Morphometric estimation of pulmonary diffusion capacity. I. Model and method, *Respir. Physiol.*, **11**:54–75 (1970).
48. Schultz, H., *Die Submikroskopische Anatomie und Pathologie der Lunge.* Heidelberg, Springer, 1959.
49. Schulz, H., Elektronenoptische Untersuchungen der normalen Lunge und der Lunge bei Mitralstenose, *Virchows Arch. [Pathol. Anat.]*, **328**:582–604 (1956).
50. Wagenvoort, C. A., Morphologic changes in intrapulmonary veins, *Hum. Pathol.*, **1**:205–213 (1970).
51. Edwards, C., and D. Heath, Pulmonary venous chemoreceptor tissue, *Br. J. Dis. Chest*, **66**:96–100 (1972).
52. Korn, D., K. Bench, A. A. Liebow, and B. Castleman, Multiple minute pulmonary tumors resembling chemodectomas, *Am. J. Pathol.*, **37**:641–672 (1960).
53. Kuhn, C., and F. B. Askin, The fine structure of so-called minute chemodectomas, *Hum. Pathol.*, **6**:681–691 (1975).
54. Churg, A. M., and M. L. Warnock, So-called "minute pulmonary chemodectoma"—A tumor not related to paragangliomas, *Cancer*, **37**:1759–1769 (1976).
55. Karrer, H. E., The striated musculature of blood vessels. II. Cell interconnections and cell surface, *J. Biophys. Biochem. Cytol.*, **8**:135–150 (1960).
56. Nathan, H., and M. Eliakim, The junction between the left atrium and the pulmonary veins, *Circulation*, **34**:412–422 (1966).
57. Samuelson, A., A. E. Becker, and C. A. Wagenvoort, A morphometric study of pulmonary veins in normal infants and infants with congenital heart disease, *Arch. Pathol.*, **90**:112–116.
58. Prinzmetal, M., E. M. Ornitz, B. Simkin, and H. C. Berman, Arterio-venous anastomoses in liver, spleen, and lungs, *Am. J. Physiol.*, **152**:48–52 (1948).
59. Tobin, C. E., and M. O. Zariquiev, Arteriovenous shunts in the human lung, *Proc. Soc. Exp. Biol. Med.*, **75**:827–829 (1950).
60. Rahn, H., R. C. Stroud, and C. E. Tobin, Visualization of arterio-venous shunts by cinefluorography in the lungs of normal dogs, *Proc. Soc. Exp. Biol. Med.*, **80**:239–241 (1952).
61. Niden, A. H., and D. M. Aviado, Effects of pulmonary embolism on the pulmonary circulation with special reference to arterio-venous shunts in the lung, *Circ. Res.*, **4**:67–73 (1956).
62. Florange, W., Anatomie und Pathologie der Arteria bronchialis, *Ergeb. Allg. Pathol.*, **39**:152–224 (1960).
63. Verloop, M. C., The arteriae bronchiales and their anastomoses with the arteria pulmonalis in the human lung; a micro-anatomical study, *Acta Anat.*, **5**:171–205 (1948).

64. Wagenvoort, C. A., and N. Wagenvoort, Arterial anastomoses, bronchopulmonary arteries, and pulmobronchial arteries in perinatal lungs, *Lab. Invest.*, **16**:13–24 (1967).
65. Weibel, E., Die Blutgefässanastomosen in der menschlichen Lunge, *Z. Zellforsch.*, **50**:653–692 (1959).
66. Robertson, B., *Micro-angiography of the lung in infancy and childhood.* Stockholm, Proprius, 1973.
67. Liebow, A. A., Recent advances in pulmonary anatomy. In *Ciba Foundation Symposium on Pulmonary Structure and Function.* London, Churchill, pp. 2–25, 1962.
68. Staubesand, J., and M. Stoeckenius, Zur Problematik des Nachweises arterio-venöser Anastomosen. II. Gefässinjektionen mit Wachskugeln bekannter Grösse, *Z. Anat. Entwicklungsgesch.*, **120**:115–120 (1957).
69. Parker, B. M., D. C. Anderson, and J. B. Smith, Observations on arteriovenous communications in lungs of dogs, *Proc. Soc. Exp. Biol. Med.*, **98**: 306–308 (1958).
70. Robertson, B., Postnatal formation and obliteration of arterial anastomoses in the human lung. A microangiographic and histologic study. *Pediatrics*, **43**:971–979 (1969).
71. Von Hayek, H., Über Kurzschlüsse und Nebenschlüsse des Lungenkreislaufes, *Anat. Anz.*, **93**:155–159 (1942).
72. Von Hayek, H., *Die Menschliche Lunge.* Springer Verlag, Berlin, 1953.
73. Verloop, M. C., *Over het Bloedvaatstelsel in de Longen van de Mensch en enkele Knaagdieren* (Ph.D. Thesis) Utrecht, P. Den Boer, 1946.
74. Liebow, A. A., M. R. Hales, and W. E. Bloomer, The relation of bronchial to pulmonary vascular tree. In *Pulmonary Circulation.* Edited by W. R. Adams and I. Veith. New York, Grune & Stratton, pp. 79–98, 1959.
75. Cudkowicz, L., and J. B. Armstrong, Observations on the normal anatomy of the bronchial arteries, *Thorax*, **6**:343–358 (1951).
76. Turner-Warwick, M., Precapillary systemic-pulmonary anastomoses, *Thorax*, **18**:225–237 (1963).
77. Marchand, P., J. C. Gilroy, and V. H. Wilson, An anatomical study of the bronchial vascular system and its variations in disease, *Thorax*, **5**:207–221 (1950).
78. Lauweryns, J. M., *De Longvaten. Architectoniek en Rol bij de Longontplooiing.* Brussel, Presses Acad. Europ., 1962.
79. Lauweryns, J. M., The juxta-alveolar lymphatics in the human adult lung, *Am. Rev. Respir, Dis.*, **102**:877–885 (1970).
80. Lauweryns, J. M., J. Baert, and W. De Loecker, Fine filaments in lymphatic endothelial cells, *J. Cell. Biol.*, **68**:163–167 (1976).
81. Wagenvoort, C. A., Classifying pulmonary vascular disease, *Chest*, **64**:503–504 (1973).
82. Wagenvoort, C. A., Classification of pulmonary vascular lesions in congenital and acquired heart disease, *Adv. Cardiol.*, **11**:48–55 (1974).
83. Wagenvoort, C. A., H. N. Neufeld, and J. E. Edwards, Cardiovascular system in Marfan's syndrome and in idiopathic dilatation of the ascending aorta, *Am. J. Cardiol.*, **9**:496–507 (1962).

84.   Heath, D., and J. E. Edwards, Configuration of elastic tissue of pulmonary
      trunk in idiopathic pulmonary hypertension, *Circulation,* 21:59–62
      (1960).
85.   Farrar, J. F., R. D. K. Reye, and D. Stuckey, Primary pulmonary hyper-
      tension in childhood, *Br. Heart J.,* 23:605–615 (1961).
86.   Roberts, W. C., The histologic structure of the pulmonary trunk in patients
      with "primary" pulmonary hypertension, *Am. Heart J.,* 65:230–236
      (1963).
87.   Heath, D., E. H. Wood, J. W. DuShane, and J. E. Edwards, The relation of
      age and blood pressure to atheroma in the pulmonary arteries and thoracic
      aorta in congenital heart disease, *Lab. Invest.,* 9:259–272 (1960).
88.   Deterling, R. A., and O. T. Clagett, Aneurysm of the pulmonary artery:
      Review of the literature and report of a case, *Am. Heart J.,* 34:471–499
      (1947).
89.   Lupi, H. E., T. G. Sanchez, S. Horwitz, and E. Guttierrez, Pulmonary ar-
      tery involvement in Takayasu's arteritis, *Chest,* 67:69–74 (1975).
90.   Lande, A., and R. Bard, Takayasu's arteritis: an unrecognized cause of
      pulmonary hypertension, *Angiology,* 27:114–121 (1976).
91.   Ishikawa, K., Natural history and classification of occlusive thrombo-
      aortopathy (Takayasu's disease), *Circulation,* 57:27–35 (1978).
92.   Sproul, E. E., A case of "temporal arteritis," *N.Y. J. Med.,* 42:345–352
      (1942).
93.   Planteydt, H. T., Arteritis temporalis, *Ned. Tijdschr. Geneeskd.,* 103:190–
      191 (1959).
94.   Plenge, K., Zur Frage des Syphilis der Lungenschlagader, *Virchows Arch.*
      [Pathol. Anat.], 275:572–584 (1930).
95.   Marble, H. C., and P. D. White, A case of traumatic aneurysm of the pul-
      monary artery, *JAMA,* 74:1778 (1920).
96.   Symbas, P. N., and H. W. Scott, Traumatic aneurysm of the pulmonary
      artery, *J. Thorac. Cardiovasc. Surg.,* 45:645–649 (1963).
97.   Urbanek, K., Zur Kenntnis der mykotischen und rheumatischen Aneu-
      rysmen der Lungenschlagader, *Z. Kreislaufforsch.,* 37:419–420 (1945).
98.   Davis, B. B., and C. P. Clarke, Surgical repair of a mycotic aneurysm of the
      main pulmonary artery complicated by a fistula between the left coronary
      artery and the pulmonary artery. A case report, *J. Thorac. Cardiovasc.*
      Surg., 63:380–383 (1972).
99.   Tung, H. L., and A. A. Liebow, Marfan's syndrome. Observation at
      necropsy with special reference to medio-necrosis of the great vessels, *Lab.*
      Invest., 1:382–386 (1952).
100. Bowden, D. H., B. E. Favara, and J. L. Donahoe, Marfan's syndrome. Ac-
      celerated course in childhood associated with lesions of mitral valve and
      pulmonary artery, *Am. Heart J.,* 69:96–99 (1965).
101. Fleming, H. A., Aorto-pulmonary septal defect with patent ductus ar-
      teriosus and death due to rupture of dissecting aneurysm of the pulmo-
      nary artery into the pericardium, *Thorax,* 11:71–77 (1956).

102. Shilkin, K. B., L. P. Low, and B. T. M. Chen, Dissecting aneurysm of the pulmonary artery, *J. Pathol.,* **98**:25–29 (1969).
103. Bernheim, J., and B. Griffel, A propos d'un cas d'anévrisme disséquant de l'artère pulmonaire, *Ann. Anat. Pathol.,* **17**:83–90 (1972).
104. Nellen, M., Idiopathic pulmonary hypertension, *S. Afr. Med. J.,* **21**:682–689 (1947).
105. Husson, G., M. Blackman, P. Riemenschneider, and A. S. Berne, Benign infundibular pulmonary stenosis with secondary dilatation of the main pulmonary artery, *N. Engl. J. Med.,* **269**:394–398 (1963).
106. D'Cruz, I. A., R. A. Arcilla, and M. H. Agustsson, Dilatation of the pulmonary trunk and of the pulmonary arteries in children, *Am. Heart J.,* **68**:612–620 (1964).
107. Deshmukh, M., S. Guvenc, S. Bentivoglio, and H. Goldberg, Idiopathic dilatation of the pulmonary artery, *Circulation,* **21**:710–716 (1960).
108. Ramsey, H. W., A. De La Terre, J. W. Linhart, L. J. Krovetz, G. L. Schiebler, and J. R. Green, Idiopathic dilatation of the pulmonary artery, *Am. J. Cardiol.,* **20**:324–330 (1967).
109. Burckhardt, D., and J. Moppert, Klinik und Hämodynamik der idiopathischen Dilatation der Arteria pulmonalis, *Z. Kardiol.,* **64**:57–68 (1975).
110. Thomas, G. C., D. M. Whitelaw, and H. E. Taylor, Rupture of the pulmonary artery complicating rheumatic mitral stenosis, *Arch. Pathol.,* **60**:99–103 (1955).
111. Madeloff, S. M., and D. G. Rushton, Rupture of the pulmonary artery associated with mitral stenosis and systemic hypertension, *Guys Hosp. Rep.,* **105**:320–327 (1956).
112. Levy, H., Partial rupture of pulmonary artery with lesions of medionecrosis in a case of mitral stenosis, *Am. Heart J.,* **62**:31–42 (1961).
113. Klos, I., Spontanruptur der Arteria pulmonalis bei Mitralstenose, *Z. Kreislaufforsch.,* **58**:860–868 (1969).
114. Ohela, K., and H. Teir, Rupture of the pulmonary artery (report of three cases), *Ann. Med. Intern. Fenn.,* **43**:39–44 (1954).
115. Whitaker, W., D. Heath, and J. W. Brown, Patent ductus arteriosus with pulmonary hypertension, *Br. Heart J.,* **15**:121–137 (1955).
116. Placik, B., S. Rodbard, J. McMahon, and S. Swaroop, Pulmonary artery dissection and rupture in Eisenmenger's syndrome, *Vasc. Surg.,* **10**:72–80 (1976).
117. Rawson, A. J., Incomplete rupture of the pulmonary artery based on cystic medionecrosis, *Am. Heart J.,* **55**:766–771 (1958).
118. Brettell, H. R., and R. E. Herrmann, Spontaneous rupture of the pulmonary artery in pulmonary hypertension, *Am. Heart J.,* **59**:263–276 (1960).
119. Kolin, V., Eine unvollständige Ruptur der Lungenschlagader, *Zentralbl. Allg. Pathol.,* **105**:497–500 (1964).
120. Condry, R. J., and L. H. Nefflin, Primary pulmonary arteriosclerosis with rupture of the pulmonary artery, *Ann. Intern. Med.,* **49**:1252–1257 (1958).

121. Pirani, C. L., F. E. Ewart, and A. L. Wilson, Thromboendarteritis with multiple mycotic aneurysms of the pulmonary artery, *Am. J. Dis. Child.*, 77:460–473 (1949).

122. Charlton, R. W., and L. A. DuPlessis, Multiple pulmonary artery aneurysms, *Thorax,* 16:364–371 (1961).

123. Kauffman, S. L., J. Lynfield, and G. R. Hennigar, Mycotic aneurysms of the intrapulmonary arteries, *Circulation,* 35:90–99 (1967).

124. Goh, T. H., Mycotic aneurysm of the pulmonary artery. A report of 2 cases, *Br. Heart J.,* 36:387–390 (1974).

125. Kourilsky, S., and J. M. Verley, Un cas de coarctation aortique de type infantile associée a un anévrysme pulmonaire rompu dans une bronche, *Arch. Anat. Pathol.,* 10:147–149 (1963).

126. Van Epps, E. F., Primary pulmonary hypertension in brothers, *Am. J. Roentgenol.,* 78:471–482 (1957).

127. Sevitt, S., Arterial wall lesions after pulmonary embolism, especially ruptures and aneurysms, *J. Clin. Pathol.,* 29:665–674 (1976).

128. Plokker, H. W. M., S. S. Wagenaar, A. V. G. Bruschke, and C. A. Wagenvoort, Aneurysm of a pulmonary artery branch: An uncommon cause of a coin lesion, *Chest,* 68:258–261 (1975).

129. Foord, A. G., and R. D. Lewis, Primary dissecting aneurysms of peripheral and pulmonary arteries, *Arch. Pathol.,* 68:553–577 (1959).

130. Epstein, S., and A. F. Naji, Pulmonary artery aneurysm with dissection after Blalock operation for tetralogy of Fallot, *J. Cardiol.,* 5:560–563 (1960).

131. Ravines, H. T., Dissecting hematomas of intrapulmonary arteries in a case of pulmonary hypertension associated with patent ductus arteriosus, *J. Thorac. Cardiovasc. Surg.,* 39:760–766 (1960).

132. Kapanci, Y., Médionécrose et anévrysmes disséquants des artères intrapulmonaires. Déscription d'un cas chez le nourrisson et étude morphogénétique de la médionécrose type Gsell-Erdheim, *Frankf. Z. Pathol.,* 74:425–440 (1965).

133. Olsen, E. G. J., Perivascular fibrosis in lungs in mitral valve disease. A possible mechanism of production, *Br. J. Dis. Chest,* 60:129–136 (1966).

134. Dingemans, K. P., and C. A. Wagenvoort, Ultrastructural study of contraction of pulmonary vascular smooth muscle cells, *Lab. Invest.,* 35:205–212 (1976).

135. Dingemans, K. P., and C. A. Wagenvoort, Pulmonary arteries and veins in experimental hypoxia. An ultrastructural study, *Am. J. Pathol.,* 93:353–361 (1978).

136. Wagenvoort, C. A., D. Heath, and J. E. Edwards, *The Pathology of the Pulmonary Vasculature.* Charles C. Thomas, Springfield, Ill., 1964.

137. Mahesree, M. L., R. N. Chakravarti, and P. L. Wahi, Packed cells, platelet-rich plasma and adenosine diphosphate in the production of occlusive vascular changes in lungs of rabbits, *Am. Heart J.,* 89:753–758 (1975).

138. Wagenvoort, C. A., and N. Wagenvoort, Pulmonary arteries in bronchial carcinoma, *Arch. Pathol.,* 79:529–533 (1965).

139. Wissler, R. W., The arterial medial cell, smooth muscle or multifunctional mesenchyme? *Circulation,* 36:1–4 (1967).

140. Arias-Stella, J., Human carotid body at high altitudes. *Meeting of the American Association of Pathologists and Bacteriologists, San Francisco,* abstract 150.

141. Hicken, P., D. Heath, D. B. Brewer, and W. Whitaker, The small pulmonary arteries in emphysema, *J. Pathol. Bacteriol.,* 90:107–114 (1965).

142. Wagenvoort, C. A., J. Nauta, P. J. van der Schaar, H. H. W. Weeda, and N. Wagenvoort, Effect of flow and pressure on pulmonary vessels. A semiquantitative study based on lung biopsies, *Circulation,* 35:1028–1037 (1967).

143. Wagenvoort, C. A., J. Nauta, P. J. van der Schaar, H. W. H. Weeda, and N. Wagenvoort, Vascular changes in pulmonic stenosis and tetralogy of Fallot in lung biopsies, *Circulation,* 36:924–932 (1967).

144. Wagenvoort, C. A., J. Nauta, P. J. van der Schaar, H. W. H. Weeda, and N. Wagenvoort, The pulmonary vasculature in complete transposition of the great vessels judged from lung biopsies, *Circulation,* 38:746–754 (1968).

145. Hatt, P. Y., and C. Rouiller, Les ultrastructures pulmonaires et le régime de la petite circulation. I. Au cours du rétrécissement mitral serré, *Pathol. Biol.,* 6:1371–1397 (1958).

146. Esterly, J. A., S. Glagov, and D. J. Ferguson, Morphogenesis of intimal obliterative hyperplasia of small arteries in experimental pulmonary hypertension. An ultrastructural study of the role of smooth muscle cells, *Am. J. Pathol.,* 52:325–348 (1968).

147. Backwinkel, K. P., H. Themann, G. Schmitt, and W. H. Hauss, Electronenmikroskopische Untersuchungen ueber das Verhalten glatter Muskelzellen in der Arterienwand unter verschiedenen experimentellen Bedingungen, *Virchows Arch. [Pathol. Anat.],* 359:171–184 (1973).

148. Webster, W. S., S. P. Bishop, and J. C. Geer, Experimental aortic intimal thickening. I. Morphology and source of intimal cells, *Am. J. Pathol.,* 76:245–284 (1974).

149. Stein, A. A., J. Mauro, L. Thibodeau, and R. Alley, The histogenesis of cardiac myxomas. In *Pathology Annual, Vol. 4.* Edited by S. C. Sommers. London, Butterworths, pp. 293–312, 1969.

150. World Health Organization, *Primary pulmonary hypertension,* Report of Committee, Geneva, 1975.

151. Harrison, C. V., Experimental pulmonary arteriosclerosis, *J. Pathol. Bacteriol.,* 60:289–293 (1948).

152. Harrison, C. V., Experimental pulmonary hypertension, *J. Pathol. Bacteriol.,* 63:195–200 (1951).

153. Barnard, P. J., Experimental fibrin thrombo-embolism of the lungs, *J. Pathol. Bacteriol.,* 65:129–136 (1953).

154. Rich, A. R., A hitherto unrecognized tendency to the development of widespread pulmonary vascular obstruction in patients with congenital pulmonary stenosis (tetralogy of Fallot), *Bull. Johns Hopkins Hosp.,* 82:389–401 (1948).

155.   Wagenvoort, C. A., Pathology of congestive pulmonary hypertension,
       Prog. Respir. Res., **9**:195–202 (1975).
156.   Heath, D., Longitudinal muscle in pulmonary arteries, *J. Pathol. Bacteriol.,*
       85:407–412 (1963).
157.   Heath, D., Hypoxic hypertensive pulmonary vascular disease, *Prog. Respir.
       Res.,* **5**:13–16 (1970).
158.   Wagenvoort, C. A., and N. Wagenvoort, Hypoxic pulmonary vascular
       lesions in man at high altitude and in patients with chronic respiratory
       disease, *Pathol. Microbiol.,* **39**:276–282 (1973).
159.   Wagenvoort, C. A., Die Bedcutung der Arterienwülste für den Blutkreis-
       lauf, *Acta Anat.,* **21**:70–99 (1954).
160.   Burton, A. C., Relation of structure to function of the tissues of the wall
       of blood vessels, *Physiol. Rev.,* **34**:619–642 (1954).
161.   Walton, K. W., and D. Heath, Iron incrustation of the pulmonary vessels
       in patent ductus arteriosus with congenital mitral disease, *Br. Heart J.,* **22**:
       440–444 (1960).
162.   Lie, J. T., Nosology of pulmonary vasculitides, *Mayo Clin. Proc.,* **52**:520–
       522 (1977).
163.   Sweeney, A. R., and A. H. Baggenstoss, Pulmonary lesions of periarteritis
       nodosa, *Mayo Clin. Proc.,* **24**:35–43 (1949).
164.   Bohrod, M. G., Pathologic manifestations of allergic and related mech-
       anisms in diseases of the lungs, *Int. Arch. Allergy Appl. Immunol.,* **13**:39–
       60 (1958).
165.   Fienberg, R., Pathergic granulomatosis, *Am. J. Med.,* **19**:829–831 (1955).
166.   Liebow, A. A., Pulmonary angitis and granulomatosis, *Am. Rev. Respir.
       Dis.,* **108**:1–18 (1973).
167.   Chumbley, L. E., E. G. Harrison, and R. A. DeRemee, Allergic granuloma-
       tosis and angiitis (Churg-Strauss syndrome). Report and analysis of 30
       cases, *Mayo Clin. Proc.,* **52**:477–484 (1977).
168.   Wagenvoort, C. A., The morphology of certain vascular lesions in pulmo-
       nary hypertension, *J. Pathol. Bacteriol.,* **78**:503–511 (1959).
169.   Wagenvoort, C. A., N. Wagenvoort, and H. J. Dijk, Effect of fulvine on
       pulmonary arteries and veins of the rat, *Thorax,* **29**:522–529 (1974).
170.   Wagenvoort, C. A., K. P. Dingemans, and G. G. Lotgering, Electron mi-
       croscopy of pulmonary vasculature after application of fulvine, *Thorax,*
       29:511–521 (1974).
171.   Wood, P., Pulmonary hypertension, *Mod. Concepts Cardiovasc. Dis.,* **28**:
       513–518 (1959).
172.   Downing, S. E., R. A. Vidone, H. M. Brandt, and A. A. Liebow, The
       pathogenesis of vascular lesions in experimental hyperkinetic pulmonary
       hypertension, *Am. J. Pathol.,* **43**:739–756 (1963).
173.   Harley, R. A., P. J. Friedman, M. Saldana, A. A. Liebow, and C. B.
       Carrington, Sequential development of lesions in experimental extreme
       pulmonary hypertension, *Am. J. Pathol.,* **52**:52a (1968).
174.   Saldana, M. E., R. A. Harley, A. A. Liebow, and C. B. Carrington, Ex-
       perimental extreme pulmonary hypertension and vascular disease in rela-
       tion to polycythemia, *Am. J. Pathol.,* **52**:935–981 (1968).

175. Ross, R. S., H. B. Taussig, and M. H. Evans, Late hemodynamic complications of anastomotic surgery for treatment of the tetralogy of Fallot, *Circulation,* **18**:553–556 (1958).

176. Wagenvoort, C. A., J. W. DuShane, and J. E. Edwards, Cardiac clinics. 151. Hypertensive pulmonary arterial lesions as a late result of anastomosis of systemic and pulmonary circulations, *Mayo Clin. Proc.,* **35**: 186–191 (1960).

177. Heath, D., and J. E. Edwards, The pathology of hypertensive pulmonary vascular disease. A description of six grades of structural changes in the pulmonary arteries with special reference to congenital cardiac septal defects, *Circulation,* **18**:533–547 (1958).

178. Björk, V. O., and E. F. Salén, The blood flow through an atelectatic lung, *J. Thorac. Surg.,* **20**:933–942 (1950).

179. Camishion, R. C., O. Yoshinozi, V. D. Cuddy, and J. H. Gibbon, Pulmonary arterial blood flow through an acutely atelectatic lung, *J. Thorac. Cardiovasc. Surg.,* **42**:599–606 (1961).

180. Hicken, P., D. Brewer, and D. Heath, The relation between the weight of the right ventricle of the heart and the internal surface area and number of alveoli in the human lung in emphysema, *J. Pathol. Bacteriol.,* **92**:529–546 (1966).

181. Junghanss, W., Das Lungenemphysem im postmortalen Angiogramm, *Virchows Arch. [Pathol. Anat.],* **332**:538–551 (1959).

182. Turunen, M., and L. Stjernvall, Submicroscopic structure of the pulmonary capillaries in patent ductus arteriosus, *Acta Chir. Scand.,* **117**:131–136 (1959).

183. Coalson, J. J., W. E. Jacques, G. S. Campbell, and W. M. Thompson, Ultrastructure of the alveolar-capillary membrane in congenital and acquired heart disease, *Arch. Pathol.,* **83**:377–391 (1967).

184. Kay, J. M., and F. R. Edwards, Ultrastructure of the alveolar-capillary wall in mitral stenosis, *J. Pathol.,* **111**:239–246 (1973).

185. Meyrick, B., S. W. Clarke, C. Symons, D. J. Woodgate, and L. Reid, Primary pulmonary hypertension: a case report including electron microscopic study, *Br. J. Dis. Chest,* **68**:11–20 (1974).

186. Aviado, D. M., Pharmacology of the pulmonary circulation, *Pharmacol. Rev.,* **12**:159–239 (1960).

187. Parker, B. M., B. W. Steiger, and M. J. Friedenberg, Serotonin-induced pulmonary venous spasm demonstrated by selective pulmonary phlebography, *Am. Heart J.,* **69**:521–528 (1965).

188. Braun, K., and S. Stern, Functional significance of the pulmonary venous system, *Am. J. Cardiol.,* **20**:56–65 (1967).

189. Heath, D., and J. E. Edwards, Histological changes in the lung in diseases associated with pulmonary venous hypertension, *Br. J. Dis. Chest,* **53**:8–18 (1959).

190. Wagenvoort, C. A., and N. Wagenvoort, The pathology of pulmonary veno-occlusive disease, *Virchows Arch. [Pathol. Anat.],* **364**:69–79 (1974).

191. Wagenvoort, C. A., Pulmonary veno-occlusive disease: Entity or syndrome? *Chest,* **69**:82–86 (1976).

192. Contis, G., R. H. Fung, G. R. Vawter, and A. S. Nadas, Stenosis and obstruction of the pulmonary veins associated with pulmonary hypertension, *Am. J. Cardiol.,* **20**:718–724 (1967).

193. Kelvin, F. M., J. A. Boone, and D. Peretz, Pulmonary varix, *J. Can. Assoc. Radiol.,* **23**:227–229 (1972).

194. Arntee, J. C., and R. M. Patton, Pulmonary varix, *Thorax,* **31**:107–112 (1976).

195. Hsu, I., G. A. Kelser, P. C. Adkins, and M. M. Shefferman, Pulmonary varix regression after mitral valve replacement, *Am. J. Cardiol.,* **37**:928–932 (1976).

196. Liebow, A. A., M. R. Hales, and G. E. Lindskog, Enlargement of the bronchial arteries, and their anastomoses with the pulmonary arteries in bronchiectasis, *Am. J. Pathol.,* **25**:211–232 (1949).

197. Cudkowicz, L., and J. B. Armstrong, The bronchial arteries in pulmonary emphysema, *Thorax,* **8**:46–58 (1953).

198. Delarue, J., C. Sors, J. Mignot, and J. Paillas, Lésions bronchopulmonaires et modifications circulatoires, *Presse Med.,* **63**:173–177 (1955).

199. Heath, D., and I. M. Thompson, Bronchopulmonary anastomoses in sickle-cell anaemia, *Thorax,* **24**:232–238 (1969).

200. Wagenvoort, C. A., G. Losekoot, and E. Mulder, Pulmonary veno-occlusive disease of presumably intrauterine origin, *Thorax,* **26**:429–434 (1971).

201. Blank, R. H., W. H. Muller, and J. F. Dammann, Changes in pulmonary vascular lesions after restoring normal pulmonary arterial pressure, *Surg. Forum,* **9**:356–359 (1959).

202. Blank, R. H., W. H. Muller, and J. F. Dammann, Experimental pulmonary arterial hypertension, *Am. J. Surg.,* **101**:143–153 (1961).

203. Geer, J. C., B. A. Glass, and H. M. Albert, The morphogenesis and reversibility of experimental hyperkinetic pulmonary vascular lesions in the dog, *Exp. Mol. Pathol.,* **4**:399–415 (1965).

204. Dammann, J. F., J. A. McEachen, W. M. Thompson, R. Smith, and W. H. Muller, The regression of pulmonary vascular disease after the creation of pulmonary stenosis, *J. Thorac. Cardiovasc. Surg.,* **42**:722–734 (1961).

205. Hruban, Z., and E. M. Humphreys, Congenital anomalies associated with pulmonary hypertension in an infant, *Arch. Pathol.,* **70**:766–779 (1960).

206. Kanjuh, V. I., R. D. Sellers, and J. E. Edwards, Pulmonary vascular plexiform lesion, *Arch. Pathol.,* **78**:513–522 (1964).

207. Kapanci, Y., Hypertensive pulmonary vascular disease. Endothelial hyperplasia and its relations to intravascular fibrin precipitation, *Am. J. Pathol.,* **48**:665–676 (1965).

208. Viles, P. H., P. A. Ongley, and J. L. Titus, The spectrum of pulmonary vascular disease in transposition of the great arteries, *Circulation,* **40**:31–41 (1969).

209. Lakier, J. B., P. Stanger, M. A. Heymann, J. I. E. Hoffman, and A. M. Rudolph, Early onset of pulmonary vascular obstruction in patients with aortopulmonary transposition and intact ventricular septum, *Circulation,* **51**:875–889 (1975).

210. Clarkson, P. M., J. M. Neutze, J. C. Wardill, and B. G. Barratt-Boyes, The pulmonary vascular bed in patients with complete transposition of the great arteries, *Circulation*, **53**:539–543 (1976).

211. Naeye, R. L., "Primary" pulmonary hypertension with coexisting portal hypertension. A retrospective study of six cases, *Circulation*, **22**:376–384 (1960).

212. Senior, R. M., R. C. Britton, G. M. Turino, J. A. Wood, G. A. Langer, and A. P. Fishman, Pulmonary hypertension associated with cirrhosis of the liver and with portacaval shunts, *Circulation*, **37**:88–96 (1968).

213. Segel, N., J. M. Kay, T. J. Bayley, and A. Paton, Pulmonary hypertension with hepatic cirrhosis, *Br. Heart J.*, **30**:575–578 (1968).

214. Levine, O. R., R. C. Harris, W. A. Blanc, and R. B. Mellins, Progressive pulmonary hypertension in children with portal hypertension, *J. Pediatr.*, **83**:964–972 (1973).

215. Yacoub, M. H., and V. C. Thompson, Chronic idiopathic pulmonary hilar fibrosis, *Thorax*, **26**:365–375 (1971).

216. Wagenvoort, C. A., and J. E. Edwards, The pulmonary arterial tree in aortic atresia with intact ventricular septum, *Lab. Invest.*, **10**:924–933 (1961).

217. Stanek, V., A. Oppelt, P. Jebavy, and J. Widimsky, A contribution to the mechanisms of the distribution of pulmonary blood flow in patients with mitral stenosis, *Bull. Physiopathol. Respir. (Nancy)*, **7**:913–924 (1971).

218. Carrington, C. B., and A. A. Liebow, Pulmonary veno-occlusive disease, *Hum. Pathol.*, **1**:322–324 (1970).

219. Hasleton, P. S., D. Heath, and D. B. Brewer, Hypertensive pulmonary vascular disease in states of chronic hypoxia, *J. Pathol. Bacteriol.*, **95**: 431–440 (1968).

220. Naeye, R. L., Alveolar hypoventilation and cor pulmonale secondary to damage to the respiratory center, *Am. J. Cardiol.*, **8**:416–419 (1961).

221. Heath, D., C. Edwards, and P. Harris, Post-mortem size and structure of the human carotid body, *Thorax*, **25**:129–140 (1970).

222. Naeye, R. L., Hypoxemia and pulmonary hypertension, *Arch. Pathol.*, **71**:447–452 (1961).

223. Arias-Stella, J., and M. Saldana, The terminal portion of the pulmonary arterial tree in people native to high altitudes, *Am. J. Pathol.*, **43**:30a (1963).

224. Edwards, C., D. Heath, P. Harris, Y. Castillo, H. Krüger, and J. Arias-Stella, The carotid body in animals at high altitude, *J. Pathol.*, **104**:231–238 (1971).

225. Naeye, R. L., Perinatal changes in the pulmonary vascular bed with stenosis and atresia of the pulmonic valve, *Am. Heart J.*, **61**:586–592 (1961).

2

Bronchial Arterial Circulation in Man
Normal Anatomy and Responses to Disease

LEON CUDKOWICZ

Wright State University School of Medicine
Dayton, Ohio

I.   Historical Introduction

The discovery of aortic branches entering the lung is attributed to Erasistratus (approximately 270 B.C.) [1,2] because of a reference made to him by Galen [3]. Miller [4], in his admirable review of the history of the bronchial circulation, points out that Galen (A.D. 130-201) observed systemic blood vessels to the lung, but failed to name them. Columbus [5], in 1559, disagreed with this contention and stated categorically that the aorta does not send branches to the lung. Dominico de Marchettis [6] was probably the first anatomist to renew interest in 1654 in the bronchial arteries and also noted venous radicles emerging from the lung, which fused with the systemic venous channels of the thorax. Little more, apparently, was heard of the bronchial circulation until the time of Ruyisch [7], who claimed priority for himself as discoverer of the bronchial arteries but denied the existence of bronchial veins.

The functional significance of the bronchial arteries appears to have remained unknown until 1808, when Reisseissen and von Sömmering [8] defined them as "die vasa nutritia der Lungen." Much was written before the nineteenth century regarding the dual circulations to the human lungs and the

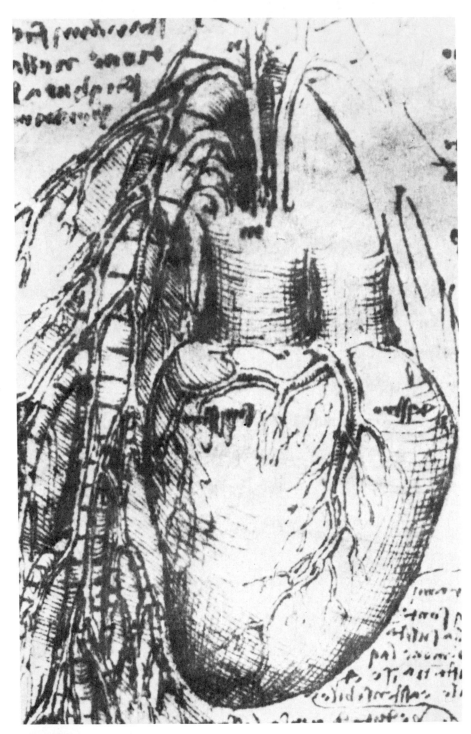

FIGURE 1

possible physiological differences between the bronchial and pulmonary arteries. No references, however, appear in the cited texts to the truly remarkable observations made on the bronchial circulation by Leonardo da Vinci nearly 500 years ago.

A. Leonardo da Vinci and the Bronchial Circulation [9]

In the Quincentenary Exhibition held in 1952 at the Royal Academy, London, and devoted to the drawings of Leonardo da Vinci, exhibit 301 showed a reproduction of a drawing from the Quaderni d' Anatomia II.I.r., Royal Windsor Library, in which Leonardo depicts the heart, the coronary arteries, the trachea, and the bronchial tree of the left lung with its accompanying bronchial arteries. The bronchial arteries are shown to arise from the aorta and to follow the individual bronchi to their termination (Fig. 1). In the same drawing is one of the earlier descriptions of a tuberculous cavity (Fig. 2) [10]. Closer scrutiny of this cavity (see Fig. 2) reveals the additional and somewhat distorted features of small bronchial arteries within its periphery.

Keele [11], in 1952 in his monograph on Leonardo's study of the heart and blood, reproduces this same drawing and quotes from Leonardo's notebooks relevant passages pertaining to the bronchial circulation:

> Why nature duplicated artery and vein in such an instrument one above the other, finding themselves for the nourishment of one and the same member (the lung).

> You may say that the trachea and the lung have to be nourished, but if you had to do with a single large venateria, this could not accompany the trachea without great interference with the movement which the trachea makes in dilatation and contraction as well as in length and thickness. Wherefore for this, nature gave a vein and artery to the trachea which would be sufficient for its life and nourishment, and somewhat removed the other large branches from the trachea to nourish the substance of the lung with greater convenience [11]. (*Author's note*: By trachea, Leonardo refers to the whole bronchial tree.)

FIGURE 1   Detail of drawing by Leonardo da Vinci of the heart, aorta, and left bronchial arteries. The aortic origin of the left bronchial arteries is depicted, as well as their course along the bronchial tree. (This is a mirror-image drawing, therefore showing the apex of the heart and the aorta on the right-hand side.) (Reproduced by gracious permission of Her Majesty Queen Elizabeth II.)

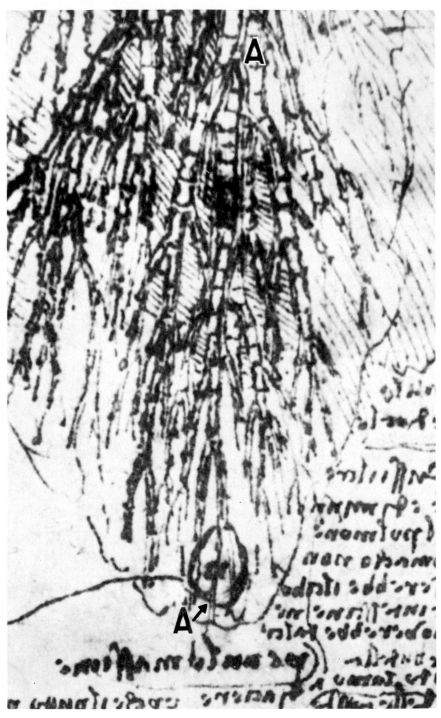

FIGURE 2

This teleological view of the function of the bronchial circulation, expressed about 300 years before Reisseissen and von Sömmering's [8] definition of the bronchial arteries as the "vasa nutritia" of the lungs, is so modern in concept that very little can really be added. It bears testimony to da Vinci's grasp of the function of organs, as much as the accuracy of his drawings emphasizes his exceptional skill as an anatomist. Without the use of contrast media to outline the intrapulmonary course of these vessels radiographically, and careful microscopy to show up the relationship of the bronchial arteries to the bronchial tree and other lung structures, modern studies of this circulation would be almost inconceivable (Fig. 3). The drawing of the bronchial circulation by Leonardo, made at a time when such methods were unknown, is therefore quite extraordinary, and ought to have pointed the way to an earlier recognition of vascular lesions in relation to lung pathology.

B.   The Nineteenth Century

With the anatomical recognition of the normal bronchial arteries in the early nineteenth century, attention began to focus on their function. The first to attack this interesting problem was probably Guillot, who in 1845 published his conclusions [12]. He injected gelatin colored yellow into the pulmonary artery, and gelatin colored red into the bronchial circulation through the thoracic aorta, then examined the lung specimens carefully for anastomotic channels and admixture of the two dyes. No arterial communication between the two systems could be demonstrated, but a venous communication existed between the bronchial arteries and the pulmonary veins.

Le Fort [13], in 1858, followed the distribution of the bronchial arteries by dissection and established some evidence that the capillaries of the bronchial arteries cease near the respiratory bronchioles, and that the capillary bed beyond is derived entirely from the pulmonary circulation.

von Luschka [14] believed that an anastomosis between the two circulations existed at the level of the capillary beds. He also first drew attention to the capillary distribution of the bronchial artery to the bronchial mucosa: ". . . that numerous bronchial arterial branches enter the walls of the finer bronchi to disappear and emerge as the capillary bed of the bronchial mucosa. During their course bronchial arterial twigs penetrate the adventitia, and furnish a capillary bed for the mucosa which, without interruption, joins the capillaries of the pulmonary arteries."

FIGURE 2   Closeup drawing by Leonardo da Vinci of a tuberculous cavity (A), left bronchial tree, and bronchial arteries. (Reproduced by gracious permission of Her Majesty Queen Elizabeth II.)

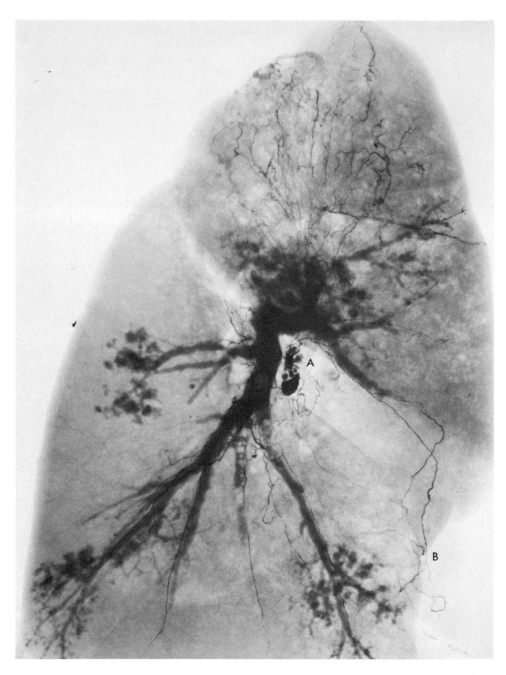

FIGURE 3 Lateral radiograph of a human left lung. The bronchial arteries and the bronchial tree have been injected with a contrast medium to outline their relationship to each other as well as the arterial blood supply to a hilar lymph node (A) and the visceral pleura (B).

Virchow [15], in 1847, occluded a lobar branch of the pulmonary artery and found that the occlusion did not result in necrosis of the dependent lobe; he concluded from this that the bronchial arteries must have maintained the nutrition of the lobe. He believed that the nutrition of some lung structures was also derived from intercostal arteries. In a subsequent publication [16] these conclusions were reiterated, and stress is laid on the enlargement of bronchial arteries resulting from the obliteration of a main pulmonary artery branch to a lobe.

Rindfleisch considered the bronchial arteries as end arteries [17]. Cohnheim and Litten [18] thought that, as end arteries, the bronchial arteries were unlikely to sustain the nutrition of a pulmonary segment deprived of its pulmonary arterial blood supply. With the classic work of Küttner [19], this contention was abandoned. He injected silver nitrate, followed by a dye which would not penetrate capillaries, into the bronchial arteries of a rabbit, and demonstrated that the bronchial arteries extended as far as the respiratory bronchioles. In a second experiment he tied the left branch of the pulmonary artery and injected a saline solution of aniline blue distal to the ligature. The right lung became blue at once, whereas the left lung showed a bluish tinge only in the bronchial mucosa. This observation led to the conclusion that capillary anastomoses existed between the two systems. From a third experiment, he concluded that ". . . the arterial divisions of the pulmonary artery . . . are end-arteries." The terminal branches of the pulmonary artery do not communicate with vessels of similar caliber derived from the bronchial arteries, and if any anastomoses exist, they must be capillary only.

Zuckerkandl [20] reviewed the problem in 1881 and in 1883 [21], and stated that the bronchial arteries are primarily nutritive to the lung. He agreed that they ramify in the bronchi, supplying the mucosa, and in addition, in the human, are the main blood supply to the pleura. He confirmed their distribution along the bronchi. He divided the venous drainage of the bronchial arteries into an upper drainage, i.e., from the larger bronchi, and a lower drainage from the smaller bronchi. The upper venous drainage leads through true bronchial veins into the azygous system of veins, and the lower joins the pulmonary veins. Zuckerkandl also found venous anastomoses between the pulmonary and systemic veins via the mediastinal veins.

C. The Early Twentieth Century

The problems of studying the bronchial circulation in the human received new emphasis by Berry in 1934 [22]. Miller had alleged that misconception regarding anastomosis between the two systems had arisen because the fluid injection materials used were too thin to resemble the behavior of blood.

Radio-opaque materials too thick to traverse capillaries were used by Berry et al. [23] in the dog and by Mathes et al. [24]

Berry concluded [22] that "Main bronchial arteries arise from the aorta or intercostal arteries at the level of T.4. They run to the posterior aspect of lung roots, giving a branch to each lung lobe which travels on the posterior wall of the corresponding bronchus. Small branches from the bronchial arteries are distributed to the esophagus and prevertebral muscles. Small anterior bronchial arteries are often seen to arise from internal mammary arteries, and pass in the mediastinal pleura to lung roots."

Radiography

No anastomosis was found to exist between the pulmonary and bronchial circulations. The injected matter could be followed as far as vessels of 14 μm in diameter. This was subsequently confirmed by histology.

Microscopy

These observations on the human lung corroborated Reisseissen and von Sömmering's [8] definition of the bronchial arteries, as the vasa nutritia of the human lung. Berry [22] also accepted Miller's findings [4] that blood supplied to capillary plexus in the walls of larger bronchi ultimately finds its way to the pulmonary veins.

Pulmonary nerves also were found by Berry [22] to receive their blood supply from the bronchial arteries. At the lung roots, twigs off the systemic vessels penetrate the epineural sheath, become distributed in the subdivision of the connective tissue, and reach the nerve fibers as discrete, tiny arterioles. Berry and Daly [25] refer in this connection to Daly and von Euler [26], who were able to maintain the excitability and conductivity of these nerves intact for over 3 hr by perfusing the bronchial vasculature in the dog.

Berry's conclusions were thus similar to Miller's, that in the human lung no anatomical anastomosis existed between the two circulations, except for the venous communication between vessels of less than 14 μm in diameter.

In the Harvey Lectures of 1935 [27], Daly presented the extant knowledge of the bronchial circulation in broad outline. He accepted Miller's anatomical description as the most reliable, and in part also favored Zuckerkandl's [20] teleological explanation of their function.

He quoted Olkon and Joanides [27], who observed lung capillaries directly below the visceral pleura through a window in the thoracic cage of a dog, and noticed that an increase in intrapulmonary pressure diminished the number of visible, open alveolar capillaries, and that the velocity of blood corpuscles in larger capillaries becomes increased. These studies support the possible existence of an arteriovenous shunt at the precapillary level. Wearn et al. [28] used a similar method and were able to observe the action of epinephrine on these superficial capillaries. Instead of a pressor effect, they witnessed the opening up of further capillaries and intermittence of flow in the already visible loops.

Daly also referred to Virchow's observation concerning the occlusion of a pulmonary artery branch to a whole lobe which led to extensive compensatory enlargement of the bronchial arteries. He paid tribute to Karsner and Ash [29], who in 1912 had shown that obstruction to small branches of the pulmonary artery appeared to have no effect on the bronchial arteries, inasmuch as the capillary anastomoses are sufficiently compensatory in such situations. The bronchial arteries dilate and form new vessels to infected areas and abscesses, where the affected area is no longer supplied by the pulmonary artery. It follows, therefore, that the bronchial vessels are principally responsible for the defense and repair of the damaged organ.

In conclusion, Daly states: "The true understanding of the role of the bronchial arteries in modifying the intrinsic pulmonary mechanism will only be possible with the added knowledge gained from the results of clinical studies correlated with histological examination of the lung."

His own later, exacting work constitutes a departure from the anatomical field into that of the highly complex physiology of the intrinsic pulmonary mechanisms [30], which has helped to usher in the current era of pulmonary pathophysiology.

II. Embryology of the Bronchial Arteries

Detailed information concerning the development of the bronchial arteries was provided by Huntingdon [31]. He showed that the primitive pulmonary plexus, destined to evolve as the capillary plexus fed by the pulmonary arteries, originates from ventral branches of the dorsal aortae and is formed before the pulmonary arteries. Subsequently, the ventral root of the sixth branchial arch grows down from the aortic bulb to fuse with a vessel growing dorsally from the pulmonary plexus. This fusion produces the pulmonary artery, which is joined at the same time by the dorsal root of the sixth aortic arch to form the ductus arteriosus. These vascular developments occur in the human embryo in the fourth to sixth week and are completed by the seventh week [32–34].

With the formation of the pulmonary artery, the blood supply of the pulmonary plexus switches and there is regression of the ventral branches of the dorsal aorta by which it was initially served. There is a stage, however, at which the primitive pulmonary plexus is supplied from both sources. This implies that during the early development of the embryo an anastomosis exists between the aortic branches and the pulmonary artery. The aortic branches do not regress completely and remain to form the bronchial arteries. The lung buds become prominent simultaneously with the development of the heart and great vessels.

Malformation of the pulmonary artery may arise from either an incomplete absorption of the bulbus cordis, resulting in pulmonary stenosis and Fallot's tetralogy, or from incomplete development of the aorticopulmonary septum, giving rise to an absent or anomalous origin of the pulmonary artery or its branches [35].

Manhoff and Howe [36] classified these anomalies according to the stage at which the normal process is interrupted. If the lungs derive their arteries from the ascending aorta (group I), a failure is implied of the aorticopulmonary septum to separate the trunks of the aorta and pulmonary arteries. The principal vessel is therefore a true persistent truncus arteriosus.

If the lungs are supplied by arteries arising from the arch of the aorta (group II), the vessels are formed from the dorsal root of the sixth arch, communicating with the primitive pulmonary plexus instead of with the ventral root of the sixth arch (the usual developmental source of the pulmonary artery).

Arteries supplying the lungs from the descending aorta (group III) are considered to represent true bronchial arteries, a persistence to an abnormal extent of the ventral branches of the dorsal aorta to the original primitive pulmonary plexus.

In group IV, the lungs are supplied by arteries having other anomalous origins, from the great vessels of the aortic arch or from vessels of the descending aorta such as the celiac plexus. True bronchial arteries require for their origin the descending aortae and the early postbranchial pulmonary plexus and its connections with the dorsal aorta [35].

A.   The Bronchial Circulation in Congenital Heart Disease

Jacobsen, in 1816 [37], gave the first description of enlarged bronchial arteries in a patient with severe pulmonary stenosis. Peacock, in 1858 [38], provided examples of bronchial arterial hypertrophy in cases of Fallot's tetralogy. East and Barnard, in 1938 [39], emphasized the gross hypertrophy of the bronchial circulation in pulmonary atresia. In addition to pulmonary stenosis [40], pulmonary atresia [35,41,42], and Fallot's tetralogy [43,44], abnormally large bronchial arteries have been described in atrial septal defects

[45], patent ductus arteriosus [46], persistent truncus arteriosus [47], and in transposition of the great vessels [48-50].

B. Clinical Features Suggestive of an Enlarged Bronchial Circulation in Congenital Heart Disease

An enlarged bronchial circulation to the lungs can be inferred in cyanotic congenital heart disease when the murmur of pulmonary stenosis and the pulmonary valve closure sounds are absent. Instead a soft, high-pitched, continuous murmur can frequently be heard under the clavicles, along the sternal borders, and to the left and right of the thoracic spine from T.2 to T.5 and along the medial borders of the scapulae.

According to Campbell and Gardner [51], subtle to obvious changes which are suggestive of an enlarged bronchial circulation are usually visible on chest radiographs. The bronchial arteries appear as a mottled mass spreading much higher than the pulmonary arteries and filling the aortic window. Occasionally, nodular peripheral shadows are visible in otherwise oligemic lung fields, suggesting vascularization via the pleura. For the study of bronchial arterial shadows the left anterior oblique view is best, inasmuch as the aortic arch and the descending thoracic aorta can be scrutinized close to the origins of most bronchial arteries. These views also are best in revealing injected bronchial arteries during retrograde aortography [52].

The first attempts at the measurement of bronchial arterial blood flow in humans were made by Bing et al. [53] in congenital heart disease. Bing et al. established a linear relationship between the age of the patient and the magnitude of precapillary bronchopulmonary anastomotic flow. The mean figure in a group of 38 patients with Fallot's tetralogy was about 1 liter min^{-1} m^{-2}. The highest flow was 2.8 liters min^{-1} m^{-2}. Flows less large were recently reported by Nakamura et al. [54] in nine patients with Fallot's tetralogy. These ranged from 0.14 to 1.27 liters min^{-1} m^{-2}. The technique used was that of Cudkowicz et al. [55].

Fishman et al. [56] adapted the Bloomer technique [57] to patients with increased bronchial circulations, including four patients with pulmonary arterial atresia. Here again, precapillary bronchopulmonary anastomotic flow was measured and flows ranging from 1.3 to 5.0 liters min^{-1} m^{-2} were reported.

C. Congenital Anomalies of the Pulmonary Arteries

Pool et al. reviewed the development of the sixth aortic arches. It is from the sixth aortic arch that the pulmonary arteries develop and reach the developing lung buds. During the seventh week of development, the sixth right dorsal aortic arch distal to the pulmonary artery atrophies and disappears. The sixth left dorsal aortic arch distal to the pulmonary artery persists as the ductus arteriosus. The definitive pulmonary artery is formed by ventral and dorsal components of the sixth arch [58].

Unilateral absence of a pulmonary artery constitutes a relatively common abnormality [59]. Wagenvoort et al. [60] summarize their experience by the inclusion of cases in which one of the two branches of the pulmonary trunk is derived from sources such as: (1) the ascending aorta; (2) a branch from the aortic arch; (3) the aortic arch itself; and (4) the descending thoracic aorta. In these situations the pulmonary trunk fails to bifurcate and continues as a single pulmonary artery to one of the lungs.

Pool et al. found 40 proved and 38 probable cases of unilateral absence of a pulmonary artery. Unilateral absence of a pulmonary artery was about equally divided between the two sides (40, left; 38, right). In 32 cases the anomaly was isolated. In 10 cases the absent right pulmonary artery became associated with patent ductus arteriosus. In 16 cases of absence of the left pulmonary artery, the association was with Fallot's tetralogy.

D.   Clinical Example of Cardiorespiratory Studies in a Patient with an Absent Left Pulmonary Artery [61]

Congenital absence of a main pulmonary artery to one lung is thus a well-documented anomaly [62,63]. Its association with unilateral cystic lung disease was emphasized in particular by Mannix and Haight [64] and Steinberg [65], and its association with unilateral emphysema by McLeod [66] and others [67,68].

Hemoptysis, usually stemming from the expanded bronchial arterial collateral circulation [69,70], is a frequent, early, and most distressing symptom [71], and pneumonectomy may be necessary. Such a decision may also be reinforced by the failure of bronchospirometry to demonstrate a significant oxygen consumption by the affected lung. Oxygen uptakes varying from 0 to 7% of the total consumption have been found [72-74], suggesting little if any participation in gas exchange by the abnormal lung.

Fishman and colleagues [56] and Tabakin et al. [72], however, improved the study of function of such lungs during bronchospirometry by the inclusion of such additional measurements as CO_2 excretion and "effective" bronchial blood flows.

A lung deprived of a main pulmonary artery and endowed with a large bronchial collateral circulation continues to possess useful respiratory functions. Elimination of CO_2 from such a lung renders it active in effective alveolar ventilation. A low oxygen consumption alone by the anomalous lung, while oxygen is respired bilaterally during bronchospirometry, is unlikely to provide full information concerning total respiratory function of that lung, particularly

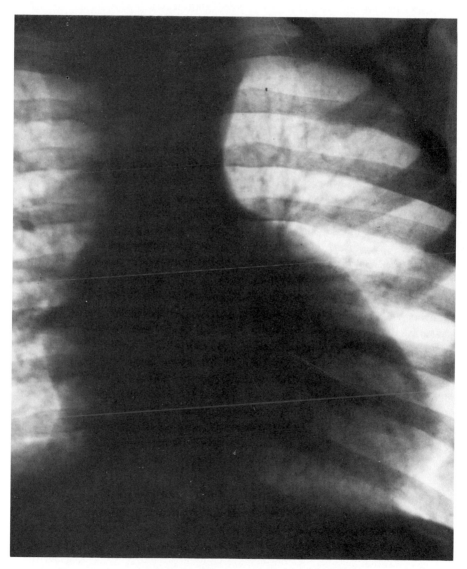

FIGURE 4 Patient with transposition of the great vessels. Chest radiograph shows oligemic lung fields with empty pulmonary bays. Cardiac silhouette suggests biventricular hypertrophy. (Reproduced from Cudkowicz and Armstrong [75], by permission of the *British Heart Journal.*)

as the oxygen consumption of that lung clearly can be increased during any deliberate reduction in arterial PO_2 tension. This maneuver in conjunction with separate CO_2 measurements seems necessary in any assessment concerning the participation of the lung in gas exchange, particularly if a pneumonectomy is contemplated as a respite from hemoptyses.

E.   Bilateral Congenital Precapillary Anastamoses in Transposition of the Great Vessels

An example of this anomaly follows in brief [75] (Fig. 4).

At autopsy, the heart was opened. A minute hole between the atria could be demonstrated. A large ventricular septal defect was present in the middle third of the septum. Both ventricular muscles were hypertrophied, and one cusp of the pulmonary valve was deformed and thickened; this caused some obstruction to the outflow. The bronchial arteries were followed from the hili along the main bronchi of each lung, and evidence of direct communication between the trunks of the bronchial and pulmonary arteries could not be found. A network of very fine arterioles, filled with the injection medium, coursed across the adventitia of the pulmonary arteries. It was thought that these vessels were dilated vasa vasorum which are normally derived from the bronchial arteries.

The *radiographs* of the injected thoracic content, taken before the heart was opened, showed that three large bronchial arteries entered the left lung hilus after emerging from the lateral aspect of the descending aorta. A large branch derived from the uppermost of the three arteries crossed the aorta posteriorly and entered the right hilus. A fourth bronchial artery arising immediately below the other three coursed directly from the aorta to the right hilus. The intrapulmonary course of the vessels became lost because of the complete superimposition of the pulmonary arterial trees, which had filled indirectly through the bronchial arteries. The injection medium, which had traversed intrapulmonary anastomoses to reach the pulmonary arteries, was conveyed to the ascending aorta and its branches through a patent subclavian-left pulmonary artery anastomosis (Fig. 5).

The postmorten radiographic and histologic studies of the injected bronchial circulation in this case suggest that bronchial artery hypertrophy occurred in the presence of patent pulmonary arteries, although some reduction in total pulmonary artery blood flow was caused by the deformed cusp of the pulmonary valve. A considerable volume of venous blood reached the pulmonary capillaries from the right-sided aorta through the bronchial arteries, and this was conveyed to the pulmonary arteries as a result of the enlargement and direct anastomoses of the vasa vasorum with the pulmonary artery lumina.

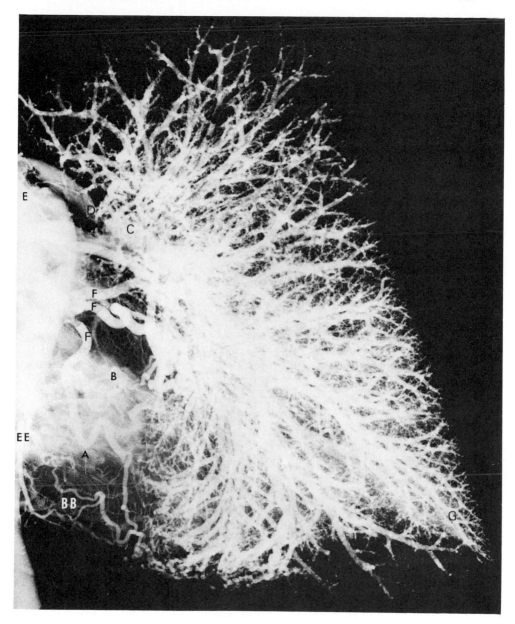

FIGURE 5 Radiograph of injected thoracic contents viewed in an antero-posterior position. (A) heart; (B) left and (BB) right coronary artery; (C) right pulmonary artery; (D) left subclavian anastomosis; (E) ligature around descending thoracic aorta; (EE) descending aorta; (F) left bronchial arteries; (G) right bronchial artery. One-third of normal size. (Reproduced from Cudkowicz and Armstrong [75], by permission of the *British Heart Journal.*)

No evidence of direct shunts between the trunks of the bronchial and pulmonary arteries could be seen, and the distribution of the bronchial arteries to the intrapulmonary structures that they normally supply was unaltered. The precapillary anastomoses between the two circulations appear, therefore, to have been brought about by the dilatation and penetration of the vasa vasorum which are normally present in the adventitia and media of the pulmonary arteries. It would appear, therefore, that these small branches of the bronchial arteries, which do not normally communicate directly with the lumina of the pulmonary arteries, can, in the presence of diminished pulmonary artery blood flow or pulmonary artery occlusion, affect precapillary anastomoses, which in turn become associated with hypertrophy of the bronchial arteries. The presence of enlarged bronchial arteries in congenital heart disease associated with patent intrapulmonary arteries suggests a predominantly systemic-to-pulmonary artery blood flow.

III. The Anatomy of
the Normal Human Bronchial Circulation

Miller [76], Hovelacque et al. [77], Nakamura [78], Berry [22], Verloop [79], von Hayek [80,81], Marchand et al. [82], Cudkowicz and Armstrong [83], and above all, Cauldwell et al. [84] have provided details concerning the origin and distribution of the bronchial arteries to normal human lungs. The methods used varied from gross inspection [83,85] to histology [79] and serial section [79,81,83,86]. Subsequent methods comprised corrosion cast techniques of the injected vasculature with different-colored plastic materials such as Vinylite, from which the lung substance can be totally excluded by treating the injected lung in an acid bath [82,86,87,88]. Postmortem angiography utilizing radio-opaque contrast media of different density, which permitted both radiological identification of the bronchial vasculature and recognition of the bronchial arteries in lung histology, was used by Cudkowicz and Armstrong [83], while postmortem angiograms in lung disease were used by Wood and Miller [89] and by Silver [90]. These techniques shed much light on the exact intrapulmonary distribution of the normal human bronchial circulation.

Miller [76] stressed that the two lung circulations could only be adequately studied if a viscid contrast medium would not penetrate the capillary beds of the respective arterial systems. Once particle size and viscosity of the fluid medium were controlled, conclusions could be drawn concerning precapillary relationships of the two circulations in the normal human lungs. Prior to discussing the intrapulmonary distribution of the bronchial arteries it is necessary to outline the extrapulmonary course of the bronchial arterial circulation and its variable origin.

A. The Extrapulmonary Course of the Bronchial Arteries

Daly and Hebb [91] cite that one of the most complete accounts of the gross anatomy of the bronchial arteries was provided by Suslov [92] in his 1895 St. Petersburg M.D. thesis. He studied 113 human cadavers and identified the origins of a total of 370 bronchial arteries as follows:

1. The aorta gave rise to 228 (62%) vessels; 160 emerged at the level between the fourth rib and the fifth intercostal space.

2. The first right intercostal artery on its dorsal surface gave origin to 84 (23%).

3. The right internal mammary artery furnished 12 (3%) bronchial arteries.

4. The second right intercostal artery 11 (3%).

5. Nine (2%) came off the right superior intercostal artery.

Suslov mentioned a common bronchial arterial trunk, arising from the aorta in 50% of cases, which divides to supply separate branches to each lung. In the remaining autopsies the number of bronchial arteries varied from 2 to 6, with the order of frequency of occurrence being 4, 3, 5, 2, and 6 arteries, respectively.

Nakamura [78] studied this variability in 150 consecutive adult necropsies. Ignoring such uncommon variations as origins from internal mammary and subclavian arteries, he showed that 68.7% of the bronchial arteries originated partly in the aorta and partly elsewhere. In 15% they arose directly from the aorta, and in only 2% did they come altogether from extraaortic sources.

Cauldwell et al. [84] provided the most extensive investigation to date concerning the variability of origin of the bronchial arteries in 150 human cadavers, and concluded that the majority of the vessels take their origin directly from the aorta (Fig. 6). The aorta: (1) in 40.67% supplied two arteries to the left and one to the right; (2) in 21.33% supplied one artery to the left and one to the right; (3) in 9.33% supplied one artery to the left and two to the right; (4) in 4.00% supplied three arteries to the left and two to the right; (5) in 4.00% supplied three arteries to the left and two to the right.

Thus, one artery to the right lung and two arteries to the left were found in just over 40% of their series. The levels of origin of these vessels

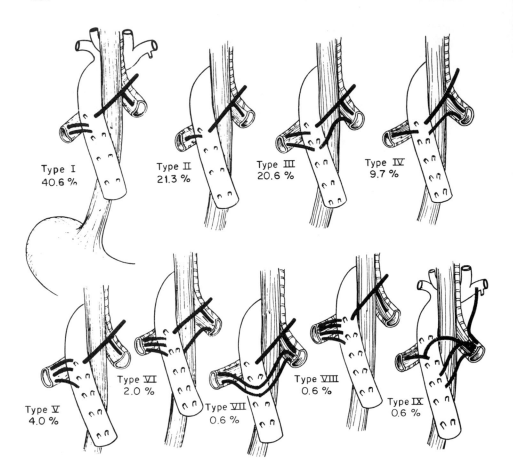

FIGURE 6   Types of bronchial arterial supply in 150 cadavers; classification based upon origin, number, and course of the vessels. Semidiagrammatic; dorsal aspect. (Reproduced from Cauldwell et al. [84], by permission of *Surgery, Gynecology and Obstetrics.*)

from the aorta varied between T.3 and T.8. In 48.4% the right-sided vessels and in 46.9% the left-sided vessels were related to the sixth thoracic segment. In 34.4% on the right side and 33% on the left side, the level of vascular origin was near the fifth thoracic segment. In 70.1% all left bronchial arteries of aortic origin emerged from the levels of T.5 and T.6. On the right side, 82.8% of the vessels originated opposite T.5 and T.6 from the aorta.

Other observers [93] have largely confirmed this extrapulmonary distribution of the bronchial arteries and have found additional minor branches which communicate with the coronary arteries [94].

B. The Intrapulmonary Course
of the Normal Bronchial Arteries

The intrapulmonary distribution of the bronchial arteries can be followed well by the corrosion method, but unfortunately this does not permit the simultaneous study of the vascular organization in relation to the morphologic structure of the lung. The most painstaking method, and probably the most rewarding, is the systematic study of both vasculature and lung structure by serial section, and this has been followed with success by Verloop [79] and Weibel [85]. For the purpose of this chapter the method employed by Cudkowicz and Armstrong [83] will be discussed in detail, because particular attention was paid to the intrapulmonary distribution of the bronchial arteries in normal lungs as a necessary and preliminary step to subsequent studies of the changes in the bronchial circulation in disease.

Derived from 10 pairs of lungs which were normal in structure and showed no histologic lesions in the lung vessels, alveoli, or bronchial tree, the radiographic appearances of these bronchial arteries were assumed to represent the normal configuration. In all 10 preparations the vascular patterns, obtained with the aid of a radio-opaque injection mass, showed uniformity and similarity of detail. The histologic sections taken from these injected lungs were deemed to represent the normal histologic equivalents of the radiological patterns.

C. The Normal Radiological Pattern
of the Human Bronchial Arteries [83]

The X-ray studies of these 10 preparations showed that the bronchial arteries emerge in varying numbers from the undersurface of the arch of the descending aorta, near the level of T.5 and T.6. These origins were inconstant, and up to three vessels were noted to enter the left hilus in one instance. There was also some variations in the respective sizes of the vessels. Before reaching the hilus they may cross the esophagus anteriorly or posteriorly, particularly the left branches. In their course from the aorta to the hilus, they send branches to the mediastinum, esophagus, hilar lymph nodes, and the vagi. On reaching the main bronchus on each side, the vessels formed an annulus surrounding the bronchus, and it is from this structure that true bronchial and pleural arteries emerge (Fig. 7).

The medial visceral pleura receives vessels directly from the annulus, but the anterior, lateral, and interlobar visceral pleurae appear to receive arteries from branches of the bronchial arteries within the fissures or lung substance. These vessels can be easily seen with the naked eye and appear over the lateral pleurae after emerging from the underlying lung (Fig. 8). They can be dis-

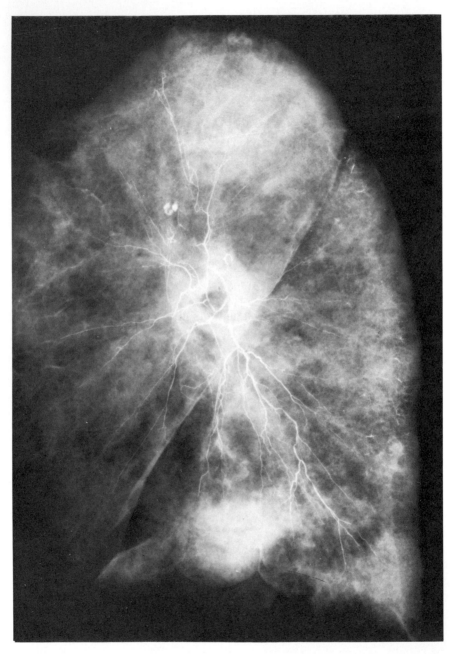

FIGURE 7   Lateral view of normal right bronchial arteriogram. Hilus faces X-ray tube. One-third of normal size. Shown are the annulus around right main bronchus and true bronchial and pleural arteries.

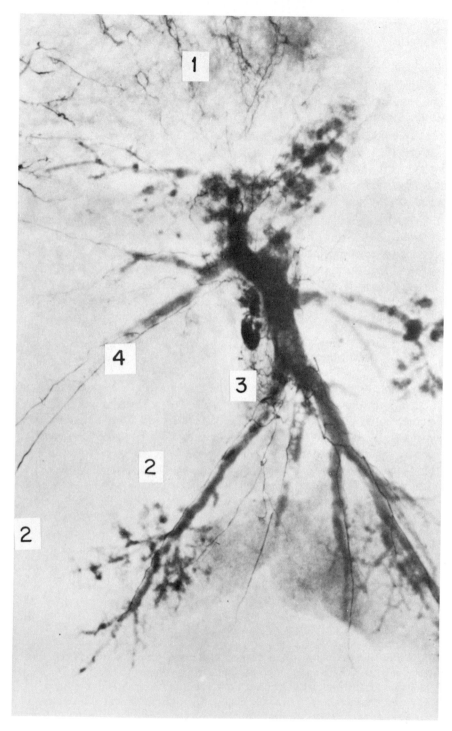

FIGURE 8   (Legend on page 132)

tinguished from the true bronchial vessels by their superficial position, which is particularly visible in lateral views, their independent course from the bronchial tree, and their relatively larger caliber at peripheral sites, where the true bronchial vessels usually disappear (Fig. 9).

The divisions in the medial pleura, which radiate from the hilus directly, might be referred to as *hilar pleural branches*; the vessels not arising from the annulus at the hilus, *lateral pleural branches*; those at the diaphragmatic surface, *basal pleural branches*; and the vessels in the fissures as *right* or *left oblique fissure*, and *right horizontal fissure branches*, respectively.

The constancy of an upper branch of the medial pleural vessels, extending to the apical pleura, has been noticed on many occasions, particularly where apical scars apparently lead to increase in its size (Fig. 10), and it is suggested that this branch might be called the *apical pleural branch*. No such constancy seems to prevail for other pleural branches, and it is therefore probably simpler to retain for these nonspecific nomenclature, i.e., the lateral and medial pleural branches already referred to.

D.   True "Bronchial Arteries"

The systemic arteries to the lungs enter the hilus to form a communicating arc around the main bronchi from which radiate the main arterial divisions along the major bronchi (Fig. 11). They adhere closely to the bronchial tree and follow the same course. They divide where the bronchi do and send at least two divisions along each bronchus, one on each side of the bronchial wall, which often tend to form an intercommunicating, horizontally oriented network in the fibrous coat of the bronchus (see Fig. 8). Smaller twigs penetrate the bronchial walls and appear as a similar network in the submucosa where this can be clearly seen with the naked eye in an opened bronchus. Under normal conditions this arrangement persists as far as the *respiratory bronchioles*. It can be categorically stated that with this technique no precapillary anastomoses with branches of the pulmonary arteries were demonstrable in any one of the 10 normal preparations. Such anastomoses were easily seen in lung disorders such as bronchiectasis.

FIGURE 8   Lateral view of left bronchial tree superimposed on left bronchial arterial pattern. The relationship of the bronchial arteries to the bronchi, visceral pleura, and lymph node at left hilus can be seen. (1) Apical pleural branch; (2) interlobar septal branches; (3) branch to hilar lymph node; (4) bronchial arteries accompanying the inferior lingular bronchus. The hilus faces away from X-ray tube. One-half of normal size. (Reproduced from Cudkowicz and Armstrong [83], by permission of *Thorax*.)

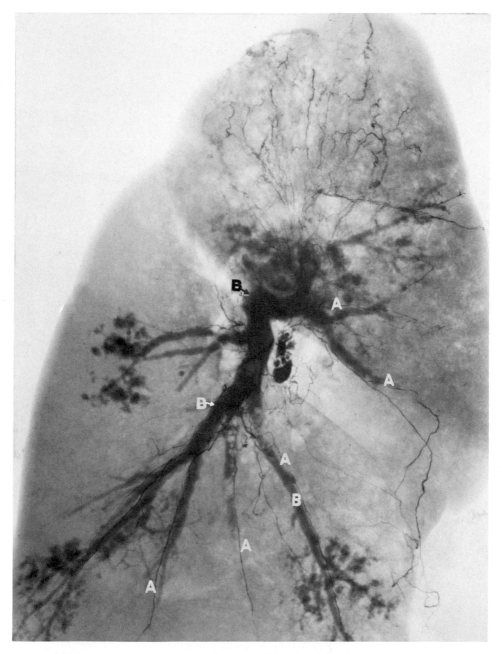

FIGURE 9 Detail of (A) bronchial arteries and (B) bronchial tree in left
bronchial arteriogram. Bronchial tree has also been filled with contrast
medium.

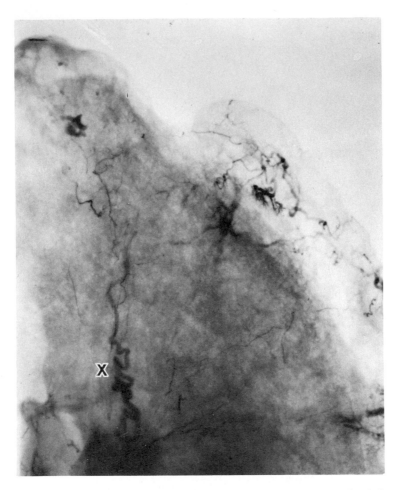

FIGURE 10   Lateral radiograph of left upper lobe of a patient with a left apical fibrocaseous tuberculous lesion. Note enlargement of left apical pleural branch (X). Approximately normal size. (Reproduced from Cudkowicz, L., and J. B. Armstrong, *Thorax,* 7:270 (1952), by permission of the journal [83].)

The normal radiological pattern just described produces a clear silhouette of the bronchial tree (Fig. 12), which permits the adoption of the accepted nomenclature of the bronchial tree (Thoracic Society, 1950 [95]) for labeling of the bronchial arterial divisions which accompany the respective major bronchi.

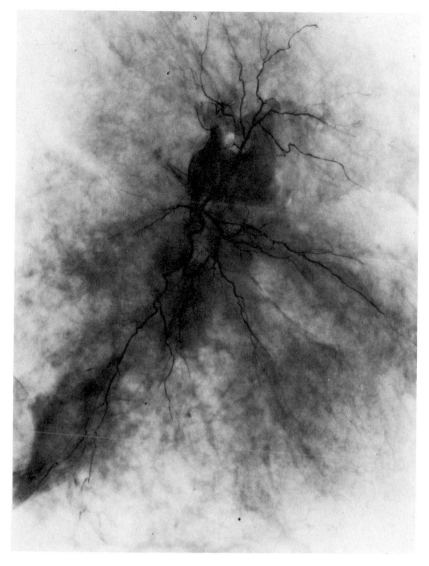

FIGURE 11 Normal pattern of left bronchial arteries seen in a lateral view of a left lung. Hilus faces X-ray tube. One-half of normal size.

The bronchial arterial divisions as seen in a right and left lateral postmortem bronchial arteriogram are shown in Figures 13 and 15, respectively. The pattern in a posteroanterior view of both lungs is depicted in Figure 17. The bronchial tree nomenclature will be applied to each set of arteries accompanying a major bronchus.

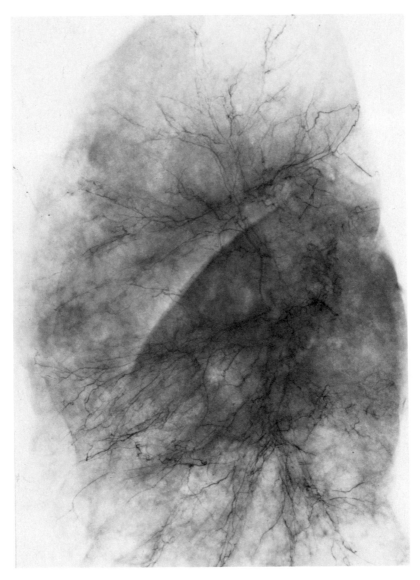

FIGURE 12 The distribution of the bronchial arteries as seen in an antero-posterior view of a right lung. The bronchial tree becomes silhouetted in this view by the bronchial arteries. (Reproduced from Cudkowicz and Armstrong [83], by permission of *Thorax.*)

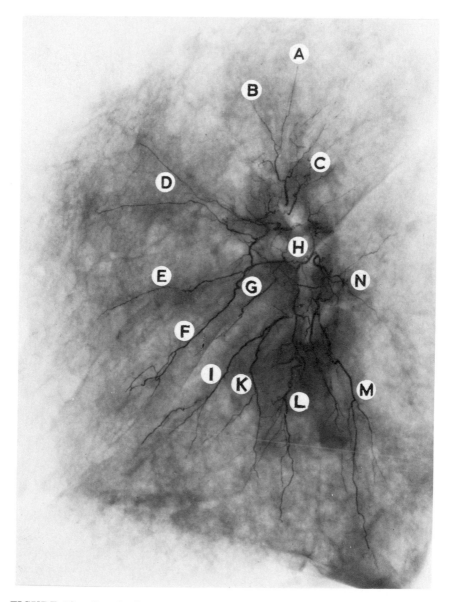

FIGURE 13 Standard pattern of right bronchial arteries seen in a lateral view of a right lung. Hilus faces X-ray tube. For details see Figure 14. For explanation of symbols, see text. (Reproduced from Cudkowicz and Armstrong [83], by permission of *Thorax*.)

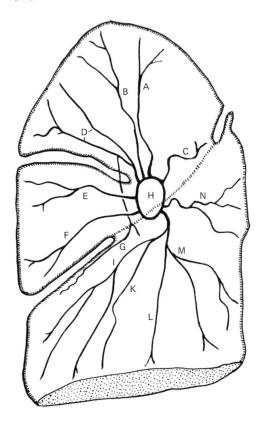

FIGURE 14   Tracing of Figure 13. The nomenclature of the bronchial arteries as seen in a lateral view of the right lung. For explanation of symbols, see text.

Figures 13 and 14 show a right lateral bronchial arteriogram demonstrating the following branches:

Right upper lobe: (A) apical pleural branch; (B) apical branches; (C) posterior branches; (D) anterior branches

Right middle lobe: (E) lateral branches; (F) medial branches; (G) interlobar pleural branches; (H) annulus

Right lower lobe: (I) anterior basal branches; (K) cardiac branches; (L) lateral basal branches; (M) posterior basal branches; (N) apical (superior) branches

Figures 15 and 16 provide a left lateral bronchial arteriogram. The arterial divisions arising from the left annulus are identifiable as follows:

Left upper lobe: (A) apical pleural branches; (B) posterior branches; (C) apical branches; (D) anterior branches; (E) superior lingular branches; (F) inferior lingular branches; (G) annulus

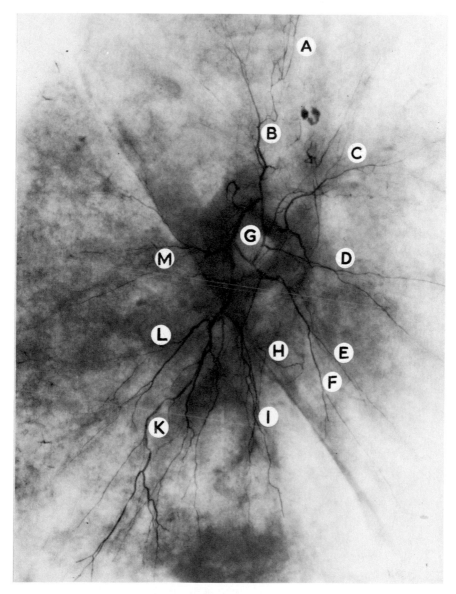

FIGURE 15 Standard pattern of left bronchial arteries seen in a lateral view of a left lung. Hilus faces X-ray tube. For details see Figure 16. For explanation of symbols, see text. (Reproduced from Cudkowicz and Armstrong [83], by permission of *Thorax*.)

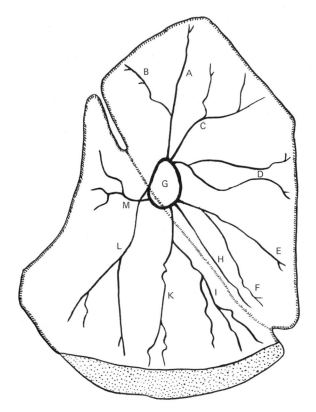

FIGURE 16 Tracing of Figure 15, with the nomenclature of the left bronchial arteries seen in a lateral view. For explanation of symbols, see text.

Left lower lobe: (H) interlobar pleural branches; (I) anterior basal branches; (K) lateral basal branches; (L) posterior basal branches; (M) apical (superior) branches

Figures 17 and 18 depict bronchial arteriograms to both lungs viewed from the posteroanterior aspect. The branches are named as follows:

Left upper lobe: (A) apical branch; (B) anterior branch; (C) superior lingular branch; (D) inferior lingular branch; (E) posterior branch

Left lower lobe: (F) lateral basal branch; (G) anterior basal branch; (H) posterior basal branch; (I) apical (superior) branch

Right upper lobe: (J) apical pleural branch; (K) apical branch; (L) anterior branch (the posterior division is not readily visible in the right upper lobe preparation)

Right middle lobe: (M) lateral branch; (N) medial branch; (O) interlobar pleural branch

Right lower lobe: (P) anterior basal branch; (Q) cardiac branch (medial basal); (R) posterior basal branch (the apical or superior division is not visible)

A finer division of this nomenclature would not serve a useful purpose, and the tracings represented by Figures 14, 16, and 18 provide the fairly standard pattern within normal lungs by means of this technique. This vascular configuration is relatively simple to follow and is fairly constant in the 10 normal sets of lungs thus examined. Variations were, however, frequent in connection with the pleural divisions. Pleural branches which appeared most frequently in the 10 normal studies have been included in Figures 14, 16, and 18. It seems of particular interest that the upper medial or apical pleural

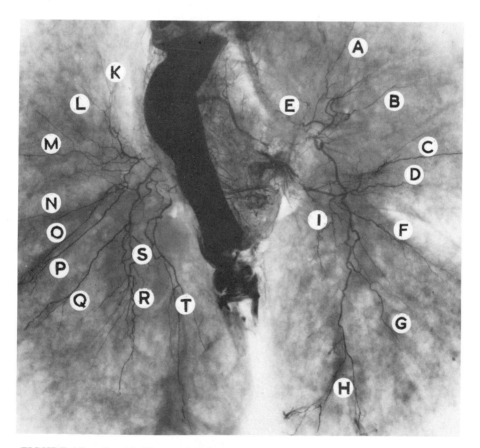

FIGURE 17 Case 1, X-ray of right and left lungs with trachea and aorta attached to show origin of bronchial arteries from aorta and their distribution in the lungs as seen in a posteroanterior view. Distortion of vessels at hili is caused by ligature around main bronchi. For details see Figure 18. For explanation of symbols, see text. (Reproduced by Cudkowicz and Armstrong [83], by permission of *Thorax*.)

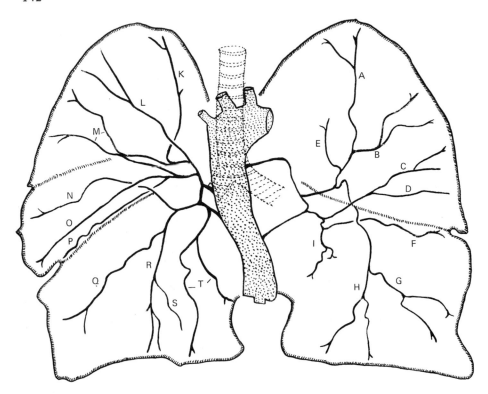

FIGURE 18   The nomenclature of the bronchial arteries. A tracing of Figure 17 to show the bronchial arterial branches in the anterolateral position. For explanation of symbols, see text.

branch varies less than the other pleural division and was demonstrable in 9 of the 10 sets of normal lungs examined.

E.   The Normal Intrapulmonary Bronchial Arterial Distribution in Histologic Section

The 10 sets of normal lungs, following angiography, provided the additional useful information concerning the normal intrapulmonary distribution of the bronchial arteries in histologic sections.

Lymph Nodes

In all instances, bronchial arteries were seen in the capsule and stroma of lymph nodes (Fig. 19). The vessels in the stroma were smaller than the

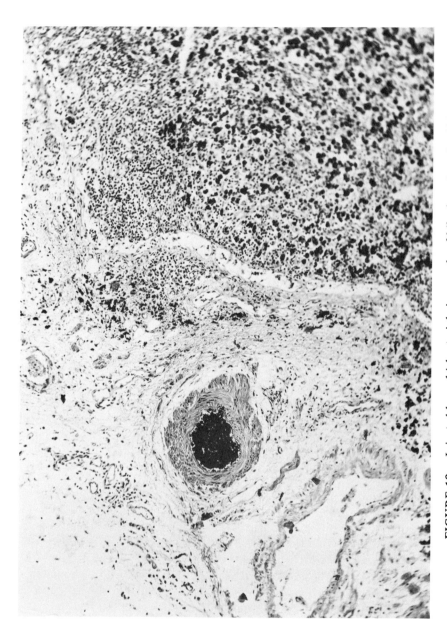

FIGURE 19 Injected bronchial arteriole in capsule of hilar lymph node. ×90.

capsular vessels and tended to run in the septa separating the lymph follicles. The caliber of the vessels varied directly with the size of the lymph nodes. Lymph nodes situated near the adventitial coat of a major bronchus received their bronchial arterial blood supply from the vessels supplying the adjacent bronchus.

Pulmonary Artery

In seven instances the vasa vasorum to the pulmonary arteries could be easily identified. They were vessels of more than 100 μm in diameter and appeared in the adventitial coat of the pulmonary artery (Fig. 20). At no time were the lumina of the vasa vasorum in communication with the lumen of a pulmonary artery. In these normal lungs they were totally confined to the adventitia, in contrast to similar vessels communicating freely with the lumina of pulmonary arteries in diseased lungs.

Vagus

In five sections of the vagi from the region of the major bronchi, well-filled bronchial arterioles were seen in the perineurium (Fig. 21). On two occasions the vessels were seen to penetrate the perineurium and to arrange themselves between the nerve fibers. No uninjected arterioles were visible near the nerve trunks, suggesting therefore that in the region of the lung hili, the bronchial arteries are nutritive to the pulmonary vagosympathetic trunks.

Main Bronchi

The main bronchi in transverse section usually revealed three to four large bronchial arteries in the peribronchial coat. Branches from there passed through the cartilaginous gaps and, after supplying the perichondrium, entered the tunica propria as small but very obviously injected vessels. Considerable numbers were seen within the glandular elements and adjacent to the basement membrane of the ciliated epithelium (Fig. 22).

Smaller Bronchi

In the smaller bronchi the bronchial arterial arrangements were the same as in the larger, but the vessels were naturally of a smaller caliber. The distribution to the structures of the bronchial walls was also the same. In the region of the bronchioles, small bronchial arterioles were seen within and without the bronchiolar walls (Fig. 23). Those which lay outside the wall ran in the fibrous septum between the accompanying pulmonary arterioles and the bronchiole. The pulmonary veins lay in the alveolar septa a little further away from the bronchiole and were duplicated at this level.

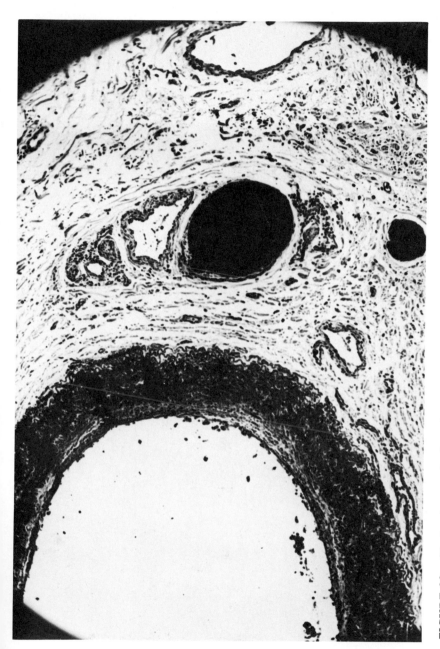

FIGURE 20 Photomicrograph of a pulmonary artery (lumen white). Bronchial arterioles (lumen black) are visible as vasa vasorum in the adventitia of the pulmonary artery (X65). (Reproduced from Cudkowicz and Armstrong [83], by permission of *Thorax*.)

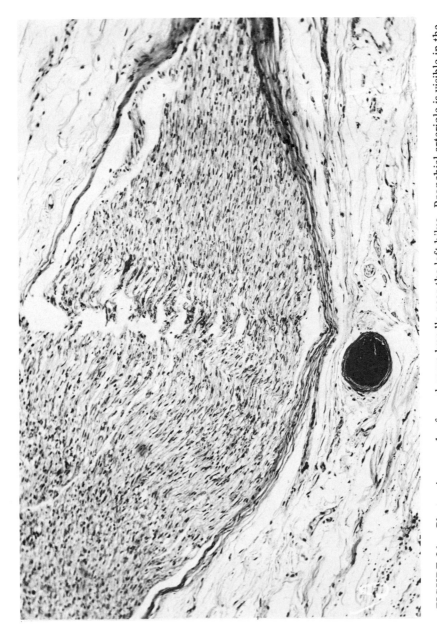

FIGURE 21   Photomicrograph of vagal nerve bundle near the left hilus. Bronchial arteriole is visible in the perineurium (X105). (Reproduced from Cudkowicz and Armstrong [83], by permission of *Thorax*.)

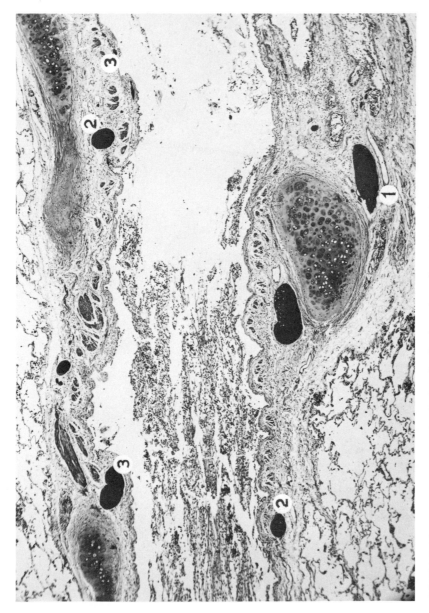

FIGURE 22 Photomicrograph of a longitudinal section of a medium-sized bronchus showing bronchial arterioles in (1) tunica fibrosa; (2) tunica propria; (3) submucosa (X35). (Reproduced from Cudkowicz and Armstrong [83], by permission of *Thorax*.)

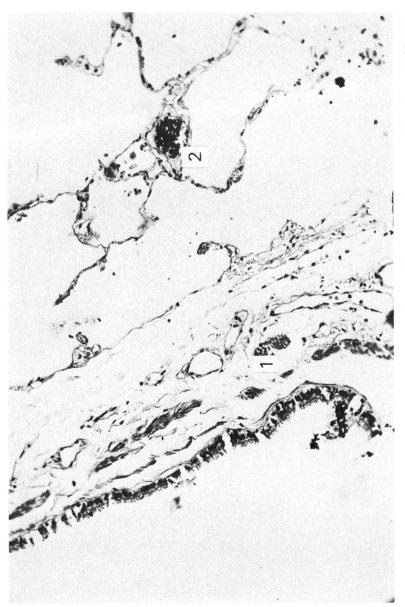

FIGURE 23 Bronchial arteriole (1) near bronchiolus and (2) in supporting tissue of alveolar wall (×175). (Reproduced from Cudkowicz and Armstrong [83], by permission of *Thorax*.)

Lung Parenchyma

Random sections of lung from the periphery showed normal anatomical features of the lobules. The capillaries were not distended as a result of the large amounts of saline which had been flushed through the preparation before injection with bismuth. Well-injected bronchial arterioles were seen in the interlobular septa (Fig. 24). Near the alveolar ducts the smallest bismuth-filled arterioles were seen adjacent to the mucosa. Their diameter was probably just over 80 μm. The corresponding pulmonary arterioles and venules were larger and free from bismuth. Larger, well-filled bronchial arterioles were, however, visible in the supporting framework of the alveolar epithelium, and they appeared to surround the air sacs with trabeculae of elastic tissue which insinuated themselves between the alveoli as outgrowths of the interlobular septa (Fig. 25).

Bronchial arteries emerging from the aorta have a wide concentric media and a well-developed internal elastic lamina. In lung sections these characteristics are evident, as is a longitudinal muscle in the intima which, occasionally and eccentrically, considerably reduces the lumen. This muscle is of interest inasmuch as Weibel, in 1958 [96], presented some evidence which indicates that these longitudinal muscle bundles of the intima develop as a result of the constant movement and stretching of these vessels and their bronchi during the phases of respiration. It is also likely that these muscle bundles, which occasionally give the impression of total occlusion of the vessel in histologic section, could have given rise to the concept of *Sperrarterien,* or blocking arteries between the two arterial circulations of the lung. This concept has been elaborated by von Hayek [80,81] and Verloop [79], who suggested that *Sperrarterien* are the site of bronchial artery and pulmonary artery precapillary anastomoses.

Pleura

Sections of the visceral pleura showed that the systemic arteries lay within the subserosal coat. Occasional vessels penetrated the pleura from the underlying lung. More frequently, and particularly at the apex, the vessels appeared to lie entirely in the pleural membrane, which would accord with the macroscopic observation that the pleural arteries of the medial pleura, and the apical pleural branch, coursed from the hilus superficially. All visible arteries in the pleura of these normal lungs were fully injected, indicating they were all derived from the bronchial arteries (Fig. 26).

The difficulty of differentiating between pulmonary and bronchial arterioles in lung sections was well recognized by Brenner in 1935 [95]. The method used at the time failed to demonstrate precapillary anastomoses

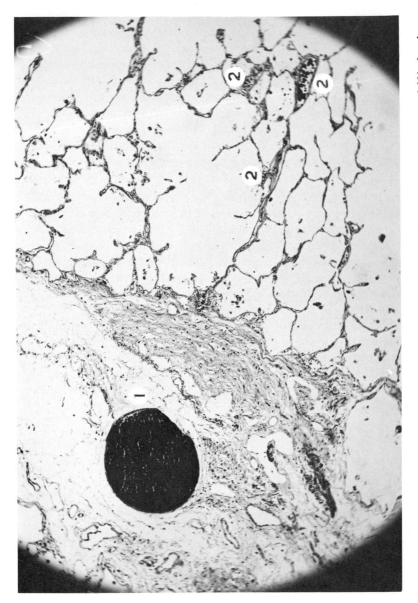

FIGURE 24 Photomicrography showing bronchial arterioles in (1) interlobular septum and (2) alveolar septum (×75). (Reproduced from Cudkowicz and Armstrong [83], by permission of *Thorax*.)

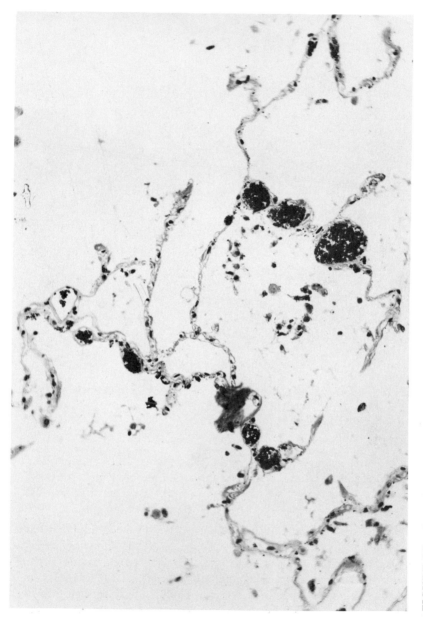

FIGURE 25 Bronchial arterioles near alveolar walls (AW) and air sacs (AS) (×205). (Reproduced from Cudkowicz and Armstrong [83], by permission of *Thorax*.)

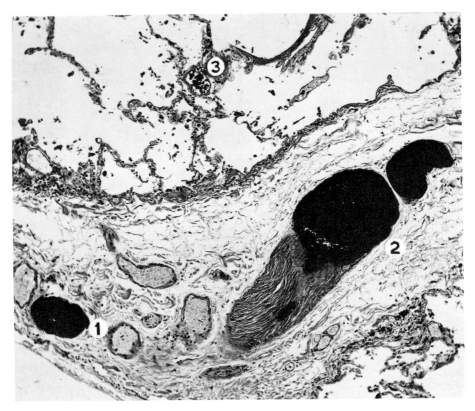

FIGURE 26   Photomicrograph of bronchiole arterioles in (1) visceral pleura;
(2) interlobular septum; (3) alveolar wall (X88). (Reproduced from Cudkowicz
and Armstrong [83], by permission of *Thorax*.)

between the bronchial and pulmonary arteries in normal lungs proximal to
vessels of 60 μm in diameter. It would appear that the bronchial artery bed
is independent of the pulmonary artery bed in health, and that true precapillary communications of the two systems are of pathologic significance.

   Finally, there are numerous bronchial arterioles in the interlobular septa
which course along trabeculae of elastic tissue to reach the interstitial tissue of
the alveoli. These interlobular arterioles are derived, not from arteries accompanying the bronchi, but from the pleural arterial system. The arterioles embedded in the interstitial tissue of the air sacs could be distinguished from the
pulmonary arterioles only by their bismuth-filled lamina and the absence of an
accompanying bronchiole. The actual supporting framework of the alveoli
therefore has its own systemic arterial blood supply.

It must be stressed that this technique does not permit the examination of the bronchial vasculature and its own capillary bed beyond vessels of 60 μm in diameter and fails to rule out precapillary, capillary, or venous anastomoses distal to this level in the normal human lung. The elegant studies by Weibel [85] have fairly conclusively shown that the bronchial arteries act as end arteries to their own major capillary territories, particularly within the bronchial walls, and that probably anastomoses have to be sought between bronchial and pulmonary venules. Töndury and Weibel [97], by careful serial sections, were able to demonstrate infrequent bronchopulmonary anastomoses at the level of small bronchioles and, in two instances, in the visceral pleura. Similar were more recent findings by Lauweryns [98]. Thus, areas of potential normal capillary anastomoses must be sought near the terminal alveolar ducts and outside the pulmonary capillary bed, namely, close to the vasa vasorum of the pulmonary arteries. In recent years, studies of the pulmonary capillaries have been undertaken by a number of investigators [99,100].

Reid and Heard [101], using a new method of injecting the pulmonary capillaries in human lungs, found that the pulmonary arterioles lead to enormous numbers of different-sized capillaries. The smallest ones supply immediately adjacent alveoli, and the largest often give off more branches to supply more distant alveoli. At a higher magnification, arterioles of about 12 μm in diameter spring from the parent arteriole, which is 75 μm in diameter, and run across the field and divide into two or three intermediate-sized branches before joining the alveolar capillary network. This network has a polygonal meshwork, in contrast to a larger bronchiolar network which has an elongated mesh and thus a directional character. The bronchiolar network comes in contact with the network derived from the bronchial arterial system near the alveolar ducts. Large pulmonary veins are sometimes seen originating in the bronchial capillary plexus.

Other excellent descriptions of the lung capillaries emerge from the studies of Boren [102], Knisely [103], Krahl [104], Liebow [105], Staub and Schultz [106], and Weibel [107].

F.   The Bronchial Veins

The venous bronchial circulation is divided into two major zones, depending on the directional flow of the bronchial venous return. Miller [108] regarded the peripheral bronchial venous drainage channels, which unite with those of the pulmonary venules near the alveolar ducts to form the pulmonary veins, as the only true anastomoses between the two circulations to the lung. These peripheral and mainly submucosal venous channels were visualized by injection techniques [109] and referred to as true bronchial veins by Marchand et al. [82].

Zuckerkandl distinguished these channels from recurrent veins draining the larger bronchi [21]. According to Wagenvoort and Wagenvoort [110] and Florange [111], the larger bronchi have a double bronchial venous network, one in the mucosa and one external to the bronchial cartilage. These networks are connected [112]. The bronchial venous system in the lung center and at the hili have their own channels, which also anastomose with the pulmonary veins [83,113].

The main direction of bronchial venous return from the larger bronchi is towards the venous plexus of the trachea, mediastinum, and periesophageal and hilar lymph node venous radicles. These tend to merge with the azygous and hemiazygous systems of veins which terminate in the superior vena cava or the coronary sinus [113]. It is assumed that approximately *one-third* of the normal bronchial venous flow returns to the right side of the heart and that the major component of the venous return reaches the left atrium by the pulmonary veins [114].

Wagenvoort and Wagenvoort [110] showed that the walls of bronchial veins are thin and contain a distinct internal elastic layer, as well as a media with some muscle fibers. In addition, valves can be observed infrequently, particularly near the hilus.

In the absence of obvious precapillary anastomoses between the normal bronchial and pulmonary arteries proximal to vessels of 60 μm in diameter it is difficult to explain some of the observations, particularly those of Prinzmetal et al. [115], who were able to follow the passage of beads with diameters up to 390 μm from the pulmonary artery to the pulmonary veins. Similar observations were made by Tobin and Zariquiev [116], who also demonstrated anastomoses between the pulmonary artery and pulmonary veins by means of corrosion techniques. It is unlikely that the bronchial circulation is involved in these anastomoses, and in the opinion of Gordon et al. [117], as well as Weibel [107], the assumption has to be made that pulmonary capillaries are *distensible* enough to permit the passage of beads of at least 17 to 30 μm in diameter.

IV. The Measurement of Bronchial Arterial Blood Flow in Humans

Measurement of bronchial arterial blood flow in the human evolved from an application of the indirect Fick's principle, and Bing et al. [53] used this method in 1947 for the assessment of bilateral bronchial arterial flows in children with Fallot's tetralogy.

Bloomer et al. [57], in 1949, introduced the now well-known method for the calculation of effective unilateral bronchial arterial anastomotic flows. The method was used in dogs after ligation of one pulmonary artery, and required bronchospirometry. Effective bronchial arterial minute flow to that lung was obtained from the direct Fick method. The uptake of oxygen by the ligated lung is measured while the contralateral normal side respires air. Pre- and postcapillary arteriovenous oxygen differences are established by arterial oxygen contents obtained in this state and subsequently while both lungs are respiring oxygen. Thus:

$$\dot{Q}_{precap}BF/min \; = \; \frac{\dot{V}O_2/min \text{ ligated lung}}{CPVO_2 \; - \; Ca_{O_2}} \tag{1}$$

$\dot{V}O_2/min$ = minute oxygen consumption. $CPVO_2 = O_2$ content of pulmonary venous blood while both lungs respire oxygen. $Ca_{O_2} = O_2$ content of arterial blood while the ligated lung respired oxygen alone. In 10 operated dogs, 19 observations revealed a stepwise rise in $\dot{Q}_{precap}BF/min$ with time after ligation. After about 4 months, the effective flow to such lungs usually exceeded 1.0 liter $min^{-1} \, m^{-2}$ and increased the left ventricular minute volume by about one-third over that of the right.

Using this technique, Madoff et al. [118] found, in a girl with a congenitally absent right pulmonary artery, an effective right bronchial precapillary minute flow of 950 ml/min.

Fishman et al. [56] also used the direct Fick method for the measurement of bilateral bronchial arterial flow in four patients with atresia of the pulmonary arteries in whom the precapillary flow constituted the entire circulation through the alveoli. The oxygen content of the precapillary bronchial arterial flow was assumed to be the same as in a systemic artery. The application of the Fick method to this type of bronchial arterial flow remains unsatisfactory. If the oxygen content of precapillary and postcapillary anastomotic bronchial blood is identical with that of systemic arterial blood, the direct Fick method would merely provide a measure for right ventricular minute flow, provided that a true, mixed venous sample, uncontaminated by systemic arterial blood, can be obtained from the pulmonary artery. Thus,

$$\dot{Q} \; Fick/min \; = \; \frac{\dot{V}O_2/min}{Ca_{O_2} \; - \; C\bar{v}_{O_2}} \tag{2}$$

would equal right ventricular output ($\dot{Q}RV$) only if $Ca_{O_2} = CPVO_2$ and $C\bar{v}_{O_2} = C_{precap}O_2$. An increase in the latter and a reduction in the former

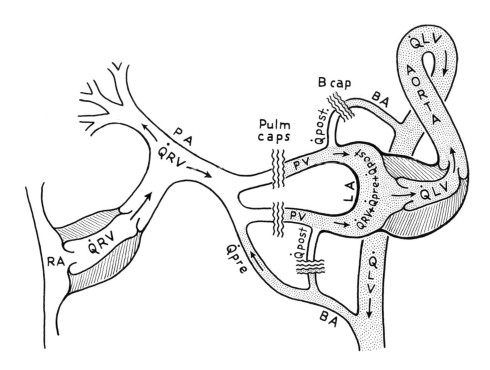

FIGURE 27   Diagram showing components of left ventricular output (minute flow). RA = right atrium; PA = pulmonary artery; LA = left atrium; BA = bronchial arteries; $\dot{Q}$RV = right ventricular output; $\dot{Q}$LV = left ventricular output; $\dot{Q}$ = precapillary anastomosis flow; $\dot{Q}$ = postcapillary anastomosis flow; B cap = bronchial postcapillaries; Pulm caps. = pulmonary capillaries. Vessels normally containing venous blood are white; those normally containing arterial blood are shaded. (Reproduced from Cudkowicz, L., et al., *American Heart Journal,* **58**:732 (1959) by permission of the journal [123].)

will both reduce the arteriovenous oxygen difference and measure a cardiac output in excess of $\dot{Q}$RV/min.

An alternative approach to the measurement of the bronchial arterial flow ($\dot{Q}$BF) is offered by the simultaneous determination of right and left ventricular outputs by an indirect dye dilution technique. Dye dilution curves obtained from the pulmonary artery after injection of an indicator close to the right atrium have been found to give accurate measure of the right ventricular output [119].

Although bronchopulmonary anastomoses may not be the only communication between the pulmonary and bronchial circulations, for the purpose of this technique it is assumed that in the steady state and in absence of other known shunts, an excess in left over right ventricular output is a measure of the bronchopulmonary circulation. Figure 27 gives a diagramatic representation of the components of the left ventricular minute flow. The bronchial venous blood returning to the right atrium through the azygous system is not specifically included.

It is assumed that the bronchial arterial minute flows ($\dot{Q}BF$) derived indirectly from estimates of the difference between simultaneously recorded minute flows of the right and left ventricles, measure postcapillary components of the bilateral, normal bronchial arterial blood flow, as well as that which reaches the lungs through precapillary anastomoses between the bronchial and pulmonary arteries in abnormal states, both of which return to the left side of the heart through the pulmonary veins. Thus, the main portion of the normal bronchial arterial flow is a bronchial-pulmonary venous anastomotic flow which is added to the right ventricular minute flow ($\dot{Q}RV/min$) to make up the left ventricular minute flow ($\dot{Q}LV/min$).

$$\dot{Q}LV - \dot{Q}RV = \dot{Q}B_{precap} + \dot{Q}B_{postcap}$$
$$\dot{Q}B_{precap} + \dot{Q}B_{postcap} = \dot{Q}BF$$

(3)

Additional flows from other systemic arteries to the lungs, such as the intercostal and pericardiophrenic arteries, are included in this measurement, but not that component of $\dot{Q}BF/min$ entering the azygous system of veins, estimated by Bruner and Schmidt in 1947 [120] in dogs at one-third of the total $\dot{Q}BF/min$.

Fritts et al. [119], in 1957, and Fox and Wood [121], in 1957, established that $\dot{Q}RV/min$ could be calculated from dye curves in blood withdrawn from the pulmonary artery after the injection of an indicator fairly close to the right atrium. With the same indicator bolus, $\dot{Q}LV/min$ can be simultaneously obtained from a peripheral arterial dye curve.

In this technique, a small amount of dye indicator is withdrawn during the inscription of the pulmonary artery curve before the blood carrying the indicator to the left heart is further diluted to form the peak of the systemic arterial curve. Apart from this effect on the $\dot{Q}LV/min$ curve peak, unsuspected early recirculation is also likely to distort the downslope of the systemic curve. Such small and probable errors greatly affect the $\dot{Q}BF/min$ derived in this manner. Nevertheless, the densitometric recordings of Evans blue by Fritts et al. [122] in 13 studies of nine patients with normal cardiorespiratory systems established a difference between the right ventricular volume and the Fick output of ±1.5%.

In another study [123], three of five patients without lung disease showed a mean difference between left and right ventricular minute flows of 1.5%. In one subject no difference could be demonstrated, and in another the $\dot{Q}RV/min$ exceeded that of $\dot{Q}LV/min$. In the study by Fritts et al. [122], the average difference between $\dot{Q}RV/min$ and $\dot{Q}LV$ in nine normal subjects was 0.9% but there was a considerable variation in the individual patients. The method is thus not yet sufficiently precise to permit the estimate of $\dot{Q}BF/min$ in the normal human.

However, differences well in excess of 10.25% have been recorded between the left and right ventricular minute volumes in patients with bronchiectasis, pulmonary neoplasms, and occluded pulmonary arteries, suggesting that this method may be useful in the presence of a large bronchial arterial minute flow. In disorders suspected of particularly poor systemic blood flows to the lungs, such as pulmonary emphysema [123] or pulmonary bilharzia, this indirect method clearly would not be sufficiently sensitive [124].

The results of published measurements of bronchial arterial flow in the human by the indirect method are shown in Table 1. Normal $\dot{Q}BF$ varies from 0.9 to 1.43% of left ventricular output. In bronchiectasis this figure appears to be much higher. Cudkowicz [125] found a mean of approximately 17.9%. Fritts [122] reported a mean of 9.7%, and Nakamura et al. [126] found a mean of 25%. In tuberculosis and primary lung cancer this problem is of considerable interest inasmuch as one would like to know if the bronchial venous blood returns to the right or to the left side of the heart. In pulmonary tuberculosis, with the indirect technique, the reported difference varies from 2.9 to 8.4% [119,123,125,127]. In silicosis, Nakamura et al. [126] observed a mean $\dot{Q}BF$ of 8.8% of $\dot{Q}LV$. In emphysema the right ventricular output seems to be almost invariably higher than that of the left [125,127]. In primary carcinoma of the lung the difference is higher [128]; this was also found by Nakamura [126] and by Ryan and Abelmann [129]. Observations on secondary carcinoma of the lung are few [128]. Postmortem injection studies [130] showed that no bronchial arterial blood supply could be demonstrated in secondary cancers, and measurements of $\dot{Q}BF$ show insignificant differences from normal controls. Nakamura et al. [126] were, however, able to demonstrate an increase in bronchial arterial blood flow in one patient with a secondary lung tumor. In lung abscess he found a similar increase. The indirect method cannot account for the azygous component of the bronchial venous flow which returns to the right heart (Fig. 28).

TABLE 1 Estimates in Humans of $\dot{Q}BF$/min by the Indirect Technique[a]

Authors	References	Normals	Bronchi-ectasis	Tuber-culosis	Silicosis	Emphy-sema	Primary lung cancer	Secondary cancer	Pulmonary bilharziasis
						Means % $\dot{Q}LV$/min			
Cudkowicz et al. (1959–1965)	123, 125, 127, 128	$N=28$ 1.43	$N=9$ 17.9	$N=24$ 4.15		−6.5	$N=9$ 6.5	$N=6$ 3.0	
Fritts et al. (1961)	119, 122	$N=9$ 0.9	$N=11$ 9.7	$N=6$ 2.9					
Nakamura et al. (1961)	126		$N=8$ 25.0	$N=8$ 8.4	$N=14$ 8.8	−0.3	$N=5$ 21.1	$N=3$ 3.3	
Abdel-Fattah et al. (1966)	124	$N=5$ 1.13							$N=15$ −1.48

[a]$\dot{Q}BF = \dot{Q}LV - \dot{Q}RV$; $\dot{Q}BF = \dot{Q}B_{precap}$; mean of $\dot{Q}BF$/min expressed as *percentage* of $\dot{Q}LV$/min.

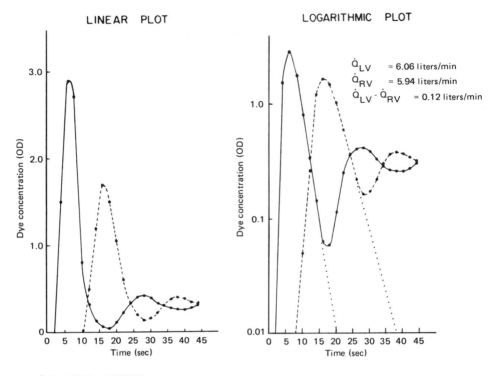

INJECTION INTO SUBCLAVIAN VEIN

—— PULMONARY ARTERY COLLECTION
---- BRACHIAL ARTERY COLLECTION

LINEAR PLOT LOGARITHMIC PLOT

$\dot{Q}_{LV}$ = 6.06 liters/min
$\dot{Q}_{RV}$ = 5.94 liters/min
$\dot{Q}_{LV} \cdot \dot{Q}_{RV}$ = 0.12 liters/min

Dye concentration (OD)

Time (sec)

T.C. 46 M. NORMAL

FIGURE 28 Normal bronchial arterial blood flow (indirect technique). Representative normal examples of simultaneously measured right and left ventricular outputs from dye dilution curves and their semilogarithmic plots (Evans blue). OD = optical density units.

V. The Bronchial Circulation in Lobar Pneumonia: The Pulmonary Arteries in Lobar Pneumonia

The behavior of the pulmonary vasculature in lobar pneumonia has been studied in life by such techniques as lung scans with microaggregates of radio-iodinated albumin, pulmonary angiography [131], and cinedensigraphy [132]. Wagner et al. [133] stressed that lung scanning of patients with pulmonary parenchymatous disease consistently demonstrates avascularity in the lung segments or lobes affected. This applies in particular to the pneumonias, in which the reduction in pulmonary blood flow matches closely the area of opacification seen in the chest radiographs. Wagner also found that serial scans failed to demonstrate restoration of pulmonary blood flow to normal, several months after the apparent cure of the pneumonia as judged on clinical grounds and by radiological criteria [134].

Standertskjöld-Nordenstam [132], in 25 patients with verified pneumonia, showed that the pulmonary arterial pulse, as depicted by the technique of cinedensigraphy [135], was absent or significantly decreased over the pneumonic area. This decrease persisted for some weeks and often for months following clinical resolution of a pneumonia. Pulse disturbances by cinedensigraphy also were consistently observable in the face of radiological clearing of the consolidation. In seven cases of pneumococcal pneumonia, the average duration of pulmonary arterial pulse reduction in the corresponding lobar site was 9 weeks from the onset of the disease. The age of the patient or associated lung disorders had no effect on the time of recovery of the pulmonary arterial pulse pattern.

Additional evidence depicting a significant reduction in pulmonary arterial blood flow in pneumonia comes from pulmonary angiography. Particularly in the early phase of the disease, inadequate filling of the corresponding lobar branches has been demonstrated [136]. The pulmonary diffusing capacity for carbon monoxide was significantly reduced in the acute stages of lobar pneumonia, and did not return to normal following clinical and radiological clearing in four patients followed for 67 days [137]. This prolonged defect is compatible with a prolonged reduction in the regional perfusion or a continuing abnormality at the alveolar-capillary membrane of the recovering lung parenchyma. Central cyanosis as an acute effect of lobar consolidation has been studied for over half a century. Reductions in arterial oxygen saturation, first documented by Stadie [138] in 1919, have been repeatedly confirmed [139,140] during the acute phase of the pneumonia [141]. The arterial oxygen desaturation is thought to stem from venous admixture, is not readily correctible by oxygen breathing [140] and is usually not the result of alveolar hypoventilation. The largest value found for a shunt of venous blood through the consolidated lobe was 9% of cardiac output. Such a level of venous admixture cannot reduce the arterial oxygen saturation to less than 92% [137]. The hypoxia of lobar pneumonia requires a mechanism other than those elaborated above, particularly changes in regional $\dot{V}/\dot{Q}$ ratios affecting areas of lung not involved by the pneumonia [142,143].

Occlusive changes in the pulmonary circulation to consolidated lungs were well demonstrated radiographically in necropsy specimens by Gross in 1919 [144]. Other observations in the preantibiotic era are worthy of note. Kaufman [145] described the changes in red hepatization as follows: "The vessels are markedly filled and the exudates show many red and white blood corpuscles, as well as exfoliated, swollen, lumpy, granular, poorly staining epithelial cells, mostly without recognizable nuclei." The gray hepatization, he noted: "Since the alveoli are filled to the maximum they press against each other and on the vessels. This circumstance, in combination with the fibrinous thrombi in some of the blood vessels, contributes to the impaired although not complete interruption of the circulation."

Pulmonary arteriolar occlusion in the early phase of pneumonia poses the question of the origin of the masses of red cells in the alveoli during the stage of red hepatization. Karsner and Ash [29] proposed an augmentation of bronchial arterial blood flow distal to the reduced or absent blood flow in an occluded pulmonary artery, suggesting that the red cells in the alveoli of red hepatization stem from the high-pressure bronchopulmonary anastomoses distal to a block in the pulmonary arterioles [29].

A. The Bronchial Circulation in Lobar Pneumonia [146]

Studies concerning the part played by the bronchial circulation in lobar pneumonia in the human are scanty, and a study derived from four patients coming to autopsy with evidence of consolidation in one or more lobes will be detailed here. The postmortem diagnoses of the four patients studied are shown in Table 2. Careful study of these patients disclosed that the reaction pattern of the two circulations to the lungs in lobar pneumonia reveals a major difference. The main branches of the pulmonary arteries in the phase of red hepatization are occluded close to the consolidated area. No information is available concerning the duration of this occlusion and the precise time of its inception. Presumably, it takes place during the phase of congestion. At the time of the formation of the red stage of hepatization with the widespread extravasation of erythrocytes into the alveoli, the bronchial arteries are also intensely congested and fail to fill with contrast medium, presumably because of this congestion, which implies a reduction in bronchial arterial blood flow. Speculation alone suggests that this reduction in bronchial arterial blood flow

TABLE 2

Number	Sex	Age	Autopsy diagnosis
1	M	67	Bilateral lobar pneumonia. Right upper lobe in red stage of hepatization. Left lower lobe in gray stage of hepatization.
2	M	55	Hypertensive heart disease. Left lower lobe pneumonia in red stage of hepatization.
3	F	74	Arteriosclerotic heart disease. Right lower lobe in gray stage of hepatization.
4	M	61	Cerebral hemorrhage. Left lower lobe in gray stage of hepatization. Bilateral apical fibrocaseous tuberculosis.

attends the outpouring of red cells into the alveoli after the bronchial arterial blood flow has become diverted into the distal branches of the pulmonary segmental arterioles and thus into the pulmonary capillaries. Pulmonary capillary rupture or increased permeability must attend the change in local hemodynamics, permitting alveolar filling with red cells derived from the high-pressure, precapillary bronchial arterial communicating vessels. Once the alveoli have become so filled, the pressure gradient between the filled alveoli and the systemic arterioles communicating with the pulmonary capillaries becomes abolished and flow in the proximal bronchial arteries is reduced. This lasts for the duration of the red stage of hepatization.

With the development of the gray stage of hepatization, the local hemodynamics change, with further dilatation of the proximal bronchial arteries. Flow is restored and now proceeds not only along the normal bronchial arterial channels but also into the peripheral bed of the pulmonary arteries, causing these to be outlined retrogradely with a contrast medium introduced into the bronchial arteries.

If these local circulatory changes are correctly interpreted, it seems that the complete restoration of the pulmonary circulation, including the pulmonary capillaries, continues well beyond the resolution phase of a lobar pneumonia. This also implies that with the slow restoration of the local pulmonary circulation a corresponding and equally slow regression in the bronchial circulation takes place. Reference was made at the outset to the slow return of the pulmonary blood flow in pneumonia, as seen in life by means of lung scans with isotopes [133]. Apart from the actual changes in bronchial arterial blood flow during the different phases of pneumonia, there remains the additional problem of the oxygen uptake from the bronchial arterial blood by the pneumonic lung. In the event of a significant oxygen uptake, the bronchial venous return from the consolidated area, which presumably follows its normal route to the pulmonary veins, will contribute to the venous admixture and hypoxemia so common in lobar pneumonia.

VI. The Bronchial Circulation in Bronchiectasis

In 1949, Liebow and associates provided evidence of striking proliferation and enlargement of the bronchial arteries in the postoperative specimens of 15 patients with chronic bronchiectasis [147]. Precapillary bronchopulmonary anastomoses were clearly demonstrated by means of Vinylite casts of the pulmonary and bronchial circulations. These communications were most widespread near the third- or fourth-order bronchi and the bronchiectatic dilatations or sacs. At these levels of the bronchial tree the bronchial arteries are normally quite small.

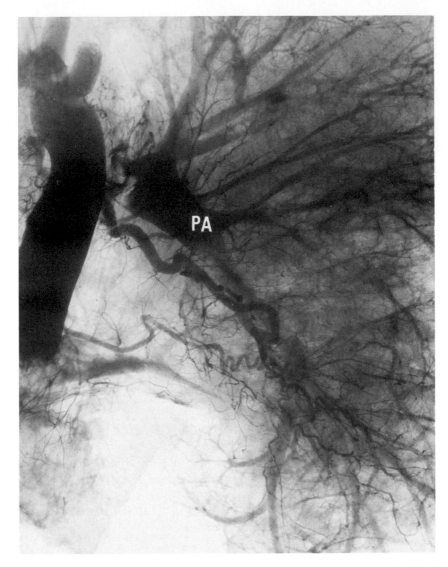

FIGURE 29   Left lower lobe bronchiectasis. Pulmonary arterial view (PA) of left lung showing large bronchial arteries conveying injection medium into left lower lobe pulmonary arteries. The left main pulmonary artery is filled retrogradely and is occluded distal to the origin of the lingular branch.

Evidence concerning the existence of large bronchopulmonary anastomoses in bronchiectatic lung segments or lobes has come from several sources [149] since the observations by Liebow [147].

Liebow et al. [148] assumed that the increase in bronchial arterial flow served the inflammatory responses and granulation tissue formation in the walls of the bronchi and peribronchial tissues. Consistent with observations of the bronchial arteries in other lung disorders, granulation tissues in the lung, as elsewhere, are fed by systemic arteries alone, and in the lung such vessels are mainly expanded bronchial arterioles.

In one of our studies, radiographs of injected lungs showed two very large bronchial arteries entering the left hilus and one artery more than 6 mm in diameter coursing to the right hilus. The left and part of the right pulmonary artery beds were also outlined. The bronchial arteries divided at the hili and followed the radicles of the pulmonary arteries very closely to the periphery. Normally distributed bronchial arteries were absent on the left side (Fig. 29).

Histologic examination showed precapillary anastomoses between the pulmonary and aberrant bronchial arteries at the periphery of both lungs (Fig. 30).

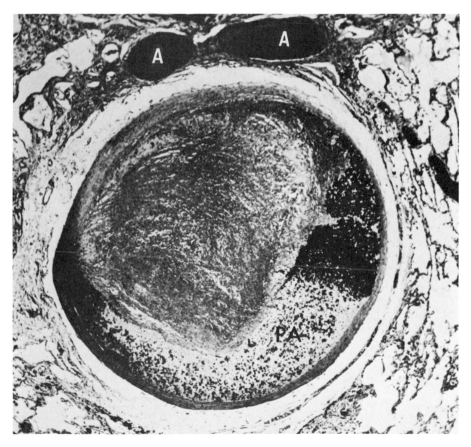

FIGURE 30 Bronchiectasis. Atheroma and intimal proliferation affect the proximal pulmonary arteries. (A) Grossly dilated vasa vasorum in the adventitial coat of the pulmonary artery not communicating as yet with the pulmonary artery lumen (PA). (Reproduced from Cudkowicz [146], by permission of *Thorax*.)

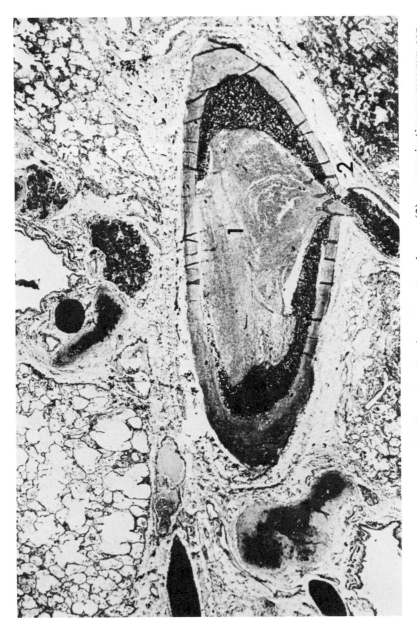

FIGURE 31   Bronchiectasis. (1) Thrombosed pulmonary artery lumen; (2) communicating vas vasorum conveys bismuth granules into patent part of pulmonary artery lumen (×100). (Reproduced from Cudkowicz [146], by permission of the *British Journal of Tuberculosis and Diseases of the Chest*.)

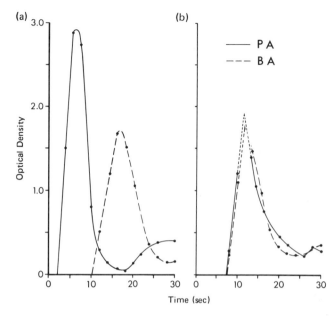

FIGURE 32 Dye dilution curves from pulmonary artery (PA) and brachial artery (BA) in (a) a normal patient; (b) a patient with severe left bronchiectasis. The appearance time and height of the curves are identical, indicating that the catheter in the pulmonary artery sampled arterial blood.

Severe intimal proliferation and atheroma of the walls of the proximal artery trunks (Fig. 31) were conspicuous.

The left ventricular output increases in patients with bilateral bronchiectasis. Figure 32 compares simultaneous right and left cardiac output curves obtained (1) from a normal patient and (2) from a patient with bronchiectasis [150].

Apart from augmenting left ventricular output, peripheral bronchopulmonary precapillary anastomoses of the type shown in Figure 29 direct flow both toward the pulmonary capillaries and, in view of systemic arteriolar pressure, toward the hilus of the main pulmonary artery. In unilateral bronchiectasis, the main pulmonary artery pressure is usually normal, and a pressure gradient therefore exists between the communicating bronchial arterioles and the pulmonary artery branch. Retrograde flow from the peripheral anastomotic site toward the right heart is not uncommon and accounts for pulmonary arterial filling defects noted sometimes during pulmonary arteriography [131] and lung scanning with macroaggregates labeled with ^{131}I in the presence of patent pulmonary arteries [133]. The high-pressure bronchial flow within these pulmonary artery branches flushes the contrast medium, or the isotope, away from the periphery and back toward the hilus (Fig. 32b), thus producing an erroneous pattern of blocked pulmonary lobar branches [150]. Unilateral bronchopulmonary precapillary anastomoses do not by themselves lead to an increase in mean pulmonary artery pressure. However, in our experience, extensive *bilateral* bronchopulmonary anastomoses, associated with bronchiectasis in particular, are usually incompatible with a normal pulmonary artery pressure. Patients with this disease frequently have mild to moderate pulmonary hypertension [151].

During cardiac catheterization of the branches of the pulmonary artery to bronchiectatic lobes, the finding of arterialized blood in an unwedged catheter position, in the presence of a normal pulmonary arterial pressure contour and without evidence of a patent ductus arteriosus, constitutes evidence of widespread precapillary bronchopulmonary anastomoses. Other investigators have found evidence of arterialized blood in branches of the pulmonary artery at surgery for bronchiectasis [152,153].

VII. The Bronchial Circulation in Pulmonary Infarction

There is a remarkable similarity between the pulmonary vascular abnormalities seen in bronchiectasis and pulmonary infarction. The similarity stems from the common denominator, namely, obstruction or occlusion of a branch of the pulmonary artery. Virchow [15] is usually credited with the observation that experimental ligation of a pulmonary artery failed to induce necrosis of the lung as long as the bronchial circulation was intact. In addition, he demonstrated that the bronchial arteries became enlarged and sustained the nutrition of the lung. Karsner and Ghoreyeb [154] concurred, and stated that pulmonary artery occlusion alone would not induce pulmonary infarction. The behavior of the bronchial circulation in this situation was elucidated by Schlaepfer [155] and Bloomer et al. [57], while Holman and Mathes [156] and Ellis et al. [157] studied the response of the bronchial circulation following experimental embolization.

Pulmonary infarction in experimental pulmonary embolization requires additional manipulations. These, according to Karsner and Ash [29], were as follows: "emboli will cause infarction even without tying the bronchial arteries if pulmonary veins are tied, or lungs are compressed from without." The lungs were compressed by an oleothorax. Such manipulations produce the requisite vascular stasis favorable for the development of experimental infarction.

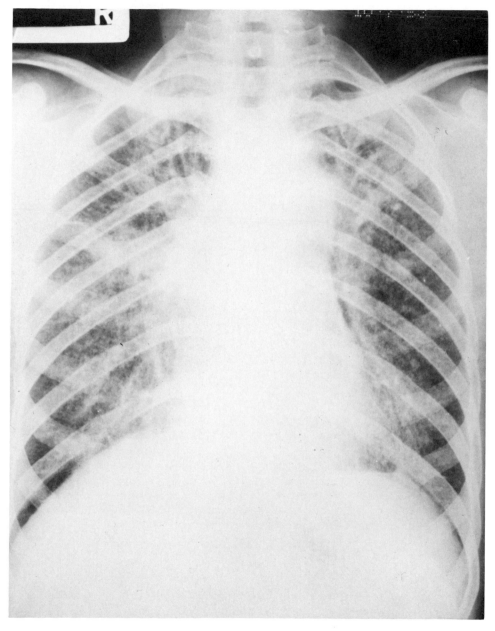

FIGURE 33   Mitral stenosis and pulmonary hypertension. Right midzone shows atelectatic shadow compatible with pulmonary infarction. Lung fields show pulmonary hemosiderosis.

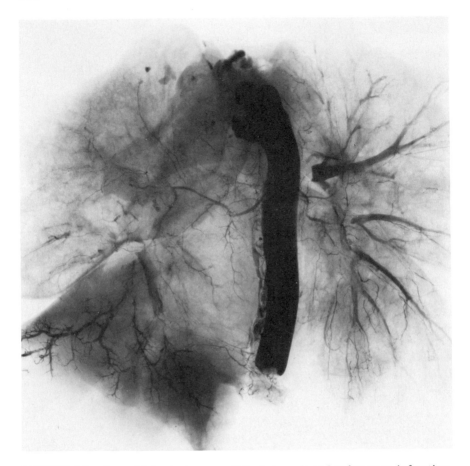

FIGURE 34   Bronchial arteriogram. Mitral stenosis and pulmonary infarction. Right lower pulmonary artery was occluded, and its peripheral bed is outlined by communicating bronchial arteries. The left lower lobe pulmonary artery was also occluded, and filling of the patent pulmonary artery took place retrogradely through precapillary bronchopulmonary anastomoses. (Reproduced from Cudkowicz [146], by permission of the *British Journal of Tuberculosis and Diseases of the Chest.*)

Holman and Mathes [156] induced necrosis in lobes by simultaneous occlusions of a pulmonary artery and corresponding bronchus. The atelectasis thus induced favored infarction. Septic emboli had the same effect.

Clinical observations indicate that pulmonary infarction in pulmonary embolic disease is the exception rather than the rule. Contemporary judgment places the overall incidence as less than 10% in pulmonary embolic episodes

[158]. Hampton and Castleman [159] examined 360 cases in the preantibiotic era, and found that 40% of pulmonary infarction occurred postoperatively, 30% in patients with heart disease and 30% in patients with diseases other than those of the heart. Gray [160] concurs and states that

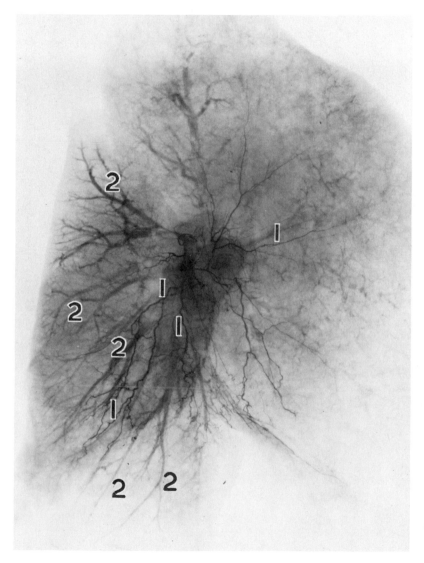

FIGURE 35 Mitral stenosis and right lower lobe pulmonary infarction. Right lateral view of bronchial arteriogram (1) showing retrograde filling of peripheral pulmonary artery bed of right lower lobe (2).

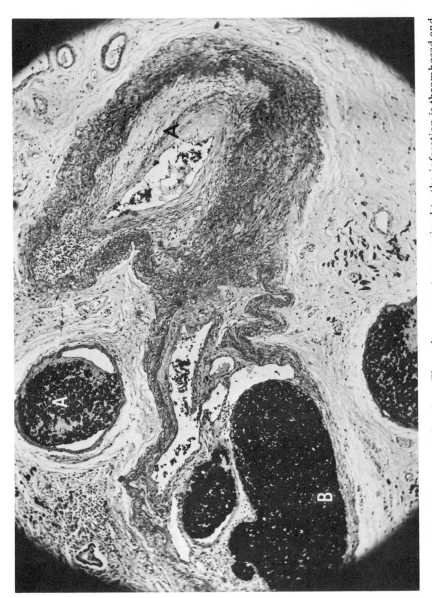

FIGURE 36   Pulmonary infarction.   The pulmonary artery proximal to the infarction is thrombosed and shows large, bismuth-filled bronchial arteries proliferating in the adventitia.   Some bismuth granules are visible in the remaining lumen of the pulmonary artery.   A = thrombosed pulmonary artery; B = proliferated bronchial artery.   ×70.

" . . . predisposing conditions appear to be of critical importance in clinical infarction. One can conclude from the available experimental and clinical data that infarction rarely follows pulmonary embolism except [in the presence of] . . . congestive heart failure, pulmonary vasculitis, blood dyscrasia (especially sickling), neoplasm, great debility, the gravid or puerperal state."

In heart disease without failure, the incidence of pulmonary infarction was found to be 33%, whereas in patients with congestive failure and low cardiac output states the incidence reached 90%. In malignancy, 47% of patients with embolism also had infarction [160].

Studies of three patients with mitral disease, pulmonary hypertension, and repeated pulmonary infarctions with frequent hemoptysis coincident with the embolic episodes are summarized.

For example, patient I had repeated distressing episodes of hemoptysis, and in spite of energetic therapy succumbed following an episode of pulmonary edema and ventricular fibrillation.

The radiography of the lungs at autopsy and after injection of the bronchial arteries showed evidence of infarction, and revealed bronchopulmonary anastomoses with retrograde filling of the distal branches of the pulmonary arteries in the infarcted areas. Figure 33 shows the chest X-ray and Figure 34 reveals occlusion of the proximal trunk of the pulmonary artery to the right lower lobe. The distal branches were patent and became heavily injected through the bronchial arteries. The left pulmonary artery tree was also outlined by widespread bronchopulmonary anastomosis. The histology of the infarcted lobes showed extravasation of red cells into the alveoli and thrombosis of the larger pulmonary arteries. The thrombosed pulmonary artery lumina were everywhere partly recanalized by the injected vasa vasorum (Figs. 35 and 36). They were dilated and conveyed the injected medium into the recanalized channels in the pulmonary arteries. At the periphery the pulmonary artery lumina were patent and filled with the injection mass which had entered them by communicating vasa vasorum. No other type of bronchopulmonary anastomosis was seen in these lungs.

It would appear that failure of the pulmonary arteries to regain patency after ordinary lobar pneumonia or following pulmonary embolization initiates dilatation and proliferation of the vasa vasorum into the lumina of the pulmonary arteries, establishing the bronchopulmonary anastomoses seen in bronchiectasis. With the diversion of the bronchial circulation from the peripheral bronchi and its other lung structures, occlusive changes in the peripheral bronchial arteries, for instance in those which supply the visceral pleura, small bronchi, and interlobular septae, can be demonstrated (Fig. 37).

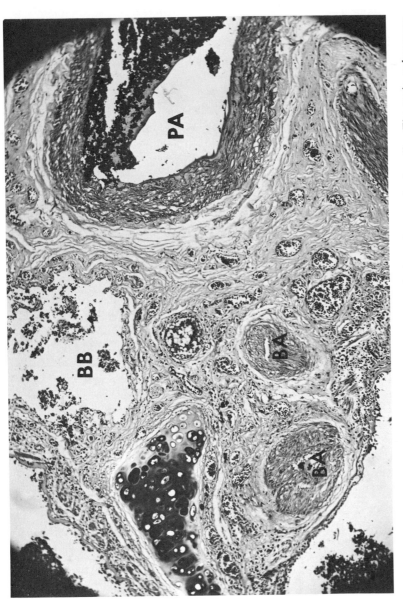

FIGURE 37   Pulmonary infarction. Section of right main bronchovascular bundle. The main pulmonary artery (PA) is patent and has become filled with bismuth by retrograde peripheral filling through broncho-pulmonary precapillary anastomoses. The bronchial arteries (BA) in their normal distribution in the wall of the adjoining bronchus (BB) are almost totally closed, suggesting diversion of bronchial arterial blood flow away from structures normally supplied by them and into the pulmonary artery bed (PA). ×75.

VIII. The Bronchial Circulation in Pulmonary Emphysema

Occlusive lesions in the pulmonary arteries of emphysematous lungs, recognized for some time, vary from an obliterative arteritis to patches of atheroma. Loeschcke [161] referred to the loss of pulmonary capillaries as the cause of the pallor of emphysematous lungs, and contended that *Kapillarschwund* preceded the development of the lung lesions. This was corroborated by Reid and Heard [101] with an India ink technique. Brenner [162], however, stressed that increasing degrees of arteriosclerosis occurred in the lungs of patients over 40 years of age irrespective of pulmonary disease, a contention challenged by Dunnill [163].

Although lesions affecting the pulmonary arteries in pulmonary emphysema have been studied, the pathology of the bronchial arteries in this disease is more obscure. In our investigations, lesions in the bronchial arteries could be demonstrated [164].

Histologic study indicates that, besides supplying arterial blood to the bronchi and bronchioles, the bronchial arteries are solely responsible for the blood supply of all intrapulmonary lymphatic structures (Fig. 19), the pulmonary nerve fibers (Fig. 21), the walls of the pulmonary arteries (vasa vasorum; Fig. 20), and to some extent the elastic framework supporting the alveoli (Fig. 25). The connective tissues supporting the air sacs derive their own bronchial arterioles from the interlobular septa (Fig. 24). From these septa, arterioles of at least 100 μm in diameter reach the alveolar supporting tissue via fibrovascular bundles which join the walls of the air sacs at right angles to the alveolar ducts. Thus, bronchial arterioles appear as muscular arterioles near the alveolar walls, where they can be distinguished only by injection methods from pulmonary arterioles of similar caliber. This suggests, therefore, that the elastic supporting framework of the alveoli possesses an arterial blood supply which is independent of the pulmonary arteries and their capillary bed.

A. Bronchial Arteriograms in Pulmonary Emphysema [164]

The changes in the bronchial arteries which were observed in 13 patients with centrilobular and 5 with panacinar emphysema can be grouped as follows.

Narrowing or Obliteration of Intrapulmonary Branches of Bronchial Arteries

A reduction in normal caliber was seen radiographically in 14 cases, and it appeared to affect the vessels already in their extrapulmonary course. On their entry into the lungs the vessels frequently failed to form an annulus around

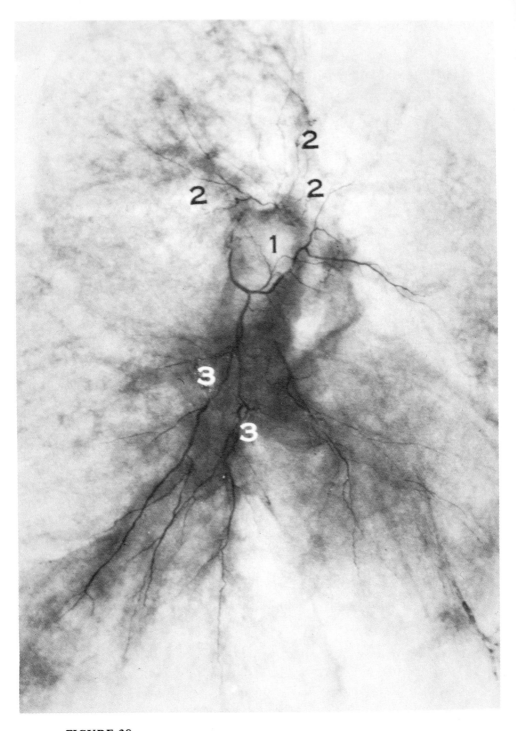

FIGURE 38

the main bronchi, and their caliber was further reduced as they spread out into the lungs (see Figs. 38 and 39). In 13 cases the bronchial arteries, following the bronchial divisions, ceased to be outlined by the contrast medium
about 5 cm beyond the lung hili, and failed to reach the periphery of the
lungs. A characteristic "pigtail" pattern of the bronchial arteries in the proximity of the hili indicated some tortuosity proximal to the occlusion of the
arterial lumina (see Fig. 39). In one case, the intrapulmonary distribution of
the bronchial arteries appeared to be normal, but their caliber was conspicuously reduced.

Serial sections of the bronchial arteries in their extra- and intrapulmonary distribution revealed progressive reduction in the lumina primarily as the
result of medial hyperplasia and intimal proliferation of varying severity (Figs.
40 and 41). This process of vascular narrowing, which led to actual occlusion
in 17 cases, extended to all branches in their distribution to the various lung
structures, and appeared to be most severe in the arterioles at the periphery
of the lungs. Medial hypertrophy often predominated in the peripheral arteries, and intimal thickening appeared to be more common in the more
proximal branches. In 16 cases with dense pleural adhesions, no extension of
the visceral pleural arteries into the adhesions could be demonstrated. The
rich pleural vascularity, which was encountered in few cases, was the result of
extension of the *parietal* pleural arterioles and their capillaries through the
adhesions to the underlying ischemic visceral pleura. The latter vessels revascularized the obliterated visceral pleural arteries. In most instances, however, the adhesions were fibrous and avascular, and in three cases no adhesions
were present in spite of the total obliteration of the visceral pleural arteries.

Anastomoses Between Bronchial and Pulmonary Arteries
with an Obliterated Peripheral Bronchial Arterial Circulation

In four instances there was radiological evidence of precapillary anastomosis in
one lung lobe between pulmonary arteries and abnormally distributed and enlarged bronchial arteries. Serial sections taken from these lobes showed on

---

FIGURE 38   *Centrilobular emphysema.* Lateral view of right bronchial arteriogram. Moderate emphysema of right upper lobe. The bronchial arteriogram
shows highly characteristic changes of emphysema. (1) Incomplete annulus
formation; (2) "pigtailing" of right upper lobe bronchial arteries quite close to
annulus with poor extension into right upper lobe; (3) normal bronchial arteries
to right lower lobe.

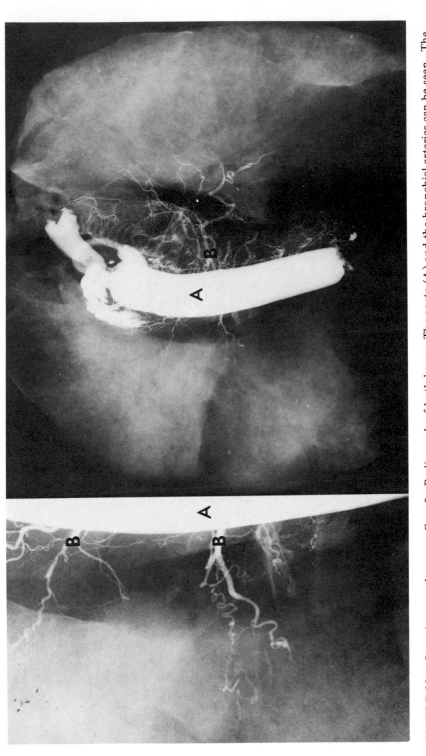

FIGURE 39 *Panacinar emphysema.* Case 8. Radiograph of both lungs. The aorta (A) and the bronchial arteries can be seen. The bronchial arteries (B) fail to penetrate beyond the hili. The appearance of "pigtailing" is well marked. No extension of the bronchial arteries into the lungs beyond the hili took place. Thus, lesions in bronchial arteries are near main bronchi (B). (Reproduced from Cudkowicz and Armstrong [164], by permission of *Thorax*.)

histologic examination that the pulmonary artery branches were occluded by organized thrombi and intimal thickening, and that the enlarged vasa vasorum in their adventitiae communicated with new channels within the thrombosed pulmonary artery lumina. The communications appeared to be more common at the periphery. Nearer the hilus, the lumina of the pulmonary arteries were reduced by the same change.

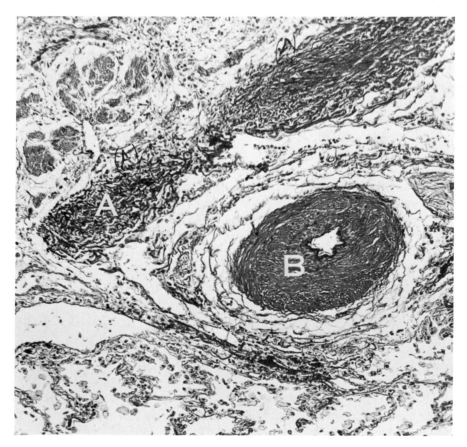

FIGURE 40   Case 2 (R.U.L., emphysema). Photomicrograph of right upper lobe bronchus: (A) cartilage of fibrosed bronchus, (B) large bronchial artery in tunica fibrosa, lumen almost totally occluded by medial hyperplasia and intimal proliferation (X135).

B.   Bronchial Arterial Lesions
in the Panacinar Type of Emphysema

The lungs at necropsy were bulky, but no bullae were seen. Adhesions were absent. The heart, weighing 335 g, was normal in size and showed no enlargement of the ventricular muscles.

After the injection of the bronchial arteries, the visceral pleural branches failed to fill. The radiographs of the injected lungs showed two fairly large bronchial arteries entering the hili and their sudden termination within 3 cm of their course along the major bronchi. The center and periphery of the lungs were devoid of bronchial arteries (Fig. 39).

Serial sections of the main bronchovascular bundles revealed dilatation of the bronchial arteries on entry into the lungs, and their subsequent occlusion within the walls of the major bronchi. The change in this case was primarily a proliferation of the intimal coat with replacement of the media by fibrosis (Fig. 41). The medium-sized bronchi showed thickening of the mucosa, degeneration of the glandular structures, fibrosis of the cartilage, and distorted, obliterated bronchial arteries in their walls. The same type of change was evident in the grossly thinned visceral pleura, which was not involved by adhesions. The visceral pleural arteries showed no recanalization. The alveolar walls appeared to be very much thickened and fibrosed in the center of the lungs; at the periphery they were thinner and collapsed. Universal occlusion of the bronchial arterioles was seen in the fibrosed structures in the lungs normally supplied by them.

C.   Correlation of Bronchial Artery Lesions
with Other Pathologic Findings

The sites of total loss of bronchial circulation corresponded with the areas in the lung where structural changes were most severe. This avascularity was particularly arresting in the fibrosed interlobular septa, visceral pleura, and smaller bronchi. The peripheral alveoli in more than half the cases showed rupture and collapse with attenuation of their epithelium. The bronchial vessels in their vicinity were occluded.

All 18 cases showed variable degrees of fibrosis of the visceral pleura, with replacement of the elastic fibers by fibrous tissue. Scarring was particu-

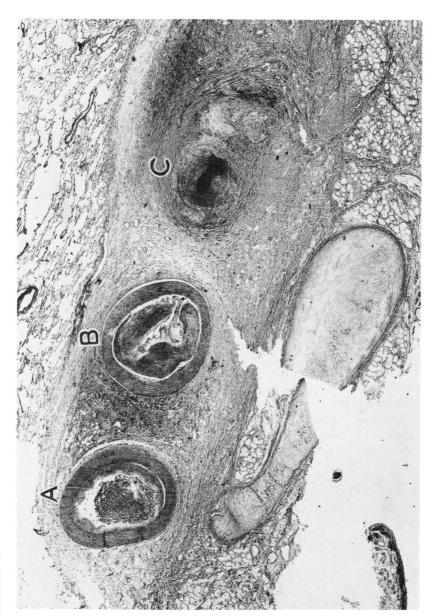

FIGURE 41 Case 8. Photomicrograph of the wall of the right main bronchus. A tortuous bronchial artery (A, B, and C) appeared three times in this section and showed progressive occlusion of its lumen by intimal proliferation. The intima and media became fully replaced by fibrosis. Hematoxylin and eosin stain (×10). (Reproduced from Cudkowicz and Armstrong [164], by permission of *Thorax*.)

larly evident in the subserous layers. In 15 instances the pleural sacs were almost totally obliterated by dense adhesions, which in all but two cases were avascular.

D. Origins of Occlusive Lesions in the Bronchial Arteries

One possible origin of these has been discussed. In most cases, however, there were no bilateral bronchopulmonary anastomoses, and the occlusive lesions must be otherwise accounted for. No satisfactory explanation for this is available. Brenner [162] described increasing degrees of arteriosclerosis in the lungs of patients over 40. Chronic sepsis as a cause of the obliteration of the bronchial arteries, and of the atrophic lesions in the periphery of the lungs and bronchi, is not very satisfactory in view of the great proliferation of the bronchial arteries uniformly seen in chronic fibrocaseous tuberculosis and acute lung infections [165,166].

It should be stressed once again that the obliterative changes, as well as the pigtailing seen more proximally in the bronchial arteriograms, occur in extrapulmonary bronchial arteries. Figure 39 shows failure of hilar annulus formation of the extrapulmonary bronchial arteries around the main bronchi. Within the emphysematous lung the distribution varies from almost normal to complete obliteration. It is exceedingly difficult to accept these occlusive changes as secondary to the distention of the lungs or high positive pressure upon the bronchial arterial vasculature. The bronchial arterial pressure far exceeds the pressures generated in the thorax even during coughing, and they are securely anchored within the adventitial coats of the main bronchi. The evidence points to a major systemic vascular change proximal to the entry of the bronchial arteries into the parenchyma of emphysematous lungs, and further experimental observations are needed.

E. Effects of Occlusive Lesions of the Bronchial Arteries

The anatomical changes seen in the lungs of the cases in this study were very variable, and lung sizes ranged from normal to true bullous emphysema. More constant was the loss of elastic tissue and the fibrosis in the interlobular septa, visceral pleura, and smaller bronchi. In nine of the cases, the pulmonary lesions predominated at the periphery; this corresponded to the occlusion of the peripheral bronchial circulation. In the remaining cases, the pulmonary changes were uniformly severe throughout both lungs and were associated with almost total occlusion of the intrapulmonary branches of the bronchial arteries. The most mobile structures of the lung, normally very rich in elastic fibers, appeared to be bereft of their arterial blood supply, and the changes seen in them could be compatible with ischemic fibrosis seen elsewhere.

IX. The Bronchial Circulation in Pulmonary Tuberculosis

A. The Vascular Pathology of Pulmonary Tuberculosis

Abnormalities of the lung vasculature in pulmonary tuberculosis derive from the original observations by Rasmussen of aneurysmal dilatations of pulmonary arteries [167]. Hemoptyses, so common in this disease, were regarded as stemming from these aneurysms. Opinion early this century differed regarding the pathology and identity of the vessels in lungs affected by pulmonary tuberculosis. Whereas Kaufmann [168] emphasized obliterative changes in the pulmonary arteries, Calmette [169] regarded the formation of small, pedunculated, pear-shaped "aneurysms of Rasmussen" in branches of the pulmonary artery which traverse the walls of tuberculous cavities as the major anomaly. Kayne et al. [170] found that younger tubercles, and even older foci, contain blood vessels. They contended that the cells participating in the formation of the tubercle are generally derived from elements of connective tissue "which have an inherent tendency to vessel formation." Thus, young tuberculous tissue is rich in capillaries and older foci are vascularized at the periphery. There is no evidence whatever that pulmonary arterioles can proliferate.

Coryllos [171] speculated on the possible clinical significance of endarteritis in the pulmonary arteries and thought this was beneficial in controlling the activity of tubercle bacilli. He considered that collapse therapy accomplished the same purpose by reducing the pulmonary artery bed. The oxygen requirements of the tubercle bacillus would thus be curtailed. Cournand and Richards [172] also attributed the benefits of collapse therapy to the reduction of oxygen and blood available to tubercle bacilli. Rich [173] presumed that the exacting oxygen requirements of the tubercle bacillus limit its multiplication in vivo and particularly within tuberculous lesions. Dubos [174] emphasized that the tubercle bacillus does not possess a glycolytic mechanism and derives its energy wholly from aerobic metabolism.

Schlaepfer [155] conjectured that ligation of a pulmonary artery in unilateral tuberculosis might delay the evolution of the tuberculous lesions, but subsequent studies [175] in the monkey showed that ligation of the pulmonary artery led to the opposite effect; namely, extensive caseous lesions contrasted with the scattered miliary lesions found in the opposite, untreated lung. The process of caseation was related to high oxygen tensions in the blood, reaching the ligated side presumably through the bronchial circulation. This accords with the observations made earlier in the nineteenth century by Guillot [176], who noted gross enlargement of the bronchial circulation in the region of the tuberculous lesion. Steinberg et al. [177] carried out angiocardiography in therapeutically collapsed lungs and noted delay in pulmonary blood flow, with crowding and obliteration of the pulmonary arteries near tuberculous areas.

It seems that the changes in the vasculature of tuberculous lungs most frequently found were lesions in the pulmonary arteries, and these appear to be mainly endarteritis or aneurysmal dilatations of the branches in contact with cavity walls [178]. Although some authors [168-179] implied that the obliterative changes in the pulmonary arteries provide an important safeguard against the occurrence of hemorrhage, the compensatory proliferation of the bronchial arteries would vitiate such a protective mechanism.

Karsner and Ash [29], during their investigations of experimental pulmonary embolization, had shown that reduction in blood flow through the pulmonary artery and reduction in pulmonary artery pressure to zero led to compensatory dilatation of the bronchial arterial bed with considerable augmentation of blood flow through that system. Calmette [169] had already considered the possibility that the aneurysmal dilatations of the vessels in the walls of tuberculous cavities could be in bronchial arterioles. Wood and Miller [180] showed that dilated bronchial arteries were present in the walls of tuberculous cavities, and that Wright [181] postulated that proliferation of pulmonary connective tissue, however caused, was accompanied by the development of new vessels derived principally from the bronchial arteries.

B.   Radiographic Studies
of Autopsied Tuberculous Lungs [178]

The most uniform feature observed in tuberculous lungs was the distortion, tortuosity, and remarkable proliferation of the bronchial arteries to frankly caseating areas. The radiograph from such a case is shown in Figure 42. An extensive plexiform network of new arteries of considerable diameter reaches the left upper lobe and bears no resemblance to the normal bronchial arterial pattern. In some vessels the caliber appears to increase towards the periphery, and one very large artery terminates in the wall of the apical cavity. Figure 43 shows similar proliferative changes in the bronchial arteries

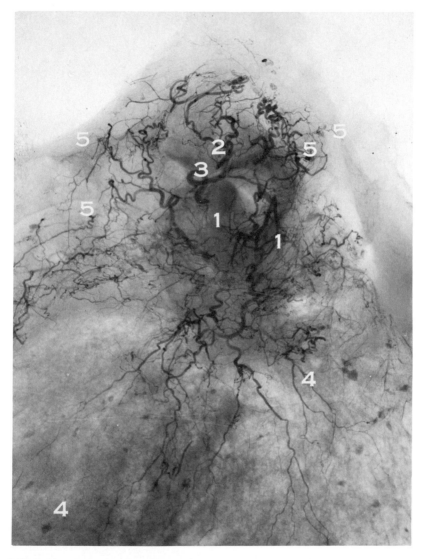

FIGURE 42   Lateral radiograph of left lung. Hilus faces X-ray tube. (1) Extensive vascularity of left upper lobe; (2) cavity; (3) termination of large bronchial artery in wall of cavity; (4) miliary tubercles; (5) thickened pleura. One-third normal size. (Reproduced from Cudkowicz [178], by permission of *Thorax.*)

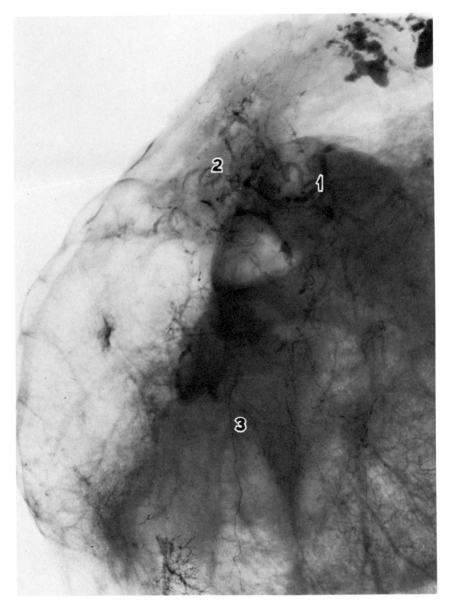

FIGURE 43   Lateral radiograph of right lung (right apical tuberculous cavitation and nontuberculous terminal bronchopneumonia). (1) Enlarged and
tortuous bronchial arteries; (2) cavity; (3) normal-sized bronchial arteries in unaffected areas. Two-thirds normal size. (Reproduced from Cudkowicz [178],
by permission of *Thorax*.)

near tuberculous lung foci in another patient. Figure 44 shows the considerable enlargement and tortuosity of the apical pleural artery in a patient in whom the tuberculous lesion was confined to the left apex.

C. Histology

Very striking histologically was the gross degree of obliteration of pulmonary artery radicles in areas of fibrocaseous tuberculosis. The lumina were occluded by intimal proliferation and thrombosis. In the branches proximal to the lesion some recanalization of the lumina had taken place by proliferation of the vasa vasorum. These arterioles are derived from the bronchial arteries, and

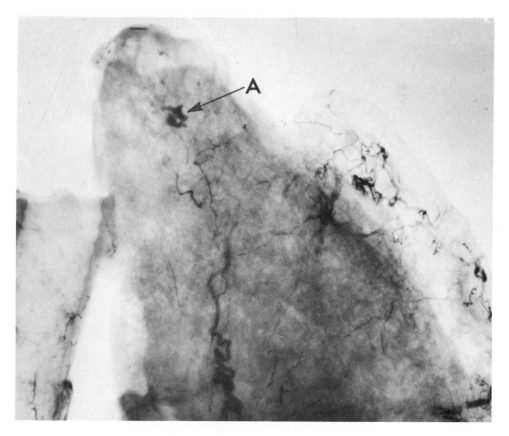

FIGURE 44   Left apical pleural branch (A) near left apical tuberculous lesion (note tortuosity). (Reproduced from Cudkowicz [178], by permission of *Thorax.*)

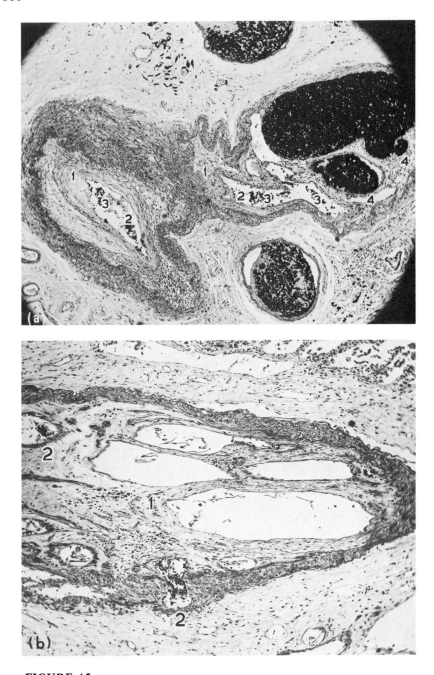

FIGURE 45

therefore conveyed the injection mass to the new lumina in the revascularized pulmonary artery branches (see Fig. 45a,b).

Associated with the presence of adhesions between the pleural surfaces were obliterative lesions in the visceral pleural arteries. The walls of these bronchial artery branches showed massive medial hyperplasia and intimal proliferation. Their occluded lumina were, however, opened up again by capillaries from the parietal pleural arteries which entered them via the adhesions (see Fig. 46).

In contrast to the endarteritic changes in pulmonary arteries and visceral pleural arteries was the dilatation of the bronchial arteries in the tuberculous areas. In many of the sections studied, the alveoli were distorted and replaced by fibrous tissue, and scarcely resembled lung tissue. The bronchi, on the other hand, often appeared quite normal, apart from the very large bronchial arteries in their coats. In the intervening connective tissue and in the interlobular septa the caliber of the bronchial arteries was very large and tended to increase even more as the vessels approached the areas of caseation. Bronchial arteries were largest in the walls of cavities, but their muscle coats appeared to be very much thinned. This conveyed the impression of dilatation of capillaries. It is possible that these dilated bronchial arterioles have in the past been considered to be aneurysmal dilatations of the pulmonary arterioles. The pulmonary arteries near caseating areas were thrombosed in these cases, and certainly appeared to have no part to play in the circulation of these lung sites (see Fig. 47a). No injected arterioles were present in the tubercles themselves, but the bronchial arterioles in their immediate neighborhood were dilated and patent (see Fig. 47b).

Thrombosis of the pulmonary artery and compensatory enlargement of the bronchial arteries accords with the postulate of Karsner and Ash [29], who had shown that this phenomenon depends on the fall in pressure in the pulmonary artery. It is also tempting to accept the teleological view of Wright [181] concerning the cause of the proliferation of the bronchial arteries. He suggested that collagen proliferation in the lungs, irrespective of the cause, demands a profuse arterial blood supply.

FIGURE 45   (a) Photomicrograph of a thrombosed pulmonary artery branch near a caseous lung focus. (1) Pulmonary artery; (2) recanalization of pulmonary artery lumen; (3) bismuth granules; (4) proliferating vasa vasorum (derived from bronchial arteries and therefore bismuth filled). ×50. (Reproduced from Cudkowicz [178], by permission of *Thorax.*), (b) Photomicrograph of a pulmonary artery some distance from tuberculous lesion showing (1) thrombosed lumen of pulmonary artery; (2) dilatation of vasa vasorum containing bismuth granules and recanalizing lumen of pulmonary artery. (Reproduced from Cudkowicz, L., *Thorax,* 8(1):46 (1953), by permission of the journal.)

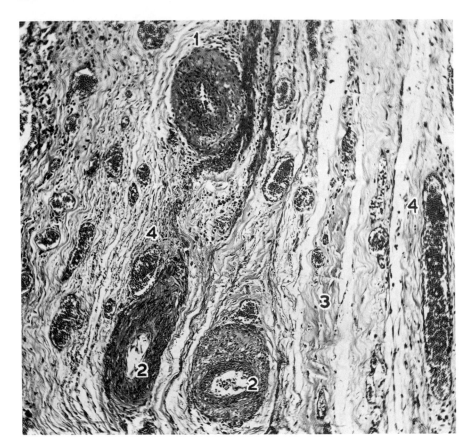

FIGURE 46   Photomicrograph of visceral pleural arteries showing (1) medial hyperplasia; (2) intimal proliferation; (3) adhesion between pleural surfaces; (4) extension of parietal capillaries into visceral pleura (X90). (Reproduced from Cudkowicz [178], by permission of *Thorax*.)

FIGURE 47   (a) Photomicrograph from edge of a tuberculous cavity (1) cavity wall; (2) bronchial mucosa; (3) occluded pulmonary artery; (4) bronchial arteries; (5) very dilated bronchial arteriole (X19). (Reproduced from Cudkowicz [178], by permission of *Thorax*.) (b) Patient 1. Photomicrograph of a miliary tubercle showing (1) dilated bronchial arteriole containing bismuth in its lumen, and situated near the tubercle; (2) giant cell (X75). (Reproduced from Cudkowicz [178], by permission of *Thorax*.)

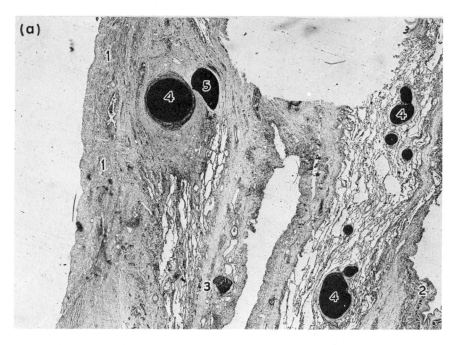

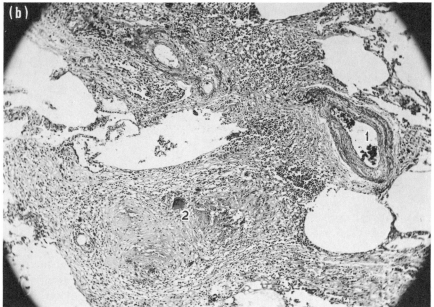

FIGURE 47

The presence of extensive arterial capillaries in the adhesions between the pleural surfaces, and the tendency of these capillaries to recanalize the obliterated pleural arteries, indicate that a profuse quantity of arterial blood is present in the neighborhood of tuberculous foci in the periphery of such lungs [178,182].

The patency of the bronchial arteries near miliary foci and their proliferation in fibrocaseous lungs should allow good concentrations of antituberculous drugs to reach the tuberculous areas. Furthermore, surgical measures to combat hemoptysis are unlikely to be successful if they are concentrated upon the pulmonary arteries alone.

Vascular abnormalities in pulmonary tuberculosis are thus common. In cases of bilateral disease, in which resectional therapy is contemplated, the question of postoperative adequacy of the remaining pulmonary vascular bed clearly arises. Cardiac catheterization is obviously necessary to allow direct measurement of pulmonary artery pressure at rest and with effort, since an abnormally high pulmonary vascular resistance under these conditions constitutes an absolute contraindication to surgery [183].

X. The Bronchial Circulation in Lung Tumors

Postmortem radiographic evidence exists of proliferation of the bronchial arteries in primary neoplasms. This systemic vascularization is responsible for the frequency of hemoptyses associated with primary bronchial carcinoma. Metastatic lung tumors do not show this pattern, a possible explanation for the absence of hemoptyses in secondary lung tumors.

By the postmortem injection technique, the bronchial arteries were studied both radiographically and histologically in cases of pulmonary neoplasms.

A. Primary Bronchial Carcinoma Radiographic Patterns [184]

A male patient, aged 61, was clinically believed to have a carcinoma of the right upper lobe bronchus, and in the radiograph a large shadow was visible in the region of the right upper lobe. The fingers and toes were clubbed. At necropsy a large secondary growth was noted in the posterior half of the right sixth rib, which had broken through the parietal pleura. The lung itself was not involved, but pressure by the tumor displaced the right upper lobe anteromedially. A mass approximately 4 X 3 cm was palpable in the right middle lobe.

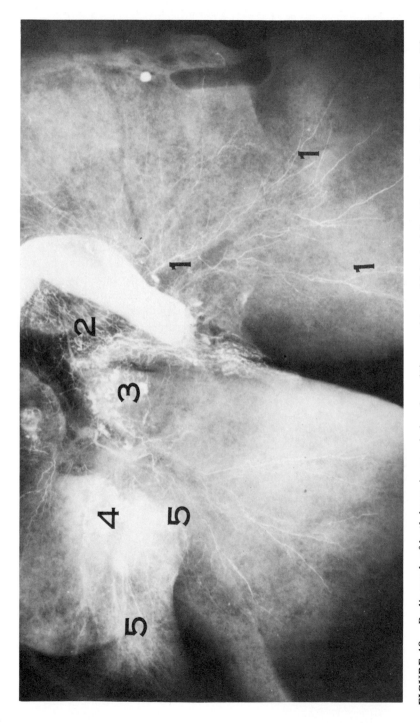

FIGURE 48 Radiograph of both lungs in case 1 showing: (1) normal bronchial arterial pattern to the left lung; (2) proliferation of the bronchial arteries to the right middle lobe with distortion of the normal pattern; (3) extravasation of the injection mass into lymph nodes at right hilus; (4) extravasation of injection mass into tumor; (5) anastomotic filling of peripheral pulmonary arteries. About one-third normal size. (Reproduced from Cudkowicz and Armstrong [184], by permission of *Thorax*.)

The radiographic appearances of the injected bronchial arteries are shown in Figure 48. A normal pattern was seen in the left lung. A dense arterial network extended from the right side of the descending aorta, and coursed to the right hilus. There, a number of lymph nodes received a profuse blood supply. The remaining irregularly spaced arteries continued to form a mesh of vessels around the tumor mass in the right middle lobe. The tumor mass itself was outlined by extravasated injection material within its substance. Anastomotic filling of the pulmonary arterioles distal to the tumor had taken place. The distribution of the bronchial arteries to the right upper and lower lobe was normal. A right bronchogram showed that the tumor arose from the medial bronchus of the right middle lobe near its inception.

Histologic examination showed secondary deposits in the pretracheal and subcarinal lymph nodes. The cells were of the "oat cell" variety. Large arterioles, filled with injection medium, were visible in the stroma and capsule of the involved lymph nodes. Large bronchial arteries were visible in the wall of the affected bronchus proximal to the tumor. At the edge of the tumor these vessels branched out and continued along strands of collagenous tissue into the tumor substance. Within the tumor itself large vascular lacunae, lined by a fine endothelium and filled with injection mass, were visible. The accompanying pulmonary artery branch showed extensive infiltration of its wall by tumor cells and occlusion of its lumen by thrombosis.

The clinical diagnosis in another male patient aged 53, before his death, was primary carcinoma of the right upper lobe bronchus, with multiple cerebral metastases. Necropsy confirmed the site of the tumor and the cerebral lesions. Radiography of the injected lungs showed good filling of the bronchial arteries, which were normal in their distribution to the left lung. Pretracheal and subcarinal lymph nodes were outlined by the injection medium. A large number of bronchial vessels entered the right upper lobe. In the radiographs two white patches indicated tumor masses in the apical and posterior segments. The pattern of the bronchial arteries in the anterior segment and in the right middle and lower lobes was normal. At the periphery of the right upper lobe, distal to the tumor masses, anastomotic filling of the pulmonary arteries was evident (Fig. 49). The histology disclosed a squamous-cell type of carcinoma in the right upper main bronchus just distal to the origin of the anterosuperior bronchial division.

FIGURE 49   Lateral radiograph of right lung of patient 2. (1) Tumor masses in apical and posterior segments of upper lobe; (2) proliferating bronchial arteries; (3) anastomotic filling of peripheral pulmonary arteries. Right hilus faces X-ray tube. One-fourth normal size.

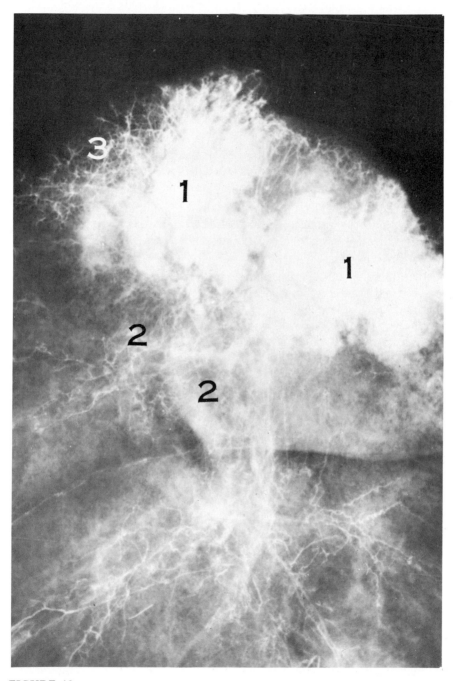

FIGURE 49

A third male patient, aged 62, had a tumor in the left upper lobe bronchus and widespread skeletal metastases. At necropsy the left upper lobe was densely adherent to the parietal pleura and a tumor was palpable in the apical segment. Radiography of the injected left lung showed considerable enlargement of the bronchial arteries running toward the tumor and extravasation of the injection medium into its substance (Fig. 50). Histology showed changes very similar to those in the previous case. The pulmonary arteries in this case were not affected, and no anastomotic filling was present.

An 85-year-old woman died from carcinoma of the stomach which had led to a fatal hemorrhage from an erosion of the lower thoracic aorta. The liver was studded with many secondary deposits, and a very large mass was palpable in the lower lobe of the right lung.

The radiographic studies of the injected lungs showed a very dense mass in most of the right lower lobe, but the bronchial artery pattern throughout both lungs was *normal*.

The histology of the mass in the right lower lobe showed a diffuse aggregate of anaplastic cells, suspended between collagenous fibrils. The pulmonary arteries in that lobe appeared to be very dilated, but were not injected. Small bronchial arteries were visible in the walls of the bronchi, and no extension of these to the tumor was seen.

Thus, primary bronchial carcinomata receive a profuse blood supply from the bronchial arteries. The pulmonary arteries accompanying the involved bronchi may be thrombosed. The contention that hemoptyses come from the bronchial arteries is well supported in view of the large- and thin-walled lacunae in the tumor substance which can be seen to be in continuity with enlarged bronchial arteries. This expanded bronchial circulation may also be of therapeutic value for the treatment of primary malignancy if it could be used for the administration of cytotoxic drugs.

On the other hand, metastatic lung tumors appear to derive their blood supply from the pulmonary arterial circulation. This difference in blood supply accounts for the infrequent association of hemoptysis with metastatic pulmonary lesions [185,186].

FIGURE 50   Anteroposterior radiograph of left lung in case 4. (1) Very large bronchial arteries; (2) tumor in apical segment of left upper lobe, showing extravasation of injection material. One-third normal size. (Reproduced from Cudkowicz and Armstrong [184], by permission of *Thorax*.)

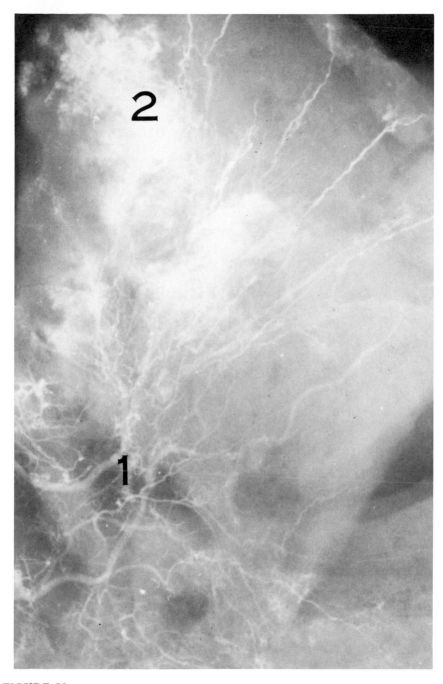

FIGURE 50

Bronchial arterial blood thus streams into the substance of a rapidly proliferating tumor. The venous drainage from these tumors is obscure, but the major proportion of blood probably returns by the pulmonary veins to the left atrium. If the oxygen extraction by neoplastic tissue is significant, a reduction in arterial PO_2 and oxygen content may be expected.

B.   Preoperative Direct Bronchial Arteriography in Patients with Lung Tumors

Recently, several studies have been published concerning aortography in lung tumors [187]. Following the aortography, Clifton and Mahajan [188] injected

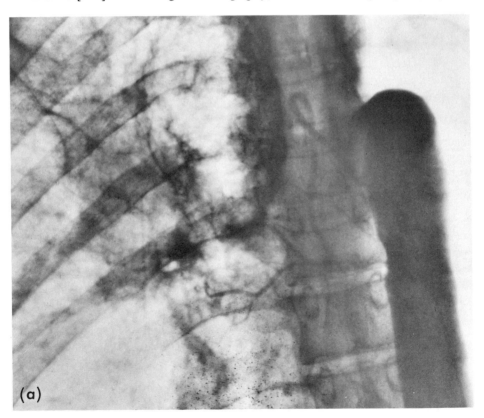

(a)

FIGURE 51   (a) Aortogram in a case of squamous cell carcinoma of the right upper lobe. (b) Same after subtraction. The bronchial artery is a branch of the first aortic intercostal artery. In the tumor region (T), several dilated small vessels are seen. (Reproduced from Groen et al. [193], by permission of *Diseases of the Chest.*)

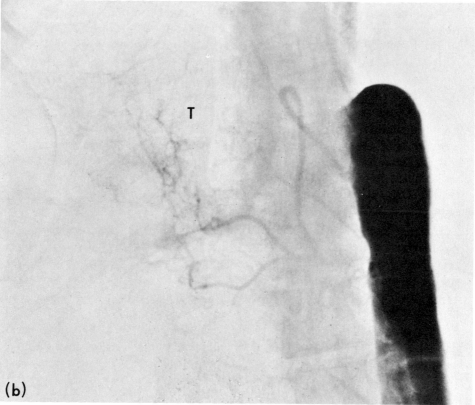

(b)

FIGURE 51b

cytotoxic drugs at the origin of the bronchial arteries with a catheter with two balloons which occluded the aorta at the levels of T.4 to T.8.

Selective bronchial arteriograms by direct catheterization have been carried out by Viamonte et al. [189] and Schober [190]. While the ostia of the bronchial arteries can be fairly easily found and entered with a suitable catheter, arteriograms are often of poor quality. With the application of the subtraction technique by des Plantes [191] and Vogelaar [192], bronchial arteriograms can be obtained in life which are nearly as clear as those derived from autopsy specimens (Fig. 51) [193].

XI. The Bronchial Circulation in the Collagen Diseases Affecting the Lungs

The unity of vascular pathology is evident in as wide a variety of clinically dissimilar conditions as disseminated lupus erythematosus, polyarteritis nodosa, dermatomyositis, scleroderma, temporal arteritis, and the rheumatic diseases [194]. The basic vascular lesion is regarded as a result of fibrinoid degeneration of the ground substance of the arterial wall leading to progressive occlusion or to aneurysmal dilatation of the vessel wall, with secondary cellular infiltration and ischemic fibrosis of the dependent structures of organs.

"Rheumatic pneumonias" have been recognized in relation to rheumatic fever [195]. von Glahn and Pappenheimer [196] found arteritis in 20% of rheumatic fever lungs, with concentric thickening of vessels and revascularization of the intima. Changes resembling those seen in rheumatic "pneumonia" were produced experimentally by Rich and Gregory [197], who considered that anaphylactic angiitis affected the pulmonary capillaries. The characteristic histologic features of the cutaneous rheumatoid nodule were established by Collins [198], and lesions of the same type were subsequently recognized in serous membranes such as visceral pleurae [199-201].

Apart from the development of rheumatoid nodules on the visceral pleura, areas of fibrinoid necrosis are thought to occur in the collagen structures of the lung parenchyma in some patients with rheumatoid disease, giving rise to the interstitial changes first reported by Ellman and Ball [202]. Caplan [203] drew attention to the increased incidence of rheumatoid disease in patients with pneumoconiosis.

Sinclair and Cruikshank [204], in an important autopsy study, compared the incidence of lung disease in 90 patients suffering from rheumatoid arthritis with 90 nonrheumatoid patients and noted that pleural lesions were twice as frequent in the former group. Similar observations were made subsequently [205].

With the recognition of the essentially systemic distribution of rheumatoid lesions by Ellman and Ball [202], evidence has gradually accumulated in favor of two distinct types of lung involvement: the formation of necrobiotic nodules on the visceral pleura and adjacent lung, which vary from 3 mm to 7 cm in diameter [206]; and the interstitial parenchymatous lesions. These lesions are not necessarily associated with pleural effusions. Horler and Thompson [207] found pleural effusions in nine patients in a series of 180 rheumatoid arthritics. Of these patients, eight were men, and all were over 40 years old.

It is not clear from the literature that a relationship exists between the development of joint swellings, parenchymatous lung disease, or the development of crops of nodules over the extremities. In the example [205] shown in Figure 52, widespread nodules preceded the pleural effusions.

The vascular changes which have been described in the lungs in all these diseases is of interest, in that the vessels involved still need to be properly identified. Matsui [208], Bevans [209], and Church and Ellis [210] believed

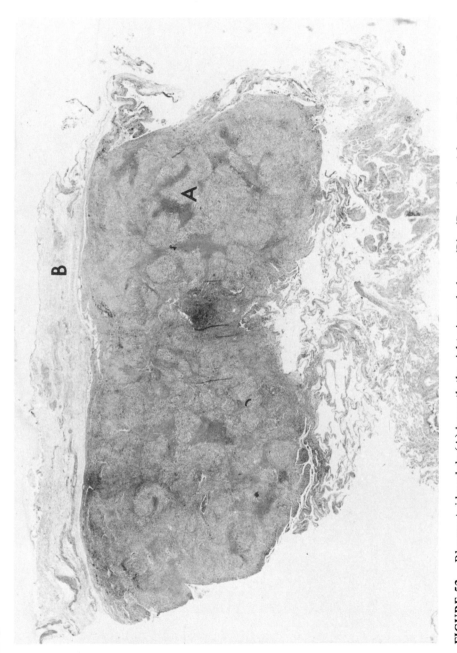

FIGURE 52 Rheumatoid nodule (A) beneath the right visceral pleura (B). (Reproduced from Cudkowicz et al. [205], by permission of the *British Journal of Diseases of the Chest.*)

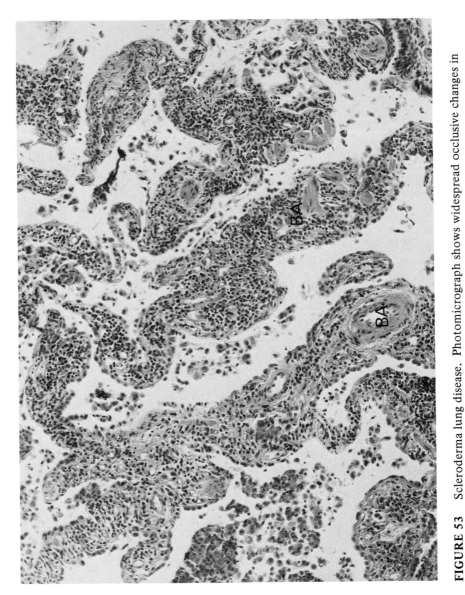

FIGURE 53   Scleroderma lung disease.   Photomicrograph shows widespread occlusive changes in peripheral bronchial arterioles (BA).   (X210).

that the vascular changes in scleroderma were in the pulmonary artery. In the same disease, Kraus [211] referred only to intimal proliferation in "small arteries" near the alveolar septa. Goetz [212] spoke of "vascular" narrowing. von Glahn and Pappenheimer [196] observed concentric thickening of "vessels" and revascularization of the intima in rheumatic pneumonias. It appears, therefore, that the identity of these vessels is by no means clear. In ordinary lung sections it is nearly impossible to distinguish between bronchial or pulmonary arterioles, unless one of these circulations has been previously injected with a contrast medium too coarse to traverse the capillary beds.

The pulmonary lesions of the systemic collagen diseases appear to be confined to the pleura, the interlobular septa and the alveolar supporting tissues, the smaller bronchi and peribronchial tissues, and to the walls of the pulmonary artery. This suggests that the wide, diffuse changes seen throughout both lung fields are in the exclusive territory of the bronchial arteries and that the lesions recorded by Bevans [209] in the walls of small bronchi do affect the bronchial arteries. Total occlusion of the bronchial arteries would deprive the lungs and the visceral pleura of their only arterial blood supply, at least until such time as it takes for pleural adhesions to form and to convey new parietal pleural arteries into the occluded bronchial artery bed. The lung lesions in these diseases, because of their characteristic pathologic localization, suggest involvement of the bronchial circulation in its widest distribution. As this circulation is responsible for the nutrition of all lung structures except the respiratory epithelium of the alveolar capillaries, it is reasonable to suppose that the variable degrees of pulmonary sclerosis, seen particularly in scleroderma, may be related to deprivation of the only arterial blood supply available to the supporting structures of the lungs (Fig. 53).

XII. The Bronchial Circulation in Pulmonary Hypertension

A compensatory enlargement of the bronchial arteries in the presence of pulmonary artery agenesis is well documented [56,61], and high bronchial arterial blood flows have been measured in Fallot's tetralogy [53,54]. The bronchial collateral blood flow is assumed to supplement the total pulmonary blood flow by proximal connections with the pulmonary arterial tree. Details of this mechanism have been discussed previously. These communicating bronchial arterioles behave like myriad small patent ducti in relation to their corresponding pulmonary arteries, permitting arterial blood to reach the pulmonary capillaries. They antedate the possible subsequent development of intrapulmonary vascular lesions in pulmonary hypertension of the six grades outlined by Heath and Edwards [213].

Goodwin [214] has demonstrated complete injection of the intrapulmonary pulmonary artery bed in the aorta in the presence of proximal pulmonary artery trunk maldevelopment (Fig. 54). Little information is available in this type of anomaly concerning the actual pressures within the distal pulmonary artery bed, catheter entry being barred by the main pulmonary artery trunk anomaly. Under experimental conditions, the pressure in a pulmonary artery branch distal to a permanent snare occlusion was found to be about the same as that proximal to the occlusion. The pressure contour distal to the occlusion, as well as blood oxygen content, were arterial in type [215]. The flows in Fallot's tetralogy attributable to the bronchial circulation seldom reach magnitudes in excess of 30% of left ventricular cardiac output, and in the example described the total flows are unlikely to exceed this value.

The demonstration of precapillary bronchopulmonary anastomoses in situations associated with a reduced or absent main pulmonary artery blood flow poses the question of the effect of persistence of such anastomoses in the presence of a normal or increased pulmonary blood flow. Evidence has been provided that in disorders such as pulmonary infarction, bronchiectasis, and lobar pneumonia, occlusive changes in the lumen of the pulmonary arterial tree usually precede the formation of such anastomoses.

Severe pulmonary hypertensive vascular disease leading to obliterative dilatation changes in the peripheral pulmonary arteries favors the development of precapillary bronchopulmonary anastomoses of a type similar to those which have already been discussed in connection with obstructive lesions in the peripheral pulmonary bed. Liebow has raised an important point concerning the angiomatoid lesions in grade IV pulmonary hypertensive vascular disease [216]. If they "are in truth new sprouts, so to speak, of pre-existing pulmonary arteries it is the first instance where pulmonary arteries have been shown to act as collaterals for occluded pulmonary arteries." Liebow then proceeded to show angiomatoid lesions associated with bronchial arterial precapillary connections in a patient with a common ventricle. Thus, the question of the identity of the vascular malformations in severe pulmonary hypertensive vascular disease remains to be resolved.

The effect of extensive bronchopulmonary precapillary anastomoses on pulmonary vascular resistance is uncertain. They are not comparable in their effect to an influx of arterial blood into the left main pulmonary artery from an uncomplicated patent ductus arteriosus. Occlusive disease in the peripheral arterial branches of the pulmonary artery is germane to their genesis. In addition to their widespread distribution, they favor retrograde flow from the periphery to the main trunks of the pulmonary artery. Such a retrograde flow is demonstrable by lung scans [133], angiography [131], selective catheterization of the branches of the pulmonary artery [151], and the shape and appearance time of a dye curve resembling that from the brachial artery,

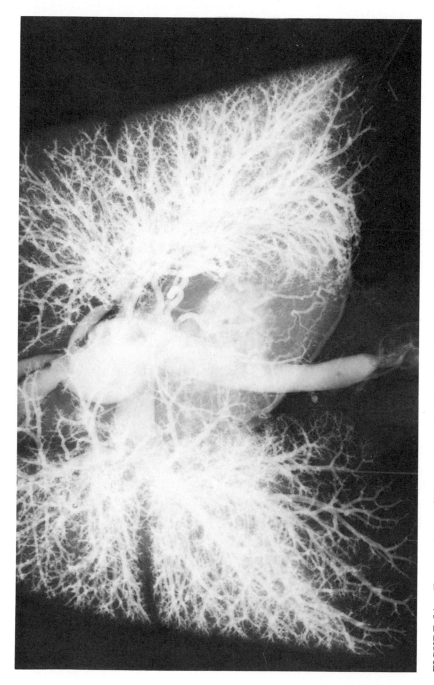

FIGURE 54 Transposition of the great vessels. Large bronchial arteries course to the left lung and completely fill the total left pulmonary artery from an aortic injection. There is no "pruning" of the distal pulmonary artery tree.

but obtained through a cardiac catheter located in the bronchial arterial stream within the left main pulmonary artery. Although such retrograde flow implies a reversed gradient of pressure from the periphery to the main pulmonary arterial trunks, the mean pulmonary artery and right ventricular pressures, particularly in unilateral disease, are unaltered. According to Spain [217], the most extensive development of bronchopulmonary precapillary anastomoses affect bronchiectatic lungs, yet pulmonary hypertension in bronchiectasis is rare.

Pulmonary hypertension is difficult to produce experimentally unless two-thirds of the pulmonary artery bed is extirpated [218]. Lesions similar to grade III pulmonary hypertensive vascular disease can be induced by experimental embolization [219] and the formation of a direct systemic to pulmonary artery anastomosis [220]. A more dramatic development of pulmonary hypertension attends the ligation of a pulmonary artery in puppies and calves soon after birth [221]. Here, presumably, the fetal type of muscular pulmonary arteries maintains its increased tone in the presence of the augmented pulmonary blood flow through the remaining patent pulmonary artery.

A. Pulmonary Hypertension in Acquired Lung Disease

In the absence of fluid retention or obvious cardiac failure, the pulmonary artery pressure of patients with even severe emphysema is virtually normal at rest, and the development of pulmonary hypertension is unpredictable [222]. The fact that pulmonary hypertension is readily reversible in patients with improvement in overall ventilation indicates that structural changes alone are unlikely to account for the pulmonary hypertension. Changes within the pulmonary arteries proximal to the capillary bed in patients with gross emphysema are seldom very striking, and seem to be restricted to the vessels close to the bronchioles [223].

There is considerable evidence that exercise in emphysematous patients leads to an increase in pulmonary artery pressure [224], as does high altitude. Overall and regional alveolar hypoventilation [225], increased arterial CO_2 tension [226], and a lowered pH of mixed venous blood [227] contribute to pulmonary hypertension. Correction of the alveolar hypoxia by instituting pure oxygen breathing does not fully correct the increase in pulmonary vascular resistance.

Although regional hypoventilation probably plays a part in the establishment of pulmonary hypertension in lung disease, other factors need to be considered. Of interest is the effect of precapillary bronchopulmonary anastomosis on pulmonary artery pressure. Unilateral anastomoses are not associated with elevations in pulmonary artery pressure. In patients with bilateral bronchiectasis and finger clubbing, where there is the widespread evidence of such anastomoses, pulmonary hypertension is frequent and independent of overall alveolar hypoventilation [228]. The relationship between the elevation in pulmonary arterial pressure and an increase in bronchial arterial blood flow remains to be elucidated.

Left ventricular enlargement [229], as well as an expansion of the bronchial circulation [230], have been observed in idiopathic pulmonary hypertension. Left ventricular hypertrophy is unlikely to be attributable to an expanded bronchial arterial flow, inasmuch as it seldom reaches levels comparable to the flow through a patent ductus. Multiple thromboses of pulmonary arteries and complex new vascular formations occur in idiopathic pulmonary hypertension which must be the consequence of the disease [213]. Bronchopulmonary anastomoses probably stem from these occlusive changes rather than exist de novo, and thus complicate pulmonary hemodynamics. Their precise effect on pulmonary artery pressure, if bilateral and extensive, is still uncertain, although earlier experimental observations [231] gave good evidence that changes in bronchial arterial blood pressure of the denervated lung produced variations in pulmonary vascular resistance. This resistance was attributed to redistribution of blood between the pulmonary and bronchial vascular systems, possibly secondary to a Venturi-like effect in the regions of anastomoses.

XIII.   Clinical Aspects of the Bronchial Circulation

To this point, we have explored the bronchial circulation in the normal lung as well as in certain cardiopulmonary diseases. Deviant patterns from the normal can be recognized both in life and at autopsy. It remains to ascribe clinical significance to these patterns, that is, the provision of reasonable proof that the human lung has an absolute need for such a blood supply.

A.   The Nutrient Role of the Bronchial Circulation

It was shown that the bronchial circulation in the human is distributed to all structures of the lung with the possible exception of the actual air sacs. This vascular territory is normally quite distinct and exclusive. It comes in communication with the pulmonary vasculature in health through a part of its venous component beyond the main bronchi. Sites of capillary anastomosis are few and occur near the alveolar ducts [101] and are probably functionally insignificant in the human. Precapillary anastomoses between arterioles more

than 60 μm in diameter could not be demonstrated in normal human lungs.
The assumption will therefore be made that the bronchial arteries in the
normal human lung behave as end arteries, feeding their own extensive capillary bed principally within the bronchial tree, pulmonary lymph nodes, pulmonary arterial walls, pulmonary nerves and ganglia, interlobular septae, and
visceral pleura. The total normal bronchial arterial flow is small and amounts
to less than 2% of the left ventricular output, but this is well within the
average range of organ blood flow when expressed in milliliters per gram unit
of dry weight of lung. Because of this relatively small, total normal bronchial
arterial blood flow and the unreliability of existing techniques in the detection
of such small flows, it has not yet been feasible to estimate critical reductions
in normal bronchial arterial flow. An additional problem arises in the selection of the groups of disease which might come under scrutiny. One reason
for this stems from the common overlap of diseases which affect the lung.
Bronchiectasis, for example, which has its own specific bronchopulmonary
anastomotic pattern, can coexist with emphysema showing a totally different
bronchial arterial pathology. Measurements in life of bronchial arterial blood
flow in these patients often yield significantly high flows [152]. Such a
finding might at first sight invalidate the concept that lung disorders so combined could possibly be complicated by a compromised nutrient blood supply.
The methods available for the estimates of bronchial arterial blood flows fail
to distinguish between bronchial arterial flow components that either traverse
the pulmonary capillary bed through precapillary anastomoses with pulmonary
arteries or augment the left ventricular output through normal postcapillary
venous shunts. Of the bronchial venous component flowing through its
normal channels, two-thirds joins the pulmonary venous flow. Demonstration
of large bronchial arterial flows therefore provides no information whatever
concerning the integrity of the normal bronchial arterial territory. In the case
of precapillary bronchopulmonary anastomoses this territory could very well
have been totally bypassed. Evidence to the effect that the bronchial arteries
in their normal distribution show occlusive changes in the presence of large
bronchial arteries communicating in an aberrant manner with precapillary
bronchopulmonary anastomoses is best represented by bronchiectasis (Fig. 55).

Can lung disorders such as emphysema induce bronchial arterial blood
vessel changes, or might the deprivation of an adequate bronchial arterial
blood supply to the bronchial tree and its glandular and nerve structures contribute to the pathogenesis of the disease? Without reliable measurements of
bronchial arterial blood flows over a significant period of the natural history
of emphysema, a definite physiological answer in favor of ischemia cannot be
provided.

In emphysema, bronchial arteries were totally occluded within a few
centimeters of their entry into the lung hilus. The corresponding serial sections
showed that the arteries already at this level, and well outside the lung

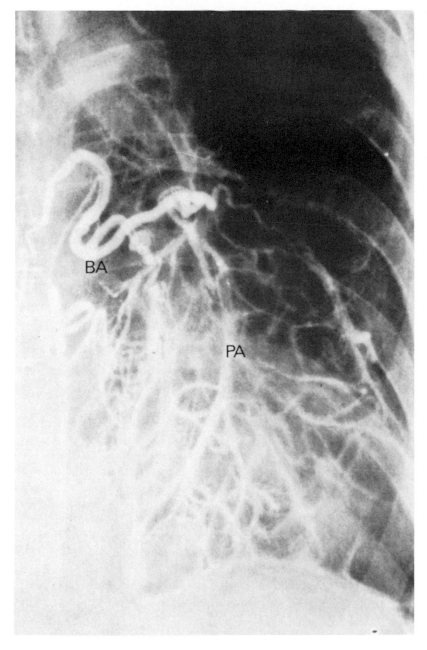

FIGURE 55 Selective bronchial arteriogram in left lower lobe segmental bronchiectasis. The very large left bronchial artery (BA) in bronchiectatic area communicates with the left lower lobe pulmonary artery (PA) through pre-capillary anastomoses and fills the left pulmonary artery tree retrogradely.

parenchyma, were obliterated by intimal proliferation. Patency of the bronchial vasculature beyond this point was absent. Such gross obliterative lesions are not the rule in emphysema, but variable reductions in caliber can usually be found. Enlargements of the true bronchial veins [232] have been found in emphysema. These drain into the azygous and hemiazygous systems of veins, and might enlarge if the pulmonary venous path for the remaining two-thirds of the total bronchial venous flow becomes blocked. The route for bronchial arterial flow from the aorta to the hilus is intact, and the extrapulmonary bronchial arteries show no reduction in caliber. The obliterative changes in the bronchial arteries beyond the hilus point to a diversion of the total bronchial arterial blood flow towards the trachea and main bronchi.

Proximal bronchial arterial occlusion constitutes a unique pattern in the lung diseases which have been studied to date. By contrast, patterns of diffuse bronchial arterial proliferation are the rule in tuberculosis and primary lung tumors. Gross increases in the size of the bronchial arteries occur with the formation of precapillary bronchopulmonary anastomoses. In the red stage of hepatization of lobar pneumonia and in the collagen diseases, the bronchial arteries show reductions in lumen size in the involved lung parenchyma and corresponding lobar or segmental bronchi. The occlusive bronchial arterial changes of pulmonary emphysema are widespread and are seen proximal to the lung parenchyma. It is difficult to conceive of the centrilobular or panacinar lobular dissolutions of emphysema producing effects on the bronchial arteries as remote as the main bronchi where the vessels are securely anchored in the scaffolding of the tunica propria.

Spain and Kaufman [233] considered the terminal bronchioles to be critically involved in emphysema, and this site has been incriminated by other observers in the pathogenesis of emphysema [234]. Wright [181] stressed that medium-sized bronchi often undergo dilatation in advanced emphysema. Atrophy of the cartilage and adventitial elastic tissue, as well as the loss of the lobular elastic fibers in the adjacent lung, render the bronchial wall unstable and permit it to collapse in early expiration. Wright [181] thought the bronchial atrophy resulted from either inflammatory or ischemic changes. Spencer and Loef [235] demonstrated that the nerve supply of the bronchial mucous glands in the human comes from the nerve plexus around the bronchial arteries. Descriptions of the changes in structure of the lung in emphysema therefore include the bronchial tree, particularly its bronchiolar component, where occlusive bronchial arterial changes are most extensive. The respiratory bronchioles are the structures which are supplied by the terminal arterioles of the bronchial arteries and which would be most vulnerable in occlusive disease of the more proximal bronchial arteries.

The nutrient role of the bronchial circulation becomes apparent in pulmonary embolism, which is rarely followed by pulmonary infarction.

Pulmonary infarction represents a very gross form of pulmonary "ischemia" and indicates absolute compromise of the nutritional blood supply to the involved lung [236]. The questions posed at the beginning of this section are concerned with specific structures such as the terminal bronchioles, the pulmonary nerves, the bronchial glandular epithelium, and smooth muscle, as well as the visceral pleura and the whole supporting framework of the lung lobule. Are these the structures most likely to suffer from a deprivation of their arterial blood supply, and, if so, which clinical manifestations depend on this combination of effects? If the peripheral structures of the lung are predictably the most vulnerable, it becomes a matter for conjecture as to which diseases should be specifically examined for ischemic effects. Spontaneous pneumothorax in the young, chronic bronchitis, and all forms of emphysema readily qualify for such scrutiny.

B. Sources of Hemoptyses

See Figure 56. Primary lung cancers have a rich bronchial arterial nutritional network, and the location of the tumor within a wall of a bronchus is favorable for development of brisk hemoptyses (see Fig. 56). In this context, hemoptyses can be attributed to leaks from the bronchial circulation into the bronchial tree. They also are of arterial origin in cavitating lung lesions and tuberculosis. In bronchiectasis, pneumonia, pulmonary infarction, and bronchial infection, *capillary* bleeding constitutes the main source. In mitral stenosis and pulmonary venous hypertension, hemoptyses derive from both capillary and bronchial venous sources. Retrograde flow from pulmonary veins into bronchial veins has been envisaged in mitral stenosis as a decompression mechanism dependent on a steep pressure gradient between the pulmonary and bronchial veins [237], rendering the valves in the pulmonary and azygous venous system incompetent. Distension and varicose dilatations of the bronchial venules have been described in mitral stenosis [238] and are thought to contribute to hemoptysis. A retrograde flow of pulmonary venous blood into the azygous system of veins would elevate the oxygen tension in azygous venous blood. Measurements in support of this concept are not available in mitral stenosis. It is perhaps relevant that a reverse of this occurs in portal hypertension, where on occasion mediastinal and periesophageal veins decompress into the pulmonary veins, reducing the systemic arterial oxygen content as a consequence of this venous admixture [239].

C. Pleural Adhesions

Pleural adhesions commonly form vascular bridges between the parietal and visceral pleurae, and are most frequently found in pulmonary tuberculosis.

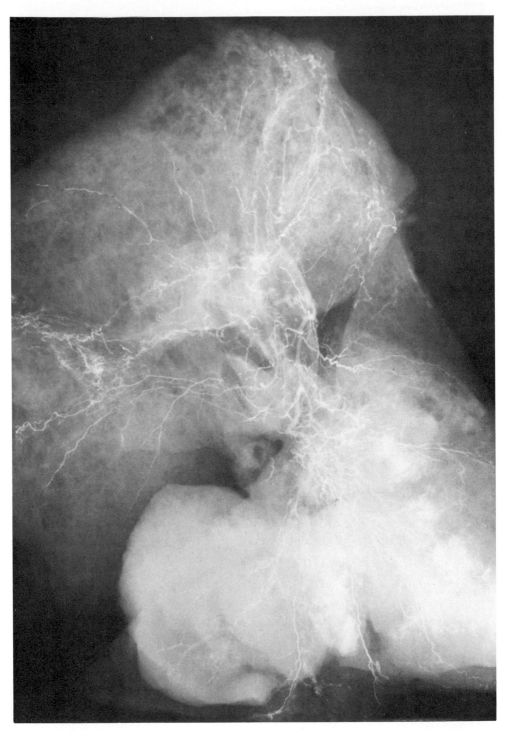

FIGURE 56   Primary lung cancer. Right lower lobe. Extensive bronchial arterial proliferation and hemoptysis.

Histologic serial sections of vascular adhesions from the parietal pleura to the lung reveal a network of fine vessels which communicate with the sparser bronchial arterial network in the visceral pleura. The vascularity is related to the inflammatory responses, which in the lung, as elsewhere, promote dilatation and proliferation of systemic arteries. The propensity of the parietal pleural arteries to augment the systemic arterial blood flow of the lung has led to the advocacy of surgical pleurodesis in pulmonary oligemia secondary to maldevelopment of the pulmonary artery trunk [240].

D. Precapillary Bronchopulmonary Anastomoses of Congenital Origin

Surgeons engaged in the correction of pulmonary stenosis, Fallot's tetralogy, or transposition of the great vessels by the open heart technique using cardiopulmonary bypass are aware of the need for venting the left atrium. Considerable quantities of blood from the aortic cannula return through precapillary bronchopulmonary anastomoses and the pulmonary veins to the left atrium. Stress has already been laid on the normally developed intrapulmonary artery bed in the presence of maldevelopments of the main pulmonary artery, particularly in Fallot's tetralogy. The intrapulmonary artery bed becomes virtually disconnected from the main trunk and functions as an alternative pathway to the pulmonary capillaries for blood flowing through precapillary bronchopulmonary anastomoses. Winship et al. [241], in a review of congenital absence and anomalous origin of the main pulmonary arteries, recommended that in addition to pulmonary angiography for the demonstration of the absent pulmonary artery, aortography should also be carried out in order to obtain adequate information of the systemic vascular connections to the affected lung.

Armed with this information, the surgeon can plan against excessive left atrial or left ventricular leakage, and make a more balanced, low-pressure functional restoration of the proximal disconnection of the pulmonary artery. This would clearly be preferable to the establishment of an additional systemic arterial anastomosis, which is ultimately calculated to compromise the intrapulmonary vasculature in a manner similar to a patent ductus.

Precapillary bronchopulmonary anastomoses in the presence of proximal pulmonary artery or valvular malformation, and probably also in regional pulmonary artery thrombosis or embolization, provide systemic arterial blood access to the alveolar capillaries for a second time. The oxygen uptake by this collateral pulmonary blood flow is low and due to its higher arterial oxygen content. This does not imply that such a lung is necessarily defective in respiratory function. If it shares adequately in overall alveolar ventilation it will participate in carbon dioxide elimination, and in the event of injury or infection of the contralateral normal lung, causing a fall in arterial oxygen content and a wider A-apO$_2$ gradient, the collateral pulmonary blood flow will accept more oxygen while traversing the pulmonary capillary bed. In this respect and through its carbon dioxide transport to the pulmonary capillaries, precapillary bronchopulmonary anastomotic flow serves a useful respiratory function.

E.   The Effects of Acquired Precapillary Bronchopulmonary Anastomoses

The striking increases in the bronchial arterial system in patients with bronchiectasis and pulmonary infarction have been noted. In both disorders the enlargement of the bronchial arteries was associated with obstructive lesions in the smaller pulmonary arteries and the formation of precapillary bronchopulmonary anastomoses. Flow through these anastomoses reach significant magnitudes after ligation of a pulmonary artery and in bilateral bronchiectasis (Fig. 57). The hemodynamic significance of these flows is still uncertain. The anastomotic channels appear to be the vasa vasorum of the pulmonary arteries, which have been shown to be richly endowed with nerve fibers and have been likened to high-resistance sphincteral vessels [235]. The evidence from studies in lobar pneumonia in the human indicates that they are relatively slow in opening up and require the period of the red and gray stages of hepatization before permitting bronchial arterial blood flow to enter the peripheral pulmonary arterial bed. Similarly, significant increases in bronchial arterial perfusion of an operated lung are not measurable until about 1 month after experimental ligation of a pulmonary artery [57,242,243].

The flows conducted through these channels in acquired lung diseases seldom exceed 25% of the left ventricular output and are usually much less. Such flows are not enough to burden the left ventricle, and striking left ventricular hypertrophy is not to be expected.

Retrograde bronchial arterial anastomotic flow towards the main pulmonary artery trunk may, on occasion, give rise to a false interpretation of a pulmonary angiogram if the contrast medium is injected proximal to the retrograde flow. Inasmuch as the contrast medium flushes mainly into the contralateral side, the appearance suggests lobar branch occlusion. This pitfall

---

FIGURE 57   Radiograph of left lower lobe bronchiectasis. The aorta (1) has been injected with a contrast medium which has entered two very large bronchial arteries (2). These convey the contrast medium through multiple precapillary anastomoses (4) into the peripheral pulmonary artery; because of its coarseness the injection medium could not enter the pulmonary capillaries but filled the whole left pulmonary artery tree (3) retrogradely. (Reproduced from Cudkowicz [127], by permission of *Medicina Thoracalis.*)

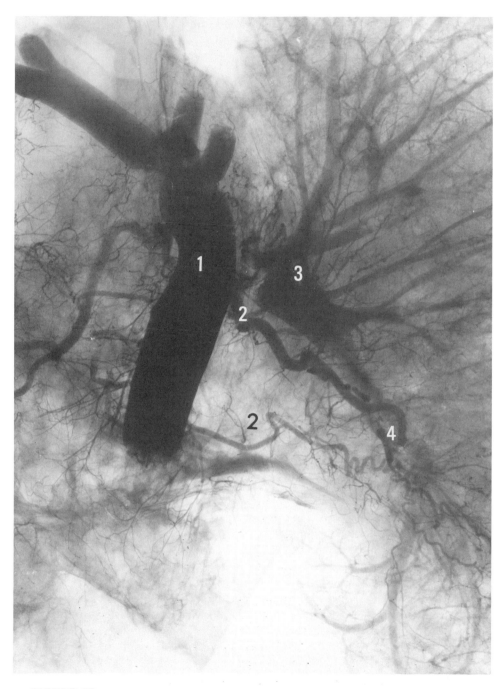

FIGURE 57

can be avoided by exploring the lobar branches of the pulmonary artery with the catheter tip and noting their patency, pressure profiles, and oxygen contents before angiography. The information to be gained from retrograde aortography is probably more valuable in these patients than that provided by pulmonary angiography alone.

Two additional problems associated with precapillary bronchopulmonary anastomoses must be mentioned because they are of considerable clinical interest. The first concerns the pathway of the bronchial anastomotic flow. The evidence in both congenital and acquired lung disease indicates that the anastomoses are effected by the vasa vasorum, which seem to be well equipped anatomically for that function and possess a rich nerve supply. In contrast with congenital bronchial arterial patterns, occlusive pulmonary arterial changes predispose to the anastomotic flow development in acquired cardiopulmonary disease. With the development of precapillary bronchopulmonary anastomoses, the bronchial feeding arteries become greatly enlarged near their origin from the aorta and then pursue an aberrant intrapulmonary course in order to link up with anastomotic channels. The normally distributed bronchial arteries within the bronchial tree in particular, fail, at least by histologic evidence, to share in the general enlargement and appear in fact to be almost occluded. This, then, suggests that the major bronchial arterial flow is an anastomotic flow which perfuses the distal pulmonary arterial bed and passes through the pulmonary capillaries into the pulmonary veins. The bronchial venous return from the major bronchi to the azygous system is then presumably also reduced, and there is no evidence to indicate that these veins are enlarged in bronchiectasis. This contrasts with observations in emphysema and mitral stenosis. With the establishment of right ventricular failure, it has been suggested that the increase in right atrial and central venous, and therefore in true bronchial venous pressure, induces a reversal of true bronchial venous flow as a result of incompetence of the bronchial venous valves. The magnitude of this reversed flow from the true bronchial veins is not known [244].

The second problem concerns clubbing of the digits, specifically, the relationship between clubbing and precapillary bronchopulmonary anastomoses. There is no obvious causal relationship between these two phenomena. Both coexist rather more frequently than any other common factor in cardiopulmonary disease. In diseases such as pulmonary tuberculosis and primary bronchial carcinoma, precapillary bronchopulmonary anastomoses are uncommon in spite of a well-developed and tortuous bronchial arterial network to the diseased lung areas. The incidence of clubbing in these two disorders has been estimated at less than 1% in tuberculosis [245,246] and at 2% in carcinoma of the lung with hypertrophic pulmonary osteoarthrophy [247-249].

According to Ginsburg [250], more recent studies show that clubbing correlated well with an increase in total bronchial arterial size and not specifically with the development of bronchopulmonary anastomoses. It is thought that the bronchial venous flow returning from the tuberculous or tumor areas and bypassing the pulmonary capillary bed could convey to the systemic circulation vasoactive substances which are normally inactivated in their passage through the pulmonary capillary bed. This concept presupposed that additional factors, other than a generalized expansion of the bronchial arterial network alone, are operative in clubbing of the digits.

Though clinical observation suggests that clubbing of the fingers is frequent in patients with arteriovenous aneurysms of the lung, subacute bacterial endocarditis, and cyanotic congenital heart lesions, the precise incidence of clubbing in these diseases still needs to be established. Hypertrophic osteoarthropathy is, however, extremely rare in congenital heart disease, and only three cases of periostitis were found in over 3000 patients with cyanotic congenital heart disease [251]. The many dissimilar diseases in which clubbing of the fingers or hypertrophic osteoarthropathy occur lack an obvious common denominator.

F. The Effects of Increased Postpulmonary Capillary Bronchial Arterial Blood Flows

An expansion in the bronchial circulation attends chronic pulmonary inflammatory disease such as tuberculosis and primary neoplasia. The new networks are extensive and are represented by Figure 58. The bronchial arteries in these diseases conform with similar systemic arterial patterns in response to inflammation and primary neoplasia elsewhere, and appear to subserve the metabolic needs of proliferating tissue. This reaction pattern seems to be an example of angiogenesis which does not compromise the bronchial circulation throughout its normal distribution. Total bronchial arterial blood flow increases in proportion to the subsequent rise of flow through the newly developed bed rather than as a result of an increased flow through preexisting normal channels. An excessively large flow through normal bronchial arterial channels beyond the metabolic needs of the normal lung structures would not be compatible with the widening in pA-aO_2 gradients found in tuberculosis and primary lung tumors. $\dot{Q}BF_{postcap}$ flows are not as large, however, as those found in bronchiectasis, and seldom exceed 10% of left ventricular output. This suggests that in spite of the extensive networks which can be demonstrated in these diseases, postcapillary bronchial flows are usually smaller than precapillary bronchopulmonary anastomotic flows which have a respiratory function to perform in pulmonary artery maldevelopment or occlusion. Postcapillary bronchial arterial flows sustain metabolic needs of diseased lung areas and do not appear to have significant effects on pulmonary hemodynamics, with the possible exception of a theoretical action on pulmonary venous tone.

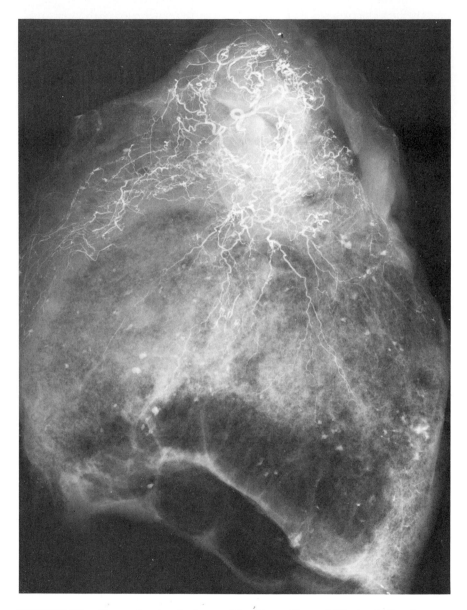

FIGURE 58   Example of exterior proliferation of bronchial circulation in tuberculosis showing increased postcapillary bronchial arterial blood flow ($\dot{Q}BF_{postcap}$).

The venous admixture from this source to the pulmonary venous flow would reduce pulmonary venous oxygen tension; a PO_2-sensitive chemoreceptor mechanism has been postulated in that vascular segment [252].

References

1. Erasistratus, cited by Claudius Galen (de affectorum locorum notita) Lib. V. cap. II (ca. 270 BC).
2. Galen, C., *Tractat. Frobeniane edit.*, Lib. 6 cap. 3., Basel (1562).
3. Galen, C. *De Venarum arterioramque dissectione*, 9. K II. 819 (ca. 180 AD).
4. Miller, W. S., *The Lung*, 2nd ed. Springfield, Ill., Thomas, 1947.
5. Columbus, R., *De Re Anatomica*. Lib. 15.2 cap. 2, 1559.
6. de Marchettis, D., *Anatomia patavii*, Padova (I. Padovii and M. Bolzetta, eds.), 1652.
7. Ruyisch, F., *Epistola anatomica*. Probl. Sexto., Amsterdam, 1732.
8. Reisseissen, F. D., and S. T. von Sömmering, *Über den Bau der Lungen*. Hecker, Berlin, 1808.
9. Cudkowicz, L., Leonardo Da Vinci and the bronchial circulation, *Br. J. Dis. Chest.*, **47**:23–26 (1953).
10. Catalogue, *Quincentenary Exhibition of Drawings by Leonardo da Vinci.* London, Royal Academy of Arts, p. 85 (1952).
11. Keele, K. D., *Leonardo da Vinci: Movement of the Heart and Blood*. London, Harvey and Blythe, 1952.
12. Guillot, N., *Arch. Gen. Med.* (Series 4) **7**(1):151–258 (1845).
13. Le Fort, L., *Recherches sur L'Anatomie du Poumon chez L'Homme* (thesis). Paris, 1858.
14. von Luschka, H., *Die Anatomie des Menschen*, Vol. I. H. Laupp, Tübingen, 1863.
15. Virchow, R., Über die Standpunkte in der wissenschaflichen Medizin, *Virchows Arch. [Pathol. Anat.]*, **1**:1–19 (1847).
16. Virchow, R., Gesammelte Abhandlungen zur Wissenschaftlichen Medizin, *Frankf. Med.*, **20**:385 (1856).
17. Rindfleisch, E., *Handbuch der Gewebelehre*, Engelmann, Leipzig, 5th ed. 1878.
18. Cohnheim, J., and M. Litten, Über die Folgen der Embolie der Lungen-arterien, *Virchows Arch. [Pathol. Anat.]*, **65**:99–115 (1875).
19. Küttner, C., Beitrag zur Kenntniss der Kreisslaufsverhältnisse der Säuge-thierlunge, *Virchows Arch. [Pathol. Anat.]*, **13**:476–523 (1878).
20. Zuckerkandl, E., Über die Anastomosen der Venaepulmonales mit den Venae Bronchiales, *Sitzungsberichte Akad. Wiss. Wien*, **3**(84):110–111 (1881).
21. Zuckerkandl, E., Verbindungen der arteriellen Gefässe der menschlichen Lunge, *Math. Nat. Klin. Sitzungsberichte Akad. Wiss. Wien. Abt.*, **2**(87): 171–174 (1883).
22. Berry, J. L., The relation between the bronchial and pulmonary circulations in the human lungs, *Q. J. Exp. Physiol.*, **24**:305–314 (1934).

23. Berry, J. L., J. F. Brailsford, and I. deB. Daly, The bronchial vascular system in the dog, *Proc. R. Soc. Lond. [Biol.]*, **109**:214–228 (1931).

24. Mathes, M. E., E. Holman, and F. L. Reichert, A study of the bronchial pulmonary and lymphatic circulation of the lung, *J. Thorac. Surg.*, **1**:339–362 (1932).

25. Berry, J. L., and I. deB. Daly, The relation between the pulmonary and bronchial vascular systems, *Proc. Soc. Lond. [Biol.]*, **109**:319–336 (1931).

26. Daly, I. deB., and U. S. von Euler, The functional activity of the vasomotor nerves to the lungs in the dog, *Proc. Soc. Med.*, **110**:92–111 (1931).

27. Daly, I. deB., The physiology of the bronchial vascular system, *Harvey Lect.*, **253**:235–255 (1935–1936).

28. Wearn, J. T., A. C. Ernstene, A. W. Bromer, J. S. Barr, W. J. German, and L. J. Zschiesche, The normal behavior of pulmonary blood vessels with observations on the intermittence of the flow of blood, *Am. J. Physiol.*, **109**:236–256 (1934).

29. Karsner, H. T., and J. E. Ash, Studies in infarction II. Experimental bland infarction of the lung, *J. Med. Res.*, **27**:205–224 (1912).

30. Daly, I. deB., Intrinsic mechanisms of the lung, *Q. J. Exp. Physiol.*, **43**:2–26 (1958).

31. Huntingdon, G. S., The morphology of the pulmonary artery in the mammalia, *Anat. Rec.*, **17**:165–202 (1919).

32. Taussig, H. B., *Congenital Malformations of the Heart*. New York, Commonwealth Foundation, 1947.

33. Pool, P. E., J. H. F. Vogel, and S. Y. Blount, Jr., Congenital unilateral absence of a pulmonary artery. A review, *Am. J. Cardiol.*, **10**:706–732 (1962).

34. Krahl, V. E., Anatomy of the mammalian lung. In *Handbook of Physiology*. Baltimore, Williams & Wilkins, 1962, pp. 213–284.

35. Allanby, K. D., W. D. Brinton, M. Campbell, and F. Gardner, Pulmonary atresia and the collateral circulation to the lungs, *Guy Hosp. Rep.*, **99**(2):110–152 (1950).

36. Manhoff, Jr., L. J., and J. S. Howe, Absence of the pulmonary artery. A new classification, *Arch. Pathol.*, **48**:155–170 (1949).

37. Jacobsen, H., cited by Christeller [40].

38. Peacock, T. B., *On Dual Formations of the Heart*. London, Churchill, 1858.

39. East, T., and W. G. Barnard, Pulmonary atresia and hypertrophy of the bronchial arteries, *Lancet*, **1**:834–837 (1938).

40. Christeller, E., Funktionelles und Anatomisches bei der angeborenen Verengerung der Lungenarterie, *Virchows Arch. [Pathol. Anat.]*, **223**:40–57 (1916).

41. Findlay, Jr., C. W., and H. C. Maier, Anomalies of the pulmonary vessels and their surgical significance, *Surgery*, **29**:604–641 (1951).

42. Jefferson, K., S. Rees, and J. Sommerville, Systemic arterial supply to the lungs in pulmonary atresia and its relation to pulmonary artery development, *Br. Heart J.*, **34**:418–427 (1972).

43. Dammann, Jr., J. F., and Ferencz, C., The significance of the pulmonary vascular bed in congenital heart disease III, *Amer. Heart J.*, 52:7–17 (1956).

44. McGoon, M. D., R. E. Fulton, G. D. Davis, D. G. Ritter, C. A. Neill, and R. White, Systemic collateral and pulmonary artery stenosis in patients with congenital pulmonary valve atresia and ventricular septal defect, *Circulation*, 56:473–479 (1977).

45. Rossall, R. E., and H. Thompson, Formation of new vascular channels in the lungs of a patient with secondary pulmonary hypertension, *J. Pathol. Bacteriol.*, 76:593–598 (1958).

46. Konn, G., Über eine Erkrankung der Sperrarterien und der arteriovenösen Anastomosen der Lunge, *Beitr. Pathol.*, 115:295–312 (1955).

47. Miller, M. K., and M. W. Lyon, Jr., Persistent truncus arteriosus, *Am. Heart J.*, 7:106–109 (1931).

48. Clarkson, P. M., J. M. Neutze, and J. C. Wardill, The pulmonary vascular bed in patients with complete transposition of the great arteries, *Circulation*, 42:131–142 (1976).

49. Robertson, B., Intrapulmonary arterial pattern in normal infancy and in transposition of the great arteries, *Acta Paediatr. Scand. [Suppl.]*, 184:1–33 (1968).

50. Aziz, K. W., M. H. Paul, and R. D. Rowe, Bronchopulmonary circulation in d-transposition of the great arteries: Possible role in genesis of accelerated pulmonary vascular disease, *Am. J. Cardiol.*, 39:432–438 (1977).

51. Campbell, M., and F. Gardner, Radiological features of enlarged bronchial arteries, *Br. Heart J.*, 12:183–200 (1950).

52. Cudkowicz, L., The localization and management of pulmonary hemorrhage. In *Critical Care Medicine*. Edited by W. Oaks. New York, Grune & Stratton, 1974, pp. 263–299.

53. Bing, R. J., L. D. Vandam, and F. D. Gray, Jr., Physiological studies in congenital heart disease II. Results of preoperative studies in patients with Fallot's tetralogy, *Bull. Johns Hopkins Hosp.*, 80:121–145 (1947).

54. Nakamura, T., R. Katori, K. Miyazawa, J. Oda, and K. Ishikawa, Measurements of bronchial arterial blood flow in tetralogy of Fallot, *Circulation*, 35:904–912 (1967).

55. Cudkowicz, L., W. H. Abelmann, G. E. Levinson, G. Katznelson, and R. M. Jreissaty, *Bronchial arterial blood flow in man, Clin. Sci.*, 19:1–21 (1960).

56. Fishman, A. P., G. M. Turino, M. Brandfonbrenner, and A. Himmelstein, The "effective" pulmonary collateral blood flow in man, *J. Clin. Invest.*, 37:1071–1086 (1958).

57. Bloomer, W. E., W. Harrison, G. E. Lindskog, and A. A. Liebow, Respiratory function and blood flow in the bronchial artery after ligation of the pulmonary artery, *Am. J. Physiol.*, 157:317–328 (1949).

58. Boyden, E. A., The time lag in the development of the bronchial arteries, *Anat. Rec.*, 166:611–614 (1970).

59. Edwards, J. E., and D. C. McGoon, Absence of anatomic origin from heart of pulmonary arterial supply, *Circulation*, 47:393–398 (1973).

60. Wagenvoort, C. A., D. Heath, and J. E. Edwards, eds. In *The Pathology of the Pulmonary Vasculature.* Congenital anomalies of the major pulmonary vessels. Springfield, Ill., Thomas, 1964, pp. 337–439.

61. Landrigan, P. L., I. E. Purkis, D. E. Roy, and L. Cudkowicz, Cardiorespiratory studies in a patient with an absent left pulmonary artery, *Thorax,* **18**:77–82 (1963).

62. Anderson, R. C., F. Char, and P. Adams, Jr., Proximal interruption of a pulmonary arch. (Absence of a pulmonary artery.) A new embryologic interpretation, *Dis. Chest.,* **34**:73–86 (1958).

63. Ferguson, A., R. Belleau, and E. A. Gaensler, Congenital absence of one pulmonary artery, *Respiration,* **26**:300–312 (1969).

64. Mannix, Jr., E. P., and C. Haight, Anomalous pulmonary arteries and cystic disease of the lung, *Medicine (Baltimore),* **34**:193–231 (1955).

65. Steinberg, I., Congenital absence of a main branch of the pulmonary artery, *Am. J. Med.,* **24**:559–567 (1958).

66. McLeod, W. M., Abnormal transradiancy of one lung, *Thorax,* **9**:147–153 (1954).

67. Reid, L., and G. Simon, Unilateral lung transradiancy, *Thorax,* **17**:230–239 (1962).

68. Darke, C. S., A. R. Crispin, and B. S. Snowden, Unilateral lung transradiancy. A physiological study, *Thorax,* **15**:74–81 (1960).

69. Blalock, A., Treatment of congenital pulmonary stenosis, *Surg. Gynecol. Obstet.,* **87**:385–409 (1948).

70. Cudkowicz, L., The blood supply of the lung in pulmonary tuberculosis, *Thorax,* **7**:270–276 (1952).

71. Linberg, E. J., Emergency operations in patients with massive hemoptysis, *Am. Surg.,* **30**:158–159 (1964).

72. Tabakin, B. S., J. S. Hanson, P. K. Adhikari, and D. B. Miller, Physiologic studies in congenital absence of the left main pulmonary artery, *Circulation,* **22**:1107–1111 (1960).

73. Oakley, C., G. Click, and R. M. McCredie, Congenital absence of a pulmonary artery, *Am. J. Med.,* **34**:264–271 (1963).

74. Darke, C. S., and T. W. Astin, Differential ventilation in unilateral pulmonary artery occlusion, *Thorax,* **27**:480–486 (1963).

75. Cudkowicz, L., and J. B. Armstrong, Injection of the bronchial circulation in a case of transposition, *Br. Heart J.,* **14**:374–378 (1952).

76. Miller, W. S., The vascular supply of the bronchial tree, *Am. Rev. Tuberc.,* **12**:87–93 (1925–1926).

77. Hovelacque, A., O. Monod, and H. Evrard, Note au sujet des artéres bronchiques, *Ann. Anat. Pathol.,* **13**:129–141 (1936).

78. Nakamura, N., Zur Anatomie der Bronchialarterien, *Anat. Anz.,* **58**:508–517 (1924).

79. Verloop, M. C., On the arteriae bronchiales and their anastomoses with the arteriae pulmonalis in the human lung, *Acta Anat. (Basel),* **5**:171–205 (1948).

80. Von Hayek, H., Über einen Kurzschluss Kreislauf und Entwicklungs geschichte in der menschlichen Lunge, *Z. Anat.,* **110**:412–422 (1940).

81. von Hayek, H., *Die Menschliche Lunge.* Berlin, Springer Verlag, 1953.

82. Marchand, P., V. C. Gilroy, and V. A. Wilson, An anatomical study of the bronchial vascular system and its variations in disease, *Thorax,* **5**:207–221 (1950).

83. Cudkowicz, L., and J. B. Armstrong, Observations on the normal anatomy of the bronchial arteries, *Thorax,* **6**:343–358 (1951).

84. Cauldwell, E. W., R. G. Siekert, R. E. Lininger, and B. J. Anson, An anatomic study of 150 human cadavers, *Surg. Gynecol. Obstet.,* **86**:395–412 (1948).

85. Weibel, E., Die Blutgefässanastomoses in der menschlichen Lunge, *Z. Zellforsch.,* **50**:653–692 (1959).

86. Nagaishi, C., *Functional Anatomy and Histology of the Lung.* Baltimore and London, University Park Press, 1972, pp. 46–81.

87. Liebow, A. A., M. R. Hales, G. E. Lindskog, and W. E. Bloomer, Plastic demonstrations of pulmonary pathology, *J. Techn. Meth.,* **27**:116–129 (1947).

88. Nakamura, T., Pulmonary circulation in silicosis, *Jpn. Circ. J.,* **19**:12 (1956).

89. Wood, D. A., and M. Miller, The role of the dual circulation in various pathologic conditions of the lungs, *J. Thorac. Surg.,* **7**:649–670 (1937).

90. Silver, C. P., The radiological pattern of injected pulmonary and bronchial arteries, *Br. J. Radiol.,* **25**:617–624 (1952).

91. Daly, I. deB., and C. Hebb, *Pulmonary and Bronchial Vascular Systems.* London, Edward Arnold, 1966.

92. Suslow, K. I., Some investigations on the anatomy of the bronchial arteries in man (trans. from Russian). M.D. Thesis, University of St. Petersburg, 1895.

93. Delarue, J., R. Abelanet, G. Chomette, and M. Levame, Recherches sur les Interpendence entre le Reseaux Arteriels Coronariens et mediastinaux chex l'homme, *C.R. Soc. Biol. (Paris),* **154**:937–938 (1960).

94. Hudson, C. L., A. R. Moritz, and J. T. Wearn, The extracardiac anastomosis of the coronary arteries, *J. Exp. Med.,* **56**:919–925 (1932).

95. Thoracic Society, Nomenclature of broncho-pulmonary anatomy: International nomenclature accepted by Thoracic Society, *Thorax,* **5**:222–228 (1950).

96. Weibel, E., Die Entstehung der Längsmuskulature in den Ästen der arteria bronchialis, *Z. Zellforsch.,* **47**:440–468 (1958); Weibel, E., *Morphometry of the Human Lung.* New York, Academic Press, 1963.

97. Töndury, G., and E. Weibel, Über das Vorkommen von Blutgefässanastomosen in der menschlichen Lunge, *Schweiz. Med. Wochenschr.,* **86**:265–269 (1956).

98. Lauweryns, J., *De Longvaten.* Bruxelles Presses Academiques Europeenesse, 1962.

99.   Policard, A., A. Collet, and L. Giltaire Ralyte, Ètude au microscope elec-
      tronique des capillaries pulmonaires chez les mammiferes, *C.R. Acad. Sci.
      [D] (Paris)*, **239**:687–689 (1954).
100. Staub, N. C., Microcirculation of the lung utilizing very rapid freezing,
      Angiology, **12**:469–472 (1961).
101. Reid, A., and B. E. Heard, Preliminary studies of human pulmonary capil-
      laries by india ink injection, *Med. Thorac.*, **19**:215–219 (1962).
102. Boren, H. G., Alveolar fenestrae (relationship to the pathology and patho-
      genesis of pulmonary emphysema), *Amer. Rev. Respir. Dis.*, **85**:328–344
      (1962).
103. Knisely, W. H., In vivo architecture of blood vessels supplying and drain-
      ing alveoli, *Am. Rev. Respir. Dis.*, **81**:735–736 (1960).
104. Krahl, V. E., Microscopic anatomy of the lungs, *Am. Rev. Respir. Dis.*,
      80:24–44 (1959).
105. Liebow, A. A., Pulmonary emphysema with special reference to vascular
      changes, *Am. Rev. Respir. Dis.*, **80**:67–93 (1959).
106. Staub, N. C., and E. Schultz, Pulmonary capillary length in dog, cat and
      rabbit, *Respir. Physiol.*, **5**:371–378 (1968).
107. Weibel, E., On pericytes, particularly their existence on lung capillaries,
      Microvasc. Res., **8**:218–235 (1974).
108. Miller, W. S., Study of the nerves and ganglia of the lung in a case of pul-
      monary tuberculosis, *Am. Rev. Tuberc. Pulmon.*, **2**:123–139 (1918).
109. Ferguson, F. C., R. E. Kobilak, and J. E. Dietrick, Varices of bronchial
      veins as a source of hemoptysis in mitral stenosis, *Am. Heart J.*, **28**:445–
      456 (1944).
110. Wagenvoort, C. A., and N. Wagenvoort, *Pathology of Pulmonary Hyper-
      tension*. New York, Wiley & Sons, 1977.
111. Florange, W., Anatomie und Pathologie der arteria bronchialis, *Ergeb.
      Allg. Pathol.*, **39**:152–224 (1960).
112. Schoenmackers, J., Über Bronchialvenen und ihre Stellung zwischen
      grossen und kleinem Kreislauf, *Arch. Kreislaufforsch.*, **32**:1–86 (1960).
113. Liebow, A. A., Bronchopulmonary venous collateral circulation with
      special reference to emphysema, *Am. J. Pathol.*, **29**:251–289 (1953).
114. Cudkowicz, L., *The Human Bronchial Circulation in Health and Disease*,
      Baltimore, Williams & Wilkins, 1968, p. 57.
115. Prinzmetal, M., E. M. Ornitz, Jr., B. Simkin, and H. C. Bergman, Arterio-
      venous anastomoses in liver, spleen and lungs, *Am. J. Physiol.*, **152**:48–52
      (1948).
116. Tobin, G. E., and M. O. Zariquiev, Arteriovenous shunts in the human
      lung, *Proc. Soc. Exp. Biol. Med.*, **75**:827–829 (1950).
117. Gordon, D. B., J. Flasher, and D. R. Drury, Size of largest arterio-venous
      vessels in various organs, *Am. J. Physiol.*, **173**:275–281 (1953).
118. Madoff, I. M., E. A. Gaensler, and J. W. Strieder, Congenital absence of
      the right pulmonary artery; diagnosis by angiocardiography with cardio-
      respiratory studies, *N. Engl. J. Med.*, **247**:149–157 (1952).
119. Fritts, Jr., H. W., P. Harris, C. A. Chidsey, III, R. H. Clauss, and A.

Cournand, Validation of a method for measuring the output of the right ventricle in man by inscription of dye dilution curves from the pulmonary artery, *J. Appl. Physiol.,* **11**:362–364 (1957).

120. Bruner, H. D., and D. F. Schmidt, Blood flow in the bronchial artery of the anesthetized dog, *Am. J. Physiol.,* **148**:648–666 (1947).

121. Fox, I. J., and E. H. Wood, Application of dye dilution curves recorded from the right side of the heart or venous circulation with the aid of a new indicator dye, *Mayo Clin. Proc.,* **32**:541–550 (1957).

122. Fritts, Jr., H. W., P. Harris, C. A. Chidsey, III, R. H. Clauss, and A. Cournand, Estimates of flow through bronchial-pulmonary vascular anastomoses with use of T-1824 dye, *Circulation,* **23**:390–398 (1961).

123. Cudkowicz, L., M. Calabresi, R. G. Nims, and F. Gray, Jr., The simultaneous estimation of right and left ventricular outputs applied to a study of bronchial circulation in dogs, *Am. Heart J.,* **58**:732–742 (1959).

124. Abdel-Fattah, M. M., H. Badawi, and M. Sala, The simultaneous right and left ventricular outputs in bilharzial cor pulmonale, *Am. Heart J.,* **71**:473–480 (1966).

125. Cudkowicz, L., Bronchial arterial blood flow in man, *Med. Thorac.,* **19**: 582–597 (1962).

126. Nakamura, T., R. Katori, K. Miyazawa, S. Ohtomo, T. Watanabe, Y. Miura, and T. Takizawa, Bronchial blood flow in patients with chronic pulmonary disease, *Dis. Chest,* **39**:193–206 (1961).

127. Cudkowicz, L., Cardio-respiratory studies in patients with pulmonary tuberculosis, *Can. Med. J.,* **92**:111–115 (1965).

128. Cudkowicz, L., Cardio-respiratory studies in patients with lung tumors, *Dis. Chest,* **51**:427–432 (1967).

129. Ryan, T. J., and W. H. Abelmann, Response of bronchial blood flow to tissue proliferation in the human lung, *J. Clin. Invest.,* **40**:1077 (1961).

130. Cudkowicz, L., and J. B. Armstrong, The blood supply of malignant pulmonary neoplasms, *Thorax,* **8**:152–156 (1953).

131. Bolt, W., W. Forssmann, and H. Rink, *Selektive Lungenangiographie.* Stuttgart, Thieme Verlag, 1957, p. 72.

132. Standertskjöld-Nordenstam, C. G., The pulmonary circulation during pneumonia. A cinedensigraphic study, *Acta Radiol. [Ther.] (Stockh.),* Suppl. 239 (1965).

133. Wagner, Jr., H. N., D. C. Sabiston, Jr., M. Iio, J. G. McAfee, J. K. Meyer, and J. K. Langan, Regional pulmonary blood flow in man by radio isotope scanning, *JAMA,* **187**:601–603 (1964).

134. Wagner, Jr., H. N., *Principles of Nuclear Medicine.* Philadelphia, Saunders, 1968.

135. Marchal, M. M., De L'enregistrement des pulsations invisibles du parenchyme pulmonaire ainsi que des pulsations cardiovasculaires par la ciné-densigraphic, *Arch. Mal. Coeur,* **39**:345–359 (1946).

136. Alexander, J. K., H. Takezawa, H. J. Abu-Nassar, and E. M. Yow, Studies on pulmonary blood flow in pneumococcal pneumonia, *Cardiovasc. Res. Cent. Bull.,* **1**:86–92 (1963).

137. Colp, C. R., S. S. Park, and H. M. Williams, Jr., Pulmonary function studies in pneumonia, *Am. Rev. Respir. Dis.,* **85**:808–815 (1962).
138. Stadie, W. C., The oxygen of the arterial and venous blood in pneumonia and its relation to cyanosis, *J. Exp. Med.,* **30**:215–240 (1919).
139. Herzog, H., H. Staub, and R. Richterich, Gas analytical studies in severe pneumonia observed during the 1957 influenza epidemic, *Lancet,* I:593–596 (1959).
140. Andrial, M., Influenzal pneumonia and blood gas analysis, *J. Thorac. Cardiovasc. Surg.,* **40**:79–89 (1960).
141. Berven, H., Studies on cardio-pulmonary function in the post-infectious phase of "atypical" pneumonia, *Acta Med. Scand. [Suppl.],* **382**:1–78 (1962).
142. Smoak, W. M., and M. Viamonte, Jr., Pulmonary investigation with radionuclides. In *Pathophysiology of Perfusion in Pulmonary Disease.* Edited by A. Y. Gibson and W. M. Smoak. Springfield, Ill., Thomas, 1970.
143. Ueda, H., M. Iio, and S. Kaihara, Determination of regional pulmonary blood flow in various cardio-pulmonary disorders, *Jpn. Heart J.,* **5**:431–444 (1964).
144. Gross, L., Preliminary report on reconstruction of circulation of liver, placenta and lung in health and disease, *Can. Med. Assoc. J.,* **9**:632–634 (1919).
145. Kaufmann, W., *Pathology for Students and Practitioners,* Vol. I. London, Lewis, 1929, pp. 352–359.
146. Cudkowicz, L., Some observations of the bronchial arteries in lobar pneumonia and pulmonary infarction, *Br. J. Dis. Chest,* **46**:99–102 (1952).
147. Liebow, A. A., M. R. Hales, and G. E. Linkskog, Enlargement of the bronchial arteries and their anastomoses with the pulmonary arteries in bronchiectasis, *Am. J. Pathol.,* **25**:211–231 (1949).
148. Liebow, A. A., M. R. Hales, W. B. Harrison, W. E. Bloomer, and G. E. Lindskog, The genesis and functional implications of collateral circulation of the lungs, *Yale J. Biol. Med.,* **22**:637–650 (1950).
149. Cudkowicz, L., and D. G. Wraith, A method of supply of the pulmonary circulation in finger clubbing, *Thorax,* **12**:313–320 (1957).
150. Cudkowicz, L., The collateral circulation of the lung and finger clubbing. A review, *Prog. Respir. Res.,* **5**:436–449 (1970).
151. Cudkowicz, L., *The Human Bronchial Circulation in Health and Disease.* Baltimore, Williams & Wilkins, 1968, Chap. 13, p. 314.
152. Alley, R. D., L. H. S. van Mierop, A. S. Peck, H. W. Kausel, and A. Stranahan, Bronchial arterial collateral circulation, *Am. Rev. Respir. Dis.,* **83**:31–37 (1961).
153. Vaccarezza, R. F., A. R. Viola, D. A. Vaccarezza, V. A. Ugo, D. J. Vacario, and E. A. Zuffardi, Verification of the collateral systemic circulation in pulmonary pathology, *Dis. Chest,* **49**:130–138 (1966).
154. Karsner, H. T., and A. A. Ghoreyeb, Studies in infarction III. The circulation in experimental pulmonary embolism, *J. Exp. Med.,* **18**:507–511 (1913).

155. Schlaepfer, K., The effect of the ligation of the pulmonary artery of one lung with and without resection of the phrenic nerve, *Arch. Surg.,* **13**: 623–629 (1926).

156. Holman, E., and M. E. Mathes, The production of intrapulmonary suppuration by secondary infection of a sterile embolic area. An experimental study, *Arch. Surg.,* **19**:1246–1261 (1929).

157. Ellis, Jr., F. H., J. H. Grindlay, and J. E. Edwards, The bronchial arteries; their role in pulmonary embolism and infarction, *Surgery,* **31**:167–179 (1952).

158. Sasahara, A. A., Current problems in pulmonary embolism, *Prog. Cardiovasc. Dis.,* **17**:161–165 (1974).

159. Hampton, A. O., and B. Castleman, Correlation of postmortem chest teleroentgenograms with autopsy findings with special reference to pulmonary embolism and infarction, *Am. J. Roentgenol.,* **43**:305–326 (1940).

160. Gray, Jr., E. D., *Pulmonary Embolism.* Philadelphia, Lea & Febiger, 1966.

161. Loesche, H., In *Handbuch der speziellen pathologischen Anatomie und Histologie,* Vol. 3. Edited by F. Henke and O. Lubarsch. Berlin, J. Springer, Part I, 1928, pp. 599–790.

162. Brenner, O., Pathology of the vessels of the pulmonary circulation, *Arch. Intern. Med.,* **56**:211–237 (1935).

163. Dunnill, M. S., Fibrinoid necrosis in the branches of the pulmonary artery in chronic non-specific lung disease, *Br. J. Dis. Chest,* **54**:355–358 (1960).

164. Cudkowicz, L., and J. B. Armstrong, The bronchial arteries in pulmonary emphysema, *Thorax,* **8**:46–58 (1953).

165. Cockett, F. B., and C. C. N. Vass, The collateral circulation to the lungs, *Br. J. Surg.,* **38**:97–103 (1950).

166. Delarue, J., C. Sors, J. Mignot, and J. Paillas, Lesions bronchopulmonaires et modifications circulatoires, *Presse Med.,* **63**:173–177 (1955).

167. Rasmussen, V. Om Haemoptyse. Navnlig den Lethale in tuberculosis, *Hospitalstidende II,* **33**:37 (1868).

168. Kaufmann, E., *Pathology for Students,* Vol. I. London, Lewis, 1929, Chap. 3.

169. Calmette, A., *Tuberculosis in Man and Animals.* Baltimore, Williams & Wilkins, 1923, p. 191.

170. Kayne, G. G., W. Pagel, and L. O'Shaughnessy, *Pulmonary Tuberculosis,* 2nd ed. London, Oxford Univ. Press, 1948, p. 210.

171. Coryllos, P. N., How do rest and collapse therapy cure pulmonary tuberculosis? *JAMA,* **100**:480–482 (1933).

172. Cournand, A., and W. D. Richards, Pulmonary insufficiency, *Am. Rev. Tuberc.,* **44**:123–172 (1941).

173. Rich, A. R., *The Pathogenesis of Tuberculosis.* Springfield, Ill., Thomas, 1944.

174. Dubos, R. J., Biologic and immunologic properties of tubercle bacilli, *Am. J. Med.,* **9**:573–590 (1950).

175. Scott, Jr., H. W., C. R. Hanlon, and B. J. Olson, Experimental tuberculosis (2). Effects of ligation of pulmonary arteries on tuberculosis in monkeys, *J. Thorac. Surg.,* **20**:761–773 (1950).

176. Guillot, N., Recherches anatomique et pathologiques sur les amas de charbon products pendant la vie dans les organes respiratoires de l'homme, *Arch. Gen. Med.,* **7**(4):151–284 (1845).

177. Steinberg, I., H. I. McCoy, and C. T. Dotter, Angiocardiography in artificial pneumothorax, *Am. Rev. Tuberc.,* **62**:353–359 (1950).

178. Cudkowicz, L., The blood supply of the lung in pulmonary tuberculosis, *Thorax,* **7**:270–276 (1952).

179. Plessinger, V. A., and P. N. Jolly, Rasmussen's aneurysms and fatal hemorrhage in pulmonary tuberculosis, *Am. Rev. Tuberc.,* **60**:589–603 (1949).

180. Wood, D. A., and Miller, M., The role of the dual pulmonary circulation in various pathologic conditions of the lung, *J. Thorac. Surg.,* **7**:64 (1937).

181. Wright, R. D., The blood supply of abnormal tissues in the lung, *J. Pathol. Bacteriol.,* **47**:489–499 (1938).

182. DeCamp, P. T., and H. B. Hatch, Jr., Massive systemic pulmonary arterial shunt through multiple pleural adhesions, *AMA Arch. Surg.,* **78**:206–211 (1959).

183. Uggla, L. G., Indications for and results of thoracic surgery with regard to respiratory and circulatory function tests, *Acta Chir. Scand.,* **111**:197–213 (1956).

184. Cudkowicz, L., and J. B. Armstrong, The blood supply of malignant pulmonary neoplasms, *Thorax,* **8**:152–156 (1953).

185. Cudkowicz, L., The localization and management of pulmonary hemorrhage. In *Critical Care Medicine.* Edited by W. W. Oaks. New York, Grune & Stratton, 1974, pp. 263–300.

186. Cudkowicz, L., Cardiorespiratory studies in patients with lung tumors, *Dis. Chest,* **51**:427–432 (1967).

187. Miyazawa, K., R. Katori, K. Ishikawa, M. Yamaki, Y. Kobayashi, K. Tsuiki, A. Matsanuga, and T. Nakamura, Selective bronchial arteriography and bronchial blood flow. Correlative study, *Chest,* **57**:416–422 (1970).

188. Clifton, E. E., and D. R. Mahajan, Technique for visualizing and perfusion of the bronchial arteries. Suggested clinical and diagnostic applications, *Cancer,* **16**:444–452 (1963).

189. Viamonte, Jr., M., R. E. Parks, and W. M. Smoak, III, Guided catheterization of bronchial arteriography, *Radiology,* **85**:205–229 (1965).

190. Schober, R., *Selektive Bronchialis arteriographie, Fortschr. Geb. Roentgenstr. Nuklearmed.,* **101**:337–348 (1964).

191. des Plantes, Z., *Subtraktion.* Thieme Verlag, Stuttgart, 1961.

192. Vogelaar, P., Subtraction technique for bronchial arteriography, *Dis. Chest,* **50**:336 (1966).

193. Groen, A. S., Z. des Plantes, and D. Westra, Angiography of the bronchial circulation in bronchial carcinoma by means of the subtraction technique, *Dis. Chest,* **48**:634–640 (1965).

194. Banks, B. M., Is there a common demonimator in scleroderma, dermato-myositis, disseminated lupus erythematosus, Libman-Sack's syndrome and polyarteritis nodosa? *N. Engl. J. Med.,* **225**:433–444 (1941).

195. Cheadle, W. B., Clinical lecture on an outbreak of rheumatic pneumonia, *Lancet,* **1**:861–863 (1888).

196. von Glahn, W. C., and A. M. Pappenheimer, Specific lesions of peripheral blood vessels in rheumatism, *Am. J. Pathol.,* **2**:235–249 (1926).

197. Rich, A. R., and J. E. Gregory, Experimental evidence that lesions with basic characteristics of rheumatic carditis can result from anaphylactic hypersensitivity, *Bull. Johns Hopkins Hosp.,* **73**:239–264 (1943).

198. Collins, D. H., Subcutaneous nodule of rheumatoid arthritis, *J. Pathol. Bacteriol.,* **45**:97–115 (1937).

199. Baggenstoss, A. H., and E. F. Rosenberg, Visceral lesions associated with chronic infectious rheumatoid arthritis, *Arch. Pathol.,* **35**:503–516 (1943).

200. Gruenwald, P., Visceral lesions in a case of rheumatoid arthritis, *Arch. Pathol.,* **46**:59–67 (1948).

201. Ellman, P., L. Cudkowicz, and J. S. Ellwood, Widespread serous membrane involvement by rheumatoid nodules, *J. Clin. Pathol.,* **7**:239–244 (1954).

202. Ellman, P., and R. E. Ball, "Rheumatoid disease" with joint and pulmonary manifestations, *Br. Med. J.,* **2**:816–820 (1948).

203. Caplan, A., Certain unusual radiological appearances in chests of coal miners suffering from rheumatoid arthritis, *Thorax,* **8**:29–37 (1953).

204. Sinclair, R. J. G., and B. Cruikshank, A clinical and pathological study of 16 cases of rheumatoid arthritis with extensive visceral involvement, *Q. J. Med.,* **25**:313–332 (1956).

205. Cudkowicz, L., I. M. Madoff, and W. H. Abelmann, Rheumatoid lung disease, *Br. J. Dis. Chest,* **53**:35–40 (1961).

206. Christie, G. S., Pulmonary lesions in rheumatoid arthritis, *Aust. Ann. Med.,* **3**:49–58 (1954).

207. Horler, A. R., and M. Thompson, The pleural and pulmonary complications of rheumatoid arthritis, *Ann. Intern. Med.,* **51**:1179–1203 (1959).

208. Matsui, S., Pathology and pathogenesis of widespread scleroderma, *Mitt. Med. Fakult, Univ. Tokyo,* **31**:55–116 (1924).

209. Bevans, M., Pathology of scleroderma, *Am. J. Pathol.,* **21**:25–51 (1945).

210. Church, R. E., and A. R. P. Ellis, Cystic pulmonary fibrosis in generalized scleroderma, *Lancet,* **1**:392–394 (1950).

211. Kraus, E. J., Zur Pathogenese der diffusen Sklerodermie, *Virchows Arch. [Pathol. Anat.],* **253**:710–734 (1924).

212. Goetz, R. H., Pathology of progressive systemic sclerosis, *Clin. Proc. (Cape Town),* **4**:337–392 (1945).

213. Heath, D., and J. E. Edwards, The pathology of hypertensive pulmonary vascular disease. A description of six grades of structural changes in the pulmonary arteries, *Circulation,* **18**:533–547 (1958).

214. Goodwin, J., Congenital heart disease. In *Clinical Disorders of the*

Pulmonary Circulation. Edited by R. Daley and J. Woodwin. London, Churchill, 1960.

215. Cudkowicz, L., Pressure and oxygen content measurements distal to temporary and permanent unilateral occlusion of a pulmonary artery in dogs, *Circ. Res.,* **6**:728–734 (1958).

216. Liebow, A. A., Discussion of structural alterations of pulmonary vessels in response to pulmonary hypertension. In *Pulmonary Circulation.* Edited by W. Adams and I. Veith. New York, Grune & Stratton, 1959, pp. 124–125.

217. Spain, D. M., Pulmonary diseases. Structural effects on the pulmonary vascular tree. In *Pulmonary Circulation.* Edited by W. Adams and I. Veith. New York, Grune & Stratton, 1959, pp. 99–108.

218. Lategola, M. T., Pressure-flow relationships in the dog lung during acute, subtotal pulmonary vascular occlusion, *Am. J. Physiol.,* **192**:613–619 (1958).

219. Heptinstall, R. H., The effects of high blood cholesterol on the pulmonary arterial changes produced by the injection of blood clot, *Br. J. Exp. Pathol.,* **38**:438–445 (1957).

220. Damman, J. F., J. P. Baker, and W. H. Muller, Pulmonary vascular changes induced by experimentally produced pulmonary arterial hypertension, *Surg. Gynecol. Obstet.,* **105**:16–20 (1957).

221. Pool, P. E., K. H. Averill, and J. H. K. Vogel, Effect of ligation of left pulmonary artery at birth on maturation of pulmonary vascular bed. In *Normal and Abnormal Pulmonary Circulation.* Edited by R. F. Grover. New York, Karger, 1963, pp. 170–177.

222. Harvey, R. M., M. I. Ferrer, D. W. Richards, Jr., and A. Cournand, The influence of chronic pulmonary disease on the heart and circulation, *Am. J. Med.,* **10**:719–738 (1951).

223. McLean, K. H., The significance of pulmonary vascular changes in emphysema, *Aust. Ann. Med.,* **7**:69–84 (1958).

224. Bühlmann, A., F. Schaub, and P. Luchsinger, Die Hämodynamik des Lungenkreislaufes während Ruhe und körperlicher Arbeit, *Schweiz. Med. Wochenschr.,* **85**:253–258 (1955).

225. Briscoe, W. A., and A. Cournand, The degree of variation of blood perfusion and of ventilation within the emphysematous lung. In *CIBA Foundation Symposium on Pulmonary Structure and Function.* Edited by A. V. S. de Reuck and M. O'Connor. London, Churchill, 1962, pp. 304–334.

226. Enson, Y., G. Guintini, M. L. Lewis, and R. M. Harvey, The influence of hydrogen ion concentration and hypoxia on the pulmonary circulation, *J. Clin. Invest.,* **43**:1146–1162 (1964).

227. Harvey, R. M., Y. Enson, and M. I. Ferrer, A reconsideration of the origin of pulmonary hypertension, *Chest,* **59**:82–94 (1971).

228. Cudkowicz, L., Bronchial arterial blood flow in man. In *Normal and Abnormal Pulmonary Circulation.* Edited by R. F. Grover. New York, Karger, 1963, pp. 390–405.

229. Fluck, D. S., R. G. Chandresekar, and F. V. Gardner, Left ventricular hypertrophy in chronic bronchitis, *Br. Heart J.,* **28**:92–97 (1966).

230. Evans, W., D. S. Short, and D. E. Bedford, Solitary pulmonary hypertension, *Br. Heart J.,* **19**:93–116 (1957).

231. Daly, I. deB., and B. A. Waaler, The effect of bronchial vascular system perfusion on the pulmonary vascular resistance in isolated lung lobes of the dog, *Q. J. Exp. Physiol.,* **46**:272–282 (1961).

232. Liebow, A. A., The broncho-pulmonary venous collateral circulation with special reference to emphysema, *Am. J. Pathol.,* **29**:251–289 (1953).

233. Spain, D. M., and G. Kaufman, The basic lesion in chronic pulmonary emphysema, *Am. Rev. Tuberc.,* **68**:24–30 (1953).

234. Leopold, J. G., and J. Gough, The centrilobular form of hypertrophic emphysema and its relation to chronic bronchitis, *Thorax,* **12**:219–235 (1957).

235. Spencer, H., and D. Loef, The innervation of the human lung, *J. Anat.,* **98**:599–609 (1964).

236. Dalen, J. E., C. I. Haffajee, J. S. Alpert, J. P. Howe, I. S. Ockene, and J. H. Paraskos, Pulmonary embolism, pulmonary hemorrhage and pulmonary infarction, *N. Engl. J. Med.,* **296**:1431–1435 (1977).

237. Gilroy, J. C., P. Marchand, and V. H. Wilson, The role of bronchial veins in mitral stenosis, *Lancet,* **2**:957–959 (1952).

238. Ferguson, F. C., R. E. Kobilak, and J. E. Deitrick, Varices of bronchial veins as a source of hemoptysis in mitral stenosis, *Am. Heart J.,* **28**:445–456 (1944).

239. Calabresi, P., and W. H. Abelmann, Portocaval and portopulmonary anastomosis in Laennec's cirrhosis and in heart failure, *J. Clin. Invest.,* **36**:1257–1265 (1957).

240. Barrett, N. R., and R. Daley, A method of increasing the lung blood supply in cyanotic congenital heart disease, *Br. Med. J.,* **1**:699–702 (1949).

241. Winship, W. S., W. Beck, and V. Schrire, Congenital "absence" and anomalous origin of the pulmonary arteries, *Br. Heart J.,* **29**:34–43 (1967).

242. Williams, M. H., and E. J. Towbin, Magnitude and time of development of the collateral circulation after occlusion of the left pulmonary artery, *Circ. Res.,* **3**:422–424 (1955).

243. Fishman, A. P., The clinical significance of the pulmonary collateral circulation, *Circulation,* **24**:677–690 (1961).

244. Horisberger, B., and S. Rodbard, Direct measurement of bronchial arterial flow, *Circ. Res.,* **8**:1149–1156 (1960).

245. Poppe, J. K., Diagnostic significance of clubbed fingers, *Dis. Chest,* **13**:658–662 (1947).

246. Roodenburg, A. E., Secondary hypertrophic osteoarthropathy, *N.Y. J. Med.,* **58**:3635–3640 (1958).

247. Clagett, O. T., J. R. McDonald, and H. W. Schmidt, Localized fibrous mesothelioma of the pleura, *J. Thorac. Surg.,* **24**:213–230 (1952).

248. Wierman, H., O. T. Clagett, and J. R. McDonald, Articular manifestations in pulmonary diseases: An analysis of their occurrence in 1024 cases in

which pulmonary resection was performed, *JAMA,* **155**:1459–1463 (1954).

249.   Jack, G. H., Pulmonary osteoarthropathy in lung cancer, *Lancet,* **1**:750 (1952).

250.   Ginsburg, J., Clubbing of the fingers. In *Handbook of Physiology,* Vol. 3. Edited by W. Hamilton and P. Dow. City, Publisher, 1965, pp. 2377–2389.

251.   Trevor, R. W., Hypertrophic osteoarthropathy in association with cyanotic congenital heart disease, *Ann. Intern. Med.,* **48**:660–668 (1952).

252.   Rudolph, A. M., Pulmonary venomotor activity, *Med. Thorac.,* **19**:184 (1962).

3

Active Control of
the Normal Pulmonary Circulation

EDWARD H. BERGOFSKY

State University of New York at Stony Brook
Stony Brook, New York

I. Introduction

Of all the regional circulations, the pulmonary vascular bed appears to have
the most exquisite and perhaps unusual set of controls for its regional and
local distribution. This conclusion is at least partly due to the revelations
which are possible in this special circulation where, unlike other vascular beds,
regional ventilation-perfusion studies permit an excellent estimate of the precise relation between the local function of a tissue (in this case, its ventilation
rate) and its perfusion [1]. Moreover, simple descriptive observations over the
past two decades have demonstrated that many of the vasoactive responses of
the pulmonary circulation are diametrically, but logically, opposite to those of
the systemic circulations [2–4].

   The genesis of the interest in the control of the pulmonary circulation
had its basis in observations made only several decades ago. The first observation affirmed in the human the low pressure, low resistance characteristics of

   The original work cited in this chapter was supported by research grants
from the United States Veterans Administration and from the National Heart,
Lung and Blood Institute, NIH, DHEW, Washington, D.C. (HL-17711).

the circulation and questioned the likelihood of a steady state of tone elicited by the constant play of the autonomic nervous system and lung vascular smooth muscle receptors bathed in a set of regulating humoral agents. A second type of observation suggested a series of paradoxical responses of the pulmonary circulation to alveolar hypoxia and hypercapnic acidosis, so that vasoconstriction occurred in the pulmonary circulation, rather than the vaso-dilatation expected from experience with the systemic vascular bed. A third type of observation suggested that sources of humoral mediators which could act as regulating agents were uniquely available to the pulmonary circulation. Two such sources explored have been (1) the perivascular mast cell and (2) the conversion of precursors to active agents by tissue within the pulmonary cir-culation, such as the endothelium.

The effect of these lines of investigation in elucidating the mechanisms of control of the normal pulmonary circulation have been enormous. Many of these lessons seem transferable to humans with certain acute and chronic physiological derangements, such as residence at high altitude, as well to patients with diseases of the lung or pulmonary vessels. The development of these observations into firm ideas regarding pulmonary circulatory control is set forth below. In the course of this description, several major questions will be addressed. (1) Is the pulmonary circulation under close autonomic control, as is the systemic circulation? (2) Is control set or tone in the pulmonary cir-culation achieved by other mechanisms, such as the interplay of circulating humoral vasoactive agents, as in the control of uterine smooth muscle? (3) What are the mechanisms underlying the hypoxic and hypercapnic pul-monary vasoconstrictor responses? (4) Are these responses adjustable in disease states for therapeutic purposes?

II. Control of the Normal Pulmonary Circulation

A. Autonomic Innervation

The anatomical distribution of the parasympathetic system to the pulmonary circulation has not been accurately mapped, if it exists at all. In fact, almost the sole reason for entertaining any idea of its existence stems from electrical stimulation experiments of single bundles, which are admittedly difficult to pick out from the coexistent sympathetic fibers in the thoracic nerves. How-ever, some experiments with nerve stimulation [5] do report a vasodilator response which, because of its unusual nature, is distinguished from sympathe-tic responses and attributable to parasympathetics. Little is known about the possible interplay of parasympathetics and sympathetics in a push-pull (or vasodilator-vasoconstrictor antagonism) relationship as exists for the rhythmi-city of the heart. Attempts to shed light on these responses with the parasympathetic mediator, acetylcholine, have revealed a paradoxical reaction, wherein pulmonary *vasodilatation* occurs to the infused mediator in doses of 0.1 mg kg^{-1} min^{-1} and smooth muscle *contraction* to this same mediator in similar concentrations in a muscle bath containing a spiral of pulmonary vascular smooth muscle media. Thus, no good anatomical evidence, and only sparse and conflicting physiological evidence, suggests the existence or any role for the parasympathetic nervous system in pulmonary circulation control.

The precise regulatory role of the sympathetic nervous system in the lung circulation is equally unclear, but its anatomical and physiological responses are far less subtle. Tracing the anatomical distribution of these fibers, particularly by fluorescent stain techniques for catecholamines, has revealed a substantial nerve supply appearing to impinge on the large conducting pulmonary arteries, on the veins, and to a lesser extent, on the small resistance vessels of the lung. Stimulation of the cervical ganglia in most animal species tested produces a remarkable rise in pulmonary arterial pressure and vascular resistance. Indirect evidence indicates that the sympathetics are activated by systemic hypoxia [6,7], and, although they may not mediate the rise in pulmonary vascular resistance during hypoxia, they do appear to stiffen the wall of the larger pulmonary conductance vessels. The latter effect would be expected to elevate *systolic* pulmonary artery pressure and so increase the topographic level at which perfusion takes place in the upright, gravity-dependent lung.

Much additional evidence indicates that the sympathetic nervous system has little role in the moment-to-moment regulation of the pulmonary circulation. First, the vasoconstrictor response to acute alveolar hypoxia is little reduced by surgical sympathectomy (in the human), by depletion of norepinephrine at nerve endings in the dog, by pharmacologic sympathetic blockage by bretylium tosylate in the animal, or by chemical sympathectomy with a dopamine analogue. Indeed, removal of the lung from the body (and hence from any relation to a reflex or central nervous-mediated sympathetic response) also fails to affect the pulmonary vasoconstrictor response to alveolar hypoxia [8–11].

None of the foregoing experience necessarily excludes the sympathetic system from a secondary or auxiliary role in the intact animal, particularly during prolonged or chronic hypoxia: (1) As will be shown below, a complete sympathetic system not only exists, but active α- and β-adrenergic receptors are abundantly present on pulmonary vascular smooth muscle. (2) Afferent, probably sympathetic, nerve fibers which may have baroreceptor capability emanate from at least large pulmonary arteries [6]. (3) Norepinephrine, traditionally located at sympathetic nerve endings, is a potent α agonist and contractor of pulmonary vascular smooth muscle. Thus, although the complete system is present in the pulmonary circulation, and although it may serve to store or enhance production of norepinephrine to moderate the

hypoxic vasoconstrictor response, no function resembling its role in the systemic circulation in moderating blood pressure and moment-to-moment vascular resistance within and between individual organs has yet been evidenced for
the pulmonary circulation.

B.   Gaseous Regulators of Pulmonary Circulation

Hypoxia

In virtually every mammal tested, and these now include, besides the human
[12,13], the cat, dog, guinea pig, rat, cow, goat, and others, alveolar hypoxia
produces a substantial rise in pulmonary arterial pressure. Not all of these
rises, however, can be attributed to pulmonary vasoconstriction. At least five
factors can potentially affect pulmonary arterial pressure during hypoxia:
vascular caliber, pulmonary blood flow, alveolar pressure or left atrial pressure,
and blood viscosity. The approximate relation of these variables indicates that
pulmonary arterial pressure is a *direct,* but not simple, function of pulmonary
blood flow and blood viscosity, and an *inverse function* of a power of the
vascular radius, plus the outflow pressures from the lung. These pressures, in
turn, vary with the zone of the lung and may be alveolar or pulmonary
venous. This relationship obviously resembles Poiseuille's law, but this law is
only remotely applicable to the pulmonary circulation where the flow is
pulsatile and vascular elements are *expansile.* Moreover, the simple, direct relationship of alveolar pressure or venous pressure to pulmonary arterial pressure, which is implied in the above relationship, is not true for the pulmonary
circulation where special relationships due to venous sluicing and parallel
vascular recruitment are present. Fortunately, some of the major variables
listed above do not change during hypoxia, and the role of the remaining
factors are considerably simplified. Thus, increased blood viscosity is a factor
in more chronic forms of hypoxia when blood hematocrit increases, but, during acute hypoxia (which may provoke large rises in pressure and pulmonary
blood flow), an instantaneous increase in blood viscosity does not occur, short
of one which might theoretically be due to some platelet-protein macroaggre-
gate [14]. Similar considerations apply to the two pressures which represent
the outflow pressure from the pulmonary vasculature, i.e., the alveolar pressure
and the left atrial pressure. With respect to alveolar pressure, no alterations in
lung compliance and airway resistance occur in the normal human or intact
animals during the normal pulmonary pressor response to hypoxia [12]. The
same is true of airway pressure in constantly ventilated animal preparations.
In disease states with airway obstruction, however, the ventilatory response to
induced or naturally occurring hypoxia may increase alveolar pressure considerably. Clear examples of this effect are seen in acute episodes of bronchial
asthma where markedly increased alveolar pressures occur independently of

hypoxemia or hypercapnia and appear to be direct causes of marked increases in pulmonary arterial pressure [15]. In a similar manner, left atrial pressure is not grossly altered by the induction of acute hypoxia in the normal human or the experimental animal. Moreover, very few cases of increased left heart pressure have been discovered in the more chronic hypoxia of patients with chronic obstructive lung disease or of the human living at high altitude, even though some subjects fall into older age groups with higher incidences of heart disease.

Only two factors affecting pulmonary artery pressure are known to consistently change during hypoxia, namely, pulmonary blood flow and the radius of the vascular bed. In each case, the effects on pulmonary arterial pressure are complex and could only be surmised prior to recent critical analyses of the mechanics of the pulmonary circulation. Even now, when both variables are changing simultaneously, as they tend to do during acute hypoxia, a complicated digital computer simulator of the pulmonary circulation is necessary to predict the ultimate effect on pulmonary arterial pressure (see Fig. 1).

From the many experimental studies of the past, we are left with the problem of appraising the contribution of the increase in pulmonary blood flow, usually between 10 and 25%, which attends tolerable levels of alveolar hypoxia induced acutely in normal unanesthetized humans and animals. Greater increases have occasionally been noted in the normal situation and in patients with chronic lung disease. The above pulmonary arterial pressure relationship predicts that a given increment in pulmonary blood flow will be attended by the same increment in pulmonary arterial pressure as would occur in a rigid pipe system. Indeed, in some forms of chronic lung or heart disease where the pulmonary arterial pressure is already high [16-18], measurements during exercise-induced increases in cardiac output indicate such a one-to-one relationship between increments in pulmonary blood flow and pressure. But in the *normal* pulmonary circulation, rises in pulmonary blood flow which tend to increase pulmonary arterial pressure are accompanied by pressure-induced recruitment of additional parallel segments of the pulmonary vascular bed, and these act to increase the overall vascular radius and reduce the overall vascular resistance [1]. Thus, the component of the pulmonary arterial pressor response to hypoxia in the normal pulmonary circulation which is due to increments in blood flow appears to be offset by its distending effect on the blood vessels.

The interplay of these multiple factors can be appreciated best when increases in pulmonary blood flow and decreases in vascular bed radius occur simultaneously. Thus, the pressor response to acute hypoxia is 6 torr in the intact cat (Fig. 2b) when the blood flow increases by 35% (from 0.32 to 0.45 liter/min). When this same lung is isolated from the cat (Fig. 2a) with blood

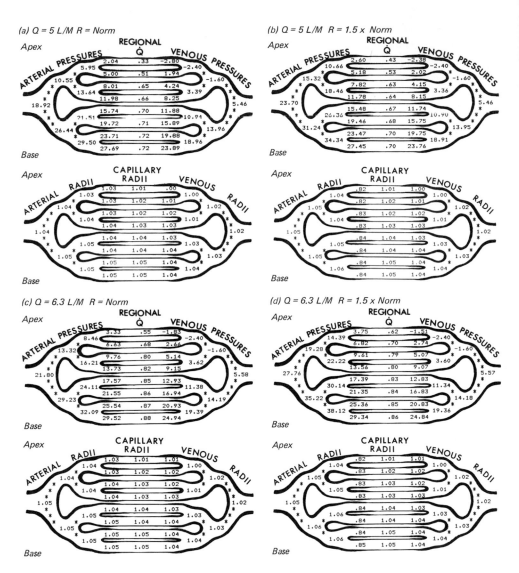

FIGURE 1a–d

(e)   **VASCULAR   RESISTANCE**

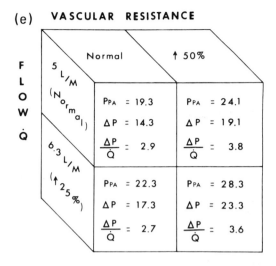

FIGURE 1e

FIGURE 1   Theoretical alterations in regional pulmonary blood flow patterns are shown which tend to minimize the pressure rises during hypoxic vasoconstriction. These were derived from a computer-based pulmonary circulatory model utilizing four arterial and four venous generations producing eight capillary levels from the apex to the base of an upright lung.

Panel (a)   The control showing, generation by generation, arterial and venous pressures and regional blood flow (upper panel) and vascular radii (lower panel), based on a normalized value of 1.0 at 0 transmural vascular pressure. Pulmonary vasoconstriction was stimulated in (b) to produce a 50% overall increase in vascular resistance (all of which is concentrated in the fourth arterial generation, which originally contained arbitrarily one-third of the total resistance) by decreasing the 0-pressure radius at this generation from 1.0 to 0.80 units (resulting in a 2.5-fold resistance increase at this generation when radii to the fourth power are translated into reciprocals of resistance).

Panel (b)   The increase in apical blood flow (from 0.33 to 0.43 liter/min in top sector) resulting from the pressure rise; and **Panel (e)**. The caliber change producing a 50% rise in resistance attended by a 33% rise in pulmonary vascular driving pressure ($\Delta P = P_{pa} - P_{pv}$) and calculated pulmonary vascular resistance ($\Delta P/\dot{Q}$).

Panels (c) and (d)   These panels illustrate the effects of 25% increments in pulmonary blood flow without and with the simulated decrease in radius to produce the 50% rise in vascular resistance; the 25% increment as shown in **Panel 1c** is attended by a 20% increment in driving pressure and a fall in calculated resistance, and the combination results in a lower calculated resistance than in **Panel 1b**, that is, a 20% rise when flow is also increased as compared with a 33% rise when flow is constant. Thus, recruitment during elevations of pulmonary artery pressure, together with pressure-induced vascular distension, comprises the perception of the vasoconstriction induced by a decrease in vascular caliber [19,20].

Part (e)   See legend for **Panel (b)**.

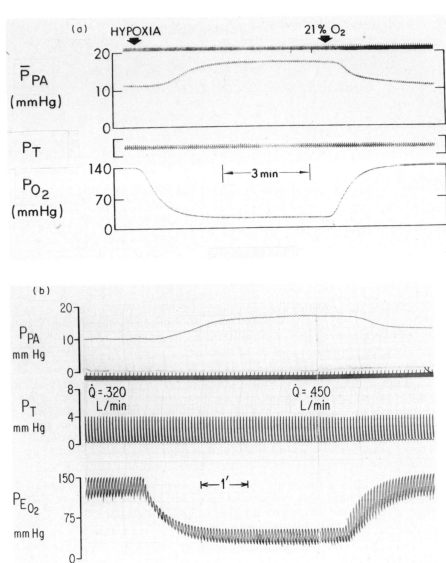

FIGURE 2 Magnitude and timing of pulmonary vasoconstrictor responses to
hypoxia in the cat. In the upper panel (a), the isolated lung perfused at constant
flow rate by autologous blood shows a similar vasoconstrictor response in terms
of magnitude and timing of onset and offset of the response as in the intact animal, where small increases in pulmonary blood flow occurred (b). PT = tracheal
pressure during assisted ventilation; PO_2 and PE_{O_2} = end-tidal PO_2 during onset
and offset of induced alveolar hypoxia.

flow *constant* (and with similar left atrial and alveolar pressures and similar pulmonary blood flow), the pressor response to hypoxia is still about the same, in the absence of the countervailing distension due to increased blood flow. Similar considerations apply to the effect of vasoconstriction-induced rises in pulmonary arterial pressure when zone I pulmonary blood vessels become fully perfused and afford additional conductance by means of these vessels. Figure 1 shows computer simulations of the distribution of pulmonary blood flow during hypoxia in the pulmonary circulation [19,20].

Hypercapnia

In the intact animal, such as dog, cat, rat, and guinea pig, the breathing of 5 to 10% CO_2, particularly when anesthesia blunts ventilatory drive and substantial rises in alveolar and arterial PCO_2 are permitted to occur, can elicit rises of 4 to 6 torr in the mean pulmonary arterial pressure [21,22]. Prior to such studies, considerable controversy existed regarding the influence of hypercapnia because experimental work in the human never fulfilled the necessary conditions for demonstrating the response clearly. The unanesthetized human, usually hyperventilated to prevent significant rises in PCO_2, and patients with chronic lung disease, though powerless to hyperventilate adequately, produced such great pressure changes in the thorax that pulmonary vasoconstriction could not easily be isolated from other variables affecting pulmonary arterial pressure [23]. Furthermore, responses in the isolated perfused lungs were not always predictable [24] before the era of excellent temperature and perfusate control [25].

Much attention has been leveled at the separation of the two possible factors affecting pulmonary vasomotion during hypercapnic acidosis, i.e., elevated levels of blood, interstitial or intracellular PCO_2, and elevated levels of hydrogen ion in the same locations. The experimental data favor the preeminent role of the hydrogen ion as the major vasoactive stimulus. For instance, acidoses produced by lactic acid, hydrochloric acid, or CO_2 breathing, which are associated with either high or low PCO_2 levels, invariably elicit rises in pulmonary vascular resistance related to the drop in blood pH, not the PCO_2 level [22]. In a similar manner, increments in blood PCO_2 accompanied by buffering conditions which do not permit a pH change (extracellularly at least) produce, if anything, a pulmonary vasodilatation [26] in dogs; experience in humans may differ [27].

Much less certainty exists regarding the extracellular or intracellular location of the molecular target sensitive to the hydrogen ion. However, an extracellular target is favored at present, because comparable degrees of extracellular acidosis from either fixed acidoses (lactic, hydrochloric) or respiratory acidosis (hypercapnic) produce the same pulmonary vasoconstrictor responses, even though much greater intracellular acidosis would be expected from the hypercapnic acidosis [22]. Utilizing the hydrogen ion alteration produced by hypercapnia, it is possible to assess the magnitude of its pulmonary vaso-constrictor response. In the anesthetized dog, a rise in pulmonary arterial pressure of 3 mmHg (or a 40% rise in pulmonary vascular resistance) accom-panies a fall in blood pH of 0.1 units. These values are not dissimilar from data in the awake human, and appear to apply over the range of pH from 7.40 to 7.10. pH values higher than 7.40 do not in themselves appear to decrease pulmonary arterial pressure in the normal human, although precise predictions regarding pulmonary vascular resistance are not possible because of some alterations in blood flow [22]. In patients with chronic obstructive lung disease, the effect of induced alkalosis is more striking, with real decre-ments in pulmonary arterial pressure occurring even in the face of rises in cardiac output [28].

Although there may be some skepticism regarding the importance of the role of the H^+ alone in the regulation of pulmonary circulation, most in-vestigators agree that this stimulus has a synergistic vasoconstrictor function in combination with alveolar hypoxia. For instance, in the isolated dog lung, the vasoconstrictor response to an alveolar PO_2 of 40 mmHg doubled when the pH was reduced to 7.20 and halved when it was raised to 7.55 [25]. In the intact dog, this synergy is not clearly obvious [22], but, in patients with lung disease, the greatest degrees of pulmonary hypertension occur with the lowest pH values for the same level of arterial hypoxemia; in the few cases where acidosis has been directly induced in patients with chronic obstructive lung disease, the pulmonary vascular responses to hypoxia have also been aug-mented [29]. The most remarkable degree of synergy between hypoxia and acidosis occurs in the pulmonary circulation of the newborn calf [30].

Figure 3 collates data from several sources which studied the interrela-tion between hypoxia and acidosis, and, as indicated, the majority of studies demonstrates an amplification of the pulmonary vasoconstrictor response by acidosis which is more than the sum of the separate responses.

However, the implications for the synergistic effect on local control of regional ventilation-perfusion ratios in the normal lung are obscure. This con-clusion stems from the very small increments in PCO_2 which can occur in badly ventilated alveoli, no matter how low the alveolar PO_2 has fallen. Since both are limited by their levels in the mixed venous blood perfusing these ab-normal alveoli, alveolar PO_2 may fall to 40 mmHg or lower and thus evoke hypoxic vasoconstriction in some alveoli, but mixed venous pH or PCO_2 is fixed at 7.37 or 46 mmHg, respectively, and would not be expected from the experimental data alone to materially augment the hypoxic vasoconstrictor response when it occurs locally.

When no limit exists to the mixed venous PCO_2 and pH, as in rapidly fluctuating ventilation states during the course of chronic respiratory diseases,

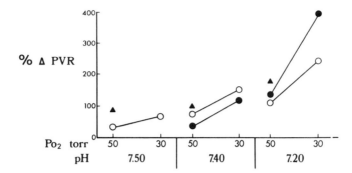

FIGURE 3 Effect of acidosis in modifying the pulmonary vasoconstrictor response to two levels (PO_2 = 50 or 30 torr) of hypoxia. ▲ = man with lung disease [28]; ○ = excised dog lobes [25]; ● = newborn intact calf [30].

the synergy between the vasoactive effects of these two gases should be more evident. Finally, little is known regarding the molecular interactions or respective receptor activity of these two gaseous stimuli which would lead to synergy. Indeed, the data are not sufficiently precise to be certain that the term *synergy* applies, i.e., that the response to the two stimuli exceeds that of the sum of each separately, rather than some mechanical enhancement of the rise in pulmonary arterial pressure to one agent, once the radius of the blood vessel has been reduced by the other, an expected result when the rise in pulmonary arterial pressure may be related to the fourth power of the radius.

Localization of Hypoxic and Hypercapnic Pulmonary Vasoconstrictor Responses

The Case for Localization to the Lung

Localization to the lung is a term incorporating the concept that the entire stimulus-response mechanism resides in the lung, not just the final motor unit, i.e., the pulmonary vascular smooth muscle. The alternative hypotheses, which do not require localization to the lung for portions of the stimulus-response limb, can be divided into several categories. These are (1) receptors for the hypoxic or hypercapnic stimulus, (2) intermediate mechanism (or humoral agent) between extrapulmonary receptor and pulmonary vessels, and (3) motor effectors of pulmonary vascular resistance, other than pulmonary vasoconstriction.

While the bulk of evidence indicating the ease with which pulmonary hypertensive responses are elicited by hypoxia or hypercapnia in the isolated lung appears to exclude extrapulmonary participation, it may still be possible that extrapulmonary factors may operate in more subtle ways in the intact animal. Some of the discredited, as well as uncertain, mechanisms are summarized as follows. A peripheral receptor, in organs such as brain or adrenal which might exert their effect on the lung circulation through autonomic nerves or a released mediator, has not been found in experiments which produce extrapulmonary isolated organ hypoxia [31]. The intermediate role of the autonomic nervous system, either as a hypoxic sensor in the lung or as a motor afferent to the pulmonary smooth muscle, has also been extensively considered. A long line of evidence or hypothesis has been used [5] to invoke the involvement of the autonomic nervous system; some of the propositions are: (1) a well-known nervous pathway exists to convey the sensory stimulus of arterial hypoxemia to the central nervous system via the carotid-aortic chemoreceptors and their respective afferent nerves, and the efferent sympathetic innervation of the pulmonary vasculature is well established; (2) hypoxemia sensed at the peripheral chemoreceptors is well known to use sympathetic pathways to excite the heart and provoke the hypoxic augmentation of cardiac output; (3) direct electrical stimulation of cervical sympathetic ganglia evokes a clear-cut pulmonary vasoconstrictor response in a lung where all mechanical influences on the pulmonary circulation have been controlled; (4) the experiments of Daly [6] have been able to establish that the reflex system enumerated above can respond to local hypoxia at the chemoreceptor under some circumstances, although it elicits only feeble pulmonary vasoconstrictor responses, and (5) sympathetic denervation in some animal preparations decreases the hypoxic pulmonary pressor response [32]. Against this line of reasoning, there is a formidible array of counterevidence to consider, summarized in the previous section, which makes important participation of the sympathetic nervous system remote. Even fanciful hypotheses of special reflexes (e.g., an alveolo-arterial [33] or a venoarterial reflex which would persist even after removal of the lung from the organism, using local axon fibers to convey the sensation of hypoxia from its origin to its effector within the lung) have never been subject to experimental support; and recent data utilizing agents designed to damage sympathetic motor endings argue against the involvement of the particular system in this process [11,34]. Finally, motor effectors for the increases in pulmonary vascular resistance, other than pulmonary vasoconstriction, have been postulated in the form of reversible cellular macroaggregates, which could be elicited by hypoxia within the pulmonary circulation and be readily reversible by normal oxygenation. Some counterpart for this mechanism has been observed, in the aggregations during hypertonic infusions [14]. However, no direct evidence exists for this mechanism in connection with hypoxia, and the hypoxic hypertensive process has been elicited in the pulmonary circulation perfused by cell-free plasmas. The role of humoral agents which originate in precursor form elsewhere but are activated by the lung itself during hypoxia or hypercapnia is discussed below.

Localization of the Hypoxic
and Hypercapnic Vasoconstrictor Responses Within the Lung

Although a subsequent section makes clear that the entire pulmonary vasoconstrictor response to hypoxia and hypercapnia is a multistage process involving several steps between application of the stimulus and the blood vessel
response, the present state of knowledge has permitted questions of localization on only two stages of the response to be successfully pressed. (1) Where
is the sensor(s) to hypoxia and hypercapnic acidosis located? (2) In which
type of vessel is the motor component of the vasoconstrictor process localized?
These two questions are not necessarily the same. For instance, the arterial
side of the pulmonary vascular bed seems, in principle, the best possibility as
the *site* of the vasoconstriction: the choice of the arterial side of the bed is
supported by the anatomical fact that the arteries are equipped with much
more musculature than the veins, and their position is such, that, unlike the
veins, their vasoconstriction will not elevate capillary hydrostatic pressure and
upset the balance between intravascular and interstitial fluid. On the other
hand, a venous site sensitive to hypoxia or hypercapnia also seems logical for
purposes of local control within the lung because of the ability of the alveolar
gaseous composition to be imposed on blood being immediately delivered to
individual veins. Thus, the original teleological purpose of the pulmonary
vasoconstrictor response to hypoxia, the regulation of blood flow to individual
air space elements to produce the optimal ventilation-perfusion ratios, is superficially best fulfilled by a venous site sensitive to the stimulus. This paradox
created the need for a hypothesis involving an alveolo-arterial or venoarterial
reflex wherein a hypoxic or hypercapnic signal from alveolus or venous blood
would be relayed back to the arterial vessel. Such an idea has never progressed
beyond the stage of hypothesis. However, an important step in unlocking this
puzzle occurred when experimental evidence suggested that the smaller pulmonary arteries were close enough to their adjacent air spaces that the prevailing
gas tensions surrounding their vascular smooth muscle, as well as the blood inside these vessels, could be affected by the alterations in alveolar gas composition. These conclusions are supported by the immediate sensing of abrupt
alterations in alveolar PO_2 by wedged pulmonary arterial catheters before recirculation could have occurred [35], and by quick-freeze methods whereby
the blood in small pulmonary arteries was observed to be at O_2 tensions
similar to those of alveolar gas rather than of mixed venous blood or pulmonary arterial blood [36].

The identification of the route of communication of the gaseous stimulus
from air space directly to small arteries within the lung afforded a firm foundation for much of the previous and subsequent experimental work. Thus, an
earlier approach used wedged pulmonary venous catheters of various sizes to

show that much, but not all, of the pressure drop across the pulmonary vascular bed during hypoxia occurred between the pulmonary arteries and veins 0.4 mm in diameter [37]. Moreover, with the exception of one author who names the capillaries as the site sensitive to hypoxia [38], the bulk of present-day evidence points to the *arterial segment alone* as both the site sensitive to hypoxia and as the segment undergoing the actual vasoconstriction in response to the hypoxia. For instance, two techniques for indirect measurement of the volume of the pulmonary vascular segments have shown that alveolar hypoxia decreases mainly the arterial volume: these include volatile gas methods as well as rapid freeze drying and anatomical counting of the red cell contents of the pulmonary blood vessel [39,40]. With regard to the site sensitive to hypoxia, much of the evidence has come from the selective induction of localized hypoxia or hypercapnia at various points throughout the pulmonary vascular bed. An early study [31] demonstrated that exaggerated hypoxemia produced by deoxygenated blood infused into the right heart of the intact dog could elicit a pulmonary vasoconstrictor response. The induction of hypoxia localized to individual segments of the vascular bed has now been precisely performed, and some recent data are illustrated by Figure 4. When the isolated lung is perfused from the arterial or the venous side of the circulation with blood equilibrated with hypoxic gas and with an adjustable alveolar gas tension, hypoxia localized to only a small portion of the vascular bed, i.e., the arteries of less than 200 μm in diameter, produces the largest pulmonary vasoconstrictor response of any form of selective hypoxia. This localization in vessels immediately adjacent to air spaces seems characteristic for hypoxia. Hypercapnic acidosis (PCO_2 = 60 mmHg, pH = 7.20), in the same sort of preparation, produces pulmonary vasoconstriction when it is applied over a much longer length of the pulmonary arterial bed [41].

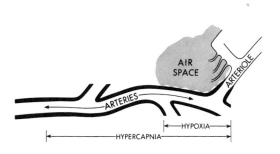

PRESSURE RESPONSES (%)			
	PRECAP	ALVEOLAR	POSTCAP	GENERAL
HYPOXIA	+12	+28	+5	+49
HYPERCAPNIA	+23	+16	+5	+40

FIGURE 4 Localization of the pulmonary vascular sites sensitive to alveolar hypoxia and hypercapnic acidosis. The largest pressor response ($^+$28%) occurred in the isolated perfused lung while alveolar hypoxia was delivered, holding perfusing blood from either the arterial or venous side of the circulation at a high O_2 tension. Hypercapnic acidosis showed predominance of the response at the arterial side [41].

All this experimental evidence is compatible with the idea that the small-to moderate-sized pulmonary artery (100 to 500 μm) is regulated by the level of O_2 and [H^+] in its immediate milieu. The O_2 level of the milieu (either intima, media, or adventitia) can be altered by either alveolar hypoxia or exaggerated mixed venous or pulmonary arterial hypoxemia. The [H^+] level in this milieu may be regulated not only by that in the inflowing pulmonary arterial blood, but also by the balance between the pulmonary arterial and the alveolar PCO_2 with which the [H^+] tissue level is in equilibrium. According to these principles, localized or generalized hypoxia of the air spaces (as in-dicated, a PA_{O_2}, about 70 mmHg or less) will elicit localized or generalized pulmonary arterial constriction. Some clinical states which produce exaggerated mixed venous hypoxemia may have pulmonary vasoconstriction which originates in this mechanism; the apparently reversible pulmonary vasocon-striction seen in mitral stenosis may represent an example of this process. An equally important clinical state, exercise, may have any hypoxemic vaso-constriction obscured by the concomitant huge increments in pulmonary blood flow which push open the pulmonary vascular bed. With respect to the [H^+] level, uncompensated metabolic or respiratory acidosis would elevate this level and, either alone weakly, or if combined with hypoxia strongly, in-crease pulmonary vascular resistance. In a similar manner, on a local level, underventilation of an air space and elevation of its PCO_2 would cause CO_2 to dissolve into the periarterial tissues and alter the equilibrium between CO_2 and [H^+], elevating the latter and hence elevating the [H^+] of the entire blood vessel.

Studies to localize the sites of the hypoxic and hypercapnic responses have led to several preliminary deductions regarding the mechanism involved. The hypercapnic stimulus may act through a mechanism different from the hypoxic stimulus, since the response occurs in large and small arteries, rather than small arteries alone. Moreover, anatomical or functional adaptation of the smaller pulmonary arteries is present which mediates the vasoconstrictor response to hypoxia. This adaptation could take the form of (1) an attached neuroreceptor, (2) a nearby cell capable of secreting humoral agents locally, or (3) specific adaptation of the membrane or excitation-contraction coupling mechanism of this portion of the vessel.

C. Humoral Agents and Their Effect on the Pulmonary Circulation

Agents Affecting Vasoactivity Through Mechanisms Susceptible to Conventional Pharmacologic Blockades

These include the catechols, i.e., the internally occurring catecholamines, some of their precursors and metabolites, and certain therapeutically effective synthetic catecholamines, as well as histamine. Although their actions on the pulmonary circulation appear to be sensitive to blockade or enhancement by pharmacologic blocking agents which are conventional for the systemic circulation, their ultimate performance in the two circulations may differ, and these differences may be used to map the relative distribution of receptors in these two circulations.

The Catecholamines

The endogenous catechols, norephinephrine and epinephrine, often have had controversial effects on the pulmonary circulation, in good measure because of their associated effects on cardiac output, pulmonary venous–left atrial back-pressure and bronchial smooth muscle and airway resistance. An intravenous injection of epinephrine may or may not cause a visible rise in pulmonary vascular resistance, since the concurrent rises in cardiac output and decreases in left atrial pressure produce mechanical effects on the pulmonary circulation that alter pulmonary vascular resistance by recruitment of parallel vascular channels, and obscure changes in resistance due to vasoactivity. This problem is analogous to the one seen in hypoxia, except that epinephrine is unique in its ability to lower left atrial pressure. Thus, various reports of pulmonary vasodilatation, vasoconstriction, and nonreactivity from the sympathomimetic amines have been reported and reviewed by Aviado [32]. Studies in isolated pulmonary vascular muscle strips or in constantly perfused lung preparations produce much clearer relationships between these agents [42]. A low concentration of epinephrine (10^{-6} g/ml) in a water bath only slightly contracts or often dilates a strip of pulmonary vascular smooth muscle. Doses of 10^{-5} g/ml elicit larger contractions and produce an additional degree of tension elicitable from this muscle by supramaximal electrical stimulus. Similar effects are seen in the femoral arterial specimen so that, for both, the tension elicitable by supramaximal stimulation is 50% greater with epinephrine in the bath solution. In the constantly perfused lung of the intact animal, infusions of 10^{-5} g produce slight vasoconstriction which amounts to more than a 10 to 20% increase in pulmonary vascular resistance. These data are consistent with an adrenergic system in which α (constrictor) and β (dilator) receptors are present, as in many types of vascular smooth muscle [43]; thus, the action of an agent such as epinephrine, which possesses both α- and β-stimulatory activity, seems attributable to a greater binding affinity for the β-dilator system, but a numerical predominance of α over β receptors. In other tissues, such as coronary artery, where epinephrine is a substantial dilator, the predominance of β over α receptors is presumed.

A comparison between phenylephrine, norepinephrine, and isoproterenol reveals further information on the adrenergic system of pulmonary arterial smooth muscle of blood vessels in perfused animal lungs [38–40]. Norepine-phrine and phenylephrine, considered dominant α stimulators, regularly produce pulmonary vasoconstriction and, as would be expected on a weight-for-weight basis, elicit a greater vasoconstrictor effect than epinephrine with its α- and β-agonist effects. Isoproterenol, a predominantly β-adrenergic stimulator, regularly produces pulmonary vasodilatation.

Histamine

A great deal of controversy surrounds the performance of histamine in the pulmonary circulation. In the bulk of reports, histamine emerges as a pulmonary pressor agent of considerable potency. In infused doses of 10^{-5} g over a 2-min period, a substantial and highly repeatable pulmonary pressor response occurs in the pulmonary circulation of dogs, cats, rats, guinea pigs, and primates [44]. If the intravenous infusion is slow enough, this pressor response can be shown to be entirely vasoconstrictive in nature, since the histamine is inactivated too rapidly to elicit increases in cardiac output or bronchoconstriction. When infusions are more rapid or confined to the systemic circulation, the very opposite response occurs in the systemic circulation, i.e., vasodilatation. Thus, histamine resembles hypoxia: both elicit pulmonary vasoconstriction and systemic vasodilatation.

The mechanism of action on vascular smooth muscle and the reasons for the paradoxical effects in the two major circulations are unfortunately still unclear. In the case of the pulmonary circulation, a consensus exists that the direct effect of a histamine bath on isolated slips of vascular smooth muscle, both arterial and venous, and the indirect effect of the infusion of histamine in the intact animal, is a contractile or vasoconstrictive one. Moreover, considerable evidence exists that both pulmonary arteries and veins are constricted in the intact animal; this evidence is based on the multiple wedged venous catheter technique [37] and the method using red cell concentrations of vascular segments [40]. Both suggest that, for a given plasma concentration of histamine, the veins constrict somewhat more than do the arteries.

In some reports, histamine appears to be dilator to the pulmonary circulation. The species include the newborn calf, as well as certain adult dogs residing at an altitude of 5000 feet; a series of comparisons of these same species at sea level and high altitude apparently demonstrates that a pulmonary circulation with considerable tone, such as with high altitude or experimental hypoxia, reacts with dilation to histamine, and this response would be consistent with the high tone believed to exist in the neonatal circulation [45,46].

The mechanism whereby histamine acts in the constrictive process is still uncertain. A direct effect of histamine on the cell membrane may cause loss

of intracellular potassium and the resulting depolarization and activation of
electrical spikes in the smooth muscle; this conjecture is based on observations
of increased serum potassium levels after histamine [47,48]. Another possibility is a direct effect of histamine on calcium movement or calcium com-
partmentalization in the vascular smooth cell. Perhaps the simplest mechanistic
principle to explain these doubly paradoxical results is the existance of a push-
pull system of vasoconstrictor-vasodilator receptors sensitive to histamine and
analogous to the α- and β-adrenergic receptors. These have now been identified
and labeled H-1 and H-2, respectively, on the basis of the responses to histamine
after the use of agents such as chlorpheniramine (H-1 blockade) or metiamide
(H-2 blockade) [49–51]. Their implications and their potential interrelationship with the adrenergic receptor system is discussed below for the pulmonary
circulation. With respect to the systemic circulation, a push-pull receptor
mechanism may be the simplest available explanation for the dichotomy in
the action of histamine on large and small blood vessels. In the systemic circulation, it is quite clear that the usual effect in the intact animal is generalized systemic vasodilatation, even though strips of aortic, carotid, and femoral
arterial smooth muscle are regularly constricted by the same concentrations of
histamine. It is thus uncertain what agency converts a clearly contractile
effect on large systemic vessels into a dilatation of the small resistance vessels
when the organism is intact. Differences in the qualitative receptor mechanisms of vascular smooth muscle at varying levels of the vasculature, the
presence of axon reflexes, and the stimulated release of other neurohumorals,
such as prostaglandins of the E or I series, have all been advanced as explanations for this additional dichotomy of the effect of histamine in the systemic
circulation [52,53].

Pharmacologic Blockade and Its Effects
on Adrenergic and Histamine Responses

The adrenergic receptor system may be characterized and quantified by the
use of specific pharmacologic blocking agents developed against α- and β-
adrenergic activity. These reactions, compared with those of the systemic
circulation, are summarized in Figure 5, which compares the effects of α
(phentolamine) with β (propranolol) blockade on norepinephrine and epinephrine responses of the pulmonary circulation of the cat. The responses are
comparable, because the perfused left lower lobe with measurable pulmonary
venous and alveolar pressures was used to compare a variety of agents. For
epinephrine, a control rise in pulmonary vascular resistance of 30% is converted to a vasodilatation equal to a 10% reduction in pulmonary vascular
resistance by the α-adrenergic blocker, phentolamine. The vasoconstrictor
response to norepinephrine is greatly reduced, in fact mostly abolished, by
α blockade, but never converted to a vasodilatation. When the β-blocking

agent, propranolol, is administered, the 30% rise in pulmonary vascular resistance to epinephrine is converted to a 100% increase, a phenomenon which well illustrates the effect of β blockade on the properties of a combined α and β stimulator such as epinephrine. Such data not only indicate that an adrenergic system exists in the pulmonary circulation, but have generated renewed interest in the effects of pharmacologic blockade on histaminic, hypoxic, and hypercapnic pulmonary vasoconstrictor responses. Figure 5 shows the extent to which α- and β-adrenergic blockade affect responses to histamine in the pulmonary circulation. β Blockade with propranalol almost doubles the constrictor response to histamine, while α blockade reduces the usual 60% increase in pulmonary vascular resistance to 10%. Unlike norepinephrine and epinephrine,

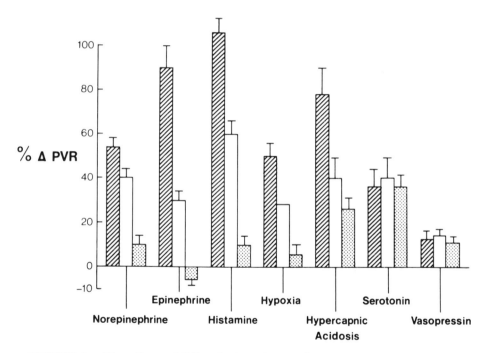

FIGURE 5 The effects of β (hatched area) and α (dotted) pharmacologic blockade on the increase (above baseline) or decrease (below baseline) in pulmonary vascular resistance on exposure to seven gaseous or humoral agents. The clear central histogram represents the average increase in pulmonary vascular resistance to the respective agonist under control conditions. The dose of each humoral agent was 10 μg. Alveolar hypoxia was produced by exposure to 8% O_2 in N_2; hypercapnic acidosis, by 10% CO_2 in air. As indicated, the pulmonary vascular effects of all agonists except serotonin and vasopressin are substantially altered by adrenergic blockade.

to which no response, or vasodilatation, occured after α blockade, histamine after such blockade evokes a mild response in some though not all animals. Responses to hypoxia and hypercapnia are also susceptible to α and β blockade: the vasoconstriction is considerably enhanced by β blockade, and markedly reduced, but not completely abolished, by α blockade. This adrenergic pharmacologic profile for hypoxia and hypercapnia somewhat resembles that of norepinephrine and also of histamine, but not serotonin, vasopressin, or (not shown) angiotensin II. The reason why α and β blockade appear to affect hypoxic and hypercapnic vasoconstrictor responses so clearly in the perfused in situ lobe, and not in the intact calf, is unclear, unless differences in applicable dose of blocking drugs and species variation account for the disparity.

Another set of receptors which may play a role in the pulmonary vascular bed is the histamine H-1 constrictor and H-2 dilator system [52]. The system has been characterized by use of H-1 and H-2 blocking agents, such as chlorpheniramine and metiamide, respectively. In other organs, chlorpheniramine prevents smooth muscle constriction induced by histamine, and metiamide prevents gastric acid secretion induced by histamine. In the pulmonary circulation, chlorpheniramine will completely prevent the vasoconstrictor effect of infused histamine and induce some degree of vasodilatation; metiamide enhances the pulmonary vasoconstrictor effect of histamine. These two responses, coupled with the usual vasoconstrictor response to histamine, have led to the supposition that the pulmonary circulation has more H-1 than H-2 receptors, and, in the systemic circulation, that the reverse is true, i.e., H-2 receptors outnumber H-1 receptors. These H-1 and H-2 blockers have moderate specificity for histamine. For instance, chlorpheniramine and metiamide [54] do not appear to affect pulmonary circulatory responses to epinephrine or norepinephrine, although older H-1 blocking agents, such as diphenhydramine, appear to have α-adrenergic blocking characteristics.

Effect of Agents Stored in the Lung
on Pulmonary Circulation

Storage of humoral agents in a depot close by pulmonary blood vessels would be an ideal mechanism of regulating the pulmonary circulation. The known depots available in the lung include nerve endings, both sympathetic and parasympathetic; specially differentiated epithelial cells, such as the bronchial neuroepithelial body; mast cells; type II epithelial cells; and wandering macrophages, neutrophils, and eosinophils. Some of these depots, by virtue of their anatomical location, are most likely to influence bronchi. Others, because of their perivascular location, are good candidates for control of the pulmonary circulation, specifically, mast cells and nerve endings and their respective contents.

A major constituent of the mast cell, histamine, has been considered above. Recent evidence indicates that it is continuously secreted in concentrations low enough to avoid detection by analytic techniques in pulmonary venous blood, but high enough to impart a tonic vasoconstriction to the pulmonary vascular bed. Data supporting this regulatory role are the effects noted with administration of the inhibitor of mast cell secretion, disodium cromoglycate, namely, a drop in pulmonary vascular resistance when this agent is given, but a greatly enhanced sensitivity of the vasoconstrictor mechanisms to infused histamine [54].

Another constituent of mast cells in many species, and of platelets in most species, is serotonin (5-hydroxytryptamine) [55]. This agent is also of interest because of the disturbances in the right heart and pulmonary circulation produced by elevated levels of serotonin in metastatic carcinoid. Serotonin is one of the most potent pulmonary constrictors known, with the same effectiveness and repeatability of histamine and even more consistency from species to species [56–58]. Its effect is also consistent in terms of the various experimental preparations utilized: isolated lungs perfused with Ringer's solution, in situ left lower lobes perfused with autologous blood, and the intact animal all behave in the same way, and in the intact animal, only modest increments in cardiac output occur so that the vasoconstrictive effects are clearly observable. In infused doses of 10^{-5} g in the perfused lung, serotonin elicits a pulmonary vasoconstriction at least 75% greater than similar doses of histamine. As Figure 5 indicates, α- and β-adrenergic blockade have no effect on the pulmonary circulatory effects of serotonin. Moreover, certain lysergic acid analogues act to depress the pulmonary circulatory responses to serotonin, but chlorpheniramine does not. Such data indicate that the action of serotonin is not mediated by any known adrenergic or histaminic receptors, but has its own receptor or other membrane or contractile effects.

Slow-reacting substance of anaphylaxis (SRS-A), which is released from the mast cell by cobra venom [59], is known by its contractile activity on the guinea pig ileum and is apparently a mild bronchoconstrictor. Its effects on the pulmonary circulation have not been experimentally worked out, but it is assumed to be a vasoconstrictor, and its potential role as a pulmonary circulatory regulator can only be surmised. Other constituents of mast cells have also only superficially been characterized. High-energy phosphate compounds, such as ATP and its analogues, are contained in several cellular elements including red cells and platelets; they all appear to be massive systemic vasodilators which produce increases in cardiac output that preclude a simple assessment of their effects on pulmonary vasoactivity. A relatively weak vasoconstrictor-effect action may be demonstrated when blood flow is held constant in the perfused lung [28], or in the very sensitive neonatal circulation of the calf, but even these effects are dissociated with difficulty from the mechanical effects on pulmonary vascular resistance of induction of platelet aggregation by these high-energy phosphates [60].

Effect of Agents Converted in the Lung on Pulmonary Circulation

These agents include angiotensin, bradykinin and kallidins, and prostaglandins.

Angiotensin

Angiotensin II, the octapeptide formed from the decapeptide, angiotensin I, by endothelial cell converting enzymes (see Aviado [44] for review) is a pulmonary vasoconstrictor with great reproducibility. Unlike histamine and serotonin, however, angiotensin is as consistently vasoconstrictor in the systemic circulation as it is in the pulmonary vasculature. Slips of vascular smooth muscle from the large vessels of virtually all vascular beds contract in response to this agent. The magnitude of the vasoconstrictor effect of angiotensin II is best seen in the isolated lung of the cat where, without the drawbacks of fluctuating systemic pressure, angiotensin on a molar basis is at least an order of magnitude more effective than histamine or serotonin in evoking pulmonary vasoconstriction [34].

In the pulmonary circulation of the unanesthetized human, when angiotension is infused in small doses (0.03 μg kg^{-1} min^{-1}) to minimize the potent systemic pressor effects, the pulmonary circulation still reacts with considerable vasoconstriction [13]. Because of its consistent vasoconstrictor effect on all vascular beds, it has been assumed that the effect of angiotensin II on all vascular smooth muscle is a "direct" one and that neither release of intermediate substances nor use of the α-adrenergic system, which is highly variable from bed to bed, need to be invoked. However, these two factors may play some role in the response to angiotensin, since α and β blockade can increase and decrease, respectively, the pulmonary vasoconstrictor effects of angiotensin II, but not nearly to the same degree as with histamine or, of course, epinephrine. Thus, angiotensin may use α receptors for part of its vasoconstrictor effect, or it may, like tyramine and other pharmacologic agents, release norepinephrine at sympathetic endings close to the pulmonary resistance vessels [61]. A vascular receptor mechanism which may be blockaded by pharmacologic agents has not been identified. However, inhibition of converting enzyme itself by potent pharmacologic agents is not only feasible, but will be introduced as a new therapeutic option in the management of systemic hypertension.

Angiotensin II was once thought to be a humoral agent "necessary" for the pulmonary vasoconstrictor response to hypoxia, although not the direct mediator [62]. Indeed, it appears to be in a good position to influence some position of the pulmonary vascular bed, in that it is converted from angiotensin I by the endothelial cell, the prevalence of which is most prominent at the capillary level (although some conversion must occur at arterial and venous portions also), and diffusion of the agent outward at the capillary or venular level may occur to a considerable extent. However, the formation site of this agent is at an anatomical disadvantage, since the hypoxic pulmonary vasoconstrictor response appears almost entirely arterial. Recent evidence has demonstrated again, however, that the depletion of angiotensin during acute hypoxia does not blunt the pulmonary vasoconstrictor response. Moreover, acute alveolar hypoxia, rather than augmenting the conversion of inactive angiotensin I to active angiotensin II, profoundly depresses this process and simultaneously prevents the inactivation of the general vascular dilator, bradykinin [63,64]. These developments diminish the importance of angiotensin in the regulation of the pulmonary circulation, but advance the idea that the frequent occurrence of systemic vasodilatation during hypoxia may be due to diminished converting-enzyme activity and the resultant predominance of systemic vasodilators.

Bradykinin and the Kallidins

These agents comprise a system of polypeptides, requiring activation by plasma factors called kallikreins. They presently have no known or suspected function in the normal pulmonary circulation. Usually, bradykinin is considered a pulmonary vasodilator [65], but in the rat it appears to be a pulmonary vasoconstrictor [66], at least after the use of the mast cell depletor, 48/80. Although its role in normal physiological function is unclear, whenever a circulating humoral agent exists in both an inactive and active form and can be activated by plasma factors, future investigation may find a function for this agent in the pulmonary circulation [67]. Its possible role in the mediation of systemic vasodilatation during alveolar hypoxia has been included above, but it should be emphasized here that it fits such a role by virtue of its known systemic vasodilator capability [64].

Prostaglandins

Three prototypic prostaglandins have received extensive attention with respect to control of the pulmonary circulation and have been periodically implicated in the hypoxic pulmonary vasoconstrictor responses [68]. These are the prostaglandins E (PGE_1 and PGE_2), a group of systemic and pulmonary vasodilators; prostaglandin $F_{2\alpha}$ ($PGF_{2\alpha}$), a systemic and pulmonary vasoconstrictor; and a prostacyclin of the I variety. Although some of these three prostaglandins, as well as others, have been found in a variety of tissues, including lung and circulating blood, their implications for the regulation of the pulmonary circulation are as yet unclear.

The two prostaglandins of the E series have been identified mainly in the lung of the sheep. In other animals, they may be released from the splanchnic area, from which they travel to the liver and the lung where they are removed from the circulation [69]; since they are pulmonary vasodilators and bronchodilators, they may conceivably have some function when stress and autonomic nervous stimulation release them from the splanchnic bed, or during hyperventilation when they are released from the lung [70]. Their pulmonary vasoactive effects may explain the hypoxemia seen in chronic hepatic disease when their failure to be taken up by the liver could result in an excess of vasodilator influence on the lung. Such generalized pulmonary vasodilatation may lower arterial O_2 tensions by lowering the pulmonary arterial pressure and promoting gravitational overperfusion of the lower lung fields, and deranging ventilation-perfusion ratios in the lung. Alternatively, such vasodilatation may open usually closed arteriovenous anastomotic channels, thereby leading to hypoxemia.

The pulmonary vasoconstrictor and bronchoconstrictor, prostaglandin $F_{2\alpha}$, also is elaborated by the lung of many species, including the human, and prostaglandin synthetase has now been detected in the mammalian pulmonary endothelial cell [71,72]. These observations indicate that prostaglandin $F_{2\alpha}$ could function as a regulator of regional pulmonary blood flow under some circumstances. Whether pulmonary cells other than endothelial produce $PGF_{2\alpha}$ is unknown at this time, but even these cells would provide a production site sufficiently close to pulmonary arteries to affect them during regional or generalized alveolar hypoxia. As with angiotensin II, the formation of the bulk of prostaglandin $F_{2\alpha}$ in the capillary, where the highest density of endothelial cells exists, bypasses a highly selective effect on the pulmonary arteries in favor of control of pulmonary veins, unless diffusion out of the capillary endothelial cell into parenchyma is an efficient route to reach the pulmonary artery. In addition, infused $PGF_{2\alpha}$ is also a consistent bronchoconstrictor, resembling SRS-A with particular regard to its slow onset and prolonged effects, and is probably elaborated in certain anaphylactic reactions [73]. Thus, it has many deleterious effects not expected during the hypoxic or hypercapnic pulmonary vasoconstriction which would compromise attempts to accurately localize this agent to the pulmonary arterial region. Such considerations are serious drawbacks to considering $PGF_{2\alpha}$ as a humoral mediator controlling the pulmonary circulation. However, it is still uncertain whether prostaglandins of any sort are constituents of the pulmonary mast cell, which is well positioned to influence the pulmonary artery.

Another serious objection to an exclusive role for $PGF_{2\alpha}$ as the intermediary agent regulating the pulmonary vasoconstrictor response to hypoxia or hypercapnic acidosis is the reported complete resistance of its pulmonary vasoconstrictor effect to enhancement or blunting by α- and β-adrenergic blocking agents. Since the hypoxic and hypercapnic pulmonary vasoconstrictor effects are, in good measure, modifiable by both forms of adrenergic blockade, $PGF_{2\alpha}$ can at best fall into the category of an additional humoral mediator, rather than the primary one [74].

Other Pulmonary Vasodilators

Acetylcholine has quite perplexing effects on the pulmonary circulation (see Aviado for review [75]). In the intact pulmonary circulation of both humans and animals, infusion of this agent produces slight vasodilatation in the normal situation. It induces more apparent vasodilatation when the pulmonary circulation is artificially constricted by induced alveolar hypoxia or infused serotonin, or when pulmonary vasoconstriction is present in chronic obstructive lung disease, primary pulmonary hypertension, and mitral stenosis [76-80]. Acetylcholine is thus similar to vagal stimulation, and in some animals where it has been tested, atropine blocks these effects [81]. The action of this agent thus suggests an enhanced state of tone is maintained in diseases with pulmonary arterial medial proliferation.

The mechanism underlying acetylcholine-induced vasodilatation is unclear, since most isolated strips of vascular smooth muscle, including pulmonary strips, constrict when bathed in acetylcholine. Several explanations have been advanced to explain the disparity. In the in vitro situation, acetylcholine may cause release of a dilating agent from sympathetic endings or from mast cells that does not occur in the isolated muscle strip; it may provoke release of a vasodilator from other structures in the vicinity of the pulmonary arteries; or it may have a dose-dependent response related to the numbers and affinity of separate vasodilator and vasoconstrictor receptors (see above).

Other agents which are unequivocally vasodilator to the pulmonary circulation are the xanthines, particularly theophylline; the organic and inorganic nitrites, such as amylnitrite; and isoproterenol-like catecholamines. These agents, because they are not circulating humoral agents which can regularly control the pulmonary circulation, are beyond the scope of this chapter, but are summarized by Aviado [75].

III. Pulmonary Vascular Tone

Despite the fact that the normal pulmonary circulation requires an extremely low perfusion pressure, averaging only 5 to 7 mmHg, and that its resistance is only 1 mmHg liter^{-1} min^{-1} in the human at rest, or one-twentieth of the resistance in the systemic circulation, this vascular bed does not appear to be completely without tone or a steady state of low-grade vasoconstriction. This

conclusion stems from the clear-cut ability to utilize pharmacologic vasodilators to produce detectable vasodilatation even in this very low resistance
circulation. Both isoproterenol and theophylline increase pulmonary circulatory levels of cyclic adenosine monophosphate (cAMP), and these increases
correlate well with modest vasodilatations [31]. It is important to emphasize,
however, that in a low-resistance circulation in the upright human, small decreases in perfusion pressure may give a misleading view of the extent of vasodilatation: Decrements in pulmonary arterial perfusion pressure which attend
vasodilatation in the lower portions of the lung may elicit *closure* of vessels in
the upper portions of the lung, which thus minimizes the fall in vascular resistance and perfusion pressure which would otherwise occur [19].

The experience with α- and β-adrenergic blockade supports the above
contention. α Blockade with phentolamine slightly lowers pulmonary vascular
resistance, suggesting spontaneous activity of the α-receptor mechanism or an
effective level of circulating α agonists, such as norepinephrine [43], or even
an agent such as histamine, the constrictor action of which is greatly influenced by α blockade. Evidence for and against the role of histamine as a tone
setter for the pulmonary circulation is of two varieties: (1) infusions of chlorpheniramine or metiamide, H-1 and H-2 antagonists, respectively, do not appear to affect baseline pulmonary vascular resistance in the intact dog [49];
(2) on the other hand, in the controlled perfused left lower lobe of the cat,
disodium cromoglycate, the mast cell stabilizer, regularly reduces pulmonary
vascular resistance, and an infusion of histamine subsequently results in an
augmented pulmonary vasoconstrictor response. Such data may suggest that
reduction of circulating histamine level lays bare both vasoconstrictor and
vasodilator receptors in the pulmonary vascular bed which were previously
occupied by histamine and that the affinity of the constrictor receptor is
greater than that of the dilator receptor for the newly infused exogenous
histamine. Whether these receptors, however, are of the accepted H-1 and
H-2 variety, or the equally important adrenergic variety, is uncertain.

IV. Regulation of Regional Pulmonary Blood Flow
by Hypoxia and Hypercapnia

These two gaseous stimuli seem to be the only known major regulators of
regional pulmonary blood flow. For instance, accommodation of the huge
increases in cardiac output during exercise appears to be wholly by passive
dilatation of this vascular bed, and no evidence exists that regional modulation
occurs via the autonomic or other system during exercise to direct blood flow
to specific pulmonary sites. Thus, the bulk of studies attempting to elucidate
pulmonary circulatory control have dealt with the hypoxic regulatory response.

This response could be operative in normal situations on a regional basis, important throughout the lung at high altitude, and the basis for a good deal of the pulmonary hypertension seen in patients with respiratory insufficiency. Because of its relative weakness and limited occurrence in disease states, the hypercapnic vasoconstrictor response, though believed to be directed through the hydrogen ion, has received much less attention with regard to its intermediate mechanisms of action. The hypoxic vasoconstrictor response in the lung has now been studied to such a degree that at least six distinctive but linked stages seem to exist over which the mechanism may act from the origination of alveolar hypoxia to the final contraction of smooth muscle which narrows the pulmonary arteries; these are listed in Table 1.

The definition of such a complex system evolved only after a long period of investigative work in this area. Among the first hypotheses was that of Liljestrand, who suggested that an intracellular lactic acidosis resulting from tissue hypoxia might be the primary factor in the induction of the pulmonary pressor response to hypoxia. This viewpoint received considerable support when it was subsequently discovered that hypercapnic acidosis or fixed mineral acidosis also evoked pulmonary vasoconstriction [82,31] and that the acidosis in some way synergized the hypoxic pulmonary pressor response [25,28]. The observations that pulmonary arterial strips lost potassium and gained sodium and were thus partly depolarized (in contrast to systemic vascular smooth muscle) suggested that the pulmonary arterial smooth muscle membrane, i.e., its Na^+-K^+-ATPase, was especially inhibited by hypoxic levels insufficient to inhibit the contractile mechanism of the cell [83]. Thus, hypoxia could act to depolarize the cell and bring it closer to its threshold for activation of the contractile process without interfering with this process. This idea would require a specialization which would contrast with systemic arterial smooth muscle, where the relaxation which is generally observed with hypoxia is attributable to the interruption of aerobic energy sources for the contractile mechanism.

However, the single largest stumbling block to the idea that acidosis occurs within the cell or a specialized pulmonary vascular smooth muscle membrane is the failure to elicit consistent contractions of the isolated muscle strip when exposed to hypoxic conditions in a Ringer's solution bath. This failure has been most evident when direct hypoxia has been applied to freshly removed pulmonary arterial specimens of cat, rat, and guinea pig [84]. Some suggestive stiffening effects have been obtained when, in guinea pig pulmonary arteries, length-tension diagrams have been performed under normoxic and hypoxic conditions [42]. Long-term alterations have occurred in the aorta when exposed chronically to hyperoxia, so that contraction occurs when returning to conditions of normal oxygenation [85]; apparently, pulmonary arteries could react similarly. Finally, contraction of dissected pulmonary

TABLE 1   Successive Mechanisms Between Stimulus and Response in Hypoxic Pulmonary Vasoconstriction

Sensor	Storage Site	Mediator	Receptor	Vascular Smooth Muscle		
				Membrane Na$^+$-K$^+$-ATPase Ca^{2+} Permeability	Electro-mechanical	
Ca^{2+} Permeability	1. Sympathetic neuron	Norepinephrine	α-Adrenergic		Sarcolemmal Ca^{2+}	
	2. Mast cell	Histamine Prostaglandins Serotonin	Histamine, H-1		Other	
	3. Neuroepithelial body					
	4. Platelets		Other ?			
P-450 Sensor	5. Type II cell	Vasopressin				
	6. Macrophages					
Ca^{2+} Permeability P-450 Sensor	Endothelium[a]	Angiotensin Prostaglandins				

[a]Activation site.

arteries could occur during hypoxia in one set of experiments, so long as bits of lung tissue remained adherent to the specimen [86]. But, all these experiments demonstrate that the mammalian pulmonary artery does not contract spontaneously to hypoxic (or acidotic conditions) and that a more complex system to initiate and sustain responses must be present.

A keystone of this system may be a humoral mediator. The list of possible mediators is shown in Table 1, along with the relationship to storage sites or activation sites where they are known. Much evidence has now accumulated regarding histamine as a possible mediator. Among the earliest pieces of information was the demonstration that the histamine depleter, 40/80, and certain antihistamines blocked the pressor response to hypoxia in the perfused animal lung [67,87].

An exceedingly important argument in favor of an agent such as histamine is the belief that it is usually released from a storage site in the vicinity of its final action. This latter is a most important attribute in order to account for the time course of the pulmonary vasoconstrictor response to alveolar hypoxia. This response is shown in Figure 2 for the isolated perfused lung subjected to alveolar hypoxia induced by tidal dilution of the lung volume. As is indicated, despite the fact that hypoxia is of only gradual onset, the pressor response occurs *only a few seconds* after the O_2 electrode first begins to record tracheal hypoxia. Such observations indicate that a square wave of hypoxia, if it could be accomplished, would elicit a pressor response in only 1 or 2 sec and thus suggests the need, if humoral agents are to be invoked in this process, for a storage depot for this agent. If a storage depot is necessary, and if the enzymatic activation of a circulating agent could not take place in so brief a time, which is by no means certain, only a few cells known to be in the lung are likely to be possibilities. They include, among others, autonomic nerve endings, secretory epithelial cells, migrating macrophages, neuroepithelial bodies [88], platelets, and mast cells. There are persuasive reasons for considering the mast cell first, without definitively excluding the others, namely, the widespread presence of mast cells in the lungs of most species, their known content of potent humoral agents, and their ability to store these agents in quantity in preparation for an abrupt release when needed [55].

Interest in the mast cell derives also from the occurrence of this humoral depot at anatomical locations strategic for the performance of two required functions: to sense the ambient O_2 tension in the air spaces and to deliver vasoconstrictors on demand to the pulmonary vessels supplying these air spaces. Figure 6 shows the close proximity of the air spaces and a typical artery of 200 μm, so that, in terms of diffusion distances for O_2, air space has as much influence on the vascular media as the PO_2 of the blood within the arterial segment. Figure 7 shows the relation between the periarterial

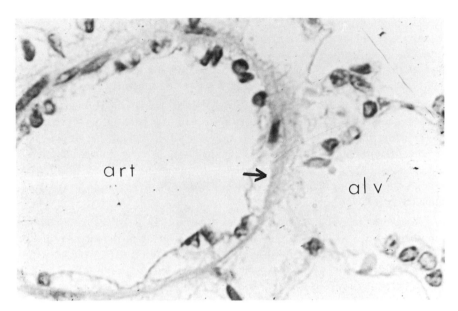

FIGURE 6   Histologic section of a small pulmonary artery, approximately 200 μm in diameter (art), in close approximation to an air space (alv) with the vascular smooth muscle of the media intervening between the two about equidistant from each.   (Cat lung; hematoxylin-eosin.)

arrangement of the mast cell and the adjacent air spaces, and other studies indicate the position of these cells to be just adjacent to the arterial adventitia. Few mast cells are seen around the veins, and, in the rat and guinea pig lung, well over half the pulmonary mast cells occur around vessels, with the remainder distributed between a peribronchial and a subpleural location [89]. The periarterial mast cells, particularly those around vessels of less than 200 μm, would sense alveolar (and to less extent pulmonary arterial) O_2 levels. The mast cells around bronchi are exposed to higher ambient O_2 levels (bronchial PO_2 varying between 100 and 150 mmHg and bronchial arterial PO_2 varying around 100 mmHg).

The pulmonary mast cell has been more directly implicated in the process [89]. Histologic techniques using special stains for mast cell granules demonstrate that the pulmonary periarterial mast cell partly degranulates during induced alveolar hypoxia in the rat and guinea pig. This acute process, occurring in the first 20 min of the hypoxic period, amounts to a 30% degranulation. Harvests of mast cells from the peritoneal cavity of the rat behave in a fashion consistent with the above response: hypoxia imposed on these cells in an in vitro preparation of Ringer's solution causes the histamine to shift from the cells to the supernatant; this shift also suggests a degranulting function for the imposed hypoxia. Moreover, radio-labeled histidine previously taken up by the lung is released into the left atrial blood during acute alveolar hypoxia as histamine and is directly proportional to the increment in pulmonary vascular resistance during hypoxia. Release of histamine into the pulmonary effluent blood has been previously demonstrated during hypoxia [90].

The mast cells do not occur as aggregates in the lung, but rather in clusters of two or three; the calculated number of mast cells in the strategic pulmonary periarterial region is very substantial and in fact for the whole lung approaches the mass of the carotid chemoreceptor. For the calculation, assumptions must include an irregular dichotomous branching of the pulmonary arterial tree and a length-diameter ratio of 3 for each vascular segment. These assumptions are then combined with experimental data [89] demonstrating that the number of mast cells per individual arterial segment from 500 to 50 μm in diameter, averages one cell for every 16 μm of vascular length. Based on the last five arterial generations of a human vascular tree (from about 16 to 20), in which the vascular diameters range from 500 to 50 μm, the total number of mast cells for each generation ranges from about 6 million at generation 16 to more than 9 million at generation 20. The total number of

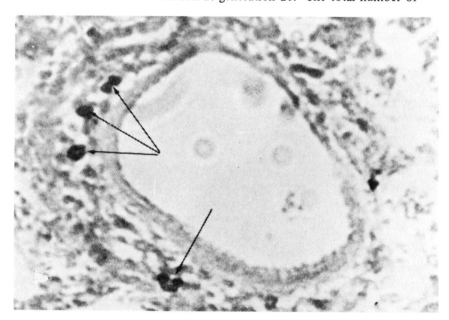

FIGURE 7   Histologic section of a small pulmonary artery showing clusters of mast cells just outside adventitia (arrows). (Cat lung, Unna's stain.)

TABLE 2 **Effect of Histaminic Blockade on Hypoxic Pulmonary Vaso-constrictor Response**

Species	Blocking agent[a]	Hypoxic pulmonary vasoconstriction	Reference
Cat	H-1 (chlor)	Inhibited	Hauge et al. [87]
Rat	H-1 (chlor)	Inhibited	Hauge et al. [67]
Dog	H-1 (chlor)	Inhibited	Sussmano et al. [91]
Dog	H-1 (pro, diph)	Inhibited	Sussmano et al. [94]
Dog	H-1 (chlor)	No effect	Tucker et al. [94]
Dog	H-2 (metiam)	Enhanced	Tucker et al. [94]
Dog	H-1 (chlor)	No effect	Hales et al. [95]
Dog	H-1 (chlor)	No effect	Howard et al. [96]
Cat	H-1 (chlor)	No effect	Barer et al. [39]

[a]histamine blocking agents, chlorpheniramine, promethazine, diphenhydramine, and metiamide.

mast cells in the lungs is about 4×10^7. Using an average mast cell diameter of 10 μm [55], a mass of the order of 1 to 2 g of tissue, i.e., similar to the carotid chemoreceptor, therefore exists in approximation to pulmonary arteries. Using estimates of the average concentration of histamine per mast cell, and the percentage of mast cell histamine released during a single episode of 20 min of alveolar hypoxia (30%) about 0.1 mg of histamine are available for this process. This quantity, when infused in a perfused left lung, is sufficient to produce a pulmonary pressor response equal to that of alveolar hypoxia in the same animal [40].

Some drawbacks exist to these interpretations of the role of histamine and its mast cell depot in the mediation of the pulmonary vasoconstrictor response to hypoxia. First, a considerable controversy now exists regarding the ability to inhibit the response with histamine antagonists. The disparate results are summarized in Table 2, where it is clear that, in more than half the reports, infused chlorpheniramine has no effect, rather than a blocking effect, on hypoxic pulmonary vasoconstriction. In one of the reports where chlorpheniramine was effective [91], its dose was at least an order of magnitude larger than in other reports, but since the species was the rat, a much smaller animal, this dose may have been appropriate for its higher metabolic ability. The other drawback is the inconsistency of the histologic degranulation seen with short-term hypoxia. Different reports, however, have used different statistical approaches and staining techniques, which make comparisons difficult [92,93]. On the other hand, these recent studies have turned up a new observation, namely, that prolonged alveolar hypoxia results in proliferation of perivascular pulmonary mast cells. The implications of this finding for the chronic hypoxic vasoconstrictor response are uncertain. However, the validity of conclusions drawn from blocking experiments is always suspect. Doses of antihistamines which are compatible with maintenance of blood pressure may not result in sufficiently high tissue concentrations to block the high levels of histamine that are secreted by the mast cells at the adventitia of the pulmonary vessel; typical chlorpheniramine doses of 1 mg/kg may not be able to block a dose of 100 μg of histamine released in the rat lung (10 to 20 g in weight) at strategic sites, where the histamine concentration might be 10- to 100-fold greater than its antagonist [94-96].

If the case for histamine as the mediator of hypoxic vasoconstriction in the lung requires substantial reservations, the case for other potential mediators is much weaker. A long list of candidates for the role of mediator appears in Table 3, along with the general characteristics which best describe this mediator, based on experimental pharmacologic work in the pulmonary circulation. With three exceptions, all the listed agents are unequivocally pulmonary vasoconstrictors; however, vasopressin, bradykinin, and acetylcholine, as indicated in the foregoing section, may be vasoconstrictors under some circumstances or in isolated pulmonary vascular strips, but are often considered vasodilators. Of the remaining unequivocal pulmonary vasoconstrictors, only three agents have the advantage of a storage depot in the lung; these are histamine, serotonin, and norepinephrine. Three others are activated or synthesized in the lung: angiotensin II, $PGF_{2\alpha}$, and SRS-A. Of these six agents, since the hypoxic and hypercapnic pulmonary vasoconstriction is so markedly affected by both α and β blockade, this pharmacologic characteristic would eliminate both angiotensin II and $PGF_{2\alpha}$ as candidates for mediator. Serotonin also suffers as a candidate, since its pulmonary vasoconstrictor effects are not only not altered, as is the hypoxic effect, by adrenergic blockade, but also because it may not exist in the human mast cell, or anywhere closer to the pulmonary artery than the bronchial neuroepithelial body [88] or the blood platelet.

The last two columns of Table 3 summarize the controversial pharmacologic studies in the field. With respect to histamine, the controversy over inhibition of hypoxic pulmonary vasoconstriction by H-1 blockade, which is summarized above, is as great as the controversy over the ability to abolish this response after histamine depletion by the mast cell degranulator 48/80 [87]. Recent evidence suggests that the degranulator itself may also act non-specifically to impair smooth muscle contractile responses to other agents [97]. The pharmacologic meaning in the norepinephrine studies is perhaps clearer: depletion of norepinephrine by sympathectomy, reserpine, or dopamine analogue does not affect the response [4,98], but α blockade does; the

TABLE 3   Comparison of Pharmacologic Characteristics of Possible Humoral Mediators of Hypoxic or Hypercapnic Pulmonary Vasoconstriction[a]

Agent	Pulmonary vasoconstrictor	Lung storage	Activated released in lung	Hypoxic α or β adrenergic response[b]	↓ Hypoxic response by inhibitor	↓ Hypoxic response by depletion
Histamine	++	++	++	+	±	+
Serotonin	++	+	+	0	unk	
Norepinephrine	++	++	++	+	+	0
Angiotensin II	++	0	++	0	0	±
PGF$_{2\alpha}$	+	0	++	0	±	0
Vasopressin	±[c]	0	0	unk	unk	unk
Bradykinin	±[c]	0	0	unk	unk	unk
SRS-A	+	0	+	unk	unk	unk
Acetylcholine	±[c]	+	+	0	0	0

[a] unk = unknown; 0 = negative; ± = conflicting reports.
[b] That is, the vasoconstrictor response enhanced and blunted by alpha and beta blockade, respectively, as occurs with hypoxia and hypercapnic acidosis.
[c] Pulmonary vasopressor response variable; often vasodilator.

hypoxic pulmonary vasoconstrictor response therefore uses the α-adrenergic receptor.

Thus, by virtue of the six characteristics listed, only three of the known agents implicated as hypoxic pulmonary vasoconstrictors remain viable candidates. These are histamine, norepinephrine, and SRS-A. In none of these is the pharmacologic profile quite complete. Histamine clearly edges norepinephrine, but studies with SRS-A are so incomplete that it may emerge as the best candidate for the mediator of this response.

Table 1 emphasizes several other possible steps in the hypoxic pulmonary vasoconstrictor response. The identification of the first step, the biophysical receptor, has only just begun. The ability to inhibit the hypoxic response with verapamil, an agent that blocks cellular Ca^{2+} influx, has been interpreted as applying to the smooth muscle cell and implying a direct effect of hypoxia on this cell [99]. However, it may be just as logical to suppose that this effect occurs at a storage or activation site of a humoral mediator within one of the specialized pulmonary cells of the second column of Table 1. More recently, inhibition of the P-450 enzymes of the electron transport chain has blunted this hypoxic response, and this enzyme may affect synthesis or release of a humoral mediator within a storage and activation site [100].

The relationship of storage and activation sites is shown, where known, for the associated mediators in the second and third columns of Table 1. The mast cell clearly contains the largest number of known potential mediators, but the contents of sympathetic nerve endings, of neuroepithelial bodies, and of type II alveolar epithelial cells have just begun to be described. In a similar fashion, although endothelial cells can synthesize angiotensin II and prostaglandins, some combination of synthesis of one type of agent and inactivation of another may provide the synergistic group of agents which is the hypoxic mediator. The relation between activation of the vasoconstrictor angiotensin and inactivation of the vasodilator, bradykinin, by a single unit, the endothelial cell, is an example of such a linked system, although hypoxia appears to inactivate, not potentiate, converting enzyme [64].

Little work has been done in the three areas specific to the pulmonary vascular smooth muscle, once a direct effect of hypoxia on the contraction of isolated vascular smooth muscle could not be consistently demonstrated. Several possible mechanisms which may link hypoxia directly to the smooth muscle cell have received attention in the past and have recently been summarized by Fishman [101]. Most of these have dealt with the cell membrane in terms of either the Na^+-K^+ pump and its inhibition by hypoxia or the Ca^{2+} permeability and its increase by hypoxia. In either case, the effect of hypoxia could be expected to decrease membrane potential, bringing the smooth muscle cell closer to its contractile threshold or to offer Ca^{2+} freely

to the smooth muscle contractile process. But, none of the effects are uniquely applicable to the pulmonary vascular smooth muscle cell. Cellular depolarization or unsequestered intracellular calcium could also act on a receptor
cell, a depot cell, or an activator cell to augment production of a neurohumoral
mediator. Thus, no proven evidence exists yet that acute alveolar hypoxia has
a specific, direct effect on the pulmonary vascular smooth muscle cells, its
membrane, its electromechanical coupling, or its contractile process. It is also
worth emphasizing that hypoxia does not, at least in the usual tolerable alveolar levels imposed, from PO_2 values of 60 down to 20 torr, affect dele-
teriously the ability of this cell to contract.

Little is known about long-term alveolar hypoxia and its effect on
physiological performance of the pulmonary vascular smooth muscle, even
though a great deal of descriptive material is available regarding the ability of
smooth muscle to proliferate to produce pulmonary vascular medial hypertrophy. In the hypertrophied state, in a series of relatively uncomplicated
clinical diseases such as scoliosis or cystic fibrosis, the pulmonary circulation
retains its ability to dilate in response to humoral vasodilators or the relief of
hypoxia and to constrict when existing hypoxia is augmented or when hypoxia is freshly introduced [16,17]. The magnitude of the vasoactivity in
these abnormal circulations is illustrated by Figure 8, which demonstrates the
decrement in pulmonary arterial pressure which occurs with the relief of

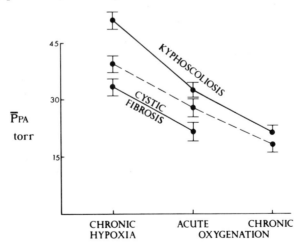

FIGURE 8   Decrease in pulmonary arterial pressure during acute or chronic
oxygenation following prolonged chronic hypoxia. For the kyphoscoliotic
group [16], oxygenation was produced acutely by 50% O_2 in N_2 for 20 min and
chronically by nasal O_2 for 2 weeks at 2 liters/min; the cystic fibrosis group received 100% O_2 for 20 min. The dashed line represents author's experience with
three cases of chronic obstructive pulmonary disease, for 1 month treated with
nasal O_2 at 2.5 liters/min.

hypoxia by high, inspired O_2 concentrations. In most cases, alterations in cardiac output were minimal and the bulk of the pressure decrease was attributable to acute pulmonary vasodilatation. The further decrements which occurred in pulmonary arterial pressure from 2 weeks to 3 months later during continuous O_2 supplementation also seem substantial. The mechanisms underlying this phenomenon, although of considerable clinical importance, are beyond the scope of this chapter, as are the effects of sea level or O_2 supplements on residents at high altitudes who have an abnormal pulmonary vascular bed.

Although hypoxic pulmonary vasoconstriction has been approached experimentally as a pulmonary arterial pressor response to generalized alveolar hypoxia, it was quickly realized that this phenomenon was an exceedingly effective controller of regional pulmonary flow down to even the smallest air sacs [82]. An underventilated air sac would have sufficient hypoxia (and hypercapnia with its synergistic effect) to minimize its own blood flow and thus restore toward normal the ventilation-perfusion balance of that region. Elevation of pulmonary arterial pressure, however, in response to generalized alveolar hypoxia, as it occurs at high altitude or in patients with alveolar hypoventilation, has been considered an entirely deleterious process, ending only in cor pulmonale. Nonetheless, generalized vasoconstriction and pulmonary arterial hypertension during hypoxia serve a significant purpose; more blood is delivered through relative dead space areas either at the top of the lung with respect to gravity or elsewhere [1,102]. The result during alveolar hypoxia is decreased dead space, decreased venous admixture, decreased alveolar-arterial PO_2 differences, and a consequently higher arterial PO_2 than might otherwise be obtained.

Thus, both local and generalized hypoxic pulmonary vasoconstriction can be regarded as useful adaptations. The disease entities where this mechanism is absent are even more illustrative of the importance of vasoactive control of regional pulmonary blood flow. One is hepatic cirrhosis, where chronic arterial hypoxemia and an absence of the pulmonary pressor response to hypoxia may occur simultaneously [103]. Whether cirrhotic patients are missing any crucial link in the complex stimulus-response circuit of the pulmonary vasoconstrictor response to hypoxia or whether some unidentified pulmonary vasodepressor, such as bradykinin or prostaglandin E, fails to be inactivated by a passage through a diseased liver and maintains a continuous state of pulmonary vasodilatation, is still uncertain. Another disease is familial dysautonomia, the hereditary defect of the autonomic motor system, as well as of many types of sensory and chemoreceptor structures [104]. In these patients, acute alveolar hypoxia induces a marked widening of the alveolar-arterial PO_2 difference [105]. In the light of present-day knowledge of pulmonary vascular mechanics, it may be deduced that alveolar hypoxia fails to elicit the pulmonary vasoconstrictor response and, in fact, bereft of its special mechanism for hypoxic vasoconstriction, this circulation dilates during hypoxia, the pulmonary arterial pressure falls, and, according to previously cited principles [1], the ventilation-perfusion balance worsens. Although the pulmonary mast cell and the neuroepithelial body and their ability to synthesize humoral agents in this entity have never been studied, the widespread sensory-receptor and motor-autonomic defects suggest a missing pulmonary vascular neuroreceptor. Although no such receptor has been anatomically demonstrated for the small pulmonary artery, this entity gives support to the idea that such a device may be discovered some day to regulate the pulmonary blood vessel. Thus, these two disease states may yield some clues to the essential links in what is no doubt a multistage process mediating hypoxic and hypercapnic-acidotic pulmonary vasoconstriction. Our present knowledge of this process suggests that no less than six stages for further experimental work may now be identified. These include (1) application of the stimulus to a special receptor; (2) release of a humoral agent and/or increased or decreased synthesis of agent; (3) diffusion of agent to arterial media; (4) activation of arterial smooth muscle receptors, and/or production of intracellular second messengers; (5) electrical activation; and (6) coupling with smooth muscle contractile mechanism (see Table 1). Identification of only the broad structure of these stages, even without a firm cellular or biochemical basis, may clarify the pathophysiology of diverse entities where vasoconstriction is carried too far, such as chronic respiratory diseases, high altitude, the noncardiac acute pulmonary edemas, chronic left heart failure, pulmonary embolism, and shock lung, as well as entities where hypoxic pulmonary vasoconstriction is not carried far enough, such as, perhaps, hepatic cirrhosis and familial dysautonomia.

V.   Summary

In summary, the pulmonary circulation is a low-pressure circulation, which is not completely without some tone. It has an extensive system of both adrenergic and histaminic receptors at the level of its vascular smooth muscle which are responsive to circulating humoral agonists, but there is very little evidence of moment-to-moment control by the autonomic nervous system. The chief controllers of regional blood flow appear to be alveolar hypoxia and, to a lesser extent, an agent synergistic to hypoxia, i.e., hypercapnic acidosis. Control by these agents persists in various cardiac, pulmonary, and vascular diseases, and, indeed in some, this control may not only dictate a generalized continuing vasoconstriction in this circulation, but also lead to proliferative changes in the pulmonary blood vessels which augment further pulmonary vascular resistance. For this reason, the intimate mechanisms underlying the pulmonary circulatory controls by hypoxia have received great attention and at present are considered to consist of a complex multistage process, probably centering around an as yet uncertain humoral mediator.

References

1. West, J. B., C. T. Dollery, and A. Naimark, Distribution of blood flow in isolated lung; relation to vascular and alveolar pressures, *J. Appl. Physiol.,* **19**:713–720 (1965).
2. Aviado, D. M., The pharmacology of the pulmonary circulation, *Pharm. Rev.,* **12**:159–239 (1960).
3. Fishman, A. P., Respiratory gases in the regulation of the pulmonary circulation, *Physiol. Rev.,* **41**:214–280 (1961).
4. Bergofsky, E. H., Mechanisms underlying vasomotor regulation of regional pulmonary blood flow in normal and disease state, *Am. J. Med.,* **57**:378–394 (1974).
5. Daley, R., The autonomic nervous system in its relation to some forms of heart and lung disease, *Br. Med. J.,* **2**:173–184 (1957).
6. Daly, I. deB., and M. deB. Daly, The effect of stimulation of the carotid body chemoreceptors on the pulmonary vascular bed in the dog, *J. Physiol. (London)*, **148**:201–222 (1959).
7. Szidon, J. P., and J. F. Flint, Significance of sympathetic innervation of pulmonary vessels in response to acute hypoxia, *J. Appl. Physiol.,* **43**: 165–171 (1977).
8. Cournand, A., The pulmonary circulation. In *Transactions of the Fourth Conference on Shock and Circulatory Hemostasis.* New York, Josiah Macy, Jr. Foundation, 1955, pp. 166–172.
9. Goldring, R. M., G. M. Turino, G. Cohen, A. G. Jamieson, B. G. Bass, and A. P. Fishman, The catecholamines in the pulmonary arterial pressor response to acute hypoxia, *J. Clin. Invest.,* **41**:1211–1221 (1962).
10. Silove, E. D., and R. F. Grover, Effects of alpha adrenergic blockade and tissue catecholamine depletion on pulmonary vascular response to hypoxia, *J. Clin. Invest.,* **47**:274–285 (1968).
11. Westphal, D., H. Kazemi, and C. Hales, Role of sympathetic nerves in alveolar hypoxic vasoconstriction, *Fed. Proc.,* **36**:611 (1977).
12. Aviado, D. M., *The Lung Circulation,* Vol. 1. London, Pergamon, 1965, Chap. 1, Table 1, p. 10.
13. Harris, P., and S. Heath, *The Human Pulmonary Circulation.* Baltimore, Williams & Wilkins, 1977, Chap. 9.
14. Eliahim, M., S. Stern, and H. Nathan, Site of action of hypertonic saline in the pulmonary circulation, *Circ. Res.,* **9**:327–332 (1961).
15. Williams, Jr., M. H., Pathophysiology and treatment of severe asthma, *N.Y. State Forum Med.,* **166**:2448–2452 (1973).

16. Bergofsky, E. H., G. M. Turino, and A. P. Fishman, Cardiorespiratory failure in kyphoscoliosis, *Medicine*, 38:263-325 (1959).
17. Goldring, R. M., A. P. Fishman, and G. M. Turino, Pulmonary hypertension and cor pulmonale in cystic fibrosis of the pancreas, *J. Pediatr.*, 65:501-524 (1964).
18. Hickam, J. B., and W. H. Cargill, Effect of exercise on cardiac output and pulmonary arterial pressures with cardiovascular disease and pulmonary emphysema, *J. Clin. Invest.*, 27:10-18 (1948).
19. Bicker, A., Computer aided non-linear modeling of the nonpulsatile aspects of the pulmonary circulation (thesis). New York University Graduate Division, 1973.
20. Bicker, A., E. H. Bergofsky, and F. J. Lupo, Non-linear mathematical simulator to predict pulmonary circulation behavior under complex conditions, *Fed. Proc.*, 33:671 (1974).
21. Ligou, J. C., and G. G. Nahas, Comparative effects of acidosis induced by acid infusion and CO_2 inhalation, *Am. J. Physiol.*, 198:1201 (1960).
22. Bergofsky, E. H., D. E. Lehr, and A. P. Fishman, The effect of changes in hydrogen ion concentration on the pulmonary circulation, *J. Clin. Invest.*, 41:1492 (1962).
23. Fishman, A. P., H. W. Fritts, Jr., and A. Cournand, Effects of breathing carbon dioxide on the pulmonary circulation, *Circulation*, 22:220-225 (1960).
24. Duke, H. N., E. M. Killick, and J. V. Marchant, Changes in pH of the perfusate during hypoxia in isolated perfused cat lungs, *J. Physiol. (London)*, 153:413-422 (1960).
25. Lloyd, T. C., The influence of blood pH on hypoxic pulmonary vasoconstriction, *J. Appl. Physiol.*, 21:358-364 (1966).
26. Malik, A. B., and B. S. L. Kidd, Independent effects of changes in H^+ and CO_2 concentrations on hypoxic pulmonary vasoconstriction, *J. Appl. Physiol.*, 34:318-323 (1973).
27. Rokseth, R., Effects of altered blood carbon dioxide tension and pH on the human pulmonary circulation, *Norwegian Monographs on Medical Science*. Oslo, Universitets forlaget, 1966.
28. Enson, Y., C. Giuntini, M. L. Lewis, T. Q. Morris, I. M. Ferrer, and R. M. Harvey, The influence of hydrogen ion and hypoxia on the pulmonary circulation, *J. Clin. Invest.*, 43:1146-1162 (1964).
29. Harvey, R. M., Y. Enson, R. Betti, M. L. Lewis, D. F. Rochester, and M. I. Ferrer, Further observations on the effect of hydrogen ion on the pulmonary circulation, *Circulation*, 35:1019-1027 (1967).
30. Rudolph, A. M., and S. Yuan, Response of the pulmonary vasculature to hypoxia and H^+ ion concentration changes, *J. Clin. Invest.*, 43:399-411 (1966).
31. Bergofsky, E. H., B. G. Bass, R. Ferretti, and A. P. Fishman, Pulmonary vasoconstriction in response to precapillary hypoxemia, *J. Clin. Invest.*, 42:1201-1215 (1963).

32. Aviado, D., *The Lung Circulation,* Vol. 1. London, Pergamon, 1965, Chap. 1, p. 3.
33. Haddy, F. J., and G. S. Campbell, Pulmonary vascular resistance in anesthetized dogs, *Am. J. Physiol.,* **172**:747–751 (1953).
34. Porcelli, R., A. Viau, M. Demeny, E. Naftchi, and E. H. Bergofsky, Relation between hypoxic pulmonary vasoconstriction, its humoral mediators and alpha-beta adrenergic receptors, *Chest,* **71S**:249–251 (1977).
35. Jamieson, A. G., Gaseous diffusion from alveoli into pulmonary arteries, *J. Appl. Physiol.,* **19**:448–452 (1964).
36. Staub, N., Gas exchange vessels in the cat lung, *Fed. Proc.,* **20**:107–109 (1961).
37. Aviado, D. M., Pulmonary venular responses to anoxia, 5-hydroxytryptamine and histamine, *Am. J. Physiol.,* **198**:1032–1036 (1960).
38. Duke, H. N., The site of anoxia on the pulmonary blood vessels of the cat, *J. Physiol. (London),* **125**:373–382 (1954).
39. Brody, J. S., E. J. Stemmler, and A. B. DuBois, Longitudinal distribution of vascular resistance in the pulmonary arterial capillaries and veins, *J. Clin. Invest.,* **47**:783 (1968).
40. Glazier, J. B., and J. F. Murray, Sites of pulmonary vasomotor reactivity in the dog during alveolar hypoxia and serotonin and histamine infusion, *J. Clin. Invest.,* **50**:2250 (1971).
41. Bergofsky, E. H., F. Haas, and R. J. Porcelli, Determination of the sensitive vascular sites from which hypoxia and hypercapnia elicit rises in pulmonary arterial pressure, from the Microcirculatory Society Symposium, April 16, 1968, *Regulation of Blood Vessel Tone. Fed. Proc.,* **27**:1420–1425 (1968).
42. Bergofsky, E. H., A study of the mechanism whereby hypoxia regulates pulmonary perfusion: Hypoxia and smooth muscle potentials. *Bull. Pathophysiol. Respir.,* **2**:297–309 (1966).
43. Porcelli, R. J., and E. H. Bergofsky, Adrenergic receptors in pulmonary vasoconstrictor responses to gaseous and humoral agents, *J. Appl. Physiol.,* **34**:483–488 (1973).
44. Aviado, D. M., *The Lung Circulation,* Vol. 1. London, Pergamon, 1965, Chap. 5.
45. Silove, E. D., and A. J. Simcha, Histamine-induced vasodilatation in the calf: Relationship to hypoxia, *J. Appl. Physiol.,* **35**:830–836 (1973).
46. Shaw, J. W., Pulmonary vasodilator and constrictor actions of histamine, *J. Physiol. (London),* **215**:34–35 (1971).
47. MacMillan, W. H., and J. R. Vane, The effects of histamine on the plasma potassium levels of cats, *J. Pharmacol. Exp. Ther.,* **118**:182–189 (1956).
48. Somlyo, A. P., and A. V. Somlyo, Vascular smooth muscle: Normal structure, pathology, biochemistry and biophysics, *Pharmacol. Rev.,* **20**:197–241 (1968).
49. Ash, A. S. F., and H. O. Schild, Receptors mediating some actions of histamine, *Br. J. Pharmacol.,* **27**:427–442 (1966).

50. Tucker, A., E. K. Weir, J. T. Reeves, and R. F. Grover, Histamine H-1 and H-2 receptors in the pulmonary and systemic vasculature of the dog, *Am. J. Physiol.*, **229**:1008–1013 (1975).

51. Black, J. W., W. A. M. Duncan, C. J. Durrant, C. R. Gannellin, and E. H. Parsons, Definition and antagonism of histamine H-2 receptors, *Nature*, **236**:385–390 (1972).

52. Flynn, S. B., and D. A. A. Owen, Vascular histamine receptors in the cat, *Br. J. Pharmacol.*, **52**:122P-123 (1974).

53. Altura, B. M., and B. T. Altura, Effects of local anesthetics, antihistamines and glucocorticoids on peripheral blood flow and vascular smooth muscle, *Anesthesiology*, **41**:197–214 (1974).

54. Porcelli, R., and E. H. Bergofsky, Histamine regulation by the lung, *Physiologist*, **20**(4):75 (1977).

55. Selye, H., *The Mast Cells*. Butterworth, Washington, D. C., 1965.

56. Porcelli, R. J., A. T. Viau, N. E. Naftchi, and E. H. Bergofsky, B-receptor influence on lung vasoconstrictor responses to hypoxia and humoral agents, *J. Appl. Physiol.*, **43**:612–616 (1977).

57. Gaddum, J. H., C. O. Hebb, A. Silver, and A. A. Swan, 5-hydroxytryptamine: Pharmacological action and destruction in perfused lungs, *Q. J. Exp. Pharmacol.*, **38**:255–270 (1953).

58. Braun, K., and S. Stern, Pulmonary and systemic blood pressure response to serotonin: Role of chemoreceptors, *Am. J. Physiol.*, **201**:369–373 (1961).

59. Vane, J. R., The release and fate of vasoactive hormones in the circulation, *Br. J. Pharmacol.*, **35**:209–222 (1969).

60. Hyman, A. L., W. C. Woolverton, D. G. Pennington, and W. E. Jacques, Pulmonary vascular responses to adenosine diphosphate, *J. Pharmacol. Exp. Ther.*, **178**:549–561 (1971).

61. Palaic, D., Effect of angiotensin on noradrenaline-^{3}H accumulation and synthesis in vivo, *Can. J. Physiol. Pharmacol.*, **49**:495–501 (1971).

62. Berkov, S., Hypoxic pulmonary vasoconstriction in the rat; the necessary role of angiotensin II, *Circ. Res.*, **35**:257–261 (1974).

63. Hales, C. A., and H. Kazemi, Failure of saralasin acetate, a competitive inhibitor of angiotensin II, to diminish alveolar hypoxic vasoconstriction in the dog, *Cardiovasc. Res.*, **11**:541 (1977).

64. Stalcup, S. A., J. S. Lipsett, R. Quenones, and R. B. Mellins, Inhibition of converting enzyme activity by hypoxia: Cardiovascular effects of circulating bradykinin in hypoxic dogs, *Am. Rev. Respir. Dis.*, **117a**:401 (1978).

65. Maxwell, G. M., R. B. Elliott, and G. M. Kneebone, Effects of bradykinin on the systemic and coronary vascular bed of the intact dog, *Circ. Res.*, **10**:359–363 (1962).

66. Hauge, A., Role of histamine in hypoxic pulmonary hypertension in the rat. I. Blockade or potentiation of endogenous amines, kinins, and ATP, *Circ. Res.*, **23**:371–383 (1968).

67. Weir, E. K., Does normoxic pulmonary vasodilatation rather than hypoxic

vasoconstriction account for the pulmonary pressor response to hypoxia? Hypothesis, *Lancet,* **232**:476–477 (1978).

68. Horton, E. W., Hypotheses on physiological role of prostaglandins, *Physiol. Rev.,* **49**:122–141 (1969).

69. Bergstrom, S., L. A. Carlson, and S. R. Weeks, Prostaglandins, *Pharmacol. Rev.,* **20**:1–37 (1968).

70. Said, S. I., S. Kitamura, and C. Vreim, Prostaglandins: Release from the lung during mechanical ventilation at larger tidal volumes, *J. Clin. Invest.,* **51**:83a (1972).

71. Okpako, D. T., The actions of histamine and prostaglandins $F_{2\alpha}$ and E_2 on pulmonary vascular resistance of the lung of the guinea pig, *J. Pharm. Pharmacol.,* **24**:40–50 (1972).

72. Ryan, J. W., R. S. Niemyer, and A. Ryan, Metabolism of prostaglandin $F_{2\alpha}$ in the pulmonary circulation, *Prostaglandins,* **10**:101–108 (1975).

73. Brocklehurst, W. E., The release of histamine and the formation of slow reacting substance (SRS-A) during anaphylactic shock, *J. Physiol. (London),* **151**:416–422 (1960).

74. Weir, E. K., A. Tucker, J. T. Reeves, and R. F. Grover, Increased pulmonary vascular pressor response to hypoxia in highland dogs, *Proc. Soc. Exp. Biol. Med.,* **154**:112–115 (1977).

75. Aviado, D. M., *The Lung Circulation,* Vol. I. Oxford, Pergamon, 1965, Chap. 6.

76. Bateman, M., L. A. G. Davidson, K. W. Donald, and P. Harris, A comparison of the effect of acetylcholine and 100% oxygen on the pulmonary circulation in patients with mitral stenosis, *Clin. Sci.,* **22**:223–231 (1962).

77. Behnke, R. H., J. F. Williams, Jr., and D. H. White, Jr., The effect of acetylcholine infusion upon cardiac dynamics in patients with pulmonary emphysema, *Am. Rev. Respir. Dis.,* **87**:56–62 (1963).

78. Bernstein, W. H., P. Samet, and R. S. Litwak, The effect of intracardiac acetylcholine infusion upon right heart dynamics in patients with rheumatic heart disease studied during exercise, *Am. Heart J.,* **63**:86–91 (1962).

79. Charms, B. L., Primary pulmonary hypertension. Effect of unilateral pulmonary artery occlusion and infusion of acetylcholine, *Am. J. Cardiol.,* **8**:94–99 (1961).

80. Fritts, Jr., H. W., P. Harris, R. H. Clauss, J. E. Odell, and A. Cournand, The effect of acetylcholine on the human pulmonary circulation under normal and hypoxic conditions, *J. Clin. Invest.,* **37**:99 (1958).

81. Bianchi, A., and G. R. de Vleeschower, Effect of various pharmacological compounds on the vagal induced lung constriction, *Arch. Intern. Pharmacodyn. Ther.,* **135**:472–480 (1962).

82. Liljestrand, G., Chemical control of the distribution of the pulmonary blood flow, *Acta Physiol. Scand.,* **44**:216–221 (1958).

83. Bergofsky, E. H., and S. Holtzman, A study of the mechanism involved in the pulmonary arterial pressor response to hypoxia, *Circ. Res.,* **20**:506–519 (1967).

84.   Lloyd, Jr., T. C., Influence of PO_2 and pH on resting and active tensions of pulmonary arterial strips, *J. Appl. Physiol.*, **22**:1101–1109 (1967).

85.   Bohr, D. F., and E. Uchida, Activation of vascular smooth muscle. In *Pulmonary Circulation and Interstitial Space.* Edited by A. P. Fishman and H. Hecht. Univ. of Chicago, 1969, pp. 133–142.

86.   Lloyd, T. C., Hypoxic pulmonary vasoconstriction: Role of perivascular tissue, *J. Appl. Physiol.*, **25**:560–565 (1968).

87.   Hauge, A., and N. C. Staub, Prevention of hypoxic vasoconstriction in the cat lung by histamine releasing agent 48/80, *J. Appl. Physiol.*, **26**: 693–699 (1969).

88.   Lauweryns, J. M., M. Cokelaere, and P. Theunynck, Serotonin producing neuroepithelial bodies in rabbit respiratory mucosa, *Science*, **180**:410–412 (1973).

89.   Haas, F., and E. H. Bergofsky, Role of the mast cell in the pulmonary pressor response to hypoxia, *J. Clin. Invest.*, **51**:3154–3162 (1972).

90.   Aviado, D. M., M. Samaneck, and L. E. Folle, Cardiopulmonary effects of tobacco and related substances. I. The release of histamine during inhalation of cigarette smoke and anoxemia in the heart-lung and intact dog preparation, *Arch. Environ. Health*, **12**:705–711 (1966).

91.   Sussmano, A., and R. A. Carleton, Effect of antihistaminic drugs on hypoxic pulmonary hypertension, *Am. J. Cardiol.*, **31**:718–723 (1973).

92.   Kay, J. M., J. C. Waymine, and R. F. Grover, Lung mast cell hyperplasia and histamine forming capacity in hypoxic rats, *Am. J. Physiol.*, **226**: 178–182 (1974).

93.   Mungall, I. P. F., Hypoxia and lung mast cells. Influence of disodium cromoglycate, *Thorax*, **31**:94–100 (1976).

94.   Sussmano, A., and R. A. Carleton, Prevention of hypoxic pulmonary vasoconstriction by chlorpheniramine, *J. Appl. Physiol.*, **31**:531–535 (1971).

95.   Hales, C. A., and H. Kazemi, Role of histamine in the hypoxic vascular response of the lung, *Respir. Physiol.*, **24**:81–88 (1975).

96.   Howard, P., G. R. Barer, B. Thompson, P. M. Warren, C. J. Abbott, and I. P. F. Mungall, Factors causing and reversing vasoconstriction in the unventilated lung, *Respir. Physiol.*, **24**:325–345 (1975).

97.   Dawson, C. A., F. A. Delano, L. H. Hamilton, and J. W. Stekiel, Histamine release and hypoxic vasoconstriction in isolated cat lungs, *J. Appl. Physiol.*, **37**:670–674 (1974).

98.   Brutsaert, D. L., Influence of reserpine and of adrenolytic agents on the pulmonary arterial pressor response to hypoxia and catecholamines, *Arch. Int. Physiol. Biochim.*, **72**:395–401 (1964).

99.   Tucker, A., I. F. McMurtry, R. F. Grover, and J. T. Reeves, Attenuation of hypoxic pulmonary vasoconstriction by verapamil in intact dogs, *Proc. Soc. Exp. Biol. Med.*, **151**:611–614 (1976).

100. Sylvester, J. T., and C. McGowan, The effects of agents which bind to cytochrome P-450 on hypoxic pulmonary vasoconstriction, *Circ. Res.*, **43**:429–437 (1978).

101. Fishman, A. P., Hypoxia on the pulmonary circulation: How and where it acts, *Circ. Res.,* **38**:221–231 (1976).

102. Haas, F., and E. H. Bergofsky, Effect of pulmonary vasoconstriction on balance between alveolar ventilation and perfusion, *J. Appl. Physiol.,* **24**:491 (1968).

103. Daoud, F. S., J. T. Reeves, and J. W. Schaefer, Failure of hypoxic pulmonary vasoconstriction in patients with liver cirrhosis, *J. Clin. Invest.,* **51**:1076 (1972).

104. Dancis, J., and A. A. Smith, Current concepts: Familial dysautonomia, *N. Engl. J. Med.,* **274**:207 (1966).

105. Filler, J., A. A. Smith, S. Stone, and J. Dancis, Respiratory control in familial dysautonomia, *J. Pediatr.,* **66**:509 (1965).

4

Mechanisms of Disease and Methods of Assessment

GABRIEL GREGORATOS
JOEL S. KARLINER
KENNETH M. MOSER

University of California, San Diego
School of Medicine
San Diego, California

I.   Classification

As is well-documented in this volume, a wide variety of pathophysiological
entities can induce abnormalities in the pulmonary vascular bed. If these abnormalities are extensive, they may lead to a final common event, namely,
pulmonary hypertension. This is the final hemodynamic expression of primary
pulmonary disorders ranging from chronic obstructive lung disease to interstitial fibrosis [1,2]. It is also a feature of many congenital and acquired
heart diseases, as well as such systemic disorders as lupus erythematosus and
scleroderma.

The physician attempting to define the basis of pulmonary hypertension
in a given patient, therefore, has a substantial list of differential diagnostic
possibilities. Indeed, he or she faces two separate challenges of significant
magnitude: (1) detection of the *presence* of pulmonary vascular disease; and
(2) pinpointing the specific location and cause of this vascular disease. These
are not tasks lightly undertaken, and, in their pursuit, it is useful to have some

TABLE 1   Pulmonary Vascular Diseases: A Pathophysiological Classification

Precapillary origin	Postcapillary origin
Pulmonary embolism (acute/chronic)	Left ventricular failure
Thromboemboli	Mitral valve obstruction
Septic emboli	Stenosis
Tumor emboli	Hypoplasia
Other types of emboli	Atresia
Pulmonary arterial thrombosis	Left atrial obstruction
Sickle cell disease	Cor triatriatum
Eisenmenger syndrome	Supravalvular stenosing ring
Tetralogy of Fallot, etc.	Thrombus
Primary pulmonary hypertension	Tumor
Idiopathic	Pulmonary venous obstruction
Toxic (aminorex fumarate)	Extrapulmonary veins: a. Normally connected (mediastinitis; tumor); b. total/partial anomalous connection
Pulmonary arteritis	
Polyarteritis	
Systemic lupus erythematosus	Intrapulmonary veins: pulmonary veno-occlusive disease
Scleroderma	
Schistosomiasis, etc.	
High altitude disease	
(hypoxic vasoconstriction)	
Persistent fetal circulation	
Intracardiac shunt lesions	
Left-to-right shunts	
Eisenmenger physiology	
Pulmonary parenchymal diseases	
COPD (emphysema/bronchitis)	
Bronchiectasis	
Pulmonary fibrosis of any cause	
(sarcoidosis; scleroderma; idiopathic)	
Skeletal thoracic defects	
Peripheral pulmonic stenosis	
Pulmonary arteriovenous fistulas	

framework to guide the diagnostic approach, i.e., some scheme for initial classification of pulmonary hypertension. Pathophysiologically, such a classification would include, classically, four types of pulmonary hypertensive vascular disease: obstructive or obliterative, vasoconstrictive, hyperkinetic, and passive [3]. However, as described elsewhere in this monograph, the pulmonary vascular bed responds, anatomically and physiologically, in a rather stereotyped manner to diverse forms of injury and stress. Thus, a vasoconstrictive element is present in many situations, including alveolar hypoventilation tion, high-altitude exposure, advanced mitral stenosis, and certain congenital heart diseases; i.e., it almost uniformly complicates the passive, hyperkinetic, and obliterative-obstructive types of pulmonary hypertension [1,4,5].

Therefore, a clinically more useful method of classifying pulmonary vascular diseases leading to pulmonary hypertension is to divide them into entities which are of "precapillary" or "postcapillary" origin. This provides a decision-making framework in which attention is focused on the question of the site of the *primary* abnormality. Table 1 lists the more common disorders leading to pulmonary hypertension according to this classification.

Naturally, no classification eliminates the need to recognize that overlap occurs because disorders which are initially purely postcapillary may be complicated by a precapillary component. For example, in advanced mitral stenosis—a clearly postcapillary entity—the initial passive pulmonary hypertension is often augmented by a variable degree of vasoconstrictive pulmonary hypertension. Similarly, in the patient with obstructive lung disease or the adult respiratory distress syndrome (precapillary entities), left ventricular failure may occur and contribute to the pulmonary hypertension [6–8].

Nevertheless, this distinction between precapillary and postcapillary serves the purpose of providing a framework for a logical approach to differential diagnosis. The remainder of this chapter is devoted to a discussion of the tools available to the clinician for the detection and classification of pulmonary vascular disease in humans. In reviewing these various diagnostic techniques, it should be recognized that the clinical detection of pulmonary vascular disease at an early stage is quite difficult, whereas the diagnosis of blatant pulmonary hypertension is easy. For example, obliteration of two-thirds of the pulmonary arterial bed by emboli or severe primary lung disease is required before significant resting pulmonary hypertension appears—a tribute to the substantial reserve capacity of the pulmonary vascular bed.

With this caveat expressed, it is appropriate that we begin this review of methods of assessment of the pulmonary vascular bed with the least costly, simplest, and most widely used approaches, namely, the history and physical examination.

II. Clinical Assessment

A. Primary Pulmonary Hypertension

The clinical manifestations of pulmonary vascular disease depend upon the
underlying etiology. Thus, patients with pulmonary hypertension secondary
to advanced mitral stenosis will present with the symptom complex of that
lesion, i.e., with progressive exercise intolerance and progressive effort dyspnea,
orthopnea, paroxysmal nocturnal dyspnea, and palpitations. If pulmonary hypertension is severe, chest pain may be included in this symptom complex. Similarly, the patient with pulmonary hypertension secondary to severe chronic obstructive pulmonary disease will complain of effort dyspnea, chronic cough,
chronic sputum production, recurrent respiratory tract infections, etc. [9].

The clinical picture of primary pulmonary hypertension will be reviewed
in some detail since this condition, despite its rarity, can serve as the prototype for many types of pulmonary vascular disease. The earliest symptom of
this insidious process is dyspnea on effort. The less advanced the vascular
disease, the more the effort required to induce dyspnea. The basis for this
effort dyspnea is not clear. It may be due to the increased ventilation man-
dated by an increased alveolar dead space, or it may result from reflex mechanisms originating in those lung zones rendered hypocapnic because of pulmonary artery obstruction. Whatever the basis for it, this effort dyspnea
easily (and often) is attributed incorrectly to poor physical conditioning.

As the disease progresses, other symptoms appear: easy fatigability,
dyspnea on modest effort or at rest, effort syncope, and angina pectoris. In
the composite series of primary pulmonary hypertension reported by Wood,
angina pectoris occurred in 20% of the patients and effort syncope in 43%
[3]. As the disease advances further, right ventricular failure supervenes and
right upper quadrant distress (due to hepatic engorgement and distension) and
peripheral edema develop.

The physical findings are related to the pulmonary hypertension, the
resultant right ventricular hypertrophy, the low cardiac output, and eventually
the development of right ventricular failure. Cyanosis is often present and is
usually peripheral in origin secondary to low cardiac output. Occasionally,
central cyanosis may be detected due to the development of a right-to-left
shunt through a patent foramen ovale. Similarly, the low cardiac output results in an arterial pulse of small volume but with a normal upstroke. At this
stage, examination of the jugular venous pulse consistently demonstrates a
giant a wave which often measures 5 to 10 cm above the jugular venous v
wave [3]. These findings are manifestations of the increased force of right
atrial contraction in an effort to provide maximum diastolic stretch of the

hypertrophied right ventricle. When right ventricular failure develops, the right atrium may also fail and the giant a wave may disappear leaving a dominant v wave in the jugular venous pulse. In this setting, functional tricuspid regurgitation will also be present, further contributing to the alterations of the jugular venous pulse.

Palpation of the precordium is both distinctive and helpful. The normally quiet (in adults) right ventricle will be palpated as a heaving systolic impulse along the left sternal border or in the subxiphoid epigastric region on full inspiration. With severe hypertrophy and dilatation of the right ventricle, rotation of the heart along its long axis may bring the right ventricle to occupy the cardiac apex. Consequently, the left ventricular impulse is not palpable. In over 50% of the cases, the pulmonary artery pulsation is palpable in the second left interspace along the left sternal edge. In the same location, pulmonic valve closure may be detected on careful palpation [3].

Careful auscultation of the heart will further confirm the diagnosis of pulmonary hypertension. Changes in the second heart sound are particularly characteristic and helpful. Recent studies, utilizing sophisticated intracardiac and intravascular micromanometry and phonocardiography [10], have shown conclusively that *normal* splitting of the second heart sound is related to the greater delay of the pulmonic incisura (pulmonic valve closure) compared to the aortic incisura (aortic valve closure) due to the longer interval separating the pulmonic incisura from the descending limb of the right ventricular pressure. This interval has been termed the "hangout time," and its duration probably reflects the compliance of the pulmonary vascular bed [10,11]. Thus, normally P_2 follows A_2. *Narrow* physiological splitting of the second heart sound due to an *earlier* pulmonic valve closure relative to aortic valve closure is a common finding in severe pulmonary hypertension [3,12]. Because of the increased amplitude and high frequency content of P_2 in pulmonary hypertension, splitting as narrow as 20 msec can be easily appreciated at the bedside, whereas in other conditions only a single sound would be heard. All patients with severe pulmonary hypertension demonstrate a marked reduction in the absolute value of the right-sided hangout time [10]. This is due to decreased capacitance and compliance of the pulmonary vascular bed, as well as the marked impedance to right ventricular ejection, which are present when significant pulmonary hypertension develops. As long as right ventricular performance is not compromised and right ventricular systole is not prolonged relative to left ventricular systole, narrow splitting of the second sound persists. When right ventricular failure develops, significant prolongation of right ventricular isovolumetric period and, therefore, right ventricular systole takes place and pulmonary valve closure is delayed relative to aortic closure. Consequently, *wide* splitting of the second sound occurs [13]. In summary, in the presence of severe pulmonary hypertension and relatively normal right ventricular function, P_2 is accentuated and S_2 is narrowly split. With the advent of right ventricular failure, wide splitting of S_2 develops.

Another distinctive auscultatory finding is a sharp, high-frequency, pulmonic ejection sound, usually detected over the dilated pulmonary artery in the second interspace at the left sternal border. A right-sided atrial diastolic gallop (S_4) is often present, usually heard best along the lower right or lower left sternal border. Accentuation of this S_4 on inspiration or during the Müller maneuver (inspiration against a closed glottis) confirms its right-sided origin. When right ventricular decompensation develops, a right ventricular diastolic gallop (S_3) may be appreciated and its right ventricular origin may be confirmed by similar maneuvers. In the composite series of 93 cases of primary pulmonary hypertension report by Wood [3], 40% of the patients demonstrated a Graham Steell's pulmonic regurgitation diastolic murmur along the upper and middle left sternal border. Loud systolic pulmonic ejection murmurs are rare. With progressive right ventricular dilatation and right ventricular decompensation, functional tricuspid regurgitation commonly develops. The murmur of tricuspid regurgitation classically is heard best along the lower left sternal border and over the xiphoid process. However, the holosystolic murmur of tricuspid regurgitation due to pulmonary hypertension may be heard well to the left of the sternum since the dilated right ventricle may occupy the entire anterior surface of the heart, including the cardiac apex. With the development of progressive right ventricular failure, signs of congestive hepatomegaly, ascites, peripheral edema, and pleural and pericardial effusions appear.

B.   Pulmonary Parenchymal Disease

The clinical recognition of pulmonary hypertension in the face of pulmonary parenchymal disease is difficult. All too frequently the clinical diagnosis of cor pulmonale is first entertained only after the right ventricle has failed and signs of systemic venous hypertension, congestive hepatomegaly, and peripheral edema are present [1]. Although cor pulmonale per se may require no treatment, there is an important reason for clinical interest in detecting pulmonary hypertension in this context before overt heart failure has set in; namely, it may allow early intervention, directed toward the underlying pulmonary disease. Unfortunately, the signs of both right ventricular enlargement and pulmonary hypertension are often obscured by the presence of pulmonary parenchymal disease, especially chronic obstructive pulmonary disease (emphysema, bronchitis) [9]. There are two reasons for this difficulty. (1) Patients with diffuse interstitial or parenchymal pulmonary disease tend to develop only moderate pulmonary arterial hypertension until late in the disease, when gas exchange becomes sufficiently deranged to cause significant hypoxia, with or without hypercapnia and acidosis [1]. (2) The hyperinflated lungs commonly seen in patients with chronic obstructive pulmonary disease tend to obscure the physical, as well as the electrocardiographic and roentgenographic, signs of right ventricular enlargement and pulmonary hypertension. Nevertheless, a careful clinical examination, even in the face of severe obstructive pulmonary disease, may be quite useful in alerting the clinician to the presence of pulmonary hypertension. Right ventricular enlargement should be looked for by seeking right ventricular pulsations in the subxiphoid region where they must be differentiated from pulsations of the abdominal aorta [9]. Similarly, auscultation of the heart in the epigastric area may disclose important heart sounds and murmurs detectable only in this region and not over the precordium. Assessment of the second heart sound is very important, and the optimal auscultatory area must be carefully looked for. Often, in cases of severe obstructive pulmonary disease, the second heart sound is heard best along the lower left sternal border and xiphoid process. Similarly, in the same setting, pulmonic systolic ejection sounds may only be heard along the xiphoid process in the epigastrium [14].

C. Pulmonary Embolism

Pulmonary embolism is recognized as a major factor contributing to the mortality and morbidity of hospitalized patients. It is covered extensively elsewhere in this monograph and will be dealt with quite briefly here. Recent studies employing radionuclide perfusion lung scans and selective pulmonary arteriograms as diagnostic screening tests suggest that fatal pulmonary embolism occurs in approximately 5 cases per 1000 inpatients and nonfatal pulmonary embolism in 20 per 1000 inpatients [15]. Diagnosis remains difficult, especially on the basis of clinical assessment alone. The prime requisite for the clinical diagnosis of acute pulmonary embolism is a high index of suspicion, particularly in those situations associated with high thromboembolic risk [16].

In terms of symptoms, almost every patient with pulmonary embolism complains of breathlessness of variable duration and severity, and most others complain of little else. The variable severity of dyspnea as a symptom is

TABLE 2   Physical Signs in Patients with Pulmonary Embolism from the Urokinase-Pulmonary Embolism Trial [17]

Tachypnea	88%
Rales	54%
↑ P_2	54%
Tachycardia > 100	43%
Temperature ≥ 37.8°C	42%
S_3 or S_4	34%
Associated thrombophlebitis	34%
Diaphoresis	33%
Arrhythmias	11%
Blood Pressure < 100 mmHg	3%
Wheezing	0%
Pleural Friction Rub	0%

probably related most closely to the extent of embolization; the mechanisms inducing dyspnea remain undefined (see Chapter 5). Pleuritic chest pain and hemoptysis are uncommon in patients without preexisting cardiopulmonary disease [15].

Table 2 lists the physical signs in patients with pulmonary embolism as reported in the Urokinase-Pulmonary Embolism Study [17]. (It should be noted that this study included only patients with extensive embolism, many of whom had preexisting cardiopulmonary disease.) The most consistent and reliable physical signs in their patient group were tachypnea and tachycardia which were almost always present. Like dyspnea, both may be transient [16]. Other physical findings which may result from bronchoconstriction and loss of surfactant include a localized decrease in breath sounds, expiratory wheezing, and fine atelectatic rales over the affected lung field.

With massive pulmonary embolism or preexisting lung disease, the cardiac findings of acute cor pulmonale may be detected. These consist of a right ventricular lift at the left sternal edge, a right ventricular diastolic gallop (S_3), a right atrial gallop (S_4), and a giant a wave in the jugular venous pulse. A systolic ejection murmur of "scratchy" quality may be heard along the upper left sternal edge. Findings relating to the second heart sound are variable. In the Urokinase-Pulmonary Embolism Study, an accentuated pulmonic component of the second heart sound was described in 54% of the patients. On the other hand, in the study of Miller and Sutton on acute massive pulmonary embolism, the pulmonic component was never thought to be louder than the aortic component of the second sound in the 18 patients in whom reliable observations of the second sound were made [18]. These findings probably relate to the fact that only modest pulmonary hypertension was recorded in these patients (pulmonary artery systolic pressures ranging from 32 to 45 mmHg). It has been suggested by these and other investigators that the acutely stressed right ventricle is unable to generate a pressure adequate to overcome resistance to ejection, so that the cardiac output is reduced and right ventricular mechanical systole is prolonged [18,19]. Wide, fixed splitting of the second heart sound results, indicating severely compromised right ventricular performance [16]. Contributing to the pattern of wide, fixed splitting of the second heart sound is early closure of the aortic valve as the left ventricular ejection time is reduced in the face of diminished venous return to the left heart.

An unusual, but characteristic, sign of pulmonary embolism is the development of a pulmonary artery stenosis murmur secondary to partial obstruction of a main branch of the pulmonary artery [20–22]. Such murmurs are usually systolic, although they may extend through the second heart sound. They have been described variously as maximal at the second to fourth left intercostal spaces, in the interscapular region, in the left or right subscapular region, and the right infraclavicular area. These murmurs have been described in cases of both acute and chronic thromboembolic occlusion of a major branch of the pulmonary artery. Disappearance or diminution of such murmurs, coincident with clot lysis or thrombectomy, has been cited as support of their proposed origin at the site of partial pulmonary arterial obstruction.

Tachycardia occurred in 43% of the 160 urokinase-pulmonary embolism patients [17]. Other rhythm disturbances, however, were distinctly unusual. Only 11% of the patients demonstrated premature atrial contractions, premature ventricular contractions, or atrial fibrillation. If only patients with preexisting cardiopulmonary disease were considered, the incidence of rhythm disturbances rose to 26%. Despite the low incidence of arrhythmias in documented pulmonary embolism, it has been suggested that atrial flutter is a frequent herald of pulmonary embolism and that this dysrhythmia, occurring without other clear-cut etiology, should initiate search for occult pulmonary embolization [23].

D. Peripheral Pulmonic Stenosis

Peripheral pulmonic stenosis is a congenital vascular malformation in which
there is narrowing of the main pulmonary artery, its bifurcation, or its primary
or peripheral branches [24]. In approximately two-thirds of the reported
cases, it is associated with other cardiovascular anomalies.

The clinical picture depends upon the degree of pulmonary arterial obstruction. Patients with mild to moderate bilateral pulmonary stenosis and
those with unilateral stenosis are usually asymptomatic. Effort dyspnea, easy
fatigability, and, eventually, symptoms of right ventricular failure may be seen
in patients with severe obstruction of either the main pulmonary artery or its
major branches. In such instances, the findings are those of central pulmonary artery and right ventricular hypertension as described in Section II.A.
However, subtle differences in auscultatory findings are present and help differentiate peripheral pulmonic stenosis from valvular pulmonic stenosis and
primary pulmonary hypertension [25,26]. The first heart sound is normal
and, in uncomplicated stenosis of the pulmonary artery or its branches, is
rarely associated with an ejection sound. A finding unique to this form of
pulmonary hypertension is that the pulmonic component of the second heart
sound is usually normal or is minimally increased in intensity. This is so
because, even in the face of significant peripheral pulmonic stenosis, the
diastolic pulmonary artery pressure is at normal or near-normal levels [25].
The second sound is usually physiologically split, with the width of the
splitting dependent upon the severity of the stenosis [26]. A systolic ejection
murmur of variable intensity is usually present at the upper left sternal border
and is unusually well transmitted to the axilla and the back. In multiple
peripheral pulmonic stenoses, long systolic or continuous murmurs may be
heard over both lung fields, the axilla, and the back, differentiating this condition from primary pulmonary hypertension.

E. Idiopathic Dilatation of the Pulmonary Artery

Idiopathic dilatation of the pulmonary artery is an uncommon anomaly that
has been ascribed to developmental defects in the pulmonary arterial elastic
tissue and to unequal division of the truncus arteriosus [25]. This usually benign condition is of interest primarily because it enters the radiographic differential diagnosis of an enlarged main pulmonary artery. The clinical picture
is usually that of an asymptomatic child or young adult with an abnormal
chest roentgenogram due to prominence of the main pulmonary artery segment. This condition may be complicated in some cases by organic pulmonic
regurgitation [25].

On physical examination the dilated main pulmonary artery may be visible and palpable in the second left intercostal space. However, there is no evidence of right ventricular overactivity, its absence differentiating this condition from pulmonary artery enlargement associated with pulmonary hypertension. On auscultation, a pulmonic ejection sound is frequently present in the second left interspace, along with a short midsystolic ejection murmur. The second heart sound varies from normal to widely split (because of increased capacitance of the dilated main pulmonary artery), and the pulmonic component may be prominent since the dilated main pulmonary artery trunk is relatively close to the anterior chest wall [27]. The clinical differential of idiopathic dilatation of the pulmonary artery from primary pulmonary hypertension or pulmonic valvular stenosis can be further aided by a recently described echocardiographic sign: fluttering of the pulmonic valve during systole [28].

F. Pulmonary Arteriovenous Fistula

Pulmonary arteriovenous fistulas are true congenital arteriovenous malformations found predominantly in the right and left lower lobes and the right middle lobe [29]. They are commonly noted as incidental radiographic abnormalities in healthy, asymptomatic, young adults. Their functional significance is that of a true right-to-left shunt, and central cyanosis may be observed if the shunt is of sufficient magnitude. It has been estimated that from one-third to three-fourths of patients with pulmonary arteriovenous fistulas also suffer from hereditary hemorrhagic telangiectasia (Rendu-Osler-Weber disease) [25]. In these cases, many of the peculiar central nervous system symptoms of vertigo, paresthesias, near syncope, visual and speech disturbances, and headaches are most likely related to the presence of intracerebral telangiectases and not to the hemodynamic burden of the pulmonary arteriovenous fistula.

Central cyanosis and clubbing are usually mild or absent when the right-to-left shunt is small, but may be impressive in the presence of a large shunt. In the presence of anemia due to bleeding from telangiectases, the cyanosis may be diminished or completely abolished [30]. Symptoms of dyspnea and fatigue are not common and appear later than cyanosis [25]. Heart failure has been reported in infancy [31], but is distinctly unusual since the hemodynamic load on the ventricles resulting from pulmonary arteriovenous fistulas is small to moderate [25]. Other symptoms include intermittent hemoptysis and recurrent bleeding from various sites secondary to the diffuse telangiectases. Hemothorax has been reported secondary to rupture of a fistula into the pleural cavity [32].

The most striking physical findings are those of the multiple telangi-
ectatic vessels which occur as clusters of small, ruby-red lesions on the face,
nasal and oral mucous membranes, tongue, lips, and cutaneous appendages of
the body. Awareness of the presence of these lesions may be the initial clue
to the diagnosis of an associated pulmonary arteriovenous fistula. As discussed above, cyanosis and clubbing depend upon the magnitude of the right-
to-left shunt. Because hemodynamic cardiac compromise is rare, the examination of the arterial pulse, jugular venous pulse, and the precordium are usually
unremarkable.

Auscultation of the chest is often helpful since the majority of pulmonary arteriovenous fistulas generate audible murmurs [25]. Frequently, these
murmurs are missed because they are faint and in unusual (nonprecordial)
sites. Since most fistulas are located in the lower lobes and the right middle
lobe, the murmurs are of maximal intensity over these lung regions [33]. The
intensity of the murmur depends upon the degree of shunting, and, since most
fistulas are relatively small, the murmurs are rarely of greater than grade III/VI
intensity. The murmurs may be either systolic or continuous [25]. An isolated diastolic murmur is rare. Since flow across the pulmonary arteriovenous malformation is dependent primarily on systemic venous return and
right ventricular output, the murmurs are altered by physiological maneuvers
which modify these parameters. For example, there is definite accentuation
of the systolic murmur on inspiration and during the Müller maneuver. A
murmur which is only systolic during quiet breathing may become continuous
during inspiration or during the Müller maneuver. Conversely, during the
Valsalva maneuver, the intensity of the murmur diminishes or may be abolished, coincident with the reduction of systemic venous return. Because of
the peripheral location of the murmur, the onset of the systolic murmur is
often delayed and the auscultatory impression of a late systolic murmur is
generated [34].

Since the capacitance of the pulmonary vascular bed in this condition is
normal or increased and the hemodynamic burden on the ventricles relatively
small, the second heart sound is usually physiologically split. Rarely, pulmonary hypertension develops in these patients for reasons not well understood
[35]. In this case, splitting of the second heart sound will be appropriately
modified, as discussed previously.

G. Pulmonary Venous Obstruction

Obstruction of the major (extrapulmonary) pulmonary veins occurs rarely
when the veins are normally connected. It is much more common with

anomalous pulmonary venous connection [36]. Anomalous connection is often associated with other developmental cardiac defects which dominate the clinical picture. Although these lesions are responsible for considerable infant mortality and morbidity, especially in the first few months of life, they also occur in older children and occasionally in adults. The clinical picture is one of pulmonary hypertension of postcapillary origin with radiographic evidence of interstitial or alveolar pulmonary edema. Detailed description of these lesions is beyond the scope of this monograph and is available in the excellent recent review by Glancy and Roberts [36].

Pulmonary veno-occlusive disease is a rare cause of postcapillary pulmonary hypertension which is characterized by severe narrowing and obstruction of the small intrapulmonary veins and venules [36–40]. Approximately 30 cases have been described in the world literature to date. Its basic etiology remains unclear. The mechanisms of obstruction include both organizing thrombi and proliferating connective tissue [40]. Wagenvoort believes that the obstructive lesions in pulmonary veno-occlusive disease are almost certainly thrombotic [38]. The inciting event is unknown, although many cases have been antedated by a febrile illness, causing speculation that an infectious agent, presumably a virus, may induce the disorder [39].

In contrast to primary pulmonary hypertension, pulmonary veno-occlusive disease appears to occur predominantly in young males [36]. The clinical picture is dominated by symptoms and signs of pulmonary arterial hypertension, with effort dyspnea being the most common early symptom [39]. Syncope and cyanosis occur late during the clinical course, with most patients dying within 2 years after onset of symptoms. Hemoptysis occurs rarely. The physical findings are those of primary pulmonary hypertension, and the diagnosis can be suspected by the chest roentgenogram which suggests a *postcapillary* origin of the hypertension. Interestingly, even cardiac catheterization often fails to distinguish between these two entities since the pulmonary artery wedge pressure is most often in the normal range in pulmonary veno-occlusive disease, presumably due to runoff of blood from the obstructed venules via collaterals [39,40]. Definitive diagnosis requires lung biopsy.

H. Central Shunts

Developmentally abnormal communications across the interatrial or interventricular septum or between the aorta and pulmonary artery result in abnormal shunting of blood between the greater and lesser circulations. The direction of shunting (left to right, or right to left) depends, in general, upon the relative pressures in the two communicating chambers. In the absence of other abnormalities, shunting is predominantly left to right since pressures in the greater circulation are higher than those of the lesser circulation. When right ventricular pressure exceeds that of the left ventricle, either due to the presence of increased pulmonary vascular resistance or right ventricular out-flow obstruction, shunt reversal through a ventricular septal defect will occur with resulting right-to-left shunting. Similar pathophysiological mechanisms govern directions of shunt flow at the atrial or great vessel level [25].

There are two reasons that central cardiac shunts are germane to a dis-cussion of pulmonary vascular disease. First, the presence of a shunt must enter the differential diagnosis of pulmonary vascular disease. Second, shunts exert definite influence on the pulmonary vascular bed. The radiographic dif-ferential diagnosis of left-to-right shunts is discussed below. The vascular responses to shunts are discussed in Chapters 1 and 5, and the clinical pre-sentations of these disorders are discussed in Chapter 8 and elsewhere [24,41].

III. The Chest Roentgenogram

The plain chest roentgenogram is a valuable tool for making the diagnosis of pulmonary vascular disease and defining its basis because a fairly good correlation exists between the roentgenographic findings and the physiological state of the pulmonary circulation [42–44]. Normally, the dependent zones of the lungs receive more perfusion than the apices in the upright position because of the relationships between pulmonary arterial, alveolar, and venous pressures [45]. Since alveolar pressure does not change from apex to base, while the vascular pressures rise due to hydrostatic effects, blood flow in the lung is gravity dependent. This tends to be reflected radiographically by dif-ficulty in visualization of upper lobe arteries in the erect position, while these vessels are progressively larger and easier to see in the midlung and bases [42]. On the plain film, the ratio of lower to upper lobe vessel caliber is 3:1 or 4:1 at locations equidistant from the pleural surface [43]. Changes in this rela-tionship in the upright posture are considered definitely abnormal [42–46]. This relationship holds only in the upright position and not for films taken in the supine position, a fact that deserves emphasis as it continues to be a source of some confusion. Similarly, during pulmonary arteriography per-formed with the patient in the horizontal position, the caliber of upper and lower lobe pulmonary vessels is normally equal.

Of additional help in assessing pulmonary hemodynamic status from the plain roentgenogram is the fact that upper lobe pulmonary *veins* are not commonly visible. In a study of 500 Army induction chest films, Milne [43] was able to clearly visualize pulmonary veins in only 30% of cases in the right upper lung field and 25% in the left upper lung field. When pulmonary venous hypertension is present, the upper lobe veins enlarge and become visible in almost all cases.

In general, different types of hemodynamic disturbances produce changes in the pattern of the pulmonary vasculature which are fairly characteristic [47]. It is useful to consider these radiographic changes under the categories of increased pulmonary blood flow, increased precapillary resistance, and increased postcapillary resistance.

Increased blood flow is typified by large, intracardiac left-to-right shunts (Fig. 1). Two characteristic changes are generally evident on the roentgenogram: first, the vessels of the upper zones become well perfused and visible in the upright position; second, there is distension and increase in caliber of the pulmonary vessels in all zones. These changes affect both arteries and veins. In the face of continued relatively normal pulmonary artery pressure, the pulmonary arterial tree retains the normal sharp, smooth vessel contours and the vessels taper normally and gradually from hilus to periphery. There is a rough correlation between the degree of enlargement of the hilar and peripheral vessels and the magnitude of the increased pulmonary blood flow [42,47]. For the changes described above to be readily apparent, the left-to-right shunt must exceed a pulmonic/systemic blood flow ratio of 2 [48].

Pulmonary arteriovenous fistulas decrease pulmonary vascular resistance and increase pulmonary blood flow. However, since pulmonary blood flow is directed primarily through the low resistance A-V fistula, the uninvolved pulmonary vessels are not engorged or distended. The fistulas are recognized on the roentgenogram as small nodules with large feeding arteries and draining veins [25].

Alterations in the pulmonary vascular pattern as a result of increased precapillary resistance are due to obstruction to flow, at the level of the major pulmonary arteries, the peripheral arteries, or the capillary bed [42]. Obstructions in these locations produce regional "oligemia" or "diminished vascularity" beyond the point of the lesion—as seen classically in pulmonary thromboembolism. Additionally, in cases of multiple peripheral pulmonic stenoses, poststenotic dilatation of the involved arteries may be seen [16,24-26,42].

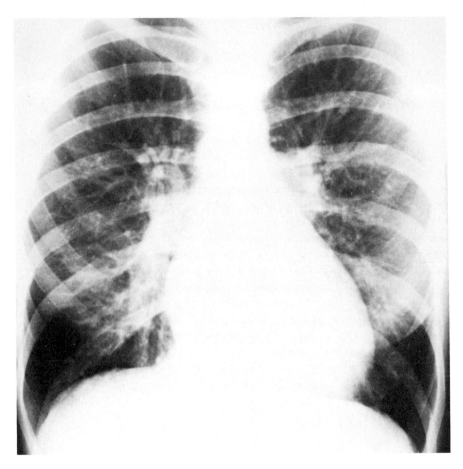

FIGURE 1   Chest roentgenogram, PA projection, 21-year-old female patient
with a large atrial septal defect and a 3.4:1 left-to-right shunt: Dilated central
pulmonary arteries and generalized engorgement of peripheral arteries and veins
are evident.

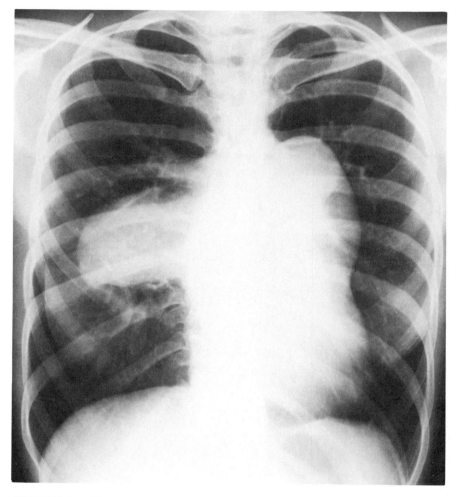

FIGURE 2 Chest roentgenogram, **PA** projection, 23-year-old female patient with a large atrial septal defect and Eisenmenger physiology. Remarkable aneurysmal dilatation of central pulmonary arteries is present associated with clear peripheral lung fields virtually devoid of vascular markings.

Increased resistance in the peripheral small pulmonary arteries occurs in primary pulmonary hypertension, pulmonary arteritis, Eisenmenger physiology, and pulmonary parenchymal disease. When pulmonary arterial hypertension is present, the roentgenogram shows marked dilatation of the central pulmonary arteries involving the main and right and left pulmonary artery branches. Constriction or obliteration of the mid- and peripheral-zone intrapulmonary arteries occurs, and, as a result, the peripheral lung fields appear relatively clear with sparse arterial and venous markings [42]. Generally, the largest central pulmonary arteries are seen in patients with severe pulmonary

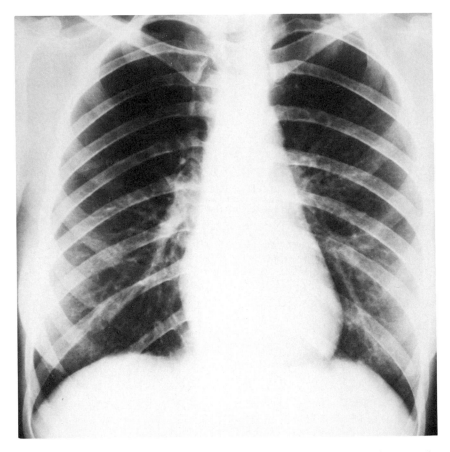

FIGURE 3   Chest roentgenogram, PA projection, 24-year-old female cyanotic patient, with common ventricle and severe pulmonary hypertension (PA pressure 104/52 mmHg): Both the cardiac silhouette and pulmonary vasculature appear normal!

hypertension superimposed on a previously large left-to-right shunt (Fig. 2). While radiographic indices have been developed [49] which correlate the size of the proximal pulmonary arteries with the presence or absence of pulmonary hypertension, these indices are not quantitatively reliable. Occasionally, severe precapillary pulmonary hypertension may exist with minimal dilatation of the central pulmonary arteries. This situation occurs especially in children with irreversible, severe pulmonary hypertension. One such case is illustrated in Figure 3.

Alterations in the chest roentgenogram as a result of increased *post-capillary* resistance to blood flow are seen in the conditions previously noted in Table 1. The typical changes resulting from elevated pulmonary venous pressure involve a redistribution of regional pulmonary blood flow which can be detected readily in the upright film [42,44,46,47]. These changes consist of constriction of the pulmonary arteries and veins of the lower lobes, associated with dilatation of the upper zone arteries and veins [44]. The basis of these changes remains unknown, although various reflex mechanisms have been proposed [42,44,50,51].

The severity of pulmonary venous hypertension can be graded radiographically more accurately than precapillary pulmonary hypertension [52]. Mild venous hypertension, on the order of 12 to 18 mmHg, is manifested as constriction of the lower zone vessels and dilatation of the upper. Moderate venous hypertension levels, on the order of 18 to 25 mmHg, produces more marked caliber changes between the lower and upper zones and, usually, early signs of interstitial pulmonary edema. Severe venous hypertension, at levels above 25 mmHg, generally produces alveolar edema. The resultant pulmonary densities tend to clear more rapidly in the peripheral lung fields, thereby producing the well-known "butterfly" or "bat wing" distribution of pulmonary edema.

The diagnosis of pulmonary venous hypertension is aided by the presence of Kerley's lines [53]. Kerley's A lines are straight, unbranching lines, extending from the hila to the upper lung zones, and are most commonly seen in acute left ventricular failure. Kerley's B lines are far more specific for pulmonary venous hypertension. They are horizontal lines seen in the lower lung zones close to the costodiaphragmatic angles and perpendicular to the pleural surfaces (Fig. 4). These lines reflect the presence of edema-thickened interlobular septa. Kerley's C lines are rarely seen and are common in a variety of interstitial pulmonary fibrotic conditions [44]. In addition to Kerley's lines, interstitial pulmonary edema may cause a diffuse loss of translucency at the bases, peribronchial cuffing, and small lamellar pleural effusions [42,44].

Evaluation of cardiac chamber size is particularly useful in differentiating the etiology of postcapillary pulmonary hypertension. For example, in

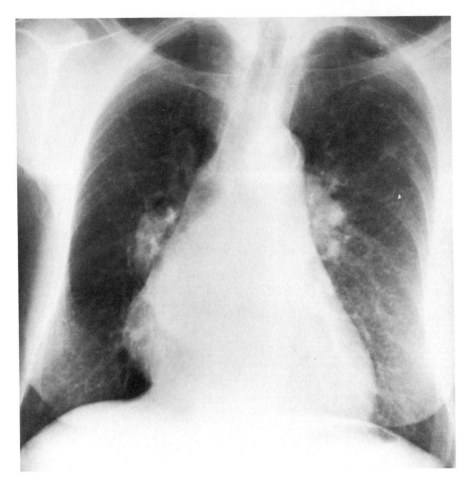

FIGURE 4   Chest roentgenogram, PA projection, 70-year-old female patient
with severe mitral stenosis. The cardiac silhouette is enlarged, and a double
density is seen representing the enlarged left atrium. The central pulmonary
arteries are dilated, and interstitial edema is present.

intrapulmonary veno-occlusive disease, signs of pulmonary edema with bilaterally increased interstitial marking and Kerley's B lines are frequently present. If,
with such findings, there are no signs of increased left atrial size, the diagnosis
of veno-occlusive disease should be strongly considered [55–57].

In evaluating pulmonary thromboembolic disease, the plain chest roentgenogram is neither sensitive nor specific [58]. (See Chapter 5.) The most
common chest roentgenogram in pulmonary thromboembolism is a negative

one [16]. During the urokinase-pulmonary embolism multicenter trial, the two most noteworthy radiographic findings were the presence of consolidation and elevation of the diaphragm on the affected side [17]. However, even these findings lose their specificity and diagnostic importance in patients with prior cardiopulmonary disease [14].

IV. The Electrocardiogram and the Vectorcardiogram

In considering the electrocardiographic diagnosis of right ventricular hypertrophy, it is useful first to understand the effects of this condition on the spatial vectorcardiogram. Because the vectorcardiogram itself is a three-dimensional construction of the instantaneous mean cardiac vector at any moment in time throughout the cardiac cycle, it is commonly displayed in 3 two-dimensional projections. For the purposes of considering right ventricular hypertrophy the horizontal plane is the most important. The horizontal plane is also the easiest to correlate with the standard precordial electrocardiographic leads, as can be seen in Figure 5. In this figure a normal, horizontal-plane vectorcardiographic loop is depicted and the projections of this loop on each of the precordial lead axes are also shown. The convention utilized is that a force moving *toward* the recording electrode produces a positive deflection on that lead axis while a force moving *away* from it produces a negative deflection. Thus, under normal circumstances, the major forces move in a counterclockwise fashion and produce progressively larger R waves across the precordium and progressively diminishing S waves.

In light of these considerations, the basis for the various patterns in right ventricular hypertrophy can be understood easily. Using the criteria of Chou and Helm [59], three types of right ventricular hypertrophy described by the vectorcardiogram can be defined (Figs. 6 through 8). In severe right ventricular hypertrophy, the horizontal loop is oriented rightward and anteriorly toward the anatomical position of the right ventricle; it is inscribed in a clockwise fashion (type A, Fig. 6). As can be appreciated, the predominant forces are directed toward the right precordial leads, and hence tall R waves will be inscribed in these leads. Prominent S waves will be inscribed in the lateral precordial leads. This pattern is often seen in congenital heart disease but can also be observed in acquired types of right ventricular hypertrophy such as those occuring in mitral stenosis.

With less severe right ventricular hypertrophy, there is less cancellation of the left ventricular forces. Thus, the vector loop is not oriented as far to the right and remains inscribed in a normal counterclockwise direction, as depicted in Figure 7 (type B). Under these circumstances, the electrocardiogram

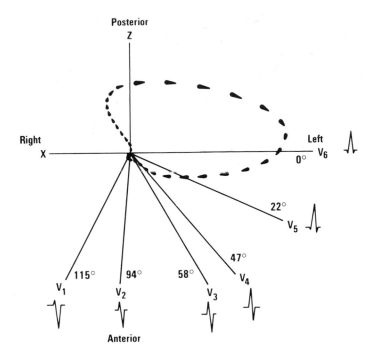

FIGURE 5   Normal horizontal plane vector loop with projections of the loop
on each of the precordial lead axes. Under normal conditions, the loop swings
initially anterior and to the right. (In this figure the heads of the "comets" indicate the direction of the loop.) As the loop turns, the major forces are directed
anteriorly and to the left and then posteriorly and to the left. The major leftward orientation, due to the normal dominance of the left ventricular muscle
mass, produces progressively larger R waves across the precordium and progressively diminishing S waves. (Modified after Chou, T. C., and R. A. Helm, *Clinical
Vectorcardiography*, New York, Grune and Stratton, 1967, p. 48.)

displays tall R waves in the right precordial leads, but usually shows a small
or no S wave in lead V_6. This type of pattern may be seen in any cause of
right ventricular hypertrophy.

The type C vectorcardiographic pattern, depicted in Figure 8, displays
forces which are initially inscribed in the normal fashion, but the remainder
of the loop is altered and displaced rightward and posteriorly. Under these
circumstances the electrocardiogram generally displays deep S waves in the
lateral precordial leads. This type of right ventricular hypertrophy is typically

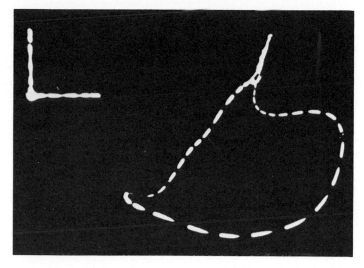

FIGURE 6 Type A right ventricular hypertrophy (horizontal plane). The initial forces are relatively normal, but the loop then swings further anteriorly and to the right as a result of predominant right ventricular forces.

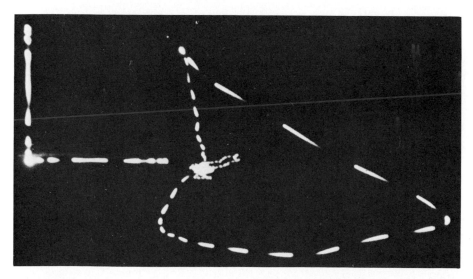

FIGURE 7 Type B right ventricular hypertrophy. The forces in the horizontal plane tend to remain predominantly anterior. In this example, more than two-thirds of the loop area is persistently anterior.

observed in patients with chronic obstructive lung disease but may also be seen in patients with mitral stenosis [60]. Presumably, this type of hypertrophy represents enlargement of the basal portion and outflow tract of the right ventricle. Because these areas of the right ventricle are posterior and are the last areas of the heart to be depolarized, only the terminal portion of the loop is altered and is oriented rightward and posteriorly.

All three types of right ventricular hypertrophy are usually associated with rightward deviation of the mean QRS axis in the frontal plane. Examples of these types of right ventricular hypertrophy in the scalar electrocardiogram are shown in Figures 9 through 11. Recently, Chou et al. suggested simple quantitative vectorcardiographic criteria for the diagnosis of right ventricular hypertrophy [61]. These include: (1) the anterior and rightward QRS loop area in the transverse plane is greater than 70% of the total; (2) the QRS loop area in the right posterior quadrant of the transverse plane is greater

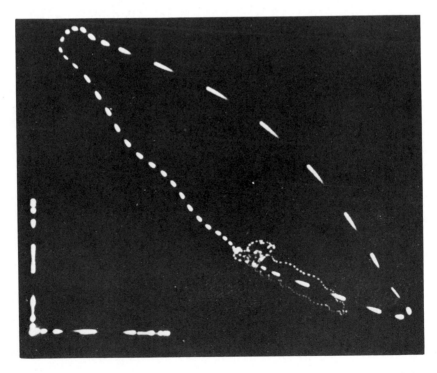

FIGURE 8   Type C right ventricular hypertrophy. The major portion of the loop in the horizontal plane is displaced posteriorly and to the right, presumably due to hypertrophy of the base and outflow tract of the right ventricle.

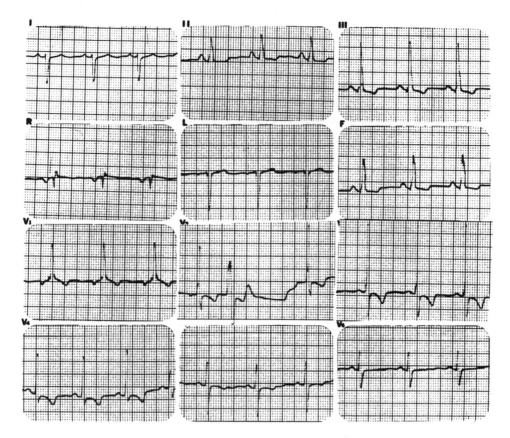

FIGURE 9   Electrocardiogram corresponding to type A right ventricular hypertrophy. The QRS axis in the frontal plane is rightward. There are tall R waves in the right precordial leads corresponding to the anterior location of the horizontal loop (see Fig. 6).

than 20% of the total; and (3) the QRS loop area in the right inferior quadrant in the frontal plane is greater than 20% of the total. Chou et al. reported that 80 of 97 patients (83%) with atrial septal defect, mitral stenosis, and chronic obstructive lung disease with pulmonary hypertension met one or more of these criteria. By contrast, the conventional electrocardiogram was suggestive of right ventricular hypertrophy in only 64 of these patients (66%).

A variety of scalar electrocardiographic criteria have previously been proposed for the diagnosis of right ventricular hypertrophy [62,63]. It should be emphasized, however, that many of these criteria were based on electrocardiograms obtained in patients with congenital heart disease. Employing these criteria and also applying the results of their own investigations to patients with cor pulmonale due to chronic obstructive lung disease, Kilcoyne and her associates proposed the following criteria for the diagnosis of cor pulmonale in the resting electrocardiogram [64]: (1) right axis deviation (> +90°), or, in serial records, the appearance of an axis shift of more than 30° to the right of the previous mean QRS axis shown; (2) R > S in lead V_{3R}, V_1, or aVR; (3) ST-segment depression in leads 2, 3, and aVF; (4) T-wave inversion or biphasic T waves in the right precordial leads; (5) abnormal R/S ratios in the left-sided V leads, i.e., marked leftward displacement of the transitional QRS complex (R = S) in the precordial lead sequence, with R < S in leads V_5 and V_6; and (6) P-wave voltage > 2.5 mm in the standard leads. However,

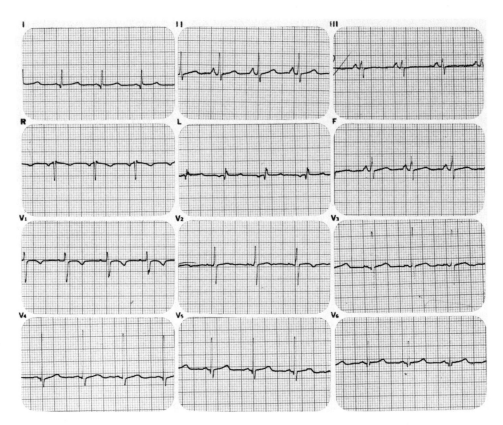

FIGURE 10   Electrocardiogram corresponding to type B right ventricular hypertrophy. In the right precordial leads the R waves are prominent but not so pronounced as in Type A. This record corresponds to the vectorcardiogram depicted in Figure 7.

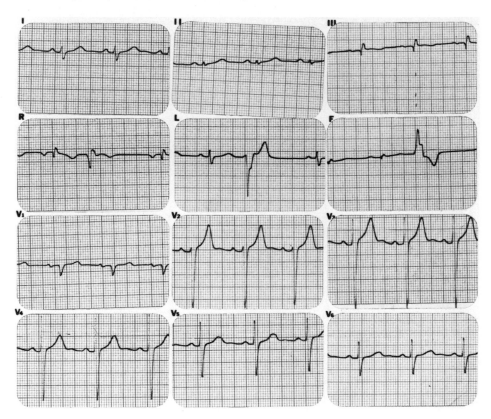

FIGURE 11 Electrocardiogram depicting type C right ventricular hypertrophy. The QRS axis in the frontal plane is rightward. There are deep S waves in the lateral precordial leads corresponding to the posterior and rightward displacement of the loop in the horizontal plane (Fig. 8).

with these criteria they reported that only 28% of 81 patients with cor pulmonale had right ventricular hypertrophy by electrocardiogram.

These investigators then analyzed certain fluctuations in the electrocardiogram which were correlated to variations in pulmonary insufficiency and evolved a dynamic electrocardiographic concept which they found useful in clinical management. These four fluctuations included: (1) a rightward shift of the mean QRS axis of 30° or more; (2) T-wave abnormalities in the right precordial leads; (3) ST depression in leads 2, 3, and aVF; and (4) transitory right bundle branch block. Fluctuations were seen when arterial oxygen saturation fell below 85% and the pulmonary artery mean pressure was 25 mmHg or greater. However, it should be pointed out that, depending on

the patient population studied, others have found the standard electrocardiographic criteria to be suggestive or diagnostic of right ventricular hypertrophy
in as many as 75% of patients having evidence of cor pulmonale [65].

It should also be noted that many patients with chronic bronchitis and
emphysema may exhibit left ventricular hypertrophy at necropsy [66]. The
most commonly associated diseases are hypertensive or arteriosclerotic heart
disease, or both. It would not be unexpected that patients with chronic obstructive lung disease might have combined ventricular hypertrophy. Such an
observation obviously applies also to patients with left-sided valvular lesions,
especially mitral regurgitation, who develop pulmonary arterial hypertension.
Thus, combined ventricular hypertrophy occurs in such individuals and at
times this may be difficult to distinguish from type C right ventricular hypertrophy by vectorcardiogram. Varriale and associates noted that the typical
horizontal loop in patients with combined ventricular hypertrophy was
counterclockwise with abnormal posterior displacement [67]. The initial
forces were always slightly anterior, either to the right or to the left. They
also observed that a significant S loop, usually involving either the entire
afferent limb or a substantial portion of afferent QRS loop, was present in all
cases. They also pointed out that it is difficult to distinguish between combined ventricular hypertrophy and cor pulmonale when the latter presents as a
posteriorly displaced counterclockwise horizontal loop. In cor pulmonale,
however, the afferent limb swings almost in a straight line, far posteriorly,
without a significant leftward extension. Furthermore, even when sophisticated
computer methods are applied to the diagnosis of biventricular hypertrophy
from the orthogonal electrocardiogram, such recognition is difficult [68].

In considering the differential diagnosis of tall R waves in the right precordial leads, the diagnosis of true posterior infarction often arises. Even if
vectorcardiograms are obtained under such circumstances, it is often difficult
to make this differentiation. Population samples show discrete differences,
but in the *individual* case this is often not possible [69]. At times it is also
difficult to distinguish the anteriorly oriented horizontal vector loop from the
normal [70]. Often the recognition of abnormal P waves (see below) along
with right axis deviation may be helpful in the diagnosis of right ventricular
hypertrophy when the transverse loop is predominantly anterior in location.
Under these circumstances, the presence of a superiorly oriented loop in the
frontal plane and significant Q waves in leads 2, 3, and aVf may help to make
the diagnosis of inferior and posterior wall myocardial infarction. Under all
these conditions, however, the history and physical examination of the patient
are often most helpful in making the proper diagnosis.

In many patients with pulmonary vascular disease, right bundle branch
block may coexist. In the presence of right bundle branch block, the type A

pattern of right ventricular hypertrophy is more common than is the type B [71]. In patients with right bundle branch block, the position of the afferent limb in the transverse plane can often be helpful, and Fedor and associates have suggested that it can be used to predict cardiac failure or severe pulmonary disease under these circumstances [71]. Recently, Chesler and associates have described a pattern resembling right ventricular hypertrophy in patients with constrictive pericarditis, and the latter must be added to the differential diagnosis of right ventricular hypertrophy [72]. In addition, "physiologic" right ventricular hypertrophy may occur in well-trained athletes [73].

Abnormal P waves also are seen in patients with pulmonary vascular disease. Pardee, in 1917 [74], and Berliner and Master, in 1938 [75], reported that tall P waves in leads 2 and 3 were found frequently in right atrial enlargement, and Kahn, in 1927, was the first to note such P waves in patients with chronic lung disease [76]. Various criteria have been employed for the diagnosis of "P pulmonale." These include a tall and peaked P wave with a height of 2.5 mm or more in leads 2, 3, and aVf and a P wave duration of 0.11 sec or less. Under normal circumstances, the P-wave axis in the frontal plane is approximately +45°; a more rightward orientation is associated with chronic obstructive lung disease [77]. However, these P-wave changes may not be related to right atrial size alone and the term "atrial abnormality" is more accurate in describing P-wave changes [78]. This concept has recently been suggested again based on the lack of correlation with abnormal P-wave morphology and left atrial size as recorded by the echocardiogram [79]. In addition, a "pseudo P pulmonale" pattern has been described by Chou and Helm in which an abnormality resembling P pulmonale may appear in patients with left atrial enlargement [80]. These authors speculated that enlargement of the left atrium, in the absence of a marked delay in intraatrial conduction, could result in an increase in the voltage of the middle and the late portions of the P wave without undue prolongation of its duration. Thus, the P wave would appear to be tall but have a normal duration and resemble the P pulmonale pattern.

In summary, the electrocardiogram and vectorcardiogram in patients with significant pulmonary vascular disease may display a number of characteristic abnormalities which can be correlated with the development of pathologic right ventricular hypertrophy. However, the sensitivity of these graphic methods is not great and it is necessary to combine them with other data to enhance their interpretation.

V. Systolic Time Intervals

Indirect measurement of the systolic time intervals (STI), and the left ventricular ejection time (LVET), have been used in patients with many

cardiac disorders to detect changes in left ventricular function. In patients
with pulmonary vascular disease it is often unclear whether pulmonary symptoms are due to left ventricular dysfunction or solely to lung abnormalities
with or without attendant right ventricular dysfunction.

Data obtained in several laboratories suggest that measurement of STI
may provide a noninvasive, yet sensitive, means for detecting depression of
left ventricular performance, particularly when applied serially in the individual patient [81–85]. It has been claimed that the STI can distinguish groups
of patients with decompensated left ventricular disease from normal subjects,
but such information is currently open to question. STI are *not* reliable for
separating patients with compensated heart disease from normal subjects,
either in the resting condition or during exercise [86]. Furthermore, the STI
can be influenced by a number of hemodynamic variables, several of which
may be operative in a given subject [87]. Thus, there is considerable controversy as to how accurately the STI reflects left ventricular performance in the
individual patient with cardiac disease [88].

The measurement of left ventricular STI requires a simultaneous recording of a high-frequency phonocardiogram, the indirect carotid arterial pulse
wave-form, and the electrocardiogram on a multichannel recorder at a paper
speed of at least 100 mm/sec. Under optimal conditions, the recordings are
obtained with the subject in the supine position and in the basal postab-
sorptive state. Calculation of the mean STI is based on the measurement of
at least 10 cardiac cycles beginning and ending with the same phase of
respiration.

As indicated above, a variety of alterations in hemodynamics influence
the STI. For example, an increase in the LVET (and its attendant measure
corrected for heart rate, the LVET-I) occurs when there is an increase in
stroke volume and an elevation in the left ventricular systolic pressure, and in
patients with hemodynamically significant aortic valve obstruction. A decrease
in the LVET occurs in patients with left ventricular failure, in individuals with
a decreased stroke volume, and when a positive inotropic drug is administered,
e.g., digitalis or isoproterenol. Unfortunately, in individual patients there may
be changes in several of these variables simultaneously with each change
having a different effect on the LVET. For example, the administration of
digitalis to a patient with left ventricular dysfunction and decreased stroke
volume would have two opposite effects on the LVET. The increase in stroke
volume resulting from the increase in inotropic state would increase the LVET,
while the increase in the velocity of contraction would tend to shorten it.

The left ventricular preejection period (PEP) is increased in the presence
of left ventricular failure, elevation in systemic diastolic arterial pressure,
diminished left ventricular filling pressure, negative inotropic influences, and
left ventricular conduction abnormalities. The PEP is decreased when the

systemic diastolic arterial pressure is diminished, when there is an increased left ventricular filling pressure and when drugs having a positive inotropic effect are administered.

As with the LVET, several simultaneous variables may affect the PEP. For example, in patients with cardiogenic shock, a high left ventricular end-diastolic pressure and a low aortic diastolic pressure result in a short PEP despite markedly depressed left ventricular performance. On the other hand, a normally or mildly elevated left ventricular end-diastolic pressure and a normal or elevated aortic diastolic pressure may be accompanied by appreciable prolongation of the PEP even if the inotropic state of the left ventricular myocardium is not depressed.

STI can be corrected for both heart rate and the patient's sex by using a regression equation derived from data on a large number of resting subjects without evidence of heart disease [81,82]. However, there are no equivalent data on the relationship of the STI to heart rate in normal subjects during supine and upright exercises. In the resting subject, the *ratio* of the PEP to the LVET varies within narrow limits and need not be corrected for heart rate or sex. Deviations of the various STI can be calculated using regression equations, as can the PEP/LVET ratio. In left ventricular failure the PEP lengthens, the LVET diminishes, and the duration of electromechanical systole remains unchanged. These altered relationships may be expressed as an increase in the PEP/LVET ratio during left ventricular failure. In the basal state, the normal ratio is 0.345 ± 0.036 (1 SD) [81,82].

Several studies have shown an inverse correlation between this ratio and the ejection fraction (stroke volume/end-diastolic volume) obtained by left ventricular cineangiography in patients with cardiac disease, but this relation does not hold well in patients with coronary artery disease [89]. We have found that serial measurements of STI are useful on occasion in following individual patients with coronary artery disease and for evaluating the effects of interventions such as coronary bypass surgery and propranolol therapy on left ventricular function [90].

In 58 patients with moderate to advanced obstructive lung disease, Hooper and Whitcomb reported significant prolongation of the PEP-I, a concurrent decrease in the LVET-I, and a significant increase in the PEP/LVET ratio [91]. They interpreted these data as indicating that subclinical left ventricular dysfunction is frequently present in such patients. Alpert and co-workers also demonstrated an alteration in left ventricular systolic time intervals in patients with chronic right ventricular failure [92]. They postulated a number of possible mechanisms for their findings, including (1) diminished left ventricular volume secondary to reduced stroke output from the failing right ventricle; (2) a relationship between left and right ventricular STI wherein the latter may be abnormal in patients with cor pulmonale (as has been demonstrated by echocardiography; see below); (3) actual alterations of contractile state of the left ventricle; and (4) a possible "reverse Bernheim phenomenon," i.e., septal encroachment on the left ventricular cavity.

The issue as to whether left ventricular performance is abnormal in patients with obstructive lung disease is not as yet completely resolved. With respect to the STI, however, it now appears that the left ventricular stroke volume frequently is reduced and this explains the decrease in left ventricular ejection times in patients with obstructive lung disease. Also, left ventricular filling pressures tend to be reduced in these patients and this may contribute to the prolonged preejection period index. Thus, the abnormalities in STI may simply reflect alterations in hemodynamic parameters without reflecting a direct depression of left ventricular inotropic state. In support of the latter contention is the observation that, in 28 patients with obstructive lung disease studied in our laboratory, the resting PEP was prolonged in 17 (65%) and the LVET-I was reduced ($<$ 408 msec) in 23 (88%) [8]. The PEP/LVET ratio was within the normal range in only 3 of 26 (12%). However, the resting mean pulmonary arterial wedge pressure was elevated in only four individuals and became abnormal with exercise in only three others. Furthermore, echocardiographic measurements of left ventricular function were normal in nine patients, seven of whom had one or more abnormal values for STI. These data suggest that reduced left ventricular filling results in abnormal values for STI in patients with obstructive lung disease. Therefore, STI values are *not* accurate indices of left ventricular performance.

It should be pointed out that both right and left ventricular systolic time intervals may be measured by echocardiography in children, in whom the pulmonary valve echogram can be readily obtained [93]. The technique, however, is not applicable to adults, in whom the pulmonary valve echogram usually cannot be measured in its entirety. Right ventricular systolic time intervals also may be assessed directly using invasive techniques, including the recording of high-fidelity pressures at cardiac catheterization. In patients with pulmonary hypertension, Curtis et al. reported that the interval between the onset of the Q wave and the pulmonic component of the second heart sound tends to remain within the normal range due to reciprocal changes in the isovolumic contraction and right ventricular ejection times [94]. Elevations of pulmonary artery diastolic pressure are associated with increases in the mean rate of isovolumic pressure rise. However, this change does not fully compensate for the widened ventriculoarterial diastolic pressure differences, and the isovolumic contraction time becomes prolonged. They also reported that factors other than stroke index depression may contribute to the decreased duration of the right ventricular ejection time, including tricuspid regurgitation and elevation of pulmonary vascular impedance.

VI. Radionuclide Techniques (Functional Studies)

It is now possible to assess ventricular function using radionuclide methods. It has been shown that, following an injection of a radioactive bolus, both right and left ventricular cavities can be imaged by using a gamma scintillation camera. The image data can be stored, together with the electrocardiogram, on magnetic tape and the left ventricle displayed selectively at end-diastole and end-systole. From these images, left ventricular end-diastolic and end-systolic volumes can be estimated using the area-length method and left ventricular ejection fraction calculated. More recently it has been shown that the ejection fraction can be obtained in a different manner, namely, by analysis of time-activity curves generated during the passage of the radioactive bolus through the left ventricle [95]. Assuming complete mixing of the radioactive tracer with the blood in the left ventricle, changes in count rate originating from this chamber during any cardiac cycle reflect changes in volume between systole and diastole. Thus, the fraction of end-diastolic blood volume ejected with each systolic contraction can be calculated from these data. Such techniques have been validated by comparison with left ventricular cineangiography [95,96].

In 120 patients with obstructive airways disease, this radionuclide technique was employed by Steele and associates to measure left ventricular ejection fraction [97]. Of 92 patients with acute respiratory failure, the left ventricular ejection fraction was normal in 60 and reduced in 32. Of the 28 patients with stable chronic obstructive airways disease, the ejection fraction was normal in 12 and reduced in 16 patients. Coronary artery disease contributed to a reduction in the ejection fraction in 18 of the patients with acute and seven of those with stable chronic obstructive airways disease. It was concluded from these data that the left ventricular ejection fraction is normal in patients with severe lung disease alone and that a reduced left ventricular ejection fraction in patients with chronic obstructive airways disease can be ascribed, in most instances, to concurrent coronary artery disease. There was no relation between the left ventricular ejection fraction and carbon dioxide or oxygen tension or arterial pH.

More recently we have developed a method for calculation of *right* ventricular ejection fraction by similar radionuclide techniques [98]. Right ventricular ejection fraction is obtained from the time-activity curves derived from the right ventricular blood pool in a manner similar to the calculation of the left ventricular ejection fraction. In 22 patients without evidence of cardiopulmonary disease, right ventricular ejection fraction ranged from 0.44 to 0.60 with a mean of 0.52 ± 0.04 (SD). Left ventricular ejection fraction in these patients ranged from 0.52 to 0.73 with a mean of 0.60 ± 0.06. Thus, right ventricular ejection fraction was moderately but significantly lower (p < 0.001). The ratio of the left to right ventricular ejection fraction was 1.17 ± 0.10 (range 1.00–1.38). This method has been applied to assess right ventricular ejection in patients with acute myocardial infarction in whom it was found that the right ventricular ejection fraction was reduced in individuals who had evidence of right ventricular infarction by [^{99m}Tc] (Sn)pyrophosphate myocardial scintigrams. The method is now being applied to the assessment of patients with obstructive airways disease. Berger et al. reported that patients with cor pulmonale and/or severe ventilatory impairment had reduced values for right ventricular ejection fraction [99]. This method appears to be a promising one, and it is hoped that it can be applied to serial studies of patients with obstructive airways disease for simultaneous evaluation of both left and right ventricular ejection fraction. In this manner it should be possible to assess the results of various interventions, including acute and chronic drug therapy, oxygen therapy, and the effect of rehabilitation programs.

VII. Echocardiography

The M-mode echocardiogram has proved to be exceedingly useful in the diagnosis of various forms of pulmonary vascular disease. Previously, in patients who had dyspnea as a major complaint without other obvious findings and without the murmur of mitral stenosis, it often was necessary to perform a cardiac catheterization to differentiate between primary pulmonary hypertension and occult mitral stenosis. Since the advent of echocardiography, this is no longer the case. A reduction in the mitral valve E-F slope plus demonstration of an enlarged left atrium, a thickened mitral valve, and anterior movement of the posterior mitral valve leaflet, all serve to make the diagnosis of mitral stenosis noninvasively. On rare occasions, patients whose symptoms mimic those of rheumatic mitral stenosis will have a left atrial myxoma producing mitral valve obstruction and pulmonary arterial hypertension. Often this diagnosis, too, can be made by routine echocardiography.

The echocardiogram also is useful in defining normal left ventricular function in patients with obstructive lung disease, as noted above. In other patients in whom left ventricular enlargement is suspected by chest X-ray, the echocardiogram can demonstrate whether left ventricular end-diastolic dimension is increased. However, it should be emphasized that it is often technically difficult to record satisfactory echocardiograms in patients with obstructive airways disease, and special transducer selection and placement may be necessary.

One feature of pulmonary arterial hypertension is paradoxical motion of the interventricular septum below its "hinge-point" [100]. Other echocardiographic features of primary pulmonary arterial hypertension have been summarized by Goodman et al. [101]. These included reduced diastolic slope of the mitral valve simulating mitral stenosis, with normal motion of the posterior leaflet; a large right ventricular dimension; and abnormal septal motion.

The pulmonary valve is technically one of the most difficult structures to record by ultrasound. The frequency of successful echo visualization of the pulmonary valve in experienced hands ranges between 20 and 50%, and this has been our experience as well. Considerably greater success is achieved in younger patients and in those with pulmonary arterial hypertension. The most common portions of the pulmonary valve usually recorded are the E-F slope, the A "dip," and the B-C slope. The remainder of systolic motion is not often seen except in patients with pulmonary arterial hypertension. In such patients, Nanda et al. [102] and Weyman et al. [103] have reported abnormalities in the E-F slope, the A wave of the pulmonary arterial tracing, the amplitude of pulmonary valve opening, and the presence or absence of midsystolic closure or fluttering of the pulmonic leaflet.

In a recent study in our laboratory, 19 patients with catheter-documented pulmonary arterial hypertension had adequate visualization of the pulmonary valve echocardiogram [104]. The data revealed that an A wave of less than 2 mm had a 69% sensitivity for the diagnosis of pulmonary arterial hypertension; a B-C slope of 450 mm/sec or greater exhibited 33% sensitivity; a B-C opening amplitude of 13 mm or greater, 45% sensitivity; a right ventricular preejection period of greater than 0.095 sec, 53% sensitivity; a right ventricular preejection period normalized for heart rate, 68% sensitivity; and the presence of midsystolic notching, a sensitivity of 38%. However, it should be emphasized that all six of these criteria are 100% specific for pulmonary arterial hypertension, although the sensitivities vary. In addition, the frequency with which the measurement can be obtained influences its applicability. Both the A wave and the right ventricular preejection period could be measured in all studies; the B-C slope, in 96%. Other parameters could be measured with decreasing frequency: B-C opening amplitude (44%); midsystolic notching was only seen in those pulmonary hypertensive patients with sinus rhythm (38%). Further, the E-F slope was highly variable and could not be routinely utilized in the assessment of pulmonary arterial hypertension from the echocardiogram [103].

As indicated earlier, right ventricular systolic time intervals can be measured from the pulmonary valve echocardiogram. Hirschfield et al. reported measurements of the right ventricular ejection time and the right ventricular preejection period in 45 normal subjects and in 64 patients with congenital heart disease who underwent cardiac catheterization. Increased pulmonary arterial diastolic pressure, augmented pulmonary vascular resistance, and elevated mean pulmonary arterial pressure resulted in an increased ratio of the right ventricular preejection period to the right ventricular ejection time [93]. Hirschfield et al. proposed that right ventricular systolic time intervals can be useful in the serial assessment of pulmonary arterial hypertension. However, it should be emphasized that this method is applicable primarily to children with congenital heart disease and is not practical in adults with various forms of pulmonary vascular disease.

VIII. Pulmonary Perfusion and Ventilation Scintiphotography

A. Perfusion Scintiphotography

Pulmonary perfusion scintiphotography (scanning) is an ideal, noninvasive method for studying the distribution of pulmonary blood flow. It has been well established that these radionuclide images faithfully reflect the distribution of pulmonary blood flow [105]. However, this is all the perfusion scan can do, i.e., demonstrate that the pulmonary blood flow distribution is normal or abnormal. If flow distribution is abnormal, this fact must be integrated with other clinical and laboratory data to define the *cause* for the abnormality.

Technical Considerations

The technique of perfusion scintiphotography warrants comment because technical errors can lead to serious misinterpretations. The agents used are rather well standardized. Macroaggregates of albumin or albumin microspheres are prepared in a size too large to traverse the pulmonary capillary bed [106]. Therefore, after intravenous injection, they lodge in the precapillary bed (transiently, because the albumin macroaggregates or microspheres dissociate over time). The particles can be radiolabeled with any one of several gamma-emitting radionuclides. The most popular currently is ^{99m}technetium.

The gamma "camera" is the imaging device which records the distribution of radioactivity (blood flow). The camera can record photographic images but also can, via magnetic tape and computer linkages, record digital information for later reproduction and quantitative analysis.

The position of the patient at the time of injection is a critical variable [107]. As noted elsewhere, pulmonary blood flow distribution is gravity dependent in the normal individual [108,109]. Therefore, injection in the erect position will result in images demonstrating increasing blood flow from apex to base—and perhaps perfusion "defects" in both apexes. Injection in the left lateral decubitus position will demonstrate reduced flow to the right (superior) lung and increased flow to the left (dependent) lung.

With injection in the supine or prone position, apex-to-base perfusion will be uniform, but on lateral scintiphotographs, a superior-to-inferior (front-to-back) gradient of flow will exist.

Applications to Detection of Pulmonary Vascular Disease: Detection of Regional Disease

Perfusion scintiphotography is an extremely sensitive technique for the detection of pulmonary vascular disease; indeed, it is possibly the most sensitive technique available. Very small vascular aberrations can be detected, aberrations that occur well before an overall increase in pulmonary resistance occurs.

As noted elsewhere in this monograph, three basic processes can alter the regional distribution of pulmonary blood flow: actual obliteration (destruction) of vessels, as in tuberculosis or emphysema; obstruction of vessels by embolic material; and vasoconstriction due to such factors as local alveolar hypoxia or hypercapnia.

Thus, the perfusion scan can detect blood flow alterations due to all the processes known to cause pulmonary vascular disease. The only requisite is that the vascular process be *nonuniform* in distribution. For example, exposure to high altitude (low inspired oxygen tensions) causes vasoconstrictive pulmonary hypertension but, because all arterioles are constricted, the lung scan will be normal. With this one caveat, the perfusion scan can detect regional flow decrements due to such diverse causes as embolism, emphysema (Fig. 12), thrombosis in the course of congenital heart disease (Fig. 13), pulmonary branch stenosis, the obliterative changes which occur early in the course of primary pulmonary hypertension, and vasoconstrictive changes due to pneumonia (Fig. 14) or bronchial obstruction (Fig. 15).

Detection of Pulmonary Hypertension

Beyond the detection of *regional* abnormalities, however, recent investigations suggest that perfusion distribution may assist in the detection of the presence of pulmonary hypertension and, further, definition as to its precapillary or postcapillary origin [110,111]. This application depends upon the fact that pulmonary hypertension alters the normal, gravity-dependent distribution of pulmonary blood flow. In precapillary pulmonary hypertension, due to the reduced capacitance of the pulmonary vascular bed, this gravity dependence is lost; that is, when the patient is injected in the erect position, there is a *failure* of the blood flow to shift toward the lung bases. There is a good

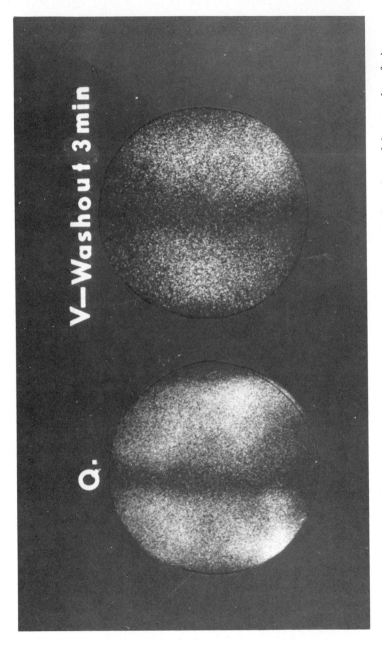

FIGURE 12 Perfusion scan (left) in patient with emphysema shows multiple regions of decreased perfusion. Ventilation scan (right) discloses multiple poorly ventilated zones which have failed to clear [133] xenon gas after 3 min of wash-out. Perfusion defects "match" ventilation defects.

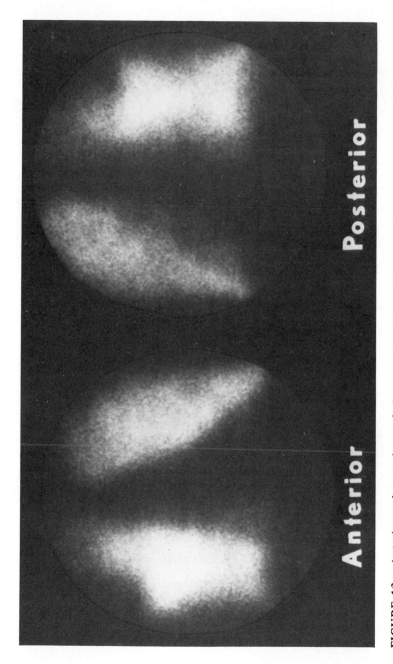

FIGURE 13 Anterior and posterior perfusion scans in patient with ventricular septal defect and pulmonary hypertension who developed multiple pulmonary arterial thrombi (emboli ?), confirmed by angiogram. Multiple perfusion defects are evident, largest in right upper lobe.

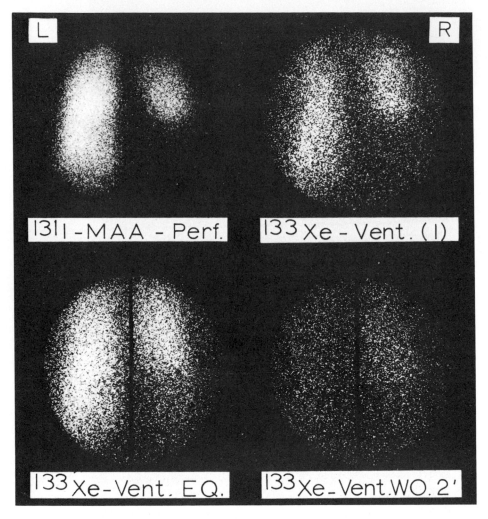

FIGURE 14   Patient with right lower and middle lobe pneumonia. There is no perfusion to these densely consolidated lobes (upper left) and no ventilation on first breath [133]xenon ventilation scan (upper right) after rebreathing to equilibrium (lower left), or during washout (lower right).

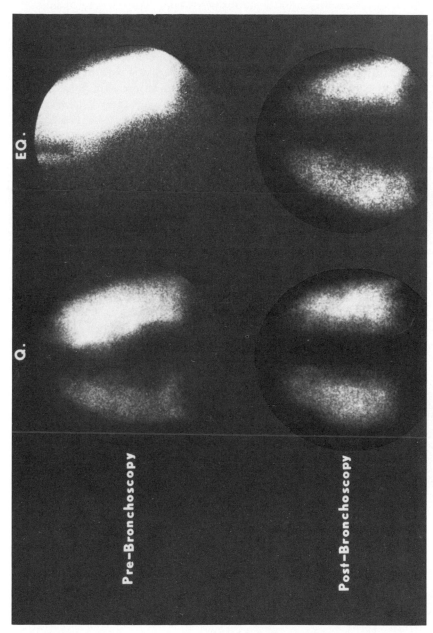

FIGURE 15 Patient with secretions blocking right mainstem bronchus. Before bronchoscopy, perfusion is markedly diminished (upper left) and essentially no ^{133}xenon is evident in the right lung on the equilibrium ventilation scan (upper right). After bronchoscopy, there is an increase in perfusion (lower left) and return of ventilation (lower right) to this lung.

correlation between the extent to which this failure to shift occurs and the magnitude of the pulmonary arterial pressure elevation. This "failure to shift" is quantified by computing an upper third/lower third (roughly apex/base) blood flow ratio.

However, when pulmonary venous hypertension exists, not only is there a failure to shift, but often there is an *upward* shift of blood flow in the erect position. As noted elsewhere in this chapter, this basal vasoconstriction has long been noted radiographically in some patients with pulmonary venous hypertension, particularly in those with mitral stenosis. This upward shift was documented by Friedman and Braunwald [112] in patients with mitral stenosis who showed an excellent correlation between the extent of the upward shift and the elevation of left atrial pressure. In our own studies of patients with postcapillary pulmonary hypertension we have found that all fail to shift perfusion downward in the erect position, but that the upward shift is an inconstant phenomenon. Patients with advanced mitral stenosis usually do demonstrate upward shift, but many with left ventricular failure as the basis for pulmonary venous hypertension do not. The reason or reasons for this difference are unknown.

B. Pulmonary Ventilation Scintiphotography

The ventilation scan permits visualization of the distribution of pulmonary ventilation. It is accomplished by having the patient inhale tracer amounts of a gamma-emitting radioactive gas. [133]Xenon and [127]xenon are the most widely used. Under the gamma camera, the wash-in and wash-out of the gas from the lungs is recorded as the patient breathes tidally. Zones of the lung which are abnormally ventilated are disclosed by observing either nonfilling (nonventilation) or slow wash-in or wash-out (diminished ventilation).

The major importance of ventilation scintiphotography in relation to the diagnosis of pulmonary vascular disease is that it allows differentiation between perfusion defects due to primary vascular disease and those due to primary parenchymal diseases [113,114]. Primary vascular disease (e.g., embolism) causes a perfusion defect, but ventilation in involved zones remains normal. Thus, a perfusion/ventilation "mismatch" results [113,114]. However, pulmonary parenchymal diseases (emphysema, fibrosis, infection) impair ventilation as well as perfusion. Therefore, ventilation and perfusion defects are "matched" [114].

Thus, mismatch of $\dot{V}$ and $\dot{Q}$ will be seen in such vascular diseases as embolism, pulmonary vasculidites in which medium- to moderate-sized arteries are involved (e.g., periarteritis), pulmonary artery agenesis, and branch stenosis.

On the other hand, $\dot{V}$ and $\dot{Q}$ both will be diminished (matched) in such disorders as emphysema, chronic bronchitis, interstitial fibrosis, pneumonia, and partial or complete bronchial obstruction (Figs. 12, 14, and 15).

Special Considerations

Even with the addition of ventilation to perfusion scintiphotography, proper interpretation of these tests requires simultaneous review of the chest X-ray. Such review is mandatory if simple interpretive errors are to be avoided.

Differentiation between perfusion defects due to obstruction and/or destruction of vessels and those due to vasoconstriction is possible if perfusion scans are repeated during intravenous infusion of a pulmonary vasodilating drug such as isoproterenol [115]. It also may be possible to differentiate between vasoconstrictive precapillary pulmonary hypertension and obstructive-obliterative hypertension by observing alterations in blood flow distribution in the erect position during pulmonary vasodilator infusion. This possibility, however, requires further investigation.

Finally, pulmonary perfusion scintiphotography is an extremely useful technique for serial follow-up of patients with known types of pulmonary vascular disease, e.g., to follow resolution rates of pulmonary emboli or alterations in blood flow distribution following cardiac surgery for congenital or acquired heart disease; to determine the reversibility of defects in emphysema-bronchitis after therapy; or to define the residual vascular impairment following infections such as tuberculosis or bacterial pneumonia.

IX. Cardiac Catheterization

Cardiac catheterization provides the definitive diagnosis in most cases of pulmonary vascular disease, particularly when combined with pulmonary angiography.

Since the early studies of Cournand and Ranges [116], Dexter et al. [117], and Zimmerman et al. [118], the technique of cardiac catheterization has advanced rapidly, and large numbers of such procedures are performed daily throughout the United States with minimal morbidity. The recent advent of balloon flotation catheters has added a new dimension to cardiac catheterization, especially in critically ill patients at the bedside [119].

Generally, in patients with pulmonary vascular disease, only catheterization of the right side of the heart is necessary. This is frequently combined with the insertion of an in-dwelling brachial artery needle for recording of arterial pressure, arterial blood sampling, and indicator dilution studies. However, when there is a question of coexisting disease of the left side of the heart, combined right and left heart catheterization is often necessary. Probe patency of the foramen ovale exists in 50% of individuals up to 5 years of age and in more than 25% over the age of 20 years [41]. In this case, catheterization of the left atrium and the left ventricle may be accomplished across the patent foramen ovale, obviating the need for retrograde left heart catheterization.

During a typical right heart catheterization in a patient with pulmonary vascular disease, the following data are obtained. (1) Pressures are recorded in the right atrium, right ventricle, main pulmonary artery, right and left main pulmonary artery branches, and from at least two pulmonary "wedge" locations. (2) Blood samples are obtained simultaneously from the main pulmonary artery and a systemic artery for blood gas analysis, including calculation of the arteriovenous oxygen content difference. Ideally, these samples should be obtained while the patient is in a near-basal condition, and they should be combined with expiratory gas collection to permit the calculation of oxygen consumption and cardiac output via the Fick principle. (3) If a left-to-right shunt is suspected, its presence is usually confirmed by an indicator dilution study. The most commonly employed indicator is the single-breath inhalation of hydrogen gas (H_2) and the detection of its appearance in the pulmonary artery by a platinum-tip catheter electrode. The introduction of ascorbic acid in a chamber distal to the location of the suspected shunt also serves the same purpose. Right-to-left shunts are diagnosed by the employment of other indicators, most commonly indocyanine green, by injection in the right atrium or right ventricle with sampling from a systemic artery through a densitometer. Cineangiographic procedures help visualize the location of the shunt and in many catheterization laboratories have supplanted indicator dilution curves. (4) If the presence of a shunt is confirmed by the indicator dilution procedure, quantitation is achieved by serial, rapid blood sampling from the right and left pulmonary arteries, the main pulmonary artery, the right ventricular outflow and inflow regions, the right atrium, the superior vena cava, the inferior vena cava, and a systemic artery. If a probe-patent foramen ovale is present, introducing the catheter into a pulmonary vein and obtaining a pulmonary venous blood sample completes this procedure. If a probe-patent foramen ovale is not present, the pulmonary venous hemoglobin oxygen saturation is assumed to be 95% in the awake patient breathing ambient air. The procedure is usually concluded with the performance of the necessary angiographic studies. Further details regarding catheterization techniques and calculation of data may be obtained from several excellent monographs [120,121].

Probably the two most important determinations obtained during right heart catheterization are the pulmonary artery pressure and the pulmonary wedge pressure. The pulmonary arterial pressure confirms or denies the presence of resting pulmonary hypertension. The wedge pressure assists in the differentiation between a precapillary and a postcapillary cause for the hypertension. Total pulmonary resistance may then be calculated by dividing the mean pulmonary artery pressure by the cardiac output; pulmonary arteriolar resistance, by subtracting the wedge pressure prior to division [120].

In general, severe pulmonary hypertension may be expected in patients with pulmonary veno-occlusive disease [122], severe mitral stenosis (mitral valve orifice area less than 0.7 cm^2), primary pulmonary hypertension, multiple or massive pulmonary emboli, and diffuse pulmonary arteritis [1]. Patients with chronic bronchitis and emphysema or diffuse interstitial pulmonary disease most often demonstrate moderate levels of pulmonary arterial hypertension until late in the course of their disease, when gas exchange abnormalities develop (see Chapter 6). Patients with large left-to-right intracardiac shunts, especially at the ventricular level, may demonstrate pulmonary arterial hypertension approaching systemic levels. However, since pulmonary blood flow may equal two or three times systemic blood flow, pulmonary arteriolar resistance may be only moderately elevated. The importance of these considerations in terms of operability is discussed in Chapters 1 and 8.

It is worth reemphasizing, however, that vasoconstriction of the pulmonary vascular bed must be considered before patients are rejected for surgery on the basis of an elevated pulmonary vascular resistance [120]. Additional maneuvers should be employed to help differentiate pulmonary vasoconstriction from fixed pulmonary vascular obstruction. These maneuvers have included the inhalation of 100% oxygen [123], and infusions of acetylcholine [124], tolazoline (Priscoline) [125,126], or isoproterenol (see Chapters 6-10). Failure of the pulmonary artery pressure and pulmonary vascular resistance to decrease with such maneuvers suggests the presence of fixed, obstructive vascular disease without a significant vasoconstrictive element [127].

The pulmonary artery wedge pressure is used widely, both in the catheterization laboratory and at the bedside, as an index of left atrial pressure. It is generally considered to accurately reflect mean left atrial pressure and, therefore, in the absence of mitral valve disease, to be a useful and reliable indicator of left ventricular diastolic dynamics [120]. However, it is well recognized that there are intrinsic limitations in interpretation of the pulmonary artery wedge pressure. Walstone and Kendall, in a retrospective analysis of 700 patients with various forms of cardiac disease, compared the pulmonary artery wedge pressure with the left atrial pressure measured directly by transseptal left atrial puncture [128]. An overall correlation coefficient of 0.93 was found. However, it was also found that scatter increased as the wedge and left atrial pressures rose. At mean wedge pressures above 25 mmHg, statistically significant differences ($p < 0.05$) were found between the pulmonary artery wedge and left atrial pressures. This progressive loss of correlation at higher levels may in part be explainable by the findings of Caro et al. [129]. They demonstrated in the experimental animal that high transcapillary pressures produced an alteration in the ratio of pulmonary arterial and pulmonary venous compliance, thereby promoting asymmetric transmission of pressure waves across the pulmonary vascular bed. Other investigators have recorded similar discrepancies between mean wedge and mean left atrial pressures and have recommended the employment of a correction factor [130], which, however, is rarely used in clinical practice.

In the presence of severe pulmonary arterial hypertension, a number of investigators have noted technical difficulties in obtaining a satisfactory pulmonary artery wedge wave-form [131-133]. The advent of flow-directed balloon-tip catheters has obviated some of these difficulties, although experienced observers note that phasic characteristics of wedge pressures obtained in patients with pulmonary hypertension may be suboptimal.

Patients with obstructive and fibrotic pulmonary diseases may demonstrate substantial alterations in pleural pressure during respiration which can influence the recorded absolute wedge pressure. Rice and coworkers [134] have recommended the use of the "effective pulmonary wedge pressure" to obviate this problem, i.e., the difference between the pulmonary wedge pressure and the simultaneous recorded esophageal pressure via an esophageal balloon. However, in ill and supine patients, even this approach presents technical and interpretive problems.

The authors of this chapter agree with the position of Kaplan [135], namely, that the pulmonary artery wedge pressure is usually a satisfactory approximation of the left atrial pressure although it is frequently affected by artifacts and respiratory variation. In our opinion, the clinical utility of the pulmonary artery wedge pressure is great. However, careful analysis of wedge pressures obtained in patients with pulmonary vascular disease, especially at the bedside, is essential, as is constant recognition of the pitfalls and problems of this measurement [136].

The pulmonary arterial end-diastolic pressure is also thought to reflect the mean left atrial pressure accurately, except in patients with preexisting pulmonary hypertension [120]. Investigations have indicated that a pressure gradient of 5 mmHg or less between pulmonary artery diastolic and mean pulmonary artery wedge pressure indicates normal pulmonary arteriolar resistance [137]. Whether, in fact, pulmonary artery end-diastolic pressure faithfully reflects left ventricular end-diastolic pressure is disputed by several investigators [138,139]. It is therefore necessary to ascertain the relationship between pulmonary arterial end-diastolic pressure and pulmonary wedge pressure in the individual patient before relying on the pulmonary artery end-diastolic pressure as a precise indicator of left atrial mean pressure.

The increased risk of cardiac catheterization in patients with severe pulmonary hypertension, particularly in the face of a low, fixed cardiac output, has been stressed by several investigators [41]. This is particularly true in patients with primary pulmonary hypertension [120]. There appears to be a significantly increased risk of a major vasovagal event leading to severe bradycardia and hypotension. Keane and Fyler [140] have reported the hazards of cardiac catheterization in children with pulmonary hypertension due to primary pulmonary vascular obstruction. During 30 catheterizations in 22 patients, five major and six minor complications were encountered. Three major complications consisted of sudden, severe bradycardia and hypotension, with one resulting death. In our experience, however, when cardiac catheterization is performed by an experienced operator, gently and expeditiously, the risks are minimized. We, therefore, do not withhold this important diagnostic procedure from any patient with severe pulmonary hypertension who requires it. This problem is further discussed in Section X.

Balloon flotation catheters carry the additional risk of injury to the pulmonary parenchyma [119]. The most common form of pulmonary injury is infarction secondary to persistent, undetected wedging of the catheter tip during long-term catheterization of the pulmonary artery. Other injuries have been reported, including a fatal intrapulmonary hemorrhage secondary to tear of a distal pulmonary arterial radicle by a balloon-tipped catheter in an anticoagulated patient [141].

Finally, it should be emphasized that hemodynamic measurements made only in the *resting* state may provide misleading information, particularly in the patient with early pulmonary vascular disease—either precapillary or postcapillary. For example, in the patient with early primary pulmonary hypertension or modest chronic pulmonary thromboembolic obstruction, right-sided pressures may be normal at rest and calculated resistance may be marginally elevated. However, with exercise augmentation of the cardiac output, significant pulmonary hypertension may appear. Similarly, handgrip or other forms of exercise may be required to elevate the wedge pressure in patients with borderline left ventricular function. Therefore, in the problem case, evaluation is incomplete (and may be misleading) unless observations are made during exercise.

Clearly, cardiac catheterization is the most definitive means for differentiating precapillary from postcapillary forms of pulmonary hypertension, a distinction which is critical to clinical decision making and often may not be possible on clinical grounds [8].

X. Pulmonary Angiography

The accumulated experience of the last 15 years has clearly documented that pulmonary arteriography is a valuable and safe procedure even in critically ill patients [142]. This procedure, particularly when the selective technique is

used [143,144], remains the most sensitive and specific diagnostic procedure
in detecting pulmonary emboli despite recent improvements in the specificity
of pulmonary ventilation-perfusion scanning techniques [145-147].

The technique of pulmonary arteriography has been adequately described
elsewhere [120,148-152]. Catheter introduction is accomplished via either an
incision and venotomy in the right or left antecubital fossa or percutaneously
(Seldinger technique) through the right femoral vein. A special pigtail catheter with a reverse curve has been developed to be used sprcifically in the percutaneous transfemoral approach [148]. However, most cardiologists and
radiologists continue to employ standard, closed-end, woven Dacron NIH or
Eppendorf catheters. Pulmonary arteriography should be combined with a full
hemodynamic study of the right side of the heart [120]. The argument that
obtaining hemodynamic data prolongs the procedure is not valid; in experienced hands, these data may be obtained rapidly with no increase in risk.
Filming may be carried out by serial cut films, or cineangiographic techniques.
Cineangiographic filming is preferable when the pulmonary angiogram is performed for reasons other than acute pulmonary embolism [120].

Originally, pulmonary angiography was carried out by injecting a large bolus
of radiographic contrast material in the main pulmonary artery and filming
the right and left hemithoraces simultaneously in the posteroanterior projection. More recently, selective injections in the right and left main pulmonary
artery branches [149], and even segmental [151] injections in lobar or segmental pulmonary arteries, have further extended the diagnostic capabilities of
this procedure. Segmental and selective injections offer several advantages
over main pulmonary artery injection. (1) There is less dilution of contrast
material during cardiac systole. (2) There is less loss of detail by overlapping
vessels. (3) Contrast material is injected directly into the vessel being examined, thereby avoiding diversion from the areas of embolization [151].
When examination of segmental or subsegmental pulmonary arterial branches
is required, magnification techniques can be employed to good advantage.

Pulmonary angiography is often performed in patients with primary pulmonary hypertension in an effort to exclude thromboembolic etiology. In
these cases, tortuosity and dilatation of the central pulmonary arteries is
demonstrable, along with uniform slowing of blood flow throughout all portions of both lungs. There is usually marked reduction in size and number of
peripheral vessels, and in most patients, discrete obstructions are not seen.
Abrupt tapering and a sparse branching pattern ("pruning") of pulmonary
arterial radicles are frequently present (Fig. 16).

In pulmonary veno-occlusive disease, the main value of the pulmonary
angiogram rests in excluding other causes of precapillary or postcapillary pulmonary hypertension [38]. In this condition, the pulmonary angiogram

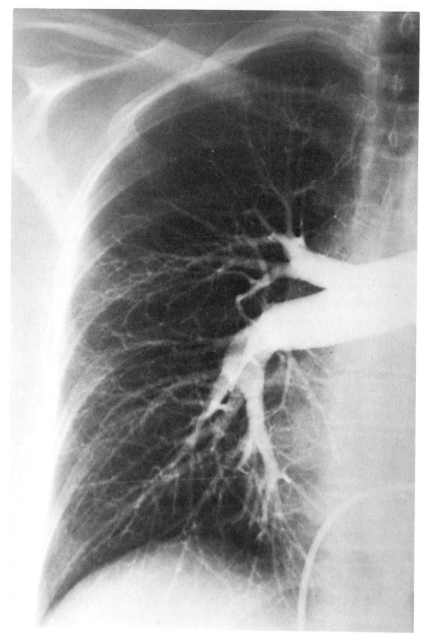

FIGURE 16   Selective right pulmonary arteriogram: Primary pulmonary hypertension in a 39-year-old female patient: The RPA and primary branches are dilated, with abrupt tapering and sparse branching of peripheral vessels.

demonstrates dilated proximal pulmonary arteries and slow pulmonary circulation similar to the findings in primary pulmonary hypertension [39,122].

Selective pulmonary arteriography, usually in the biplane mode, is the single most valuable diagnostic tool in peripheral pulmonic stenosis [41,153]. The extent, severity, distribution, and exact location of the lesions, along with presence or absence of poststenotic dilatation, can be well visualized. In some cases, selected oblique views may be necessary. If peripheral pulmonic stenosis coexists with other cardiac defects, delineation of the stenotic lesions becomes an important part of the preoperative assessment [154].

Pulmonary arteriography is also the definitive diagnostic procedure in cases of congenital pulmonary arteriovenous fistulas [155]. Because of the relative lower vascular resistance offered by the fistula compared to the unaffected portions of the pulmonary vascular bed, blood flow through the lesion is increased at the expense of the remaining pulmonary lobe or segment. As a result, angiographic visualization of the lesion is extremely simple because of preferential streaming of the contrast material through the fistula. Since multiple arteriovenous fistulas occur in perhaps 30% of patients, it is important that pulmonary angiography include both lung fields in their entirety.

In cases of chronic obliterative pulmonary vascular disease, pulmonary angiography is of little value in elucidating the underlying etiology. Generally speaking, the pulmonary vasculature appears similar in cases of chronic fibrotic upper lobe tuberculosis, postradiation fibrosis, schistosomiasis, etc. [156]. Furthermore, pulmonary arteriography does not distinguish between reduced vascularity due to obliterative anatomical changes as opposed to functional reductions in blood flow. However, pulmonary angiography remains an excellent technique for delineating the extent and severity of disease and helping plan pulmonary resection.

Pulmonary angiography is often employed as a "forward technique" in an attempt to visualize the large pulmonary veins, left atrium, and left ventricle [120]. In these cases, cineangiographic technique is preferable to static serial cut films. This forward technique is particularly useful in the diagnosis of congenital stenosis of the pulmonary veins, total and partial anomalous pulmonary venous return, and cor triatriatum. If a left atrial myxoma or left atrial thrombus is suspected, forward pulmonary angiography is the preferred technique to visualize the left atrium. It is generally agreed that catheterization of the left ventricle should not be undertaken in these cases because of the risk of precipitating systemic embolism.

Recently, pulmonary wedge angiography has been employed as a method to assess peripheral circulation in the lung in patients with parenchymal disease. It is performed by wedging an end-hold catheter and injecting a small amount of contrast material while filming. Normally, a distinct capillary

TABLE 3   Incidence of Complications of
Pulmonary Angiography [158]

Type of complication	Number
Cardiac perforation	3
Pyrogenic reaction	7
Arrhythmia	5
Bronchospasm	3
Pulmonary edema	1
Hypotension	1
Angioneurotic edema	1
Anaphylaxis	1
Shock	2

"blush" will be recorded. Schrijen and Jezek have concluded that the total or partial absence of the normal capillary blush when several wedge angiograms are performed in different locations represents a reduction in the pulmonary vascular bed [157].

Pulmonary angiography is a safe procedure with minimal morbidity. The complications occurring in 544 consecutive studies at the Peter Bent Brigham Hospital during the years 1964 through 1973 are listed in Table 3 [158]. It must be noted that the period during which these data were collected encompasses the early days of pulmonary arteriography. The three cardiac perforations all occurred during the first 100 cases. Complications related to the angiographic contrast material also have decreased in frequency with improvements in contrast media. In the face of primary pulmonary hypertension, all catheterization and angiographic studies carry an increased risk [120]. Main pulmonary artery injection of a large bolus of contrast material in such patients should be avoided. With the increasing reliance placed on selective and segmental pulmonary arterial injections, the risks associated with pulmonary angiography have been minimized.

References

1. Fishman, A. P., Chronic cor pulmonale, *Amer. Rev. Respir. Dis.,* **114**:775–794 (1976).
2. Heath, D., Pulmonary hypertension in pulmonary parenchymal disease, *Cardiovasc. Clin.,* **4**:79–96 (1972).
3. Wood, P., *Diseases of the Heart and Circulation,* 3rd ed. Philadelphia, Lippincott, 1968.

4. Ferrer, M. I., Cor pulmonale (pulmonary heart disease): Present day status, *Am. Heart J.,* **89**:657–664 (1975).
5. Reeves, J. T., and R. F. Grover, High altitude pulmonary hypertension and pulmonary edema, *Prog. Cardiol.,* **4**:99–118 (1975).
6. Davies, H., and H. R. Overly, Left ventricular function in cor pulmonale, *Chest,* **58**:8–14 (1970).
7. Burrows, B., J. J. Kettel, A. H. Niden, M. Rabinowitz, and C. F. Diener, Patterns of cardiovascular dysfunction in chronic obstructive lung disease, *N. Engl. J. Med.,* **286**:912–918 (1972).
8. Unger, K., D. Shaw, and J. S. Karliner, Evaluation of left ventricular performance in acutely ill patients with chronic obstructive lung disease, *Chest,* **68**:135–142 (1975).
9. Phillips, J. H., and G. E. Burch, Problems in the diagnosis of cor pulmonale, *Am. Heart J.,* **66**:818–832 (1963).
10. Shaver, J. A., R. A. Nadolny, J. D. O'Toole, M. E. Thompson, P. S. Reddy, D. F. Leon, and E. I. Curtiss, Sound pressure correlates of the second heart sound: An intracardiac sound study, *Circulation,* **49**:316–325 (1974).
11. Shaver, J. A., J. D. O'Toole, E. I. Curtiss, M. E. Thompson, P. S. Reddy, and D. F. Leon, Second heart sound: Role of altered greater and lesser circulation. In *Physiologic Principles of Heart Sounds Murmurs,* American Heart Association monograph 46. Dallas, American Heart Association, 1975.
12. Perloff, J. K., Auscultatory and phonocardiographic manifestations of pulmonary hypertension, *Prog. Cardiovasc. Dis.,* **9**:303–340 (1967).
13. Slodki, S. J., A. T. Hussain, and A. A. Luisada, The Q-II interval: III. A study of the second heart sound in old age, *J. Am. Geriatr. Soc.,* **17**:673–679 (1969).
14. Phillips, J. H., and G. E. Burch, Selected clues in cardiac auscultation, *Am. Heart J.,* **63**:1–8 (1962).
15. Sharma, G. V. R. K., and A. A. Sasahara, Diagnosis of pulmonary embolism in patients with chronic obstructive pulmonary disease, *J. Chron. Dis.,* **28**:253–257 (1975).
16. Moser, K. M., Pulmonary embolism, *Am. Rev. Respir. Dis.,* **115**:829–852 (1977).
17. The urokinase pulmonary embolism trial: A national cooperative study, *Circulation,* **47**:Suppl. II (1973).
18. Miller, G. A. H., and G. C. Sutton, Acute massive pulmonary embolism. Clinical and haemodynamic findings in 23 patients studied by cardiac catheterization and pulmonary arteriography, *Br. Heart J.,* **32**:518–523 (1970).
19. Shaver, J. A., and J. D. O'Toole, The second heart sound: Newer concepts. Part I: Normal and wide physiological splitting, *Mod. Conc. Cardiovasc. Dis.,* **46**:7–12 (1977).
20. Houk, V. N., C. A. Hufnagel, J. E. McClenatham, and K. M. Moser, Chronic thrombotic obstruction of major pulmonary arteries. Report on a case successfully treated by thrombendarterectomy and a review of the literature, *Am. J. Med.,* **35**:269–282 (1963).

21. Chertow, B. S., L. J. Hertko, and R. A. Carleton, Pulmonary artery stenosis murmurs, *Arch. Intern. Med.,* **121**:97–100 (1968).
22. Cohen, S. I., H. Hecht, J. Cantor, and E. Morkin, Flow murmur associated with partial occlusion of the right pulmonary artery, *Am. Heart J.,* **90**: 376–379 (1975).
23. Johnson, J. C., N. C. Flowers, and L. G. Horan, Unexplained atrial flutter: A frequent herald of pulmonary embolism, *Chest,* **60**:29–34 (1971).
24. Franch, R. H., and B. B. Gay, Jr., Congenital stenosis of the pulmonary artery branches, *Am. J. Med.,* **35**:512–529 (1963).
25. Perloff, J. K., *The Clinical Recognition of Congenital Heart Disease.* Philadelphia, Saunders, 1970.
26. Emmanouilides, G. C., Obstructive lesions of the right ventricle and the pulmonary arterial tree. Edited by A. J. Moss, F. H. Adams, and G. C. Emmanouilides. In *Heart Disease in Infants, Children and Adolescents,* 2nd ed. Baltimore, Williams & Wilkins, 1977.
27. Criscitiello, M. G., and W. P. Harvey, Clinical recognition of congenital pulmonary valve insufficiency, *Am. J. Cardiol.,* **20**:765–772 (1967).
28. Asayama, J., T. Matsuura, N. Endo, T. Watanabe, H. Matsukubo, K. Furukawa, and H. Ijichi, Echocardiographic findings of idiopathic dilatation of the pulmonary artery, *Chest,* **71**:671–673 (1977).
29. Anabtawi, I. N., R. G. Ellison, and L. T. Ellison, Pulmonary arteriovenous aneurysms and fistulas. Anatomic variations, embryology and classification, *Ann. Thorac. Surg.,* **1**:277–285 (1965).
30. Foley, R. E., and D. P. Boyd, Pulmonary arteriovenous aneurysm, *Surg. Clin. N. Am.,* **41**:801–806 (1961).
31. Hall, R. J., W. P. Nelson, H. A. Blake, and J. P. Geiger, Massive pulmonary arteriovenous fistula in the newborn; a correctable form of "cyanotic heart disease;" an additional cause of cyanosis with left axis deviation, *Circulation,* **31**:762–767 (1965).
32. Brummelkamp, W. H., Unusual complication of pulmonary arteriovenous aneurysm: Intrapleural rupture, *Dis. Chest.,* **39**:218–221 (1961).
33. Sahn, S. H., I. Bluth, and H. Schub, Pulmonary arteriovenous fistula, *Dis. Chest,* **44**:542–546 (1963).
34. Waldhausen, J. A., and H. B. Schumacker, Jr., Pulmonary arteriovenous fistulas, *Heart Bull.,* **14**:57–60 (1965).
35. Sperling, D. C., M. Cheitlin, R. W. Sullivan, and A. Smith, Pulmonary arteriovenous fistulas with pulmonary hypertension, *Chest,* **71**:753–757 (1977).
36. Glancy, D. L., and W. C. Roberts, Congenital obstructive lesions involving the major pulmonary veins, left atrium or mitral valve: A clinical, laboratory and morphologic survey, *Catheter and Cardiovasc. Diagnosis,* **2**:215–252 (1976).
37. Carrington, C. B., and A. A. Liebow, Pulmonary veno-occlusive disease, *Hum. Pathol.,* **1**:322–324 (1970).
38. Wagenvoort, C. A., Vasoconstrictive pulmonary hypertension and pulmonary veno-occlusive disease, *Cardiovasc. Clin.,* **4**:97–113 (1972).

39. Schackelford, G. D., E. J. Sacks, J. D. Mullins, and W. H. McAlister, Pulmonary venoocclusive disease: Case report and review of the literature, *Am. J. Roentgenol.,* **128**:643–648 (1977).

40. Chawla, S. K., C. F. Kittle, L. P. Faber, and R. J. Jensik, Pulmonary venoocclusive disease, *Ann. Thorac. Surg.,* **22**:249–253 (1976).

41. Moss, A. J., F. H. Adams, and G. C. Emmanouilides, *Heart Disease in Infants, Children and Adolescents,* 2nd ed. Baltimore, Williams & Wilkins, 1977.

42. Simon, R., The pulmonary vasculature in congenital heart disease, *Radiol. Clin. N. Am.,* **6**:303–317 (1968).

43. Milne, E. N. C., Correlation of physiologic findings with chest roentgenology, *Radiol. Clin. N. Am.,* **11**:17–47 (1973).

44. Basta, L. L., P. T. Lerona, and L. E. January, Physical and radiologic examination of the lung in the evaluation of cardiac disease, *Am. Heart J.,* **90**:255–264 (1975).

45. West, J. B., *Frontiers of Pulmonary Radiology.* New York, Grune & Stratton, 1968.

46. Meszaros, W. T., Lung changes in left heart failure, *Circulation,* **47**:859–871 (1973).

47. Simon, M., The pulmonary vessels: Their hemodynamic evaluation using routine radiographs, *Radiol. Clin. N. Am.,* **1**:363–376 (1963).

48. Fouche, R. F., W. Beck, and V. Schrire, The roentgenologic assessment of left to right shunts in atrial septal defects, *Am. J. Roentgenol.,* **89**:254–260 (1963).

49. Lupi, E., C. Dumont, V. M. Tejada, S. Hurwitz, and F. Galland, A radiologic index of pulmonary arterial hypertension, *Chest,* **68**:28–31 (1975).

50. Herles, F., J. Kolar, and J. Kozena, Regional activity of the lung vessels to minute changes in acidity of perfusing fluid, *Cardiovasc. Res.,* **6**:641–647 (1972).

51. Iliff, L. D., R. E. Greene, and J. M. B. Hughes, Effect of interstitial edema on distribution of ventilation and perfusion in isolated lung, *J. Appl. Physiol.,* **33**:462–467 (1972).

52. Simon, M., A. A. Sasahara, and J. E. Cannilla, The radiology of pulmonary hypertension, *Semin. Roentgenol.,* **2**:368–388 (1967).

53. Milhem, R. E., J. D. Dunbar, and R. W. Booth, The "B" lines of Kerley and left atrial size in mitral valve disease. Their correlation with the mean left atrial pressure as measured by left atrial puncture, *Radiology,* **76**:65–69 (1961).

54. Felson, B., The hila and pulmonary vessels. In *Chest Roentgenology.* Philadelphia, London, Toronto, Saunders, 1973.

55. Wagenvoort, C. A., Pulmonary venoocclusive disease. Entity or syndrome? *Chest,* **69**:82–86 (1976).

56. Scheibel, R. L., K. L. Dedeker, D. F. Gleason, M. Pliego, and S. A. Kieffer, Radiographic and angiographic characteristics of pulmonary venoocclusive disease, *Radiology,* **103**:47–51 (1972).

57. Liebow, A. A., K. M. Moser, and M. T. Southgate, Rapidly progressing dyspnea in a teenage boy, *JAMA,* **223**:1243–1253 (1973).

58. Moses, D. C., T. M. Silver, and J. J. Bookstein, The complementary roles of chest radiography, lung scanning and selective pulmonary angiography in the diagnosis of pulmonary embolism, *Circulation,* 49:179–188 (1974).

59. Chou, T. C., and R. A. Helm, *Clinical Vectorcardiography.* New York, Grune & Stratton, 1967.

60. Mershon, J. C., J. R. Medina, R. W. Evans, J. W. Edgett, J. M. Kioschos, F. W. Kroetz, and W. P. Nelson, Use of the vectorcardiogram to recognize right ventricular hypertrophy in mitral stenosis, *Chest,* 64:173–181 (1973).

61. Chou, T. C., M. P. Masangkay, R. Young, G. F. Conway, and R. A. Helm, Simple quantitative vectorcardiographic criteria for the diagnosis of right ventricular hypertrophy, *Circulation,* 43:1262–1267 (1973).

62. Meyers, G. B., H. A. Klein, and B. E. Stofer, The electrocardiographic diagnosis of right ventricular hypertrophy, *Am. Heart J.,* 35:1–40 (1948).

63. Sokolow, M., and T. P. Lyon, The ventricular complex in right ventricular hypertrophy as obtained by unipolar precordial and limb leads, *Am. Heart J.,* 38:273–294 (1949).

64. Kilcoyne, M. M., A. L. Davis, and M. I. Ferrer, A dynamic electrocardiographic concept useful in the diagnosis of cor pulmonale, *Circulation,* 52:903–924 (1970).

65. Dines, D. E., and T. W. Parkin, Some observations on the value of the electrocardiogram in patients with chronic cor pulmonale, *Mayo Clin. Proc.,* 40:745–750 (1965).

66. Murphy, M. L., J. Adamson, and F. Hutcheson, Left ventricular hypertrophy in patients with chronic bronchitis and emphysema, *Ann. Intern. Med.,* 81:307–313 (1974).

67. Varriale, P., R. J. Kennedy, and J. C. Alfenito, Vectorcardiogram of combined ventricular hypertrophy: Posterior counterclockwise loop (Frank system), *Br. Heart J.,* 31:457–461 (1969).

68. Gamboa, R., J. D. Klingeman, and H. V. Pipberger, Computer diagnosis of biventricular hypertrophy from the orthogonal electrocardiogram, *Circulation,* 39:72–82 (1969)

69. Mathur, V. S., and H. D. Levine, Vectorcardiographic differentiation between right ventricular hypertrophy and posterobasal myocardial infarction, *Circulation,* 42:883–894 (1970).

70. Ha, D., D. I. Kraft, and P. D. Stein, The anteriorly oriented horizontal vector loop: The problem of distinction between direct posterior myocardial infarction and normal variation, *Am. Heart J.,* 88:408–416 (1974).

71. Fedor, J. J., A. Walston, II, G. S. Wagner, and J. Starr, The vectorcardiogram in right bundle branch block, *Circulation,* 53:926–930 (1976).

72. Chesler, E., A. S. Mitha, and R. E. Matisonn, The ECG of constrictive pericarditis—Pattern resembling right ventricular hypertrophy, *Am. Heart J.,* 91:420–424 (1976).

73. Roeske, W., R. A. O'Rourke, A. Klein, G. Leopold, and J. S. Karliner, Non-invasive evaluation of ventricular hypertrophy in highly trained athletes, *Circulation,* 53:286–292 (1976).

74. Pardee, H. E. B., The electrocardiogram as an aid in the diagnosis of cardiac valvular disease, *JAMA,* **68**:1250–1252 (1917).

75. Berliner, K., and A. M. Master, Mitral stenosis: A correlation of electro-cardiographic and pathological observations, *Arch. Intern. Med.,* **61**:39–59 (1938).

76. Kahn, M. H., The electrocardiogram in bronchial asthma, *Am. J. Med. Sci.,* **173**:555–562 (1927).

77. Calatayud, J. B., J. M. Abad, N. B. Khoi, W. W. Stanbro, and H. M. Silver, P-wave changes in chronic obstructive pulmonary disease, *Am. Heart J.,* **79**:444–453 (1970).

78. Saunders, J. L., J. B. Calatayud, K. J. Schulz, V. Maranhao, A. S. Gooch, and H. Goldberg, Evaluation of ECG criteria for P-wave abnormalities, *Am. Heart J.,* **74**:757–765 (1967).

79. Josephson, M. E., J. A. Kastor, and J. Morganroth, Electrocardiographic left atrial enlargement. Electrophysiologic, echocardiographic and hemo-dynamic correlates, *Am. J. Cardiol.,* **39**:967–971 (1977).

80. Chou, T. C., and R. A. Helm, The pseudo P pulmonale, *Circulation,* **32**: 96–105 (1965).

81. Weissler, A. M., and C. L. Garrard, Jr., Systolic time intervals in cardiac disease – 1, *Mod. Conc. Cardiovasc. Dis.,* **40**:1–4 (1971).

82. Weissler, A. M., and C. L. Garrard, Jr., Systolic time intervals in cardiac disease – 2, *Mod. Conc. Cardiovasc. Dis.,* **40**:5–8 (1971).

83. Garrard, Jr., C. L., A. M. Weissler, and H. T. Dodge, Relationship of altera-tions in systolic time intervals to ejection fraction in patients with cardiac disease, *Circulation,* **42**:455–462 (1970).

84. Martin, C. E., J. A. Shaver, M. E. Thompson, P. S. Reddy, and J. J. Leonard, Direct correlation of external systolic time intervals with internal indices of left ventricular function in man, *Circulation,* **44**:419–431 (1971).

85. Ahmed, S. S., G. E. Levinson, C. J. Schwartz, and P. O. Ettinger, Systolic time intervals as measures of the contractile state of the left ventricular myocardium in man, *Circulation,* **46**:559–571 (1972).

86. McConahay, D. R., C. M. Martin, and M. D. Cheitlin, Resting and exercise systolic time intervals: Correlations with ventricular performance in patients with coronary artery disease, *Circulation,* **45**:592–601 (1972).

87. Ross, J., Jr., R. A. O'Rourke, K. L. Peterson, P. Ludbrook, M. H. Craw-ford, G. R. Leopold, J. S. Karliner, B. E. Sobel, and W. L. Ashburn, Non-invasive methods for the assessment of cardiac function, *Calif. Med.,* **119**: 21–37 (1973).

88. Perloff, J. K., and N. Reichek, Value and limitations of systolic time in-tervals (preejection period and ejection time) in patients with acute myo-cardial infarction, *Circulation,* **45**:929–932 (1972).

89. Eddleman, Jr., E. E., R. H. Swatzell, Jr., W. H. Bancroft, Jr., J. C. Baldone, Jr., and M. S. Tucker, The use of systolic time intervals for predicting left ventricular ejection fraction in ischemic heart disease, *Am. Heart J.,* **93**: 450–454 (1977).

90. Johnson, A. D., R. A. O'Rourke, J. S. Karliner, and C. Burian, Effect of

myocardial revascularization on systolic time intervals in patients with left ventricular dysfunction, *Circulation,* **40, 41** (Suppl. 1):91–96 (1972).

91. Hooper, R. G., and M. E. Whitcomb, Systolic time intervals in chronic obstructive pulmonary disease, *Circulation,* **50**:1205–1209 (1974).

92. Alpert, J. S., F. D. Rickman, J. P. Howe, L. Dexter, and J. E. Dalen, Alteration of systolic time intervals in right ventricular failure, *Circulation,* **50**:317–323 (1974).

93. Hirschfeld, S., R. Meyer, D. C. Schwartz, J. Korfhagen, and S. Kaplan, Measurement of right and left ventricular systolic time intervals by echocardiography, *Circulation,* **51**:304–309 (1975).

94. Curtiss, E. I., S. Reddy, J. D. O'Toole, and J. A. Shaver, Alterations of right ventricular systolic time intervals by chronic pressure and volume overloading, *Circulation,* **53**:997–1003 (1976).

95. Schelbert, H. R., J. W. Verba, A. D. Johnson, G. W. Brock, N. P. Alazraki, F. J. Rose, and W. L. Ashburn, Nontraumatic determination of left ventricular ejection fraction by radionuclide angiocardiography, *Circulation,* **51**:902–909 (1975).

96. Steele, P. P., D. van Dyke, R. S. Trow, H. O. Anger, and H. Davies, Simple and safe bedside method for serial measurement of left ventricular ejection fraction, cardiac output, and pulmonary blood volume, *Br. Heart J.,* **36**:122–131 (1974).

97. Steele, P., J. H. Ellis, Jr., D. van Dyke, F. Sutton, E. Creagh, and H. Davies, Left ventricular ejection fraction in severe chronic obstructive airways disease, *Am. J. Med.,* **59**:21–28 (1975).

98. Tobinick, E., H. Schelbert, H. Henning, M. LeWinter, and J. S. Karliner, Right ventricular ejection fraction assessed by radionuclide angiography in patients with acute and chronic ischemic heart disease, *Circulation,* **57**:1078–1084 (1978).

99. Berger, H. J., R. A. Matthay, J. Loke, R. C. Marshall, A. Gottschalk, and B. L. Zaret, Assessment of cardiac performance with quantitative radionuclide angiocardiography: Right ventricular ejection fraction with reference to findings in chronic obstructive pulmonary disease, *Am. J. Cardiol.,* **41**:897–905 (1978).

100. Hagan, A. D., G. Francis, D. Sahn, J. S. Karliner, W. Friedman, and R. A. O'Rourke, Ultrasound evaluation of systolic anterior septal motion in patients with and without right ventricular volume overload, *Circulation,* **50**:248–254 (1974).

101. Goodman, D. J., D. C. Harrison, and R. L. Popp, Echocardiographic features of primary pulmonary hypertension, *Am. J. Cardiol.,* **33**:438–443 (1974).

102. Nanda, N. C., R. Gramiak, T. I. Robinson, and P. M. Shah, Echocardiographic evaluation of pulmonary hypertension, *Circulation,* **50**:575–581 (1974).

103. Weyman, A. E., J. C. Dillon, H. Feigenbaum, and S. Chang, Echocardiographic patterns of pulmonic valve motion with pulmonary hypertension, *Circulation,* **50**:905–910 (1974).

104. Lew, W., H. Henning, H. Schelbert, and J. S. Karliner, Assessment of E-point septal separation as an index of left ventricular performance in patients with acute and previous myocardial infarction, *Am. J. Cardiol.*, **41**:836–845 (1978).

105. Tisi, G. M., G. A. Landis, A. Miale, Jr., and K. M. Moser, Quantitation of regional pulmonary blood flow: Validity and potential sources of error, *Am. Rev. Respir. Dis.*, **97**:843–850 (1968).

106. Taplin, G. V., E. K. Dore, D. E. Johnson, and H. S. Kaplan, Suspension of radioalbumen aggregates for photoscanning of the liver, spleen, lungs and other organs, *J. Nucl. Med.*, **5**:259–275 (1964).

107. Moser, K. M., and A. Miale, Jr., Interpretive pitfalls in lung photoscanning, *Am. J. Med.*, **44**:366–376 (1968).

108. West, J. B., *Ventilation/Blood Flow and Gas Exchange.* Oxford, Blackwell, 1965.

109. Kaneko, K., J. Milic-Emili, M. B. Dolovich, A. Dawson, and D. V. Bates, Regional distribution of ventilation and perfusion as a function of body position, *J. Appl. Physiol.*, **21**:767–777 (1966).

110. Giuntini, C., M. Mariani, A. Barsotti, F. Fazio, and A. Sautolicandro, Factors affecting regional blood flow in left heart valvular disease, *Am. J. Med.*, **57**:421–436 (1974).

111. Brach, B., V. Sgroi, and K. Moser, Postural changes in pulmonary blood flow as an indicator of pulmonary hypertension, *Am. Rev. Respir. Dis.*, **115**(4–11):308 (1977).

112. Friedman, W. F., and E. Braunwald, Alterations in regional pulmonary blood flow in mitral valve disease by radioisotope scanning, *Circulation*, **34**:363–376 (1966).

113. DeNardo, G. L., D. A. Goodwin, R. Ravasini, and P. A. Dietrich, The ventilatory lung scan in the diagnosis of pulmonary embolism, *N. Engl. J. Med.*, **282**:1334–1336 (1970).

114. Moser, K. M., M. Guisan, A. J. Cuomo, and W. L. Ashburn, Differentiation of pulmonary vascular from parenchymal diseases by ventilation/perfusion scintiphotography, *Ann. Intern. Med.*, **75**:597–605 (1971).

115. Goldzimer, E. L., R. G. Konopka, and K. M. Moser, Reversal of the perfusion defect in experimental canine lobar pneumococcal pneumonia, *J. Appl. Physiol.*, **37**:85–91 (1974).

116. Cournand, A. F., and H. S. Ranges, Catheterization of the right auricle in man, *Proc. Soc. Exp. Biol. Med.*, **46**:462–466 (1941).

117. Dexter, L., F. W. Haynes, C. S. Burwell, E. C. Eppinger, R. R. Sagerson, and J. M. Evans, Studies of congenital heart disease. II. The pressure and oxygen content of blood in the right auricle, right ventricle, and pulmonary artery, with observations on the oxygen saturation and source of pulmonary "capillary" blood, *J. Clin. Invest.*, **26**:554–560 (1947).

118. Zimmerman, H. A., R. W. Scott, and N. D. Becker, Catheterization of the left side of the heart in man, *Circulation*, **1**:357–359 (1950).

119. Swan, H. J. C., and W. Ganz, Use of balloon flotation catheters in critically ill patients, *Surg. Clin. N. Am.*, **55**:501–520 (1975).

120. Grossman, W., *Cardiac Catheterization and Angiography.* Philadelphia, Lea & Febiger, 1974.
121. Yang, S. S., L. G. Bentivoglio, V. Maranhao, and H. Goldberg, *Cardiac Catheterization Data to Hemodynamic Parameters,* 2nd ed. Philadelphia, Davis, 1978.
122. Thadani, V., C. Burrow, W. Whittaker, and D. Heath, Pulmonary veno-occlusive disease, *Q. J. Med.,* **44**:133–159 (1975).
123. Fishman, A. P., Respiratory gases in the regulation of the pulmonary circulation, *Physiol. Rev.,* **41**:214–280 (1961).
124. Wood, P., E. M. Besterman, M. K. Towers, and M. B. McIlroy, The effect of acetylcholine on pulmonary vascular resistance and left atrial pressure in mitral stenosis, *Br. Heart J.,* **19**:279–286 (1957).
125. Grover, R. F., J. T. Reeves, and S. G. Blount, Jr., Tolazoline hydrochloride (Priscoline): an effective pulmonary vasodilator, *Am. Heart J.,* **61**:5–15 (1961).
126. Brammel, H. L., J. H. K. Vogel, R. Pryor, and S. G. Blount, Jr., The Eisenmenger syndrome, *Am. J. Cardiol.,* **28**:679–692 (1971).
127. Abdel-Fattah, M. M., A. Abou-Zeina, A. M. Nomeir, H. Badawi, and M. Saleh, Intrapulmonary acetylcholine in bilharzial cor pulmonale, *Am. Heart J.,* **95**:141–145 (1978).
128. Walston, A., and M. E. Kendall, Comparison of pulmonary wedge and left atrial pressure in man, *Am. Heart J.,* **86**:159–164 (1973).
129. Caro, C. G., D. H. Bergel, and W. A. Seed, Forward and backward transmission of pressure waves in the pulmonary vascular bed of the dog, *Circ. Res.,* **20**:185–193 (1967).
130. Luchsinger, P. C., H. W. Seipp, Jr., and D. J. Patel, Relationship of pulmonary artery-wedge pressure to left atrial pressure in man, *Circ. Res.,* **21**:315–318 (1962).
131. Fowler, N. O., B. Black-Schaffer, R. C. Scott, and M. Gueron, Idiopathic and thromboembolic pulmonary hypertension, *Am. J. Med.,* **40**:331–345 (1966).
132. Yu, P. N., Primary pulmonary hypertension: Report of six cases and review of the literature, *Ann. Intern. Med.,* **49**:1138–1161 (1958).
133. Trell, E., Pulmonary hypertension in disorders of the left heart, *Scand. J. Clin. Lab. Invest.,* **31**:409–418 (1973).
134. Rice, D. L., R. J. Awe, W. H. Gaasch, J. K. Alexander, and D. E. Jenkins, Wedge pressure measurement in obstructive pulmonary disease, *Chest,* **66**:628–632 (1974).
135. Kaplan, S., *Pressure Curve Analysis in Intravascular Catheterization,* 2nd ed. Edited by H. A. Zimmerman. Springfield, Ill., Thomas, 1966, pp. 288–357.
136. Bernstein, W. H., E. M. Fierer, M. H. Laszlo, P. Samet, and R. S. Litwak, The interpretation of pulmonary artery wedge (pulmonary capillary) pressures, *Br. Heart J.,* **22**:37–44 (1960).
137. Manjuran, R. S., J. B. Agarwal, and S. B. Roy, Relationship of pulmonary artery diastolic and pulmonary artery wedge pressures in mitral stenosis, *Am. Heart J.,* **89**:207–211 (1975).

138. Bouchard, R. J., J. H. Gault, and J. Ross, Jr., Evaluation of pulmonary arterial end-diastolic pressure as an estimate of left ventricular end-diastolic pressure in patients with normal and abnormal left ventricular performance, *Circulation,* **44**:1072–1079 (1971).

139. Rahimtoola, S. H., H. S. Loeb, A. Ehsani, M. Z. Sinno, R. Chuquimia, R. Lal, K. M. Rosen, and R. Gunnar, Relationship of pulmonary artery to left ventricular diastolic pressures in acute myocardial infarction, *Circulation,* **46**:283–290 (1972).

140. Keane, J. F., and D. C. Fyler, Hazards of cardiac catheterization in children with pulmonary hypertension due to primary pulmonary vascular obstruction, *Lancet,* **1**(8016):863 (1977).

141. Golden, M. S., T. Pinder, W. T. Anderson, and M. D. Cheitlin, Fatal pulmonary hemorrhage complicating use of a flow-directed balloon-tipped catheter in a patient receiving anticoagulant therapy, *Am. J. Cardiol.,* **32**: 865–867 (1973).

142. Dalen, J. E., Pulmonary angiography in pulmonary embolism, *Bull. Physiopathol. Respir.,* **6**:45–63 (1970).

143. Williams, J. R., and W. C. Wilcox, Pulmonary embolism: Roentgenographic and angiographic considerations, *Am. J. Roentgenol.,* **89**:333–342 (1963).

144. Sasahara, A. A., M. Stein, M. Simer, and D. Littman, Pulmonary angiography in the diagnosis of thromboembolic disease, *N. Engl. J. Med.,* **270**: 1075–1081 (1964).

145. Szucs, M. M., H. L. Brooks, W. Grossman, J. S. Banas, S. G. Meister, L. Dexter, and J. E. Dalen, Diagnostic sensitivity of laboratory findings in acute pulmonary embolism, *Ann. Intern. Med.,* **74**:161–166 (1971).

146. Linton, D. S., E. M. Bellon, J. F. Bodie, and A. M. Rejali, Comparison of results of pulmonary arteriography and radioisotope lung scanning in the diagnosis of pulmonary emboli, *Am. J. Roentgenol. Radium Ther. Nucl. Med.,* **112**:745–748 (1971).

147. Gilday, D. L., K. P. Poulose, and F. H. DeLand, Accuracy of detection of pulmonary emboli by lung scanning correlated with pulmonary arteriography, *Am. J. Roentgenol. Radium Ther. Nucl. Med.,* **115**:732–738 (1972).

148. Grollman, J. H., J. E. Price, and R. K. Granf, Percutaneous transfemoral right heart catheterization—the pulmonary wedge catheter, *Am. J. Cardiol.,* **30**:646–647 (1972).

149. Johnson, B. A., A. E. James, Jr., and R. I. White, Oblique and selective pulmonary angiography in diagnosis of pulmonary embolism, *Am. J. Roentgenol. Radium Ther. Nucl. Med.,* **118**:801–808 (1973).

150. Kattan, K. R., Angled view in pulmonary angiography—a new roentgen approach, *Radiology,* **94**:79–82 (1970).

151. Bookstein, J. J., Segmental arteriography in pulmonary embolism, *Radiology,* **93**:1007–1012 (1969).

152. Bookstein, J. J., and T. M. Silver, The angiographic differential diagnosis of acute pulmonary embolism, *Radiology,* **110**:25–33 (1974).

153. Gay, B. B., R. H. Franch, W. H. Shuford, and J. V. Rogers, Roentgenologic features of single and multiple coarctations of the pulmonary artery and branches, *Am. J. Roentgenol.,* **90**:599–613 (1963).

154. Gregoratos, G., R. C. Jones, and E. J. Jahnke, Unilateral peripheral pulmonic stenosis complicating tetralogy of Fallot, *J. Thor. Cardiovasc. Surg.,* **50**:202–209 (1965).

155. Dotter, C. T., Congenital abnormalities of the pulmonary arteries. In *Angiography,* Vol. I, 2nd ed. Edited by H. L. Abrams. Boston, Little, Brown, 1971, pp. 463–476.

156. Dotter, C. T., Acquired abnormalities of the pulmonary arteries. In *Angiography,* Vol. I, 2nd ed. Edited by H. L. Abrams. Boston, Little, Brown, 1971, pp. 477–482.

157. Schrijen, F., and V. Jezek, Haemodynamics and pulmonary wedge angiography findings in chronic bronchopulmonary disease, *Scand J. Respir. Dis.,* **58**:151–158 (1977).

158. Alpert, J. S., and J. E. Dalen, Pulmonary angiography in the diagnosis of pulmonary embolism, *Intern. Med. Digest,* **9**:17–22 (1974).

5

Pulmonary Vascular Obstruction Due to Embolism and Thrombosis

KENNETH M. MOSER, M.D.

University of California, San Diego
School of Medicine
San Diego, California

I.   Introduction

One of the often overlooked functions of the pulmonary circulation is to serve as a "sieve" for any particulate materials which gain entry into the venous blood. If such particles are too large to traverse the pulmonary capillary bed, they lodge in the lung as emboli. Furthermore, "sticky" materials of smaller size, for example, tumor cells or leukocytes, also may attach to the pulmonary vessels. In addition, the pulmonary circulation is the potential recipient of other nonparticulate noxious agents introduced into the venous blood, such as irritant drugs capable of inducing vasculitis and/or vasospasm. In these modern days, the list of particulate and irritant agents capable of assaulting the pulmonary circulation mounts with regularity.

Certainly, however, the most common material filtered by the lung is the bland thromboembolus which has detached from its origin as a thrombus somewhere in the venous circulation. Thus, venous thromboembolism will be the major focus of attention in this chapter, with more minor treatment being afforded the other embolic entities.

341

II. Venous Thromboembolism

Pulmonary embolism ranks as the most common acute pulmonary disease
among hospitalized patients in the United States, accounting for some 50,000
deaths each year [1]. As such, it also is the pulmonary vascular disease most
frequently encountered by the practicing physician. The disorder does not
respect subspecialty lines in medicine. Virtually all physicians must be concerned with it—the generalist, the surgeon, the internist, the obstetrician and,
all too often, the pathologist. Only the pediatrician rarely is involved with
embolism, for it is uncommon in children (except those with severe cardiorespiratory disease).

Embolism attracts special interest among physicians not only because of
its ubiquity but also because of the manner in which it occurs. Previously
healthy individuals suddenly and unexpectedly succumb to it or suffer an
acute, frightening bout of cardiopulmonary compromise. Patients recovering
uneventfully from minor surgical procedures or medical illnesses, and women
in the postpartum period, suffer a similar fate. Physicians naturally abhor
such sudden, apparently unpredictable catastrophes.

Yet the interest and concern with the diagnosis and treatment of pulmonary embolism is actually misdirected [2]. Embolism is not a *disease.* It is
simply a *complication* of venous thrombosis. Therefore, clinical and investigative attention is more appropriately directed to venous thrombosis. If
venous thrombosis can be prevented, pulmonary embolism will not occur. If
venous thrombosis is promptly detected and treated, the incidence of pulmonary embolism will be reduced. Venous thrombosis lacks the clinical drama
and excitement of pulmonary embolism. But this "mundane" entity is the
problem, and better understanding of venous thrombosis can sharply lessen
the frequency with which the physician encounters the largely preventable
dramatic embolic episode.

A. Deep Venous Thrombosis

It has generally been agreed since the last century that the three factors which
can promote deep venous thrombosis (DVT) are stasis, injury to the intima of
the venous wall, and coagulation changes. The nature of the "coagulation
changes" promoting thrombosis (the so-called hypercoagulable state) has not
been defined, despite substantial investigative effort. Indeed, except for
rather rare conditions such as antithrombin III deficiency [3], there are as yet
no reliable or specific tests available to detect a hypercoagulable state in a
given patient. This may stem from the fact that, experimentally, a transient
hypercoagulable state can be induced by injection of amounts of coagulation

factors so small that they cannot be detected except by the ease with which thrombosis is induced by coexistent stasis [4]. Because "risk" cannot be measured directly, it is derived assessing the "risk profile" on a clinical basis [5]. There are certain clinical contexts in which stasis and/or intimal injury are common: surgery, pregnancy and the postpartum state, congestive heart failure, prolonged bed rest, burns, and trauma, particularly trauma to the pelvis and lower extremities. There are other factors known to increase the risk of DVT, such as advancing age, obesity, use of high-estrogen oral contraceptive pills, prior DVT, marked varicosities, and cancer. Thus, assessment of these

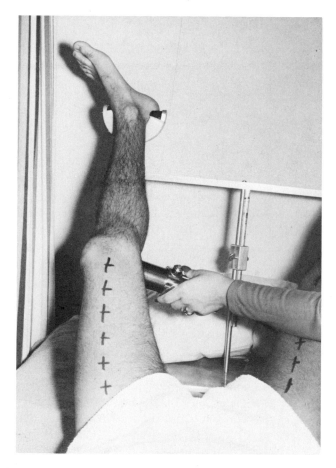

FIGURE 1   Radiofibrinogen leg scanning being performed. Leg is elevated, to drain blood and improve "target to background" ratio, either by device pictured or by elevation of bed.

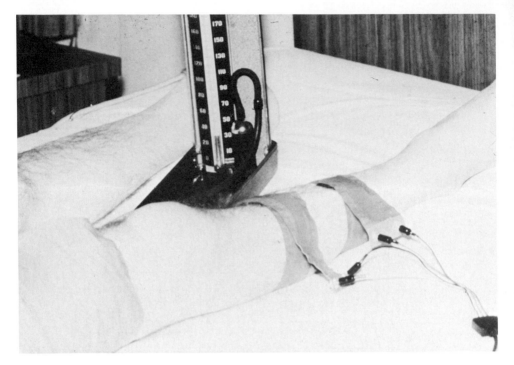

FIGURE 2 Impedance phlebography. Inflation and deflation of blood pressure cuff on thigh alters calf impedance; the impedance changes are detected by the circumferential electrodes.

factors is the basis for establishing the degree of risk in a given patient. For example, the obese patient with a prior history of DVT who faces abdominal surgery is at "high risk."

The development of new, noninvasive techniques for the detection of deep venous thrombosis has provided additional insight into the risk factors, incidence, and natural history of DVT [6-12]. Such methods, particularly leg scanning after injection of radio-labeled fibrinogen and impedance phlebography, also are useful in *monitoring* patients at high risk of DVT (Figs. 1 and 2). Indeed, the combination of radiofibrinogen leg scanning with impedance phlebography is equal in sensitivity and reliability to contrast venography in the detection of DVT (Fig. 3). These techniques have taught us much. Among the lessons learned to date is that the vast majority of deep venous thrombi which lead to significant pulmonary embolism arise in the deep veins of the lower extremities. Exceptions to this rule are patients with significant right ventricular and/or atrial dilatation, injury, or chronic

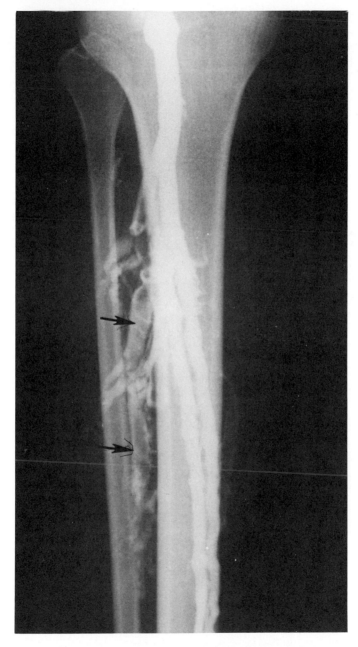

FIGURE 3a Venogram demonstrating extensive "filling defects" (arrows) in calf veins.

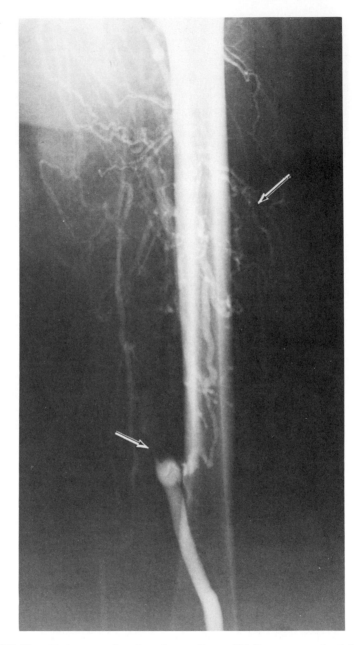

FIGURE 3b   Venogram showing abrupt "cut-off" (lower arrow) of deep
venous system in thigh and some collaterals (upper arrow).

arrhythmias, in whom intracardiac thrombi occur with some frequency. We also have learned that more than 50% of DVT of the lower extremities are not detectable even by the most careful *clinical* examination. No wonder, then, that embolism often arises so unexpectedly.

Another "lesson" is that most venous thrombi following surgery arise *during* or immediately after surgery, not several days later [6]. Furthermore, in this context and others, most venous thrombi arise in the calf, cause no or few symptoms, and resolve even without therapy [7]. Calf thrombi pose little embolic risk—either because they rarely give rise to emboli or because the emboli which do occur are small, cause few symptoms, and are difficult to detect. On the other hand, thrombi extending into or arising in the deep veins of the thigh and pelvis pose a substantial embolic risk [8,9].

These important facts have led to studies designed to assess new approaches to the prophylaxis of DVT in high-risk patients. The principal thrust of attempts to prevent DVT is clear: prevention of DVT is prevention of its major complication, embolism. Thus far, minidose heparin (5000 units subcutaneously b.i.d.) has proven to be the most effective prophylactic regimen applied, in most patient groups [7]. In patients undergoing hip replacement, and with significant lower extremity injury, prothrombinopenic drugs (and perhaps, aspirin) seem superior [10,11]. Undoubtedly, in the future, other regimens will be proposed. At least, adequate means are now available for evaluating them.

Application of minidose heparin and other prophylactic regimens to large population groups undoubtedly will have an impact upon the incidence of pulmonary embolism. However, deep venous thrombi will continue to develop in many patients and the problem of pulmonary thromboembolism will remain with us for some time to come.

B. Pulmonary Embolism

Acute Consequences

When an embolus detaches from its site of origin and lodges in the lung, a sequence of events occurs which is now rather well understood. This sequence is of importance because it conditions both diagnostic approach and management decisions. Indeed, the residual unknowns in this sequence are the bases of certain continuing diagnostic and management controversies.

When an embolus lodges in one or more pulmonary arteries, certain pathophysiological consequences occur acutely. The *respiratory* consequences may include creation of an alveolar dead space, pneumoconstriction in the embolized zone(s), hypoxemia, hyperventilation, and loss of surfactant.

The *alveolar dead space* created is simply a zone of ventilated, nonper-fused lung. In the absence of perfusion, such a zone cannot participate in pulmonary gas exchange and the ventilation to this zone is "wasted" (except to the extent that bronchial arterial flow develops). If an embolus is or be-comes *partially* occlusive, such a zone is converted into a "high V/Q" area and less of the ventilation is wasted.

Pneumoconstriction in the embolized zone is a consequence of constric-tion of smooth muscle in the distal air spaces [12]. This constriction has the effect of reducing "wasted" ventilation by shifting ventilation away from the embolized areas. This pneumoconstriction appears to be mediated by alveolar hypocapnia [12], although humoral mediators released from platelets also may play a role [13,14]. It is reversed, in the experimental animal, by inhalation of CO_2-enriched air and by lung hyperinflation. Such pneumoconstriction has not been demonstrated conclusively in the human. It may be moderated or absent because humans are free to rebreathe dead-space gas into embolized zones, thereby maintaining alveolar CO_2 at higher levels than observed in the tracheally divided, embolized animal; and because the human lung is often hyperinflated (by deep breathing) after embolization.

The mechanisms inducing *hyperventilation* are unclear. Reflexes related to mechanical changes in the embolized lung zones are the most likely candi-dates [15]. If chest pain does occur, this may contribute.

Hypoxemia is *not* an inevitable consequence of embolism. When it does occur acutely, it most likely arises from overperfusion of the remaining non-embolized lung zones so that, despite increased ventilation, low V/Q ratios occur in these zones [16,17]. The *degree* of hypoxemia tends to correlate with the *extent* of embolic occlusion, which fits with this explanation. A patent foramen ovale may serve as the site of a right-to-left shunt if acute pulmonary hypertension occurs. Pulmonary hypertension may also cause per-fusion of low V/Q zones in the patient with preexisting lung disease, zones which would receive little blood flow if the normally present hypoxic vaso-constriction were not "overcome" by pulmonary hypertension. An acute decline in cardiac output with a widening of the A-V difference also may contribute to hypoxemia. The lowered mixed venous oxygen content, passing through normal "shunt" pathways and low V/Q zones, leads to a decline in the arterial oxygen content. Finally, beyond the acute event, if thrombus lysis allows reperfusion, this blood may pass through poorly ventilated zones (pneumoconstricted, or the site of congestive atelectasis or true infarction). Thus, depending upon the prior state of the patient, the extent and hemo-dynamic consequences of embolic obstruction, and the time postembolism, the mechanism(s) responsible for hypoxemia may vary.

Surfactant loss is not an *immediate* consequence of embolic occlusion. It takes 18 to 24 hr of *total* occlusion before interruption of nutrient supply depletes surfactant [18,19]. Because total occlusion often does not persist for that period in humans and perhaps because alveolar PCO_2 is not drastically reduced [20], surfactant depletion does not occur commonly. If it does occur, that lung zone loses both alveolar stability and the integrity of the alveolocapillary membrane. The results are atelectasis and pulmonary exudation of blood into the involved areas of the lung (Fig. 4).

Hemodynamically, the consequences are straightforward. Pulmonary obstruction results in an increase in pulmonary vascular resistance, an increase in pulmonary arterial pressure, and a rise in right ventricular work. The extent of these changes reflects the magnitude of occlusion. If they are severe, the thin-walled right ventricle may be unable to accept the work load and acutely fail.

The *severity* of these acute cardiopulmonary consequences is conditioned by several factors. Clearly, one of these is the *extent* of embolic occlusion per se—the more extensive the obstruction, the more striking the immediate consequences. Another major factor is the prior cardiopulmonary status of the patient. An embolus obstructing one lobar artery is usually well tolerated by an otherwise normal individual, whereas it may cause severe symptoms in someone with significant preexisting cardiac or pulmonary disease. More controversial is the possible role of humoral and reflex factors in conditioning the severity of the cardiopulmonary response to embolism. Numerous studies in various animal models have suggested that reflex and humoral factors may cause postembolic bronchoconstriction and vasoconstriction [12-15]. Perhaps the most convincing of the animal experiments have been those demonstrating the role of bronchoactive and vasoactive amines released from platelets. It has been shown that fresh venous thrombi develop a substantial layering of platelets in situ (Fig. 5) and during passage from their venous site of origin to the lung [13,14]. Once lodged in the lung, these thrombus-attached platelets undergo aggregation and release serotonin and other amines capable of inducing bronchoconstriction and pulmonary arterial constriction. These substances, therefore, can magnify the degree of pulmonary mechanical compromise and the extent of pulmonary hypertension that would have been induced by obstruction alone. The extent to which these humoral-reflex factors participate in human embolism is unknown. If platelet-related humoral factors are operative, "fresh" (nonorganized) thromboemboli must be involved. Of course, in humans, one has no idea whether the thrombus was "fresh" or "aged" at the time it detached and became an embolus.

Natural History of Embolism

Once the patient has survived the acute episode, a new sequence of dynamic events occurs. The most important of these events is *resolution* of the embolus. The word resolution is used to describe two quite separate events by

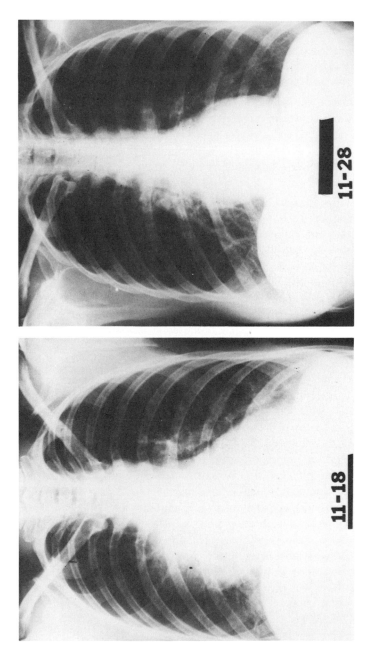

FIGURE 4   Chest roentgenogram on left of 26-year-old female with sudden onset of dyspnea 24 hr earlier. Embolic obstruction of right lower lobe was proven by angiogram. A large infiltrate due to congestive atelectasis or infarction was present. Chest roentgenogram on right taken 10 days later showed complete radiographic clearing. Perfusion scan was also normal. Absence of volume loss or scarring indicates that the original infiltrate was due to congestive atelectasis, not tissue death (see text).

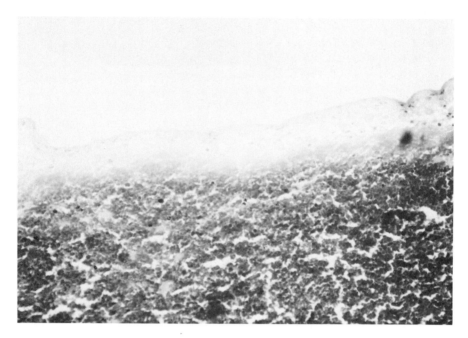

FIGURE 5 This experimental thrombus was formed in canine femoral vein by the Wessler technique, and removed 30 min after exposure to venous blood flow. Amorphous superficial layer chiefly composed of platelets is seen above the original "red" venous thrombus.

which luminal patency is restored: fibrinolysis (thrombolysis) and organization. Just as in the case of venous thrombosis, most emboli resolve rather quickly and completely via these mechanisms [21-24].

The plasminogen-plasmin system is normally activated to achieve thrombus dissolution. Activation of the proenzyme plasminogen to the active proteolytic enzyme plasmin occurs via release of plasminogen activators by mechanisms which are not well understood. Since plasminogen is contained *within* the fibrin mesh of the thrombus itself, such activation promotes thrombus dissolution from "within" as well as without. The pulmonary arterial intima is a rich reservoir of plasminogen activator, and it is likely that activator release from the intima is promoted by embolic lodgement. This is suggested by the very rapid lysis of emboli in the dog in the absence of systemic plasminogen activation. Thus, it is likely that normal thrombolysis is a local phenomenon, with release of activator from the intima of the vessel involved by thromboembolism.

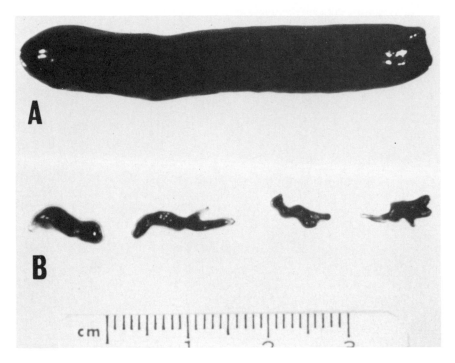

FIGURE 6   (A) Thrombus formed in inferior vena cava of dog by the Wessler technique. (B) Residual emboli recovered from lungs 4 hr after thrombus comparable to (A) was released from inferior vena cava. Extent of lysis in this short period is evident.

Whatever the mechanisms involved, the fact is that spontaneous thrombolysis occurs with great dispatch in the dog [21]. Within hours, fresh venous thrombi undergo substantial dissolution and pulmonary emboli lyse even more rapidly (Fig. 6). It appears that the dog rarely calls upon organization to complete the process of resolution.

In the human, however, thrombolysis is neither as rapid nor as uniformly effective. Precise data still are lacking, but some guidelines are available (Fig. 7). The most rapid total resolution of an embolus reported to date occurred in 51 hr [25]. Other reports indicate that resolution proceeds rapidly during the first several days after embolic lodgement, probably chiefly due to fibrinolysis [22,24]. Thereafter, resolution continues more slowly via organization, with the major portion having been completed within 2 weeks and some further clearing up to 6 weeks. Beyond 6 weeks, there appears to be little further change, because residual obstruction at this time is due to organized thrombi which persist indefinitely [26-28].

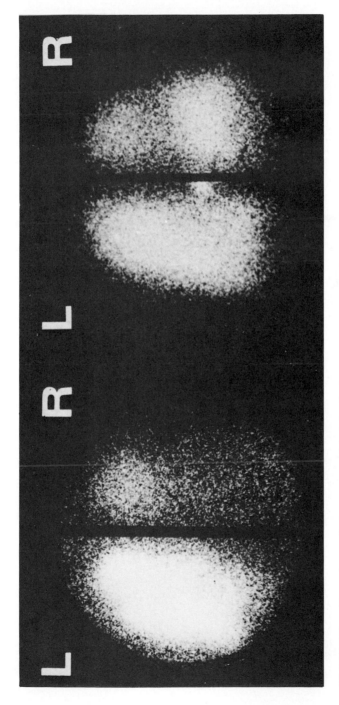

FIGURE 7a Posterior perfusion scan on left (4/17/73) shows very large perfusion defect in patient with angiographically proven embolic obstruction of right main pulmonary artery (some blood flow to apical segment of upper lobe persisted). Perfusion scan on right (5/8/73) shows extensive reperfusion after 3 weeks.

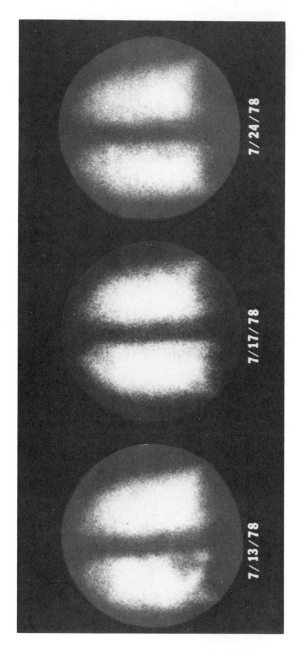

FIGURE 7b   Posterior perfusion scans in patient with embolization of left lower lobe vessels. Left, 12 hr after onset, defects are obvious. Center, 4 days later, marked reperfusion has occurred. Right, 11 days after onset, perfusion has essentially returned to normal.

One quite uncommon event in the natural history of embolism is the occurrence of pulmonary infarction (tissue death). The rarity of infarction is not unexpected because the lung is uniquely endowed with three routes by which oxygen can reach lung tissue: the tracheobronchial tree, the pulmonary arterial circulation, and the bronchial arterial circulation. Thus, obstruction of the pulmonary arterial circulation alone is not sufficient to induce hypoxic injury to the involved lung zone. Experimentally, induction of infarction in animals requires compromise of two of the three oxygenation routes [29]. There is a counterpart to this in humans. Patients with preexisting cardiac or pulmonary disease, such as the majority of those in the UK-SK national study, may have clinical-radiographic indications of infarction in 50% or more of the patients studied [27]. The incidence in otherwise normal individuals is, in our experience, rare. Furthermore, most instances of clinical "infarction" actually represent congestive atelectasis, not tissue death. Congestive atelectasis is a consequence of the surfactant depletion discussed previously. The atelectasis and increased permeability of the alveolocapillary membrane lead to volume loss and exudation of hemorrhagic fluid into the involved area(s), perhaps augmented by increased collateral blood flow via the bronchial arterial circulation. This sequence can lead to hemoptysis, pleural irritation (and pleuritic chest pain), and a roentgenographic infiltrate. However, the lung remains structurally intact. With thrombus resolution or increased bronchial arterial blood flow, surfactant production is restored, the debris is cleared by normal lung clearance mechanisms, and the lung is restored to its preembolic status (Fig. 4). Even with persistent pulmonary arterial occlusion, such restoration occurs, making removal of such chronic obstructions feasible [19,28]. True infarction, leading to fibrotic organization of the involved zone(s), and clearing by linear scarring on sequential chest X-rays, is rare indeed.

Of interest, of course, are those individuals in whom embolic resolution does *not* occur. There are probably two major reasons for resolution failure: (1) some deficiency (not yet experimentally verified) of the activation or function of the fibrinolytic system, and (2) embolic obstruction by thrombi which have aged prior to embolization or have an unusual composition. Aged thrombi are less susceptible to fibrinolysis; indeed, if *organized* prior to detachment, they are not susceptible at all. Thrombi particularly high in fibrinogen content or low in plasminogen content also are resistant to lysis. Whichever of these factors may be operative, "nonresolvers" are subject to chronic thrombotic obstruction and, if this obstruction is extensive, to the development of cor pulmonale (Fig. 8).

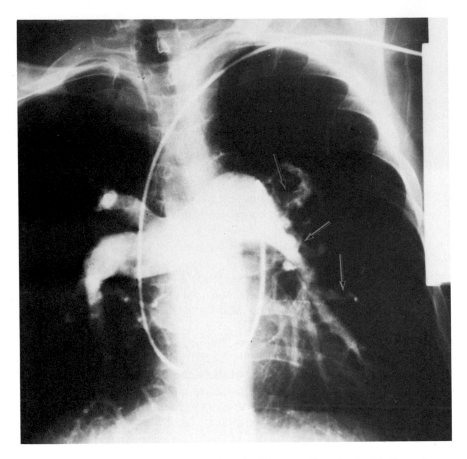

FIGURE 8a   Angiogram, anterior view, in 31-year-old patient with thromboembolic obstruction of multiple pulmonary arteries documented 3 years previously. Multiple filling defects (arrows) are present.

Diagnosis of Pulmonary Embolism

The pathophysiological consequences of embolism are such that no truly
specific historical or physical findings are available upon which a diagnosis
can be based firmly. The symptoms of embolism cover a wide spectrum from
mild, transient dyspnea to severe breathlessness and syncope [27,30,31]. The
only symptom which regularly occurs is dyspnea, usually of sudden onset.
Pleuritic chest pain and hemoptysis only occur if congestive atelectasis or infarction develop and, as already mentioned, these events develop in a minority
of patients—and in these only many hours postocclusion. Severe chest pain,
mimicking coronary insufficiency, occurs with massive embolism, as does

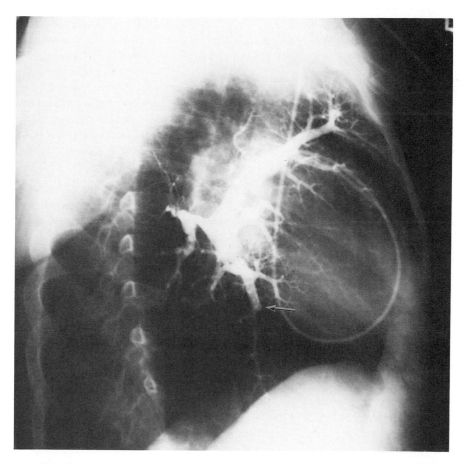

FIGURE 8b   Angiogram, different view, same patient, shows abrupt cut-off
(arrow) of segmental vessel. Cor pulmonale was present (PA pressure = 100/60).
Thrombendarterectomy was performed successfully.

syncope. But all these historical features are nonspecific and can occur in a
variety of cardiopulmonary disorders. Some diagnostic help is provided by
the context in which these symptoms present, e.g., in the postoperative period, after lower extremity trauma, or in the postpartum period.

Physical findings are, likewise, usually modest and not definitive. *The
lungs are most often clear to percussion and auscultation.* While some have
reported wheezing, indicative of pneumoconstriction [32] mediated by serotonin release [33], we have not detected this in our experience. With congestive atelectasis or infarction, evidence of consolidation or a pleural friction
rub may be present. The characteristic findings of a pleural effusion may be

noted. Cardiac findings almost invariably include tachycardia, but this is the only consistent sign. With *massive* embolism, a right ventricular lift, a third heart sound (of right ventricular origin), and a loud pulmonary closure sound may be heard. However, if right ventricular failure occurs and cardiac output falls, the closure sound may be normal or even decreased. Fixed splitting of the second sound may develop in such patients, indicative of right ventricular failure. Pulmonary ejection murmurs or clicks also may be detected. However, most emboli are not massive and, therefore, do not cause significant pulmonary hypertension or right ventricular failure. Therefore, few cardiac findings are present in the majority of patients.

Thus, it is apparent that the physical findings associated with embolism often are minimal and serve only to *suggest* the diagnosis of embolism, not to *make* the diagnosis with confidence. Only with extensive embolism in certain clinical contexts does sufficient evidence exist on the basis of the history and physical examination to make a diagnosis with reasonable confidence. Thus, laboratory tests are almost invariably required to confirm the clinical diagnostic suspicion of embolism.

Various "specific" blood tests and combinations of tests have been proposed as being useful in the diagnosis of pulmonary embolism. Such tests include measurement of specific fibrinopeptides and fibrin degradation products, of platelet behavior, and of various tissue-derived enzymes [34–36]. Unfortunately, none of these tests has proven sufficiently sensitive, reliable, or specific to serve as the basis for a diagnosis of embolism. A chest X-ray certainly should be obtained in all pulmonary emboli suspects [37]. However, its major value lies in ruling out other entities that may mimic embolism (e.g., pneumothorax) because there are no pathognomonic findings that make a diagnosis of acute embolism. Certain radiographic findings are suggestive, such as lung zones lacking in vascular markings and disparity in the size of comparable pulmonary arteries. However, none of these findings is specific. Furthermore, while congestive atelectasis or infarction may produce pulmonary infiltrates, such infiltrates have no special diagnostic configuration or location (except, perhaps, their usual abutment against a pleural surface). Pleural effusion is, similarly, a nonspecific finding. *The fact is that the most common chest X-ray in embolism is "within normal limits"* (Fig. 9).

The same label "potentially suggestive, but not diagnostic," applies to the electrocardiogram [30,38]. The EKG in pulmonary embolism usually

---

FIGURE 9   (a) Pulmonary angiogram in 28-year-old male demonstrating extensive embolic occlusion. Note filling defect in left lower lobe vessel (arrow) and abrupt cut-off of right middle lobe vessel (arrow). (b) Chest roentgenogram in this patient. It is within normal limits.

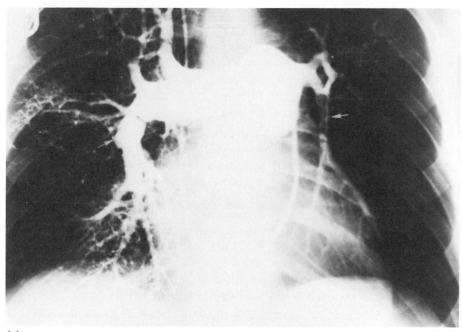

(a)

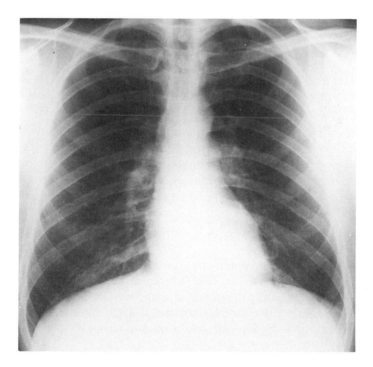

(b)

shows a tachycardia and, often, "nonspecific ST-T changes." If emboli are massive (and most are not) or induce acute cor pulmonale because they occur in a patient with preexisting cardiopulmonary disease, the EKG may show "P pulmonale," right axis deviation, an S_1-Q_3 configuration, and deeply inverted T waves across the anterior precordial leads. But, the absence of these findings in no way mitigates against the diagnosis, and other conditions (e.g., acute respiratory failure) can produce them.

Arterial hypoxemia is not an invariable finding in embolism. Furthermore, hypoxemia occurs in a variety of cardiorespiratory diseases that may mimic embolism (e.g., respiratory failure, pneumonia, granulomatous pleuritis with effusion). As noted previously, several mechanisms may cause arterial hypoxemia in embolism. The results of animal investigations [16,17] are difficult to relate to humans because patients are usually seen some hours after the event, may have other cardiopulmonary problems present, rarely totally occlude arteries with emboli, are not mechanically ventilated, and are free to rebreathe their dead-space gas. Perhaps the most important diagnostic point is that arterial hypoxemia may be absent in the patient with embolism and, therefore, a normal arterial PO_2 does not exclude the diagnosis.

Thus, the "standard" laboratory tests often provide little assistance in the diagnosis of pulmonary embolism. However, it should be noted that the diagnostic information provided by the history, physical examination, and standard laboratory tests can be substantial and persuasive. Indeed, therapy can usually be instituted after such evaluation, particularly since many other possibilities are excluded in the process. But there are only two procedures which provide a reasonable degree of sensitivity and reliability in the diagnosis of embolism: pulmonary perfusion and ventilation scintiphotography, and pulmonary angiography.

Perfusion scintiphotography faithfully reflects the distribution of pulmonary blood flow [39]. Embolism distorts this distribution by creating, through obstruction, zones of reduced or absent blood flow, commonly referred to as perfusion "defects." However, any process which *destroys* or *constricts* pulmonary arterial vessels also can diminish regional perfusion and cause perfusion defects (e.g., necrotizing infection, old or recent, or regional hypoventilation). Thus, the scan is a *sensitive* detector of changes in regional blood flow, but it lacks specificity.

Despite its inherent nonspecificity, the perfusion scan is of great value in the diagnostic evaluation of the embolic suspect. First, *a normal scan essentially rules out clinically significant thromboembolic obstruction.* Over a period of more than 5 years, we have not seen a single instance in which an embolic suspect with a negative scan was proved to have emboli by angiogram or at autopsy.

Interpretation of a *positive* scan, however, must be undertaken with caution. While various "patterns" of defects have been suggested as "high probability" or "low probability" we have not found them reliable in detecting or excluding pulmonary embolism. More useful is combining the abnormal scan with other data, particularly the history, physical examination, and chest X-ray. In the patient who is in a clinical setting in which embolic risk is high, who has symptoms strongly suggestive of embolism, who has no evidence of cardiopulmonary disease, and whose chest X-ray is unremarkable, a perfusion scan showing one or more defects (regardless of pattern) provides very strong evidence of embolism. It is certainly justifiable to treat many such patients for embolism without additional diagnostic studies, unless an identifiable risk exists with respect to anticoagulant therapy.

But if the patient does not meet the criteria noted, or if question exists about cardiopulmonary disease or the chest X-ray, a ventilation scan should be done to enhance the specificity of the diagnosis. Such increased specificity derives from the fact that embolism results in areas of high or infinite V/Q ratios in the lungs—areas with reduced to absent blood flow but normal ventilation [40–43]. Conversely, *parenchymal* disorders causing perfusion defects are invariably associated with reduced or absent ventilation in the same lung zones. Thus, embolism causes V/Q "mismatch" (Fig. 10), while parenchymal diseases cause "matched" V and Q abnormalities (see Chapter 4). Ventilation scans can be performed with several radioactive gases, the most useful for clinical purposes being ^{133}xenon and ^{127}xenon. With appropriate dose selection, a ^{133}xenon scan can be performed immediately after ^{99m}technetium perfusion scan. ^{127}Xenon has slight dose and convenience advantages over ^{133}xenon. But, whichever gas is used, the *technique* of ventilation scanning is critical to proper interpretation. Ventilation scans usually consist of a wash-in, an equilibrium, and a wash-out phase [41]. Of these phases, the most sensitive for the detection of poorly ventilated lung regions is the wash-out phase (see Chapter 4). In looking for V/Q match or mismatch, it is this *wash-out* phase of the ventilation scan that should be compared with the perfusion scan. So called single-breath ventilation scans can be particularly misleading. These are done by having the patient inhale a *single breath* of radioactive gas (from RV or FRC to TLC) and obtaining an image at TLC. Patients with severe obstructive lung disease often have "normal" ventilation scans when this insensitive technique is used (see Chapter 4).

With appropriate technical performance, the combined "V/Q" approach is highly specific for the diagnosis of embolism and other vascular obstructive entities, including pulmonary artery agenesis [44].

However, the diagnostic "standard" for embolism is *pulmonary angiography*. Even this procedure has its problems and limitations. The technique

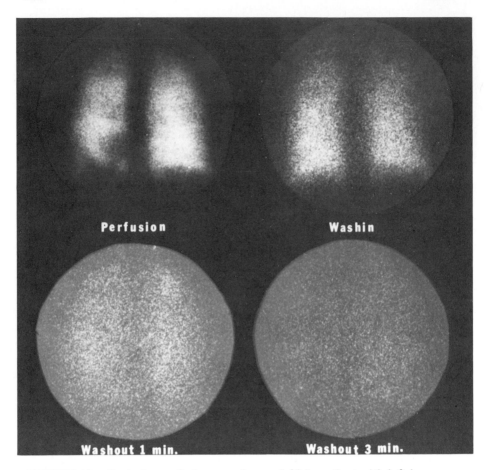

FIGURE 10 Posterior perfusion scan (upper left) in patient with left lower lobe emboli. Defects are apparent. Washin of [133]xenon (upper right) is normal, as is washout of [133]xenon from these regions at 1 min (lower left) and 3 min (lower right).

requires experience if it is to be performed properly, and skilled performance is essential to high diagnostic yield. Main pulmonary artery injection followed by selective injection into suspicious regions is the preferred approach. Main pulmonary artery injection *alone* is usually not adequate. Other specialized approaches may enhance diagnostic accuracy, such as magnification techniques and balloon occlusion of lobar or segmental arteries prior to injection of contrast medium.

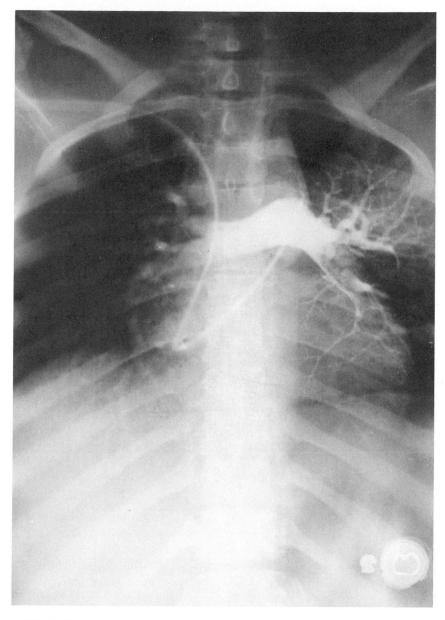

FIGURE 11   Angiogram demonstrating large filling defect in distal left main pulmonary artery, extending into left lower lobe pulmonary artery.

Even with angiograms of high technical quality, interpretation is not a simple matter. There are only two reliable diagnostic findings (Figs. 8, 9, and 11): the "filling defect" and the "cut off" [30,31,45,46]. Some experience is needed to assure that even these abnormalities are constant (seen on serial films) and not due to flow or vessel crossing artifacts.

There has been concern that very small emboli can be missed, even with ideal V and Q scans and angiograms (short of magnification). That is unquestionably the case [42]. However, it is highly doubtful that such small emboli can produce acute, clinically expressed symptoms. Therefore, the resolution limitations of current scanning and angiographic procedures are of more concern to the investigator studying embolism in animal models than to the clinician concerned with ascertaining the presence of embolism in a symptomatic patient.

On the horizon are techniques which may further assist diagnosis. Positive imaging of emboli with [^{123}I] fibrinogen, ^{111}In-labeled platelets, and other "thrombus seeking" radionuclides offer promise [47,48]. In our laboratory, we have succeeded in directly visualizing in vivo emboli in the experimental animal with a specially designed fiberoptic device [49].

Thus, there now exist excellent procedures for the detection of emboli in humans and the future holds the promise of further improvement. The perfusion scan, furthermore, provides an excellent means of following the resolution rate of emboli, as well as for assessing recurrence. In this regard, it should be noted that the perfusion scan may become normal even though an angiogram demonstrates some residual obstruction. This occurs because normal distal flow returns when 20 to 30% of the luminal diameter of the supplying artery has been restored [50]. Thus the scan, which mirrors flow, can become normal well before total resolution, as depicted by the angiogram, occurs.

Management of Thromboembolism

The last decade has been one of exciting advances in medical and surgical approaches to the prevention and treatment of venous thromboembolism. A detailed review of these management options and the controversies surrounding them is beyond the scope of this chapter, and detailed reviews of this matter are available elsewhere [31,51-54]. Certain major points are worthy of note here, however. Recent investigative and clinical emphasis has been focused chiefly—and properly—on the early detection and prevention of deep venous thrombosis. Detection and prevention go hand in hand since better detection enhances our ability to identify truly high-risk patients for DVT *and* which *types* of DVT are likely to give rise to embolism. Several preventive regimens are already available (warfarin, minidose heparin), and others are being explored (antiplatelet agents, mechanical compressive devices). Further investigation will lead to better selection of patients and more effective prophylactic options in the future.

As to the treatment of active venous thrombosis and pulmonary embolism, heparin is clearly the drug of choice. Controversy persists about the safest, most effective ways to administer and monitor this drug [51]. Similar discussion surrounds the appropriate role of the thrombolytic agents (streptokinase, urokinase) in treatment, particularly whether their benefit (as opposed to heparin) outweighs their risk and cost [27,51].

Similarly unresolved are the roles of surgical procedures such as embolectomy and vena caval obstruction. Despite long use, patient selection for these procedures remains unsettled.

III. Chronic Thromboembolic Pulmonary Hypertension

As noted above, most pulmonary emboli in humans resolve. Pathologically, webs and bands may be left in their wake (see Chapter 1), but normal perfusion and gas exchange are restored. In a minority of patients, however, emboli do not resolve and continue to obstruct, partially or totally, the affected vessels. These obstructing lesions are no longer "thrombi," subject to acute embolectomy. They are organized and endothelialized.

Despite these resolution failures, most such patients recognize no cardiopulmonary symptoms because the reserve capacity of the pulmonary vascular bed is so substantial. However, there are two groups of patients who do achieve clinical recognition (often late) because of nonresolution: those with massive "central" obstruction of main or lobar arteries; and those with obstruction of multiple, more distal vessels [55]. Both these groups, on the basis of the extent of obstruction, are pulmonary hypertensive. Their embolic event(s) may or may not have been recognized, and many carry erroneous diagnoses ranging from "hyperventilation" to "chronic lung disease" to "primary pulmonary hypertension." As noted elsewhere in this volume, precapillary forms of pulmonary hypertension are often difficult to detect early and may achieve recognition only when dyspnea on exertion, effort syncope, or overt right ventricular failure supervene.

Recognition of the massive, central form of obstruction is of particular importance because it is surgically remediable by endarterectomy [28,56]. More of these patients now are being discovered because: (1) more patients are sequentially followed beyond the acute event, and (2) perfusion scans are more widely utilized in evaluating patients with dyspnea of uncertain cause.

More than 20 such patients now have been operated upon with a success rate that has steadily risen as diagnostic, cardiac surgical techniques and intensive care management have improved (Fig. 8). It is of interest that those patients with major *central* emboli rarely have occlusion extending into the more distal vessels, presumably because of prompt establishment of bronchial arterial collateral flow to the obstructed pulmonary arteries. This same flow preserves the integrity of the pulmonary parenchyma. Unfortunately, severe, sustained hypertension can injure the pulmonary arterial bed, which remains unobstructed. Thus, these patients develop a "two-compartment" pulmonary arterial bed— a normal one beyond the obstruction and a "high-resistance" one in the nonobstructed areas. This has significance because, after thromboendarterectomy, blood flow is diverted to the newly opened, low-resistance vessels. A hemorrhagic pulmonary edema often occurs in these zones [28, 56]. Fortunately, with modern ventilator support techniques, patients now can be sustained through this difficult period.

The other type of thromboembolic hypertension, due to multiple small emboli, is not subject to surgical correction at this time. It can be distinguished from "idiopathic" primary pulmonary hypertension by angiography, though magnification techniques may be required.

IV.   In Situ Pulmonary Vascular Thrombosis

A.   In Major Arteries

Thrombotic occlusion of major pulmonary arteries, other than as a sequel of embolism, is a rare event. Furthermore, distinction between such true in situ thrombosis and that due to organization of a prior embolus is often difficult or impossible, even at the autopsy table [57–59].

In those instances in which in situ thrombosis has been well documented, it has not appeared de novo in an otherwise normal pulmonary arterial tree. In virtually every instance described, there has been evidence that one or both of two known progenitors of thrombosis was present: stasis of flow, or damage to the arterial wall [57–59]. In a number of cases, pulmonary atherosclerosis due to sustained pulmonary arterial hypertension secondary to massive right-to-left shunts has provided the apparent nidus for thrombus development (see Chapter 4). Traumatic injury to the chest and to pulmonary arterial walls seems to have been the antecedent event in other cases. We have seen one patient in whom thrombosis of the remaining major branch occurred following right lower lobe resection, perhaps due to trauma or torsion. Invasion or compression of major arteries by tumor, usually originating in the lung, has led to in situ thrombosis in some patients. A variety of other diseases capable of producing vessel wall injury also have been incriminated, including tuberculosis, measles, and syphilis.

Stasis apparently has played a major role in the development of thrombosis in patients with protracted left ventricular failure and severe mitral stenosis. Both stasis and vessel wall injury may play a role in congenital cyanotic heart disease. But, in many of these situations, differentiation from embolism is difficult [60]. Therefore, while a variety of disorders may promote in situ thrombosis, it appears to be a rather rare event, and, when it does occur, a ready explanation is usually at hand.

B. In Small Arteries

In situ thrombosis of small pulmonary arteries and arterioles, in contrast to that in major vessels, is a rather common event. One instance of particular interest is its occurrence in patients with sickle cell anemia [61]. In this situation, the inciting event appears to be tangling and sludging of the abnormally shaped cells in the smaller vessels of the lung, followed by thrombosis and, on occasion, a frank infarction. Recurrent episodes of thrombosis may lead to obstructive pulmonary hypertension in these patients over the years.

Small vessel thrombosis also occurs in the course of numerous cardiopulmonary disorders which involve the pulmonary vasculature or parenchyma [60]. In many of these situations it is difficult to determine whether the vascular occlusion has resulted from intimal proliferation or from thrombosis since the "end lesions" of both processes are so similar. For example, in scleroderma there is often advanced intimal proliferation of the small arterial vessels of the lung and small vessel thrombosis occurs in these same abnormal vessels [62,63]. Similar problems arise in sorting out the role of the obliterative vascular lesions encountered in congenital heart disease with large left-to-right shunts.

Any inflammatory, fibrotic, or destructive disease of the pulmonary parenchyma can involve the smaller arterial vessels. Again, the initial lesions may be thrombotic, or the vessel simply may be included in the fibroobliterative process obtaining in the surrounding parenchyma. Even in such a commonly benign process as sarcoidosis, invasion of the vascular wall often occurs, to the point of complete obstruction [64]. In any diffuse pulmonary disease in which loss of vascular bed is sufficient to produce pulmonary hypertension, the hypertension itself will induce further vascular injury, intimal proliferation, and thrombosis in the small pulmonary vessels. Thus, a "vicious cycle" develops leading to progressive pulmonary hypertension.

Finally, thrombosis of the small pulmonary arteries (and veins) is a common event in patients with cardiac lesions associated with sharply reduced pulmonary blood flow. Heath has noted that such thrombosis is especially likely if the pulmonary blood flow falls below 2.5 liters min^{-1} m^{-2} [65]. Pulmonary stenosis is the most common lesion involved, though some thrombotic obliteration has been seen with tricuspid atresia. If, in addition to this reduced blood flow, there are associated cardiac anomalies which produce right-to-left shunting, particularly widespread thrombosis occurs in small pulmonary vessels [66]. Such diffuse small vessel obstruction is of considerable clinical significance as it may prevent consideration of otherwise feasible surgical corrective procedures.

C. In Major Veins

Like thrombosis of major pulmonary arteries, thrombosis of major pulmonary veins is an uncommon event except with rather evident precipitating cause. Perhaps the most frequent offenders are tumors, particularly bronchogenic carcinoma, which directly invade or compress the pulmonary veins to induce thrombosis. Fibrosing mediastinitis, whatever its specific etiology, also can entrap pulmonary veins and obstruct them, with or without thrombotic assistance [67]. Obstruction of major pulmonary veins due to fibrotic entrapment may produce the radiographic picture of severe pulmonary venous hypertension, including "septal lines" and/or marked regional pulmonary edema. The focal nature of the radiographic picture may provide a clue to what has occurred. Symptoms of dyspnea and hemoptysis are often present.

The large pulmonary veins also may thrombose, though rarely, as a result of left atrial obstructive lesions. Left atrial myxoma may lead to thrombosis, and large atrial thrombi secondary to mitral stenosis may extend into the pulmonary veins.

D. In Small Veins

Thrombosis in the small pulmonary veins is extremely uncommon in the absence of an obvious cause. To be sure, the small pulmonary veins, like the small pulmonary arteries, frequently become thrombosed in the course of inflammatory or neoplastic disorders of the lung. As mentioned, they frequently are thrombosed extensively in cyanotic congenital cardiac disease in which pulmonary blood flow is reduced, and extensive intimal proliferative lesions are common in all disorders which produce chronic venous hypertension.

In recent years, attention also has been directed to a small group of patients in whom, without known cause, widespread thrombotic obstruction of small and medium-sized pulmonary veins has led to progressive pulmonary hypertension and death. "Pulmonary veno-occlusive disease" has involved all age groups, has no sex predilection, and the antecedent histories of the patients have not provided etiologic clues [68,69]. Most are initially diagnosed as mitral stenosis or primary pulmonary hypertension. The only definitive diagnostic procedure is lung biopsy. Even on biopsy, care must be taken, with elastic stains, to identify the often obliterated veins. Unfortunately, there is no known effective therapy for this disorder.

V. Septic Thromboembolism

The vast majority of emboli arise from a noninfectious focus. These bland thromboemboli induce their effects by the mechanisms previously described: obstruction, perhaps release of vasoactive amines, and inflammation of the intima. However, there are instances in which infection initiates thrombosis, with organisms actually invading the thrombus. Any embolus resulting from such a thrombus serves not only as an obstructing mass, but also as a vector of infection. Thus, the pathogenesis, clinical features, and management of septic thromboembolism differ substantially from those in bland thromboembolism.

There are two major contexts in which septic thromboembolism is encountered commonly: as a complication of intravenous drug use [70,71], and following gynecological-obstetric procedures [72]. With reference to gynecological-obstetric procedures, the classic inciting event is a septic abortion. However, this process also can occur after normal delivery and in-hospital sterile procedures such as a D & C.

To these two common causes have been added a number of other potential sources of infected emboli which are consequences of modern medical technology, namely, the array of devices left in-dwelling in a vein for any significant period of time. Catheters placed in peripheral veins and central veins, ventriculoatrial shunt catheters, transvenous pacemakers, and catheters for hemodialysis—all these may serve as a nidus for septic emboli [73,74]. Yet, as these devices have come into vogue, some previously frequent sources of septic phlebitis and embolization have essentially disappeared, namely, bacterial infection in ears, sinusitis, and mastoiditis.

In all these circumstances, the pathologic sequence of events is similar. The first event appears to be the invasion of a traumatized vein by microorganisms. In drug users, the vein is at one of the sites employed for intravenous (and occasionally subcutaneous) drug administration. In gynecological-obstetric patients, the pelvic veins are involved; in patients with catheters, the cannulated vein. Pathologically, the involved vein(s) are found to be thrombosed by mixtures of blood clot and bacteria, resembling a test tube of blood clot which has been used as a culture medium. The friable nature of this thrombotic material explains the high potential for dislodgement of small, repetitive emboli from such foci.

At this juncture, the diagnosis of septic thrombophlebitis may be obscure, presenting as a "fever of unknown origin." There may be localizing signs of inflammation directing attention to the involved vein(s). However, in septic pelvic thrombophlebitis, such signs may not be present and pelvic examination often is deceptively unremarkable [72,75].

The process may gradually resolve (with or without specific therapy) at this phase. However, if embolism develops, new features appear. The patient, already septic, becomes progressively more breathless, often with cough, sputum production, hemoptysis, and pleuritic chest pain developing [76]. The chest roentgenogram is characteristic [77]. Multiple, small, nodular densities appear, usually with slightly "fuzzy" outlines. These lesions may rapidly increase in number so that X-rays taken at 24-hr intervals often show striking worsening. This reflects the occurrence of repetitive, small, infected emboli. The lesions may be so numerous that they become confluent. Usually, *cavitation* (a rare event in bland embolism) appears within the nodules after hours or days and may rapidly progress to thin-walled cavities (Fig. 12). This extremely characteristic clinical and chest roentgenographic picture should suggest the diagnosis in any patient who has risk factors known to promote this process.

Complicating the approach to these patients is the fact that bacteremia commonly occurs. This may give rise to right-sided endocarditis (tricuspid and, rarely, pulmonary valve). The friable valvular vegetations may then embolize to the lungs, producing the same clinical and roentgenographic features. Indeed, evidence of endocarditis always should be sought in these patients.

Further complicating the problem is that these septic, immobilized patients also are candidates for *bland* venous thrombosis in the deep veins of the lower extremities and embolism from this source. We have seen several such documented instances.

Initial therapy for septic phlebitis is directed against both the infection and the thromboembolism with vigorous antibiotic therapy combined with heparinization. The positive effects of adding heparin to the antibiotic regimen have been well-documented [75]. Often, blood cultures are negative and antibiotic selection must be made empirically, usually combining drugs effective against gram-negative anaerobes with those effective against gram-positive organisms (including penicillinase-producing staphylococci). Any obviously infected focus should be drained. *Clearly, if any catheter or device is in-dwelling in the venous system, it should be removed promptly and cultured.*

There is some controversy as to whether heparin should be utilized when septic embolization occurs, particularly if right-sided endocarditis is present or suspected. The concern is with hemorrhagic risk. However, the bulk of evidence, and our own experience, suggests that heparin is an important part of the therapeutic regimen in such patients [75] and that hemorrhagic risk is quite small (unlike, perhaps, the risk in left-sided endocarditis).

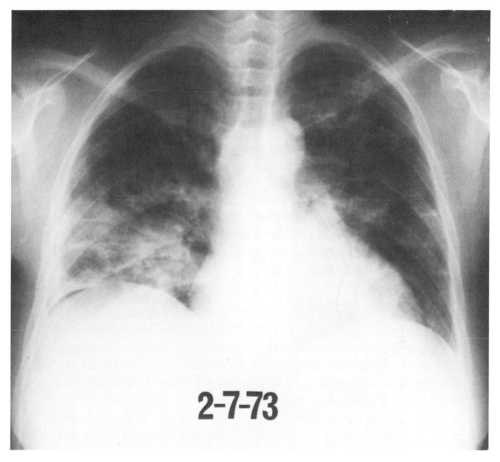

FIGURE 12   Chest roentgenogram obtained 10 days post partum in patient who had developed fever and chills 72 hr after apparently normal delivery. Characteristic picture of multiple septic emboli from pelvic source. Note multiple bilateral infiltrates, some confluent, some cavitating. A thin-walled cavity is evident above right diaphragm. Response to antibiotic-heparin regimen was excellent.

Furthermore, the efficacy of the intial regimen is crucial because repetitive embolization can lead rapidly to a fatal outcome. The key to successful therapy is prompt cessation of further embolization from the "feeding focus."

If antibiotic-heparin therapy (plus catheter removal, if present) fails to half the embolic process within 24 to 48 hr, attention turns to surgical procedures to isolate drainage from the infected area. In septic pelvic thrombophlebitis, this requires ligation of the inferior vena cava and the left ovarian vein. Other sites of venous ligation depend upon the embolic source. Ligation is often followed by dramatic improvement in a desperately ill individual [72]. Happily, ligation (and other procedures such as hysterectomy or extirpation of an infected valve) are rarely needed when combined antibiotic-heparin therapy is applied.

VI. Pulmonary Emboli Other than Thromboemboli

As stated previously, the pulmonary vessels serve as a filter for venous blood derived from all body areas and for the lymph, which gains access to them via the thoracic duct. It is not surprising, then, that a wide variety of materials have been found lodged in the smaller pulmonary vessels and that, on occasion, the "filter" is overwhelmed to the point of serious or fatal obstruction to pulmonary blood flow and compromise of gas exchange function.

Despite the many types of nonthrombotic emboli which may occur, three general principles should be borne in mind: (1) *any* substance which can gain access to the systemic veins or the thoracic duct will lodge in the pulmonary vascular bed if its size prevents passage; (2) irritative materials of *any* size which gain access may lead to obliterative or thrombotic changes in the pulmonary vascular bed; and (3) if the patient survives the embolic or irritiative-thrombotic event, which is almost always the case, the occurrence of the event may not be suspected; indeed, even if suspected, it rarely can be proven to have occurred short of lung biopsy or autopsy. This latter being the case, most instances of nonthromboembolic injury undoubtedly escape detection and, therefore, descriptions of them are based on those few instances in which their severity, or special circumstances, or death, permitted their recognition.

A. Tissue Emboli

Fat Embolism

Among the many types of tissue which embolize to the lungs, fat has attracted the widest attention [78,79]. Yet, it is a controversial type of embolism. There is *no* controversy regarding the fact that fat does embolize to the lung under certain circumstances. Fat cells and neutral fat often can be recovered from the lungs of patients dying after bone fractures (particularly of the long bones), other types of severe trauma, burns, and surgery. There has been an upsurge in interest in this type of embolism during each major war because of these associations. Fat emboli also have been observed following limited trauma—and apparently spontaneously—in some patients with fatty livers due to alcoholism, steroid therapy, or carbon tetrachloride poisoning. There also is no question that intravenous infusion of large amounts of neutral fat can induce dyspnea, pulmonary hypertension, and gas exchange abnormalities in experimental animals [80].

However, there is reason to question the relationship between these facts and the fat embolism *syndrome* observed in humans. The syndrome, well described in the literature [78,79,81,82], has a natural history as follows. A patient who has sustained bone trauma (or has one of the other inciting events noted above) is admitted to the hospital in good condition with a negative physical examination aside from the traumatized areas. The patient is alert and oriented with no evidence of cardiopulmonary abnormality. However, after a 12- to 36-hr "latent" period, the patient's condition suddenly deteriorates. Mental aberrations proceeding to delirium and coma may develop. High fever may occur. Marked dyspnea, tachypnea, and tachycardia develop. Multiple petechiae may appear, particularly over the thorax and upper extremities. The lungs may be filled with fine rales. Chest X-ray discloses a diffuse "alveolar-filling" type pattern throughout both lung fields. The patient may be cyanosed and arterial blood gas studies reveal arterial hypoxemia (of a "shunt" type) and hypocapnia. A lowered hematocrit and thrombocytopenia often develop. Fat may be recovered from sputum and urine (though fat may be absent and may occur in other conditions). The patient may succumb or slowly improve over hours to days with careful supportive therapy. If the patient succumbs, the lungs are found to be edematous and markedly congested, often with zones of frank hemorrhage. There may be fat recovered from the lungs, though usually in surprisingly limited quantity. The brain may show similar changes.

There are several "missing links" between this *syndrome* and the occurrence of fat embolism. If it is due to acute *obstruction* of lungs, brain, and skin vessels with fat, why the latent period? Why the severe vascular injury and exudation in the pulmonary vascular bed? Why the thrombocytopenia? Perhaps the explanation lies in the widely held view that the fat particles themselves are not the major culprits; rather, the picture is due to the enzymatic digestion of neutral fat by lipases, releasing free fatty acids. It is these irritating fatty acids which induce severe local capillary damage and the pathophysiological and clinical problems that ensue [83,84]. This thesis is the most tenable one advanced, though it has not been proven to occur in humans.

Treatment of suspected fat embolism is identical to that for any form of "adult respiratory distress syndrome," namely, supportive. Heparin, ethanol infusion, and corticosteroids all have been applied; the first two clearly seem ineffective, while the third has had equivocal results [81,82,85]. One problem in assessing "specific therapy" is that when the patient survives, the diagnosis must remain presumptive; when the patient dies after many hours, failure to find neutral fat may not negate the diagnosis. Thus, fat embolism syndrome remains a clinically accepted event in search of a definitive explanation of its mechanism and, indeed, its relationship to embolization of neutral fat.

Amniotic Fluid Embolism

This entity bears much resemblance to fat embolism in that it is a devastating, unexpected event whose etiology has been cloudy, and which can be proven to exist only with a meticulous postmortem examination in the patients who succumb [86,87].

Two classic sequences have been observed. Both begin shortly after membrane rupture, during spontaneous or Cesarean delivery, with sudden appearance of dyspnea, cyanosis, and systemic hypotention. One group of these patients succumbs immediately. A larger group survives for several hours, at which time massive uterine hemorrhage, hypofibrinogenemia, and perhaps increased fibrinolytic activity are discovered. Some of this latter group survive after intensive therapy.

Autopsy in those who die may disclose lodgement in small pulmonary arterial vessels of particulate amniotic fluid components (lanugo hairs, epithelial squamous cells, vernix, and mucin); and of granular, eosinophilic masses composed of agglutinated platelets and fibrin.

The sequence seems explained by a sudden infusion of amniotic fluid into the venous circulation. The fluid may gain access via placental tears, spontaneous myometrial ruptures (or surgical incision), or cervical tears. In spontaneous labor, uterine contractions may help to "pump" such fluid into veins if the fetal head is lodged in the pelvis. However entry is gained, the amniotic fluid exerts two effects. (1) Because it is a thromboplastic material, it leads to widespread intravascular coagulation. The pulmonary vessels are included in this process. Further, this diffuse coagulation consumes fibrinogen, platelets, and other coagulative components at such a rate that they are reduced to levels which promote hemorrhage ("consumptive coagulopathy"). (2) The particulate contents of the fluid lodge in the small lung vessels.

Should the patient survive the initial insult, the coagulation abnormality will lead to hemorrhage and persistence or recurrence of shock. The shock, plus intravascular coagulation, may stimulate release of endogenous fibrinolytic activity, thereby potentiating the hemorrhagic tendency.

It is likely that the severity of symptoms is directly related to the extent and speed of amniotic fluid infusion. It is known that animals survive intravenous infusion of pure thromboplastin, after a period of initial distress, so long as the infusion rate is carefully controlled [88]. Acceleration of the infusion rate leads to diffuse pulmonary thrombosis and death. It would appear that it is the thromboplastic effect of the fluid, rather than its particulate emboli, which poses the greatest threat.

The entity should be suspected whenever the symptoms described appear during or immediately following delivery. Initial treatment is supportive. Close observation of the coagulation system, particularly of fibrinogen and fibrinolytic activity, and of the need for blood replacement is mandatory. All such patients should be typed and cross matched for potential transfusion. Transfusion of fresh blood is currently the favored method of treatment. In the past, two other forms of therapy have been explored: infusion of human fibrinogen, and administration of ∈-aminocaproic acid (EACA), an inhibitor of the fibrinolytic system. Fibrinogen infusion is associated with a substantial risk of hepatitis and, further, is usually consumed rapidly if the consumptive coagulopathy is still proceeding. If the coagulopathy has subsided, fibrinogen usually returns to acceptable levels without administration of exogenous fibrinogen. Thus, fibrinogen administration is rarely indicated. EACA does block excessive fibrinolytic activity. However, such activity appears to be a *response* to diffuse coagulation, serving to lyse the thrombi which have developed. To block this response might serve to prevent this lytic removal. Therefore, EACA (like fibrinogen) is now used rarely. Blood replacement is the most efficacious therapy. With prompt detection, close observation, blood replacement, and good supportive measures, survival of patients with this dread complication of pregnancy is now the rule.

Tumor Emboli

The lung serves as a filter for tumor cells, as for the other materials already described, a fact which makes the lung a frequent metastatic target. However, in some patients true "tumor emboli," thrombi containing a variable number of neoplastic cells, occur [89,90]. Any tumor which can invade a systemic vein and produce thrombosis is capable of provoking tumor emboli, and the presence of a few such fibrin-cellular composites in the lung is not an uncommon autopsy finding in patients with malignancy.

Less common are those patients in whom the symptoms due to pulmonary tumor emboli dominate the clinical picture [90]. These patients present
with the symptoms and signs of pulmonary embolism. The striking feature is
the steady *continuance* of recurrence (or failure to resolve) despite adequate
and often prolonged anticoagulant therapy. The author has seen this sequence
in patients with hepatic carcinoma, pancreatic carcinoma, sarcoma of the
right ventricle, and right atrial myxoma, and it has been described with a
number of other tumors. The cell-thrombus foci may be in the hepatic veins,
the inferior or superior vena cava, or the cardiac chambers or valves. Steady
deterioration of the patient's status may occur due to increasingly severe pulmonary vascular obstruction. This unusual entity should be considered whenever multiple *small* to moderate-sized pulmonary emboli continue to appear
during adequate anticoagulant therapy. A decline in the patient's nutritional
status to a more striking degree than can be attributed to embolism alone
also provides a clue.

Perhaps the most common tissue source of emboli now is *bone marrow*
[91]. It has been recognized for many years that occasional marrow fragments lodge in the lungs after trauma to marrow-containing bones, or after
surgical procedures involving bone transection or compression (thoracotomy,
sternal splitting, procedures for scoliosis correction). Bone infarcts, as seen in
sickle cell anemia, also occasionally lead to marrow embolism. But the incidence of marrow embolism has been increased sharply since the introduction
of closed cardiac massage. This procedure, involving considerable sternal and rib
trauma (and often fracture), is invariably associated with autopsy evidence of
marrow embolism.

Brain tissue also has been recovered from lung under two different circumstances: in adults, following severe traumatic brain injuries; and in neonates with serious brain malformations [57]. After severe trauma, *liver cells*
also have been recovered from the lungs. *Trophoblastic tissue* has been discovered so frequently in the lungs of women dying during pregnancy or after
delivery that some observers regard it as a routine event in the pregnant female. Occasionally, in patients with hydatidiform mole, severe trophoblastic
embolization may occur.

B. Foreign Body Emboli

Foreign body embolism has increased steadily in both frequency and variety
as our environment has become more hostile, medical instrumentation more
ingenious, and drug abuse more widespread.

Iatrogenic foreign body emboli have become rather common. *Plastic
intravenous tubing* is perhaps the most frequent offender. Cracking, shearing,

or inadvertent escape of such tubing leads to its lodgement in the right cardiac chambers or the pulmonary vascular bed. If nonradioopaque tubing is involved, difficulty may be encountered in locating it by roentgenogram. Such emboli merit removal, not because of the symptoms they induce, but because of their possible role in promoting subsequent thrombosis or infection.

However, an even more common type of foreign body embolism encountered now is that observed in *narcotic addicts.* A wide variety of irritant agents are used purposely, or find their way inadvertently, into the veins and pulmonary arteries of the addict population [92-94]. For example, talcum powder, occasionally used to "cut" heroin, has a severe sclerosant action on the pulmonary vessels, as well as a minor direct embolic effect. Clearly, focal vascular injury and embolization is frequent in narcotic addicts. Abnormal perfusion scans and pulmonary functional abnormalities are commonly seen, as are thrombo-obliterative changes at autopsy [94-96]. Furthermore, these insults may be diffuse enough to cause pulmonary hypertension [97].

A special kind of foreign body embolism has been described in recent years following *lymphangiography* [98]. The oily, radioopaque material used for this procedure (Ethiodol) usually is injected in the lymphatics of the lower extremities to define the status of abdominal lymph nodes. For example, such studies are a routine part of efforts to "stage" disease in patients with Hodgkin's disease. The contrast medium gains access to the lungs via the thoracic duct and causes diffuse pulmonary microembolism [98,99]. Despite this, the patient usually remains asymptomatic because of the vast reserve capacity of the pulmonary vascular bed, though a rather startling X-ray of miliary opaque emboli may be present (Fig. 13). However, if large injections of the contrast medium are given, or if the patient has associated pulmonary disease, acute dyspnea and even death may result. When this occurs, therapy can be only supportive. Prevention is more reliable, through careful cardiopulmonary evaluation of patients *before* the procedure and use of the *smallest amount* of contrast material necessary for adequate visualization.

A similar kind of microembolism is purposely induced for other diagnostic purposes, namely, the use of radio-labeled particles of albumin (macroaggregates or microspheres) for lung photoscanning studies. While the number of particles injected is carefully controlled, and their life span in the pulmonary bed is short, caution should be exercised in using such materials after *long storage* since the *dose* is measured in terms of *radioactivity.* Therefore, to deliver the proper dose of radioactivity, a larger number of *particles* must be given of "old" materials which have undergone extensive radioactive decay. Such "old" materials should be discarded. Also, occasionally, mixing of these materials with blood has resulted in the formation of small thromboparticulate

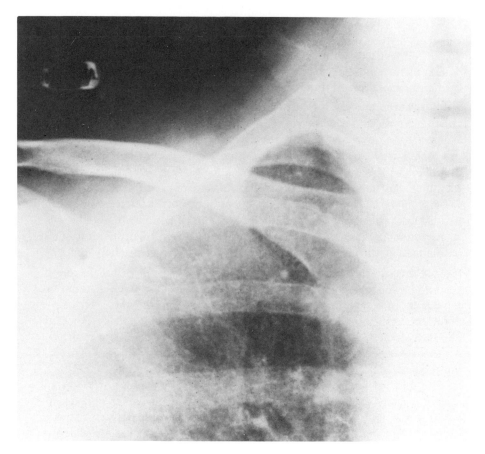

FIGURE 13 Fine (miliary) pattern in right upper lobe vessels of patient following lymphangiogram. Diffuse pattern represents embolization of contrast medium.

aggregations. The injection of such materials results in bizarre "hot spots" on the photoscan [100], although no symptoms have been noted as a result.

Air is another foreign substance which can enter the pulmonary circuit after gaining accidental access to systemic veins. This is undoubtedly a common event in modern medical practice. However, the development of symptoms depends on the amount of air reaching the lungs per unit time [101]. Small amounts of air can be removed rather rapidly from blood and lungs, so no symptoms develop although, experimentally, repetitive small air injections can induce pulmonary vascular lesions [102]. It is the substantial bolus of air entering the heart rapidly which causes difficulty. The precise mechanism by which air embolism may lead to death is not clear. It is known that the air-blood mixture is churned in the right atrium and ventricle into a "froth" which has difficulty traversing the pulmonary capillary network. The froth, on reaching the alveolocapillary bed, apparently induces vasoconstrictive-obstructive changes which lead to acute pulmonary hypertension.

Air embolism has been encountered in many contexts. Wounds of and surgery upon the head, neck, and thorax are particularly dangerous because the strong suction exerted on veins in these areas by inspiration encourages air entry. Diagnostic procedures in which air insufflation is used are also known offenders (pneumoperitoneum, insufflation of the Fallopian tubes and the bladder, retroperitoneal air studies). Carbon dioxide is the gas of choice in all such procedures because its extremely high solubility in blood makes significant embolism virtually impossible. (However, its rapid obsorption also requires that desired X-rays be obtained with dispatch.) Air embolism also may complicate cardiopulmonary bypass procedures. And, of course, it may occur whenever intravenous catheters or needles are in place.

Special forms of gas embolism may develop whenever acute decompression of the body occurs, with nitrogen bubbles the usual offender. Decompression may occur with pressure losses in tunnels under construction at depth, when divers ascend too rapidly from depth, or when aviators ascend too rapidly from sea level without protective compression [103]. Air embolism also may occur with acute decompression when asymptomatic lung cysts expand rapidly and rupture. Pneumothorax most commonly occurs in this situation, but air embolism may develop if the lung is lacerated.

The therapy of gas embolism consists of immediate action to prevent entrance of the air into the lungs and, failing this, hyperbaric compression. The former can be attempted by placing the patient promptly in the left lateral decubitus so that air collects in the superiorly placed right atrium (as is done in carbon dioxide angiography). The latter requires access to a hyperbaric chamber.

C. Parasitic Emboli

Of the many parasitic infections which may gain access to the pulmonary circulation, only one is known to produce significant embolic lesions: schistosomiasis [104,105]. While there are differences in the behavior of the three schistosomal flukes (*s. hematobium, s. mansoni, s. japonicum*), all three can produce pulmonary vascular obstruction.

Both schistosomal flukes and ova may reach the pulmonary circulation. The numbers of each reaching the lung are usually rather small. However, when diffuse hepatic fibrosis has occurred, bombardment of the lungs through collateral channels is enhanced.

Ova not only impact in small pulmonary vessels but also, because they are "sticky," may attach to the walls of large-diameter pulmonary vessels. Once in the pulmonary bed, the ova may create difficulties in three different ways: (1) by direct, physical obstruction of small arteries, (2) by release of irritating substances which induce necrosis and fibrosis of vessel walls, and (3) by serving as antigenic stimuli to induce allergic granulomatous reactions in the vessels. The latter two mechanisms are the most significant, for they may lead to severe obliterative changes in vessels of significant size.

The worms themselves can contribute to vascular obstruction by direct impaction, but apparently generate little vessel wall reaction while they are alive. However, when the flukes die (or are killed by therapy), a severe focal vascular reaction results. This is a consideration when therapy directed against the flukes is contemplated.

Through these various mechanisms, both ova and flukes can induce obliterative changes extensive enough to produce substantial pulmonary hypertension. Indeed, hypertension can become so marked that, pathologically, angiomatoid lesions appear in the small pulmonary arteries; and that, clinically, pulmonary hypertension and right ventricular failure dominate the picture [104]. Once pulmonary hypertension becomes established, obliterative changes promoted by the hypertension itself will lead to progressive stress upon the right ventricle.

References

1. Wessler, S., *Venous Thromboembolism: Scope of the Problem, in Prophylactic Therapy of Deep Vein Thrombosis and Pulmonary Embolism.* DHEW Publication No. (NIH) 76-866, 1976, pp. 1–10.
2. Moser, K. M., Pulmonary embolism: Where the problem is not (Editorial), *JAMA,* **236**:1500, 1976.
3. Egeberg, O., Inherited antithrombin deficiency causing thrombophilia, *Thromb. Diath. Haemorr.,* **13**:516 (1965).
4. Wessler, S., Studies in intravascular coagulation. IV. The pathogenesis of serum-induced venous thrombosis, *J. Clin. Invest.,* **34**:647 (1955).
5. Foster, C. S., and E. Genton, The epidemiology of venous thrombosis, *Milbank Mem. Fund Q.,* **50**:(Part 2) 1 (1972).
6. Kakkar, V. V., C. T. Hower, C. Flanc, and M. B. Clarke, Natural history of post-operative deep vein thrombosis, *Lancet,* **2**:230–233 (1969).
7. Kakkar, V. V., T. P. Corrigem, and D. P. Fossard, Prevention of post-operative embolism by low dose heparin: An international multicenter trial, *Lancet,* **2**:45 (1975).
8. Mavor, G. E., and J. M. D. Galloway, The iliofemoral venous segment as a source of pulmonary emboli, *Lancet,* **1**:871–874 (1967).

9. LeMoine, R., and K. M. Moser, Does a "safe" form of deep venous thrombosis exist? *Clin. Res.,* **26**:136A (1978).

10. Sevitt, S., Venous thrombosis and pulmonary embolism: Their prevention by oral anticoagulants, *Am. J. Med.,* **33**:703–716 (1962).

11. Harris, W. H., C. Salzman, C. Athanasoulis, A. C. Waltman, S. Baum, and R. W. DeSanctis, Comparison of warfarin, low molecular weight dextron, aspirin and subcutaneous heparin in prevention of venous thromboembolism following total hip replacement, *J. Bone Joint Surg. [Br.],* **56A**: 1552 (1974).

12. Severinghaus, J. W., E. W. Swenson, T. Finley, M. T. Lategola, and J. Williams, Unilateral hypoventilation produced by occlusion of one pulmonary artery, *J. Appl. Physiol.,* **16**:53 (1961).

13. Gurewich, V., J. L. Cohen, and D. P. Thomas, Humoral factors in massive pulmonary embolism: An experimental study, *Am. Heart J.,* **76**:784 (1968).

14. Thomas, D., M. Stein, and G. Tanabe, Mechanisms of broncho constriction produced by thrombo emboli in dogs, *Am. J. Physiol.,* **206**:1207 (1964).

15. Widdicombe, J. G., Reflex mechanisms in pulmonary thromboembolism. In *Pulmonary Thromboembolism.* Edited by K. M. Moser and M. Stein. Chicago, Yearbook Publishers, 1973.

16. Levy, S. E., and D. H. Simmons, Mechanism of arterial hypoxemia following pulmonary thromboembolism in dogs, *J. Appl. Physiol.,* **39**:41–46 (1975).

17. Dantzker, D. R., P. D. Wagner, and V. W. Tornabene, Gas exchange after pulmonary thromboembolization in dogs, *Circ. Res.,* **42**:92–103 (1978).

18. Chernick, V., W. H. Hodson, and L. J. Greenfield, Effect of chronic pulmonary artery ligation on pulmonary mechanics and surfactant, *J. Appl. Physiol.,* **21**:1315 (1966).

19. Finley, T. H., E. W. Swensen, J. A. Clements, R. G. Gardner, R. R. Wright, and J. W. Severinghaus, Changes in mechanical properties, appearance and surface activity of extracts of one lung following occlusion of its pulmonary artery in the dog, *Physiologist,* **3**:56 (1960).

20. Sanders, B. S., J. W. Shepard, Jr., A. Jobe, K. Migai, K. M. Moser, and L. Gluck, Alveolar CO_2 tension as a mediator of lamellar body release in experimental left pulmonary artery occlusion, *Chest,* **72**:411 (1977).

21. Moser, K. M., M. Guisan, E. E. Bartimmo, A. M. Longo, D. G. Harsanyi, and N. Chiorazzi, In vivo and post-mortem dissolution rates of pulmonary emboli and venous thrombi in the dog, *Circulation,* **48**:170 (1973).

22. Tow, D. E., and H. N. Wagner, Recovery of pulmonary arterial flow in patients with pulmonary embolism, *N. Engl. J. Med.,* **276**:1053 (1967).

23. Murphy, M. L., and R. T. Bulloch, Factors influencing the restoration of blood flow following pulmonary embolization as determined by angiography and scanning, *Circulation,* **38**:1116 (1968).

24. Dalen, J. D., J. S. Banas, H. L. Brooks, G. L. Evans, J. H. Paraskos, and L. Dexter, Resolution rate of acute pulmonary embolism in man, *N. Engl. J. Med.,* **280**:1194 (1969).

25. James, III, W. S., S. J. Menn, and K. M. Moser, Rapid resolution of a pulmonary embolus in man, *West J. Med.,* **128**:60–64 (1978).
26. Paraskos, J. A., S. J. Adelstein, R. E. Smith, F. D. Ruchman, W. Grossman, L. Dexter, and J. E. Dalen, Late prognosis of acute pulmonary embolism, *N. Engl. J. Med.,* **289**:55 (1973).
27. Urokinase-streptokinase pulmonary embolism trial: A national cooperative study, *JAMA,* **229**:1606 (1974).
28. Moser, K. M., and N. S. Braunwald, Successful surgical intervention in severe chronic thromboembolic pulmonary hypertension, *Chest,* **64**:29–35 (1973).
29. Karsner, H. T., and A. A. Ghoreyeb, A study of the relation of pulmonary and bronchial circulation, *J. Exp. Med.,* **18**:500–506 (1913).
30. The urokinase pulmonary embolism trial. A national cooperative study, *Circulation,* **47**(Suppl. II):1–108 (1973).
31. Moser, K. M., Pulmonary embolism: State of the art, *Am. Rev. Respir. Dis.,* **115**:829–852 (1977).
32. Webster, Jr., J. R., G. B. Saddeh, P. R. Eggum, and J. R. Suker, Wheezing due to pulmonary embolism—treatment with heparin, *N. Engl. J. Med.,* **274**:931–933 (1966).
33. Thomas, D. P., J. Gurewich, and T. P. Ashford, Platelet adherence to thromboemboli in relation to the pathogenesis and treatment of pulmonary embolism, *N. Engl. J. Med.,* **274**:953 (1966).
34. Wacker, W. E. C., M. Rosenthal, P. Snodgrass, and E. Amador, A triad for the diagnosis of pulmonary embolism and infarction, *JAMA,* **128**:8 (1961).
35. Sobel, B. E., Serum enzymes and the diagnosis of pulmonary embolism. In *Pulmonary Thromboembolism.* Edited by K. M. Moser and M. Stein. Yearbook Publishers, Chicago, 1973.
36. Wilson, III, J. E., L. J. Bynun, and C. M. Crotty, The fibrinolytic system in early and late recurrence of venous thromboembolism, *Clin. Res.,* **26**:164A (1978).
37. Torrance, D. J., *The Chest Film in Massive Pulmonary Embolism.* Springfield, Ill., Thomas, 1963.
38. Stein, P. D., J. E. Dalen, K. M. McIntyre, A. H. Sasahara, N. K. Wenger, and P. W. Willis, The electrocardiogram in acute pulmonary embolism, *Prog. Cardiovasc. Dis.,* **17**:247 (1975).
39. Tisi, G. M., G. A. Landis, A. Miale, Jr., and K. M. Moser, Quantitation of regional pulmonary blood flow: Validity and potential sources of error, *Am. Rev. Respir. Dis.,* **97**:843–850 (1968).
40. De Nardo, G. L., D. A. Goodman, R. Ravisini, and D. A. Dietrich, The ventilatory lung scan in the diagnosis of pulmonary embolism, *N. Engl. J. Med.,* **282**:1334 (1970).
41. Moser, K. M., Clinical applications of ventilation/perfusion scintiphotography. In *Textbook of Pulmonary Diseases.* Edited by G. L. Baum. Boston, Little, Brown, 1974.
42. Alderson, P. O., J. L. Doppman, S. S. Diamond, K. G. Mendenhall, E. L. Barron, and M. Girton, Ventilation-perfusion lung imaging and selective

pulmonary angiography in dogs with experimental pulmonary embolism, *J. Nucl. Med.,* **19**:164–171 (1978).

43. McNeil, B. J., A diagnostic strategy using ventilation-perfusion studies in patients suspect for pulmonary embolism, *J. Nucl. Med.,* **17**:613–616 (1976).

44. Gluck, M. C., and K. M. Moser, Pulmonary artery agenesis. Diagnosis with ventilation and perfusion scintiphotography, *Circulation,* **41**:859–867 (1970).

45. Dalen, J. E., V. S. Mathur, H. Evans, F. W. Haynes, A. A. Pur-Shahriani, P. D. Stein, and L. Dexter, Pulmonary angiography in experimental pulmonary embolism, *Am. Heart J.,* **72**:509 (1966).

46. Stein, P. D., J. F. O'Connor, J. E. Dalen, A. A. Pur-Shahriani, F. G. Hoppin, D. T. Hammond, F. W. Haynes, F. G. Fleischner, and L. Dexter, The angiographic diagnosis of acute pulmonary embolism: Evaluation of criteria, *Am. Heart J.,* **73**:730 (1967).

47. Goodwin, D. A., J. T. Bushberg, P. W. Doherty, M. J. Lipton, F. K. Conley, C. I. Diamonti, and C. F. Meares, Indium-111-labeled autologous platelets for location of vascular thrombi in humans, *J. Nucl. Med.,* **19**:626–634 (1978).

48. DeNardo, S. J., G. L. DeNardo, R. F. Carretta, A. L. Jansholt, K. A. Krohn, and N. F. Peek, Clinical usefulness of I-123-fibrinogen for detection of thrombophlebitis, *J. Nucl. Med.,* **16**:524 (1975).

49. Tulumello, J., J. H. Harrell, and K. M. Moser, Direct visualization of pulmonary emboli in the dog, *Chest,* **74**(3):352 (1978).

50. Moser, K. M., P. Harsanyi, M. Guisan, and E. Butler, Pressure-flow relationships with progressive pulmonary arterial narrowing, *Fed. Proc.,* **27**:578 (1968).

51. Moser, K. M., *Pulmonary Embolism. Current Therapy.* Philadelphia, Saunders, 1978, pp. 134–140.

52. *Prophylactic Therapy of Deep Vein Thrombosis and Pulmonary Embolism.* DHEW Publication No. (NIH) 76-866, 1975.

53. Rosenberg, R. D., Heparin action, *Circulation,* **49**:603 (1974).

54. Genton, E., Guidelines for heparin therapy, *Ann. Intern. Med.,* **80**:77 (1974).

55. Wagenvoort, C. A., and N. Wagenvoort, *Pathology of Pulmonary Hypertension.* New York, Wiley & Sons, 1977.

56. Moser, K. M., V. N. Houk, R. C. Jones, and C. C. Hufnagel, Chronic, massive obstruction of the pulmonary arteries, *Circulation,* **32**:377–385 (1965).

57. Spencer, H., *Pathology of the Lung.* Oxford, Pergamon, 1977.

58. Savacool, J. W., and R. Charr, Thrombosis of the pulmonary artery, *Am. Rev. Tuberc.,* **44**:42–57 (1941).

59. Magidsion, O., and G. Jacobson, Thrombosis of the main pulmonary arteries, *Br. Heart J.,* **17**:207 (1955).

60. Wagenvoort, C. A., D. Heath, and J. E. Edwards, *The Pathology of the Pulmonary Vasculature.* Springfield, Ill., Thomas, 1964.

61. Moser, K. M., and J. G. Shea, The relationship between pulmonary infarction, cor pulmonale, and the sickle states, *Am. J. Med.,* **22**:561–576 (1957).

62. Weiss, S., E. A. Stead, J. V. Warren, and O. T. Benley, Scleroderma heart disease, *Arch. Intern. Med.,* **71**:749 (1943).

63. Trell, E., and C. Lindstrom, Pulmonary hypertension in systemic sclerosis, *Ann. Rheum. Dis.,* **30**:390 (1971).

64. Michaels, L., N. J. Brown, and M. Cory-Wright, Arterial changes in pulmonary sarcoidosis, *Arch. Pathol.,* **69**:741 (1960).

65. Heath, D., D. E. Donald, and J. E. Edwards, Pulmonary vascular changes in a dog after aorto-pulmonary anastomosis for four years, *Br. Heart J.,* **21**: 187 (1959).

66. Harris, P., and D. Heath, *The Human Pulmonary Circulation. Its Form and Function in Health and Disease.* Baltimore, Williams & Wilkins, 1962.

67. Nasser, W. K., H. Feigenbaum, and C. Fisch, Clinical and hemodynamic diagnosis of pulmonary venous obstruction due to sclerosing mediastinitis, *Am. J. Cardiol.,* **20**:725–729 (1967).

68. Brown, C. H., and C. J. Harrison, Pulmonary veno-occlusive disease, *Lancet,* **2**:61–65 (1966).

69. Liebow, A. A., K. M. Moser, and M. T. Southgate, Rapidly progressive dyspnea in a teenage boy, *JAMA,* **223**:1243–1253 (1973).

70. Bain, R. C., J. E. Edwards, C. H. Scheifley, and J. E. Geraci, Right-sided bacterial endocarditis and endarteritis, *Am. J. Med.,* **24**:98–110 (1958).

71. Jaffe, R. B., and E. B. Koschmann, Intravenous drug abuse: Pulmonary, cardiac and vascular complications, *Am. J. Roentgenol.,* **109**:107–120 (1970).

72. Collins, C. G., E. W. Nelson, J. H. Collins, B. B. Weinstein, and E. A. MacCallum, Suppurative pelvic thrombophlebitis. II. Symptomatology and diagnosis. A study of 70 patients treated by ligation of the inferior vena cava and ovarian veins. *Surgery,* **30**:311 (1951).

73. Stein, J. M., and B. A. Pruitt, Suppurative thrombophlebitis: A lethal Iatrogenic disease, *N. Engl. J. Med.,* **282**:1452–1455 (1970).

74. Goodwin, N. J., J. J. Castronuovo, and E. A. Friedman, Recurrent septic embolization complicating maintenance hemodialysis, *Ann. Intern. Med.,* **71**:29–38 (1969).

75. Dunn, L. J., and L. W. Van Voorhis, Enigmatic fever and pelvic thrombophlebitis: response to anticoagulants, *N. Engl. J. Med.,* **276**:265–268 (1967).

76. Fred, H. L., and T. S. Harle, Septic pulmonary embolism, *Dis. Chest,* **55**: 483 (1969).

77. Jaffe, R. B., and E. B. Koschmann, Septic pulmonary emboli, *Radiology,* **96**:527–532 (1970).

78. Sevitt, S. S., *Fat Embolism.* London, Butterworth, 1962.

79. Moylen, J. A., Diagnosis and treatment of fat embolism, *Am. Rev. Med.,* **28**:85 (1977).

80. Mylea, S., and C. Sylven, Induced fat embolism by means of radioactive-labelled fat, *Acta Chir. Scand.,* 142:361–365 (1976).

81. Moylen, J. A., Fat emboli syndrome, *J. Trauma,* 16:84 (1976).

82. Herndon, J. H., The syndrome of fat embolism, *South. Med. J.,* 63:12 (1975).

83. Peltier, L. F., Toxic properties of neutral fat and free fatty acids, *Surgery,* 62:756 (1967).

84. Derks, C. M., and D. Jacobovitz-Derks, Embolic pneumopathy induced by oleic acid, *Am. J. Pathol.,* 87:143 (1977).

85. Ashbaugh, D. G., and T. G. Petty, The use of corticosteroids in the treatment of respiratory failure associated with massive fat embolism, *Surg. Gynecol. Obstet.,* 123:493–500 (1966).

86. Attwood, H. D., The histologic diagnosis of amniotic fluid embolism, *J. Pathol. Bacteriol.,* 76:211–215 (1958).

87. Ratnoff, O. D., J. A. Pritchard, and J. E. Calopy, Medical progress: Hemorrhagic states during pregnancy, *N. Engl. J. Med.,* 253:63 (1955).

88. Astrup, T., and O. K. Albrechtsen, Serum effects following tissue thromboplastin infusion, *Thromb. Diath. Haemmo.,* 21:117 (1969).

89, Morgan, A. D., The pathology of subacute cor pulmonale in diffuse carcinomatosis of the lungs, *J. Pathol. Bacteriol.,* 61:75 (1949).

90. Storey, P. B., and W. Goldstein, Pulmonary embolization from primary hepatic carcinoma, *Arch. Intern. Med.,* 110:262 (1962).

91. Garvey, J. W., and F. G. Zak, Pulmonary bone marrow emboli in patients receiving external cardiac massage, *JAMA,* 187:59 (1964).

92. Hopkins, G. B., Pulmonary angiothrombotic granulomatosis in drug offenders, *JAMA,* 221:909 (1972).

93. Wendt, V. E., H. E. Puro, J. Shapiro, W. Mathews, and P. L. Wolf, Angiothrombotic pulmonary hypertension in addicts: "Blue velvet" addition, *JAMA,* 188:755 (1964).

94. Douglas, F. G., K. J. Kafilmont, and N. L. Patt, Foreign particle embolism in drug addicts: Respiratory pathophysiology, *Ann. Intern. Med.,* 75:865 (1971).

95. Camargo, G., and C. Culp, Pulmonary function studies in ex-heroin users, *Chest,* 67:331 (1975).

96. Soin, J. S., H. N. Wagner, D. Thomashaw, and T. C. Brown, Increased sensitivity of regional lung measurements in early detection of narcotic lung disease, *Chest,* 67:325 (1975).

97. Robertson, Jr., C. H., R. C. Reynolds, and J. E. Wilson, III, Pulmonary hypertension and foreign body granulomas in introvenous drug abusers, *Am. J. Med.,* 61:657–664 (1976).

98. Gold, W. M., J. Yonder, S. Anderson, and J. A. Nadel, Pulmonary function abnormalities after lymphangiography, *N. Engl. J. Med.,* 273:519–524 (1965).

99. Tisi, G. M., W. G. Wolfe, R. J. Fallat, and J. A. Nadel, Effects of O_2 and CO_2 on airway smooth muscle following pulmonary vascular occlusion, *J. Appl. Physiol.,* 28:570 (1970).

100. Moser, K. M., and A. Miale, Jr., Interpretive pitfalls in pulmonary photo-scanning, *Am. J. Med.,* **44**:366–376 (1968).

101. Ericsson, J. A., J. D. Gottlieb, and R. B. Sweet, Closed chest cardiac massage in the treatment of venous air embolism, *N. Engl. J. Med.,* **270**: 1353 (1965).

102. Boerema, B., Appearance and regression of pulmonary arterial lesions after repeated intravenous injections of gas, *J. Pathol. Bacteriol.,* **89**: 741 (1965).

103. Behnke, A. R., Decompression sickness: Advances and interpretations, *Aerosp. Med.,* **42**:255 (1971).

104. Turner, P. P., Schistosomal pulmonary arterial hypertension in East Africa, *Br. Heart J.,* **26**:821–837 (1964).

105. Jawalurz, K. I., and C. M. Karpas, Pulmonary schistosomiasis: A detailed clinicopathological study, *Am. Rev. Respir. Dis.,* **88**:517–527 (1963).

6

Pulmonary Vascular Disease
Secondary to Lung Disease

DONALD HEATH and PAUL SMITH

University of Liverpool
Liverpool, England

I.   Introduction

There is a close interrelationship between the functions of heart and lung, so
that diseases of the one commonly affect the function of the other. The
anatomical pathway through which this mutual involvement is effected is the
pulmonary vasculature. In this chapter we shall be concerned with the manner
in which primary diseases of the lung can bring about disorder or disease of the
pulmonary circulation. It is not our purpose to present a compendium of lung
conditions which may induce changes in pulmonary blood vessels. Rather, we
shall attempt to delineate the principles which underlie the involvement of the
pulmonary vasculature by primary lung disease.

Diseases of the lung commonly lead to chronic alveolar hypoxia, which is
one of the most potent constrictors of the pulmonary arterial tree. Hence, any
pulmonary disease chronically disturbing the gaseous environment of the
terminal portion of the pulmonary arterial tree will induce in it sustained vasoconstriction and finally structural changes. On the other hand, some pathologic
components of primary lung disease, such as fibrosis, may involve the pulmonary vasculature directly and organically. As we shall see later, proximity to,

rather than involvement in, an area of fibrosis induces a different form of pulmonary vascular disease. Granulomatous diseases may also directly infiltrate the structure of the pulmonary arteries. The lung has a dual blood supply, being perfused by both the systemic and pulmonary circulations, and this anatomical circumstance sometimes allows for the development of abnormal communications between the two circulations exposing the pulmonary vasculature to unaccustomed hemodynamic conditions. Thus, hypoxia, pulmonary fibrosis, granulomatous disease, and bronchopulmonary anastomoses constitute the main factors through which primary lung pathology may induce pulmonary vascular disease, and we shall consider each of them in turn.

II. Hypoxia

Hypoxia is a potent constrictor of the terminal portions of the pulmonary arterial tree and, when this action is sustained, it leads to muscularization of this part of the pulmonary vasculature and significant pulmonary arterial hypertension. Chronic alveolar hypoxia occurs in many diseases but the commonest and most important in Western Europe and North America are chronic bronchitis and emphysema. Other lung diseases which may lead to chronic alveolar hypoxia are cystic fibrosis [1] and some forms of interstitial pulmonary fibrosis. In kyphoscoliosis the condition is caused by the small lung and chest volume [2]. Grossly obese patients may develop the Pickwickian syndrome [3-5] in which shallow breathing leads to chronic alveolar hypoxia. Finally, sustained alveolar hypoxia occurs in the absence of any predisposing disease in the large populations of people who live at altitudes exceeding 3000 m and who are thereby subjected to a diminished partial pressure of oxygen in the ambient air [6].

A. Pathology of the Pulmonary Vasculature in Emphysema

In pulmonary emphysema, longitudinally orientated smooth muscle appears in the intima of muscular pulmonary arteries [7]. It forms small fasciculi separated by broad anastomosing bands of elastic tissue (Fig. 1). This intimal longitudinal muscle may be a response to longitudinal stretching of the vessel around dilated airways [8]. It can occur in the absence of pulmonary arterial hypertension, although this hemodynamic abnormality may help to stimulate its formation [7,9]. Hypertrophy of the original media of circularly oriented muscle in muscular pulmonary arteries, if present at all, is usually slight even when there is right ventricular hypertrophy. This is probably related to the fact that the degree of pulmonary arterial hypertension in emphysema is relatively mild and intermittent, occurring during attacks of respiratory infection

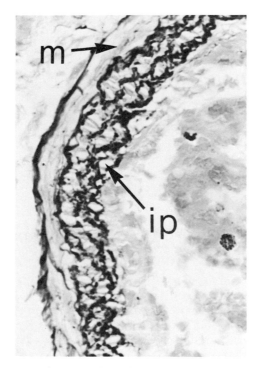

FIGURE 1   Segment of a muscular pulmonary artery from a case of emphysema. The vessel has been stained so that elastic fibers appear black. The media (m) is thin and internal to it is a proliferation of the intima (ip) comprising anastomosing elastic fibers with longitudinally oriented smooth muscle cells within its interstices. (Elastic Van Gieson, X 600.)

or fluid retention. In this respect, the pulmonary hypertension of emphysema differs from that associated with the severe forms of pulmonary vascular disease complicating congenital cardiac shunts where medial hypertrophy of pulmonary arteries is prominent and often associated with obliterative intimal fibrosis or even fibrinoid necrosis.

In some cases of emphysema there *is* muscularization of pulmonary arterioles. Normally, these vessels consist of endothelium resting upon a single elastic lamina, but when they become muscularized a layer of circularly oriented smooth muscle forms internally to the elastic lamina (Fig. 2). A new, thinner, internal elastic lamina forms subjacent to the endothelium. The result is a vessel resembling a systemic arteriole and, like it, capable of constricting and increasing the resistance to the flow of blood through the lungs. There is a relationship between the presence of muscularized arterioles and right ventricular hypertrophy in emphysema, suggesting that they are

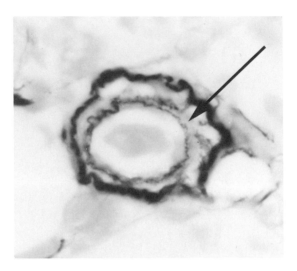

FIGURE 2   Muscularized pulmonary arteriole from a rat subjected to a pressure of 380 mmHg for 5 weeks. The external boundary of the vessel consists of the original, thick elastic lamina of the arteriole. Internal to this is a broad layer of circularly oriented smooth muscle (arrow). The inner aspect of the media is lined by a thin, newly formed, internal elastic lamina. (Elastic Van Gieson, X 1500.)

intimately concerned with the increase in pulmonary vascular resistance. The absence of occlusive fibrous or fibroelastic lesions in the pulmonary arteries or arterioles in states of chronic hypoxia is of considerable functional significance because the associated pulmonary arterial hypertension is reversible. Sometimes in emphysema one encounters acellular intimal fibrosis in muscular pulmonary arteries and arterioles but it is not occlusive. It is tempting to suggest that this is an aging process occurring to the intimal longitudinal muscle, but this has not been proven. Some of the intimal fibrosis may be secondary to organization of thrombus [10]. It seems likely that factors apart from alveolar hypoxia influence the pulmonary vasculature in emphysema.

These vascular lesions occur not only in emphysema but also in association with the other causes of chronic alveolar hypoxia referred to above. This combination of lesions is sufficiently distinct to merit a specific designation, and we have coined the term *hypoxic hypertensive pulmonary vascular disease* (hypoxic HPVD) [11]. In brief, hypoxic HPVD comprises muscularization of pulmonary arterioles, the development of longitudinal muscle in the intima of pulmonary arteries, and the absence of significant intimal fibrosis.

B. Studies on the Hypoxia of High Altitude

A useful way of examining the effects of chronic hypoxia on the pulmonary circulation, uncomplicated by lung disease, is to study native highlanders who live in high, mountainous areas. The three regions where much of this work has been carried out are the high Andes of Peru, the Himalayas, and the mountainous areas of Colorado. Only recently has it been recognized that these subjects have a moderate elevation of their pulmonary arterial blood pressure. In 1956, Rotta et al. [12] found that the pulmonary arterial mean pressure in people born and bred at Morococha in Peru, at an altitude of 4540 m, was double that of the level of 12 mmHg found in permanent residents of Lima at sea level. This concept of pulmonary hypertension induced by high altitude is now well documented following further studies in the Peruvian Andes [13]. Elevation of the pulmonary arterial pressure at high altitude is associated with right ventricular hypertrophy [14] and muscularization of the pulmonary arterioles [6,15]. In some cases there is a production of longitudinally oriented smooth muscle in the intima of muscular pulmonary arteries and muscularized arterioles [11]. These changes will also occur in a person who is born at sea level and then spends several years of continuous residence at high altitude.

The highlanders have pulmonary hypertension from birth and retain the muscularization of the pulmonary arterioles characteristic of fetal life. There are also differences in configuration of the elastic tissue in the media of the pulmonary trunk between people born and living at high altitude and people born and living at sea level. Lowlanders retain the fetal "aortic" configuration [16] for about 3 months and then the elastic tissue starts to fragment. A number of possible "transitional" configurations exist which the elastin can adopt, and one of these is called the "persistent" pattern in which only a few elastic fibers fragment [17]. At sea level the transitional configurations A [16] and B [17] do not usually persist longer than 2 to 3 years, after which the sparse, highly fragmented "adult" configuration predominates. In native highlanders the duration of these phases is prolonged by a factor dependent upon the altitude. Thus, over 4000 m the aortic configuration persists for about 9 years and is followed by the persistent pattern. Conversion to the adult type occurs very late at the age of 60 years [18]. At lower altitudes of between 3440 and 3840 m, the aortic configuration disappears after 3 years and the persistent configuration becomes converted into the adult type between 20 and 55 years of age. These effects are almost certainly produced by the incomplete fall in pulmonary arterial blood pressure from fetal levels which occurs when the high-altitude child is born. This is also reflected by the thicker media in the pulmonary trunk of highlanders [19].

Other species besides the human respond to hypoxia by developing pulmonary arterial hypertension. Cattle are highly susceptible because their pulmonary vasculature is naturally muscular and reactive. Other low-altitude species which have to acclimatize and are also vulnerable include dogs, sheep, rats, and mice. Species which have evolved in a high-altitude environment are genetically *adapted* rather than *acclimatized* to hypoxia and do not develop significant pulmonary arterial hypertension. They include the llama, alpaca, vicuña, yak, and species of mountain geese [6]. The hypoxic HPVD induced in cattle and other species which are not indigenous to altitude is similar to that in humans, except that intimal longitudinal muscle has not been reported in their pulmonary arteries so far as we are aware.

The pulmonary vascular disease of hypoxia is purely muscular in nature. Those grades of hypertensive pulmonary vascular disease secondary to cardiac shunts, in which there is no occlusive intimal fibrosis, are also muscular in nature. In them it has been shown that the pulmonary hypertension is reversible upon closure of the cardiac defect [20]. In the same way the pulmonary vascular disease of hypoxia is also reversible. Thus, when high-altitude natives move to a new home at sea level, their pulmonary hypertension declines by two stages to that of sea-level residents [13]. The initial response to the removal of the hypoxic stimulus in humans appears to be a relaxation of constricted pulmonary arteries and arterioles. This causes a rapid drop in pulmonary vascular resistance with an associated fall in pulmonary arterial blood pressure close to normal. This is followed by a gradual decline in pulmonary arterial hypertension over the next 2 years as the muscularized arterioles lose their muscle coat [6]. This reversibility of hypoxic pulmonary hypertension has been studied in experimental animals [21,22]. Thus, when rats are placed in a decompression chamber at a pressure of 380 mmHg, they develop pulmonary arterial hypertension. This is associated with right ventricular hypertrophy after a 2-week exposure. When the animals are returned to sea-level atmospheric pressure, there is a steady decline in pulmonary arterial blood pressure and a regression of right ventricular hypertrophy over a period of 5 weeks. This reversibility of hypoxic pulmonary hypertension may be of considerable importance when applied to the treatment of emphysema.

C.   The Causes of Hypoxic Pulmonary Hypertension

Alveolar hypoxia and probably hypoxemia constrict pulmonary arteries and arterioles but dilate systemic vessels. This constrictive effect is readily demonstrated in experimental animals and in lungs devoid of all neural connections. It is an intrinsic property of lung tissue and is the mechanism responsible for the generation of acute pulmonary arterial hypertension which develops soon after humans or most animal species breathe air with a low partial pressure of oxygen. The view that this acute vasoconstriction is caused more by alveolar hypoxia than by hypoxemia was recently questioned in a review by Fishman [23]. He believes that hypoxemia is probably of importance in maintaining the tone of pulmonary arteries whereas alveolar hypoxia exerts its effect primarily on the arterioles and precapillaries. An acute increase in pulmonary vascular tone is unlikely to be sustained enough to cause a chronic elevation of pulmonary vascular resistance such as occurs in the native highlander. Under these circumstances of chronic hypoxia the pulmonary arterial hypertension has an organic basis in muscularization of pulmonary arterioles. These muscular vessels are capable of constriction and exerting a more profound effect upon vascular resistance than the pulmonary arteries. The native highlander retains the fetal type of muscularized pulmonary arterioles from birth. The lowlander moving to high altitude develops such small muscular vessels after exposure to a period of alveolar hypoxia or hypoxemia.

Naeye [24] produced hypoxia in dogs and calves by constricting their bronchi. At the same time he maintained normal pulmonary arterial pressures and oxygen saturation. Both groups of animals developed hypertrophy and hyperplasia of smooth muscle in the terminal portions of the pulmonary arterial tree. Since hypoxemia was absent, Naeye concluded that alveolar hypoxia was the cause. However, other studies have demonstrated that hypoxemia will constrict pulmonary arteries and arterioles. In view of the close proximity of pulmonary arterioles to alveoli we think it likely that the direct influence of hypoxic air stimulates muscularization.

Several workers have searched for a chemical mediator which can maintain the pulmonary arteries and arterioles in a constricted state for the many years that an individual may live at high altitude or suffer from chronic bronchitis and emphysema. In 1969, Bergofsky [25] suggested that mast cells in the vicinity of pulmonary arteries release histamine, which causes vessels to constrict. This is an attractive hypothesis because the periarterial mast cell is in a strategic position to act as an intermediary, being situated between the hypoxic air and the vascular media. Numerous experiments have been performed which tend to support this hypothesis. Thus, in the isolated perfused rat lung, antihistaminic drugs diminish the pulmonary pressor response to hypoxia, whereas histaminase inhibitor potentiates it [26]. Furthermore, during hypoxia, the concentration of histamine in the venous return from the lungs increases [27]. In dogs, pretreatment with the agent disodium chromoglycate resulted in a failure to elevate their pulmonary vascular resistance when they were breathing a hypoxic gas mixture [28]. It has also been found that an increase in the number of mast cells occurs in the adventitia of pulmonary arteries of rats rendered hypoxic in a decompression chamber [29,30]. It was concluded that mast cells undergo hyperplasia as a response to increased demand for histamine in order to maintain the increased vascular tone over a prolonged period. However, working with rats, Mungall [30] failed to prevent right ventricular hypertrophy when chronically hypoxic rats were given disodium chromoglycate. Furthermore, in one series of experiments it was observed that right ventricular hypertrophy preceded rather than followed hyperplasia of mast cells. Such an observation could be interpreted as indicating that pulmonary hypertension causes a hyperplasia of mast cells and that secretion of histamine actually moderates the hypoxic pressor response rather than mediates it [31]. Experiments on calves, pigs, rats, sheep, guinea pigs, and dogs lead to a similar conclusion [32].

Even if one accepts that histamine is the hypoxic vasoconstrictor in rats and guinea pigs, it is very doubtful whether such a mechanism operates in humans. In a recent survey of the literature it was found that in all published reports histamine caused *vasodilatation* of pulmonary arteries in humans. It also produced little change in pulmonary blood pressure and reduced the pulmonary vascular resistance by almost half [33]. Also in a clinical trial, the histamine antagonist, chlorpheniramine, failed to modify the pulmonary vascular response to hypoxia in chronic bronchitis and emphysema [34]. From this evidence it would seem that mast cells and histamine are unlikely to be involved in the genesis of hypoxic pulmonary hypertension in humans.

It has been suggested that the renin-angiotensin system is involved as a chemical mediator in the development of muscularization of the pulmonary arterial tree in chronic hypoxia [35]. In the dog, infusion of angiotensin I or II caused a threefold increase in the vasoconstrictive response of the pulmonary circulation to hypoxia [36]. Also, inhibition of formation of angiotensin II in rats significantly reduced the right ventricular hypertrophy and pulmonary vascular changes in response to chronic hypoxia [37]. These studies suggest that chronic hypoxia exerts its influence by way of the renin-angiotensin system. In this respect it has been shown that there is an increased activation of the renin system of the hypoxic rat [38], and furthermore, mice exposed to hypoxia show increased granulation of their juxtaglomerular apparatus and elevated levels of angiotensin I-converting enzyme in their lungs and serum [39]. It is not yet clear whether the muscularization of pulmonary arterioles is augmented by increased levels of angiotensin II or by an increased sensitivity of pulmonary arterial smooth muscle to this compound. However, it has been shown that angiotensin-converting enzyme is located in the pulmonary endothelial cells. Thus, if this enzyme were sensitive to the partial pressure of oxygen in the alveolar air, it could conceivably mediate the hypoxic pressor response by converting angiotensin I to angiotensin II, which in turn acts upon vascular smooth muscle by stimulating muscularization and constriction [36].

Perhaps alveolar hypoxia has a direct effect on vascular smooth muscle without the involvement of a mediator. The walls of small pulmonary arteries and arterioles are so close to the airways that a chemical intermediary is theoretically unnecessary. It is unlikely that the smooth muscle responds to a deprivation of oxygen by reduced synthesis of ATP since oxidative phosphorylation can take place at a normal rate in a PO_2 of only a few millimeters of mercury. A much more sensitive mechanism is required such as occurs in the oxygen-sensitive carotid bodies. Theoretically, increased sensitivity could be obtained via the action of enzymes involved in the synthesis and catabolism of ATP, whereby a small decrease in ATP concentration in the muscle could result in large changes in the permeability of the plasmalemma to calcium ions, with resultant muscular contraction [33].

D. The Ultrastructure of Hypoxic HPVD

There is a paucity of published work on the ultrastructure of hypertensive pulmonary vascular disease, especially of the hypoxic variety. However, new data are beginning to give us a fresh insight into the effects of hypoxia on the pulmonary blood vessels. First, considering vasoconstriction, one might expect that when vascular smooth muscle cells contract, they simply become shorter and thicker. However, this is not the case. Prolonged pulmonary vasoconstriction in rats induced by the pyrrolizidine alkaloids monocrotaline and fulvine produces numerous evaginations of the vascular smooth muscle in pulmonary veins [40,41]. These project from the intimal margin of the media, traverse the basement membrane, and displace the overlying endothelial cells (Fig. 3). The muscular evaginations are pale and devoid of myofilaments and make such close contact with the endothelium that they resemble vacuoles within the endothelial cells. Closer examination reveals that these "apparent vacuoles" are attached to the underlying muscle and are lined by two membranes, the gap between them being interstitial space between muscle and endothelium. Similar vacuoles with double membranes and pale cytoplasm have been described in the pulmonary veins [42], and in the intima of the pulmonary trunk [43] of rats rendered hypoxic for 1 month. We have also seen numerous muscular evaginations in the pulmonary veins of rats which had been subjected to severe hypoxia for only 4 hr. The process of muscular evagination is a universal property of contracted smooth muscle [44] and will even occur to a lesser extent in normal pulmonary blood vessels which constrict during postmortem collapse of the lung [45]. It is not known whether muscular evaginations occur in constricted pulmonary blood vessels in humans, but since this property of smooth muscle is so widespread it is likely that it is also shared by the human pulmonary vasculature.

The pathogenesis of muscularization of pulmonary arterioles has been studied in detail in rats. Electron microscopy reveals that normal pulmonary arterioles contain a tenuous, discontinuous layer of smooth muscle subjacent to the endothelium [42]. After exposure to a reduced atmospheric pressure

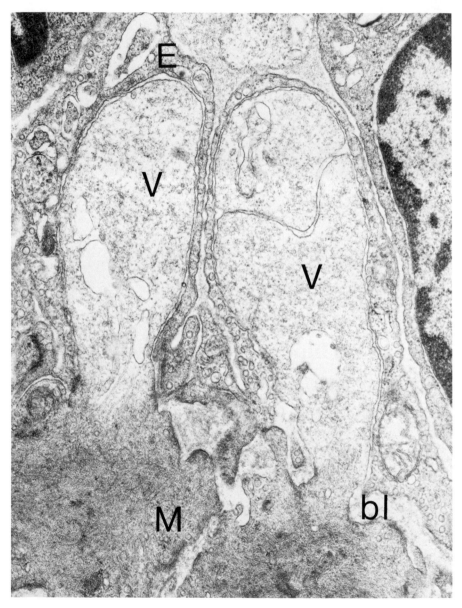

FIGURE 3   Pulmonary vein from a rat which had been subjected to a barometric pressure of 265 mmHg for 5 hr.   The vessel is constricted, and two pale evaginations (V) can be seen extending from the underlying medial smooth muscle (M).   The muscular evaginations traverse the basal lamina of the endothelium (bl) and displace the endothelial cells (E) into the lumen. Note that the evaginations lack myofilaments and appear to be surrounded by a double membrane. As such they resemble vacuoles within the endothelium. The double

of 380 mmHg for 2 weeks, these muscle cells undergo hypertrophy to produce a discontinuous layer of muscle between the elastic lamina and the endothelium (Fig. 4). At this stage there is only one elastic lamina. After 3 weeks, a hyperplasia of muscle occurs and immature smooth muscle cells appear beneath the endothelium (Fig. 5). These have abundant rough endoplasmic reticulum, mitochondria, and free ribosomes with peripherally dispersed myofilaments. By 4 weeks, most of these cells have matured and now closely resemble smooth muscle cells in arteries. At this stage there is a continuous broad media of muscle together with the early deposition of elastin in the basement membrane of the endothelium (Fig. 6). By 5 weeks, this elastin deposition is complete and forms a new elastic lamina internal to the media (Fig. 7) [42]. The process of muscularization thus involves hypertrophy of existing muscle, together with the appearance of new immature muscle from elsewhere. It is not clear whether this new muscle arises from local division of existing muscle, migrates from adjacent arteries, or is derived from transformation of fibrocytes.

There is no published work on the origin of longitudinal muscle in the intima of pulmonary arteries in hypoxic HPVD. Studies on the hyperplastic arteriosclerosis of systemic hypertension have shown that smooth muscle cells migrate from the media to the intima of mesenteric and renal arterioles [46, 47]. These smooth muscle cells contain an abundance of organelles with a relative paucity of peripherally displaced myofilaments. They are identical to the myointimal cells described by Buck [48] in the experimental intimal thickening produced by arterial ligation. Similar changes have been described in the pulmonary arteries of dogs with experimentally induced pulmonary hypertension [49]. In all these experiments the muscle cells secreted an abundance of ground substance, elastin, and collagen and with the passage of time came to resemble fibroblasts more closely than smooth muscle. One could conjecture that the intimal muscle in hypoxic HPVD is derived by a similar process, but for some reason this muscle becomes aligned in the longitudinal rather than the circumferential axis of the vessel. The ultrastructure of this interesting condition requires examination.

FIGURE 3 (continued)
membrane is in reality the single limiting membrane of smooth muscle on its inner aspect and the limiting membrane of endothelium on its outer aspect. The gap between the two membranes is interstitial space separating endothelium from smooth muscle. (Electron micrograph X 25,000.)

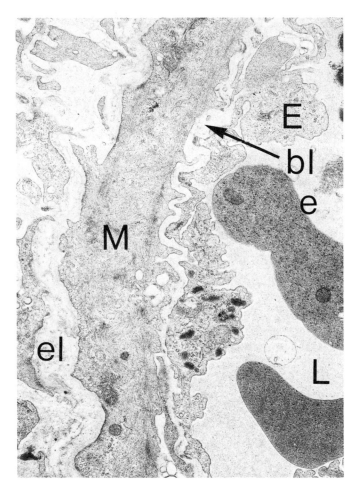

FIGURE 4 Pulmonary arteriole from a rat subjected to a barometric pressure of 380 mmHg for 1 week. The lumen of the vessel (L) contains erythrocytes (e) and is lined by a thin layer of endothelial cells (E). Beneath the endothelium is a narrow basal lamina (bl). The smooth muscle cell (M) in the media of the arteriole is much broader than normal and has undergone hypertrophy in response to the hypoxic stimulus. The exterior of the vessel is lined by a single elastic lamina (el). (Electron micrograph X 12,500.)

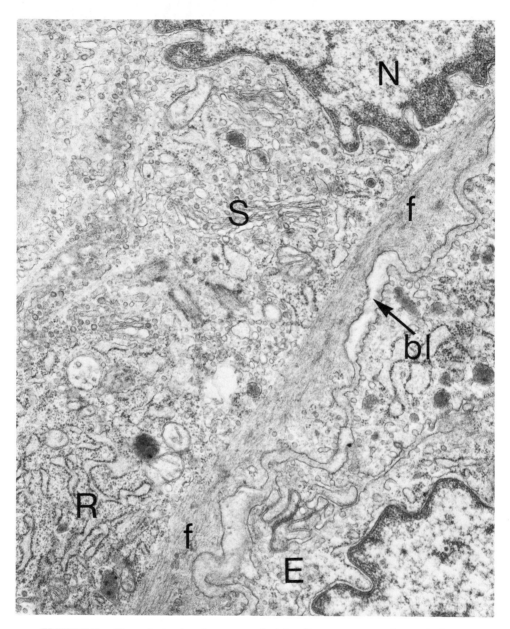

FIGURE 5 Muscularized pulmonary arteriole after exposure to hypoxia for 2 weeks. The figure shows an immature smooth muscle cell within the media. It consists of a nucleus (N) and an abundance of rough (R) and smooth (S) endoplasmic reticulum. Myofilaments are few in number and are confined to a narrow zone at the periphery of the cell (f). The smooth muscle cell is in direct contact with the basal lamina (bl) of the endothelium (E). (Electron micrograph × 25,000.)

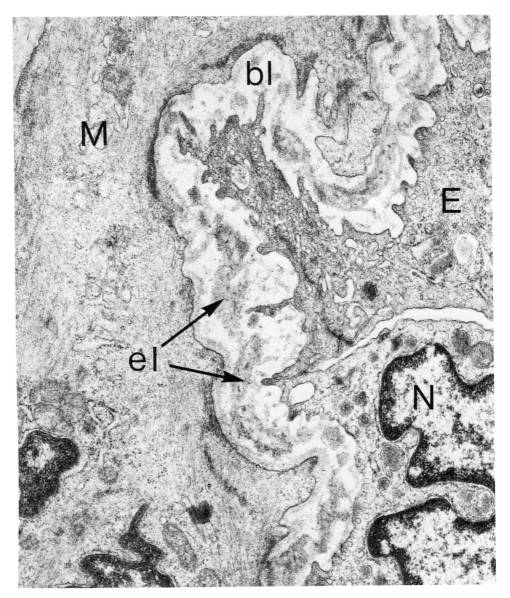

FIGURE 6 Muscularized pulmonary arteriole from a rat exposed to hypoxia for 4 weeks. The new smooth muscle (M) in the media of the arteriole is now mature and shows a reduction in cytoplasmic organelles with a corresponding increase in the extent of myofilaments. A nucleus (N) of endothelial cells (E) is shown. Beneath the endothelium the basal lamina (bl) is 3 times its normal thickness. It shows within it the deposition of dark, amorphous deposits which are immature elastin fibers (el). (Electron micrograph × 25,000.)

E.   Morphometry of the Lung in Emphysema

In the account we have given above of the development of pulmonary hypertension in states of chronic hypoxia, we have taken the view that the pathogenesis depends on the constriction and muscularization of the pulmonary arterioles. However, by its very nature, emphysema destroys lung parenchyma and its capillaries. Hence, it has been suggested that obliteration of part of the pulmonary capillary bed may cause the pulmonary hypertension. If this were the case, there should be a direct correlation between the degree of destruction of the lung and the level of pulmonary arterial hypertension as assessed by the weight of the right ventricle. This hypothesis can be tested by applying quantitative morphometric techniques.

The simplest method of assessing the extent of involvement of the lung by emphysema is to point-count slices of lung fixed in distension by instillation of formalin down the trachea or preferably inflated by the formalin-steam method of Weibel and Vidone [50]. A transparent grid is placed over the lung slice and the number of points coinciding with abnormal air space is counted. It is a fundamental assumption of the point-counting technique that these measurements in two dimensions can be applied to the volume of the lung as a whole. This method confirms the impression one gains from looking at lungs at necropsy, that centrilobular emphysema generally involves less of the lung than the panacinar form. However, when the percentage of abnormal air space is plotted against right ventricular weight, no correlation exists between them [51]. When the cases are divided into panacinar and centrilobular forms, there is a suggestion that right ventricular hypertrophy is more likely to occur with centrilobular emphysema [51,52]. This is despite the fact that centrilobular emphysema involves less of the lung. In this respect, point-counting underestimates the importance of the lesions since a percentage of abnormal air space as low as 14% with centrilobular emphysema can be associated with pronounced right ventricular hypertrophy. With panacinar emphysema there usually needs to be 40 to 70% of lung destroyed before right ventricular hypertrophy occurs [51].

More sophisticated methods of measuring the extent of emphysema involve morphometric analysis of histologic sections. Using these techniques, one can determine the total number of alveoli in the lung, the total alveolar volume, the mean alveolar volume, the internal surface area of the lung, and the internal surface area of the alveoli. The manner in which these techniques are performed need not concern us here. For further details the reader is referred to the review of Dunnill [53]. Using these methods, the total internal surface area of the lungs together has been estimated at between 45.6

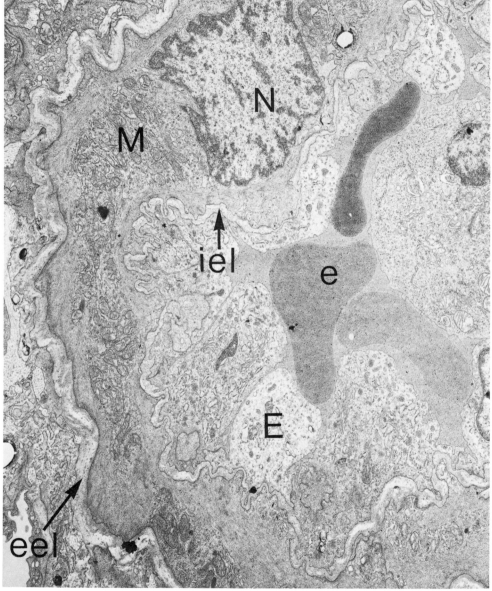

FIGURE 7   Low magnification of a muscularized pulmonary arteriole from a
rat exposed to hypoxia for 4 weeks. The nucleus (N) and cytoplasm (M) of a
large, mature, smooth muscle cell can be seen in the media. The adventitial
aspect of the media is lined by the original, thick elastic lamina of the arteriole
which now forms the external elastic lamina (eel). The intimal aspect of the
media is lined by a thinner elastic lamina which has been formed from the
deposition of elastin in the endothelial basal lamina. This now forms the in-

and 82.8 m² from three nonemphysematous lungs. Calculated for a standard lung volume of 6 liters the scatter is reduced to between 58.5 and 83.4 m², with a mean of 70 m² [54]. In four cases of panacinar emphysema the internal surface area of a standard lung volume of 6 liters was 17.2 to 40.3 m², and in three cases of centrilobular emphysema the range was 25.0 to 55.1 m² [54]. Thus, centrilobular emphysema is associated with a much smaller reduction in internal surface area than the panacinar form.

The mean value for the total number of alveoli in the two lungs added together, calculated from various publications, is 273×10^6 [33]. In panacinar emphysema this value expressed as a mean of several methods is 63×10^6 and in centrilobular emphysema it is 215×10^6 [33]. Once again, centrilobular emphysema is associated with a relatively small diminution in the numbers of alveoli.

When the weight of the right ventricle is correlated with the internal surface area of the lung no relationship exists [54]. Similarly, there is no relationship between the number of surviving alveoli and right ventricular weight. It is clear from these data that there is no relationship between the degree of lung involvement in emphysema and right ventricular hypertrophy. If a reduction in internal surface area of the lung is considered to reflect a reduction in the alveolar capillary bed, the inescapable conclusion is that the pulmonary hypertension in emphysema is not caused by loss of capillaries. It is perhaps more closely related to the *type* of emphysema regardless of the extent of tissue destruction.

F.   Factors Involved in the Pathogenesis of Pulmonary Hypertension in Chronic Bronchitis and Emphysema

Hypoxia

In the preceding section we discussed at length the effects of chronic exposure to hypoxia on the pulmonary circulation. We pointed out that hypoxic HPVD is identical to the pulmonary vascular disease found in those cases of emphysema complicated by pulmonary hypertension. We noted that these are the cases in which there is severe dyspnea and hypoxemia. It is reasonable to conclude that alveolar hypoxia is the cause of pulmonary hypertension in

---

FIGURE 7 (continued)
ternal elastic lamina (iel). This accounts for the tenous nature of the internal elastic lamina of muscularized pulmonary arterioles as viewed with the light microscope. The lumen of the vessel contains erythrocytes (e) and is lined by endothelium (E) which bulges into the lumen due to constriction of the arteriole. (Electron micrograph X 7500.)

emphysema. However, it is not immediately clear how alveolar hypoxia is produced by emphysema, especially in view of the fact that the centrilobular form of the disease is more commonly associated with the hemodynamic abnormality. The explanation lies in the increased dead space which the dilated airways create. In centrilobular emphysema, the dilated respiratory bronchioles create an increased dead space in the pathway between bronchioles and alveoli. Since such lesions tend to be diffuse, the air at each inspiration must pass through these spaces before reaching the site of gas exchange. Consequently, much of the inspired air is lost in this dead space without actually reaching the alveoli. The alveoli become underventilated and their partial pressure of oxygen falls [33]. By contrast, panacinar emphysema, although more destructive, tends to be focal in distribution. There are thus large areas of normal lung in which gas exchange can occur without an increased dead space. In addition, the destruction of alveolar capillaries and the hypoxic vasoconstriction in emphysematous regions have the effect of diverting blood to healthy parts of the lung [33]. In panacinar emphysema, therefore, extensive damage to the lung is necessary before hypoxemia and hypoxic HPVD occur.

Increased Blood Volume

The polycythemia associated with the hypoxemia of emphysema will cause an increase in total blood volume. Phases of acute respiratory failure will also have the same effect. The increased blood volume will raise the static blood pressure throughout the circulation and in particular raise the pulmonary arterial and pulmonary wedge pressures independently of any increase in pulmonary vascular resistance [33].

Increase in Blood Viscosity

The increase in hematocrit caused by polycythemia will increase the viscosity of the blood. A greater pressure will, therefore, be required to maintain a normal blood flow. In the systemic circulation this will have little effect because hypoxemia induces vasodilatation. However, in the pulmonary circulation the increased viscosity could be expected to exaggerate the increased pulmonary vascular resistance caused by vasoconstriction. Polycythemia, in the absence of hypoxia, has been induced in rats by transfusion of packed red cells. It resulted in a significant increase in right ventricular weight, suggesting that increased blood viscosity plays a role in the production of hypoxic pulmonary hypertension [55].

Increase in Airways Resistance

Chronic bronchitis and emphysema are diseases which are clinically characterized by increased airways resistance. In chronic bronchitis this is caused by bronchospasm and occlusion of bronchi by viscous, mucous plugs. In emphysema the increased airways resistance is caused by compression of bronchioles during expiration. Normally, bronchioles are held in a patent state by surrounding lung tissue. In emphysema, however, this tethering effect is lost due to destruction of lung tissue. Consequently, the increased intrathoracic pressure of expiration collapses the bronchioles, thus raising the resistance to expiration and increasing the intrathoracic pressure still further [33]. This bronchiolar collapse is detected clinically as a reduced forced expiratory volume. Furthermore, collapse of small bronchioles, such as occurs in emphysema, can raise the intrathoracic pressure sufficiently to create a secondary collapse of larger bronchi.

There is evidence to suggest that the raised intraalveolar pressure in emphysema causes compression of the pulmonary arteries during each expiration [33]. This creates an intermittent increase in pulmonary vascular resistance. Furthermore, an increase in airways resistance can create an abnormally low alveolar pressure during inspiration which will have little influence on the pulmonary arteries. This swing from abnormally high to abnormally low alveolar pressure during respiration can be associated with a normal value of the *mean* alveolar pressure. By this mechanism it should be possible to have a situation in which there is an increased pulmonary vascular resistance in the presence of a normal mean alveolar pressure [33]. In conclusion, the combined effects of alveolar hypoxia and increases in the levels of airways resistance, blood volume, and viscosity are responsible for causing pulmonary hypertension in chronic bronchitis and emphysema. The most potent of these factors is probably hypoxia.

G. The Reversibility of Pulmonary Hypertension

As we discussed above, hypoxic hypertensive pulmonary vascular disease in highlanders and in animal experiments is completely reversible. Since the pulmonary vascular pathology in emphysema is of the same type, it too should be reversible. Several studies have shown that continuous breathing of high concentrations of oxygen reduced the mean pulmonary arterial pressures of patients with emphysema [33]. However, although statistically significant, these reductions in pulmonary arterial pressure and resistance were small and did not result in normal values being reached. This inability of oxygen to bring about an immediate and total reversal of pulmonary hypertension is due to the fact that in states of chronic hypoxia the raised pulmonary arterial pressure is based on organic, muscular changes in the pulmonary arterioles, as we have demonstrated. Also to be considered is the different physiological state of the high-altitude native and the emphysematous patient. In the former there is a normal or elevated ventilation of the alveoli due to increased minute volume. Consequently, carbon dioxide is rapidly flushed out of the alveoli so that the highlanders have a diminished alveolar PCO_2. In emphysema the alveoli are underventilated so that hypercapnia and acidosis develop. Carbon dioxide may act as a vasoconstrictor and can thus cause an increase in pulmonary vascular resistance even where there is a normal alveolar PO_2 [33].

Administration of oxygen for several weeks should permit the muscular media of pulmonary arterioles to regress in the same way it does when the high-altitude native returns to sea level. Prolonged administration of 30% oxygen for 4 to 8 weeks in patients with chronic bronchitis and emphysema caused a fall in mean pulmonary arterial pressure from 43 to 32 mmHg [33]. This was a greater fall in pressure than that induced by acute inhalation of oxygen, but it still leaves a considerable residual elevation of the pulmonary blood pressure.

The advent of portable liquid oxygen systems has made the rehabilitation of patients with emphysema and severe dyspnea more practicable. Six patients who were treated by this means were studied extensively at Denver, Colorado [56]. The patients were studied for 1 month without oxygen therapy and then for 1 month with it. The quantity of oxygen administered was adjusted to maintain a normal pulmonary arterial oxygen tension. After 1 month of therapy the patients showed a greatly increased exercise tolerance, and reduced pulmonary arterial pressure and resistance. The increased exercise tolerance was not merely the result of acute exposure to oxygen, since improvement was progressive over the 4-week period. It should be noted, however, that these patients still showed a residual elevation of pulmonary arterial pressure in the region of 30 mmHg. Also, mechanical lung function did not alter with oxygen therapy. Consequently, although the clinical status of the patients was much improved, they were by no means able to live a normal life and were totally dependent upon the oxygen in order to walk or perform any form of mild physical exertion.

An investigation into the efficacy of long-term oxygen therapy in chronic bronchitis and emphysema is currently being performed in Great Britain under the sponsorship of the Medical Research Council [57]. We were fortunate to have the opportunity to examine lung tissue from two of these cases which came to necropsy. One of these was a control case who had not received oxygen treatment. He showed typical hypoxic HPVD with intimal longitudinal muscle and numerous muscularized pulmonary arterioles. There were 28 muscularized arterioles per square centimeter of lung section. The second case had received continuous oxygen therapy for 3½ years. In this case, muscularized pulmonary arterioles were scarce and occurred with a frequency of only 0.7 arteriole per square centimeter. Thus, if one can draw any conclusions from only two cases, oxygen therapy appeared to have almost totally reversed the muscularization of arterioles. However, the muscular pulmonary arteries of both cases contained intimal longitudinal muscle which had progressed in many vessels to an acellular intimal fibrosis. In fact, intimal fibrosis was more pronounced in the second case and amounted to 37.8% occlusion of the vascular lumen, whereas occlusion of arteries in the first case was only 27.8% of the lumen. Thus, prolonged oxygen therapy was not able to reverse the intimal proliferation in the pulmonary arteries of this case which could have been responsible for maintaining a residual increase in pulmonary vascular resistance.

In conclusion, pulmonary emphysema differs from high-altitude hypoxia in that it is associated with hypercapnia, mechanical resistance to the flow of air, raised intrathoracic pressure, and intimal fibrosis of muscular pulmonary arteries in long-standing cases. These factors appear to be responsible for the incomplete reversibility of pulmonary hypertension in emphysema. It remains to be seen whether they seriously embarrass attempts at obtaining long-term amelioration from the symptoms of this disease.

III.   Pulmonary Fibrosis

A.   Vessels Within Fibrotic Areas

Pulmonary blood vessels in an area of lung overtaken by fibrosis become entrapped and engulfed by it. Pulmonary arteries and veins first show severe intimal fibrosis or fibroelastosis. The intimal fibrosis is rigid and splints the underlying media, which tends to atrophy. The pulmonary vessels become progressively compressed and actively infiltrated by the surrounding fibrous tissue (Fig. 8). Sometimes a part of the circumference of the muscular media is destroyed by the fibrous tissue and is sharply delineated from the remaining healthy media. This distortion and destruction of the vessel favors intravascular thrombosis, the thrombus subsequently showing fibrous organization and perhaps recanalization. As this process reaches its conclusion the affected pulmonary blood vessel is left as nothing more than a fibroelastic mass engulfed by fibrous tissue (Fig. 8). During the early stages of this process, the elastic laminae can be recognized but they are eventually obliterated as part of a tangled fibroelastic nodule. Hence, whereas chronic hypoxia is associated with sustained pulmonary vasoconstriction, pulmonary fibrosis is characterized by physical obliteration of part of the pulmonary arterial tree. One might imagine that such an obliterative fibrotic process would lead to an irreversible pulmonary arterial hypertension of fixed organic basis. However, in the majority of cases the pulmonary fibrosis destroys only a small part of the pulmonary arterial tree so that the blood flows not through the narrowed and distorted fibrotic vessels but through the surrounding, comparatively

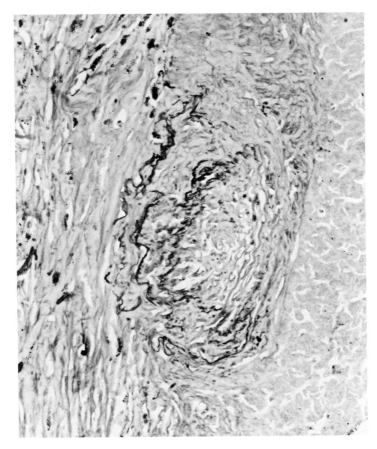

FIGURE 8   Transverse section of a muscular pulmonary artery from a case of hematite lung in which the pulmonary fibrosis is due to particles of silica inhaled with the iron sesquioxide. There has been almost total fibrous ablation of the vessel, so that remnants of elastic fibrils, seen to the left, are the only remaining traces of the media. (Elastic Van Gieson, X 315.)

normal, pulmonary arteries. Furthermore, developing pulmonary fibrosis not infrequently stimulates the formation of bronchopulmonary anastomoses which, as we shall see later, may allow retrograde flow of blood to normal lung.

The progressive fibrous obliteration of pulmonary blood vessels that we describe here is a feature of massive pulmonary fibrosis such as occurs in the pneumoconioses, as contrasted to interstitial pulmonary fibrosis. The inorganic dusts which lead to such progressive fibrosis with involvement of the pulmonary vasculature are silica, asbestos, and talc. Wells [58] studied the changes in the pulmonary blood vessels in coal-worker's pneumoconiosis. In this condition, the conducting elastic pulmonary arteries proximal to focal or massive areas of fibrosis are dilated and atheromatous. Acid mucopolysaccharides accumulate in the media of these large vessels, which thus show an intense metachromasia with toluidine blue. There may even be cystic medial degeneration, as occurs in this class of vessel in cases of congenital cardiac septal defect associated with severe pulmonary hypertension [59]. Should the elastic pulmonary arteries become attached to hard masses of lymph nodes filled with silica particles they may become ulcerated [58]. In these large conducting vessels there may be histologic evidence that two or three distinct episodes of thrombosis have taken place.

The obliterative pulmonary vascular disease produced by the pneumoconioses is often characterized histologically by specific dust particles or fibers such as asbestos bodies and dust cells containing the particulate matter concerned. One must be careful before too readily ascribing the pulmonary fibrosis and pulmonary vascular disease to the dust which can often be demonstrated and forms the most striking histopathological feature. A case in point is hematite lung, which evokes a most pronounced obliterative pulmonary vascular disease (Fig. 9) [60]. In this condition, which used to occur in miners in the Whitehaven area of Cumberland in northern Britain, large amounts of hematite dust occur in the intimal fibrous tissue, the media, and the adventitia. However, while these aggregations of iron sesquioxide and the large numbers of surrounding siderophages are so striking, it is the associated inhaled silica dust which causes the pulmonary fibrosis and vascular disease, not the iron ore.

B. Vessels Bordering Fibrotic Areas

A different set of histologic changes overtake pulmonary arteries which are in proximity to, and distorted around, areas of fibrosis but which are not physically surrounded by fibrous tissue. Such arteries show the development of longitudinally oriented smooth muscle fibers within the intima (Fig. 10). At first, isolated fibers, appearing round in transverse section, or small fasciculi, are seen. With the thickening of this intimal layer of longitudinal muscle, individual clumps of muscle fibers become delineated one from another by elastic fibrils. With the passage of time, fibrous tissue appears in the intimal layer, progressively replacing the longitudinal muscle so that eventually the appearances are those of a "nonspecific intimal fibrosis." Should one be unaware of the preceding muscular stage, the interpretation of the intimal fibrosis would probably be fallacious. These fibromuscular changes in the intima extend into

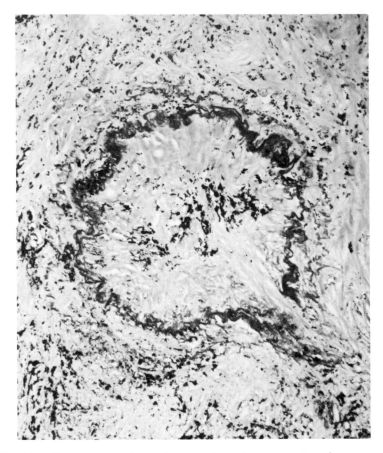

FIGURE 9 Transverse section of a muscular pulmonary artery from a case of hematite lung. The lumen is occluded by fibrous tissue in which are embedded collections of hematite dust. The internal elastic lamina has become thick and elastotic. There is almost total fibrosis of the media. (Elastic Van Gieson, X 60.)

pulmonary arterioles but are lost before the transition into precapillaries occurs. It will be appreciated how different in structure and functional potential is such a pulmonary arteriole from the muscularized pulmonary arteriole found in the states of chronic hypoxia described above. In the fibrotic lung the arteriolar vessel comprises a thick, single elastic lamina bounded on its inner aspect by longitudinal muscle admixed with fibrous tissue, whereas in chronic hypoxia, as we have seen, the pulmonary arteriole has a distinct media of circular muscle bounded by the outer, thick, original elastic lamina and an inner, thin, newly formed elastic lamina (Fig. 2). This difference in structure almost certainly implies a different functional connotation. It seems likely that the longitudinal muscle is formed as a response to elongation and stretching of the pulmonary artery as it is distorted around fibrous nodules in the lung. If this hypothesis were true, one would anticipate finding the same histologic changes whenever a pulmonary artery became distorted around nodules in the lung no matter what their nature. This is in fact precisely what is found. Thus, hyperplasia of intimal longitudinal muscle in the pulmonary arteries occurs in cases of pulmonary emphysema [7]. As noted previously, Dunnill [8] suggested that muscular pulmonary arteries in centrilobular emphysema are distorted by the abnormal air sacs in the centers of secondary lung lobules, and this stretching, associated sometimes with pulmonary arterial hypertension, may be the basis for the development of

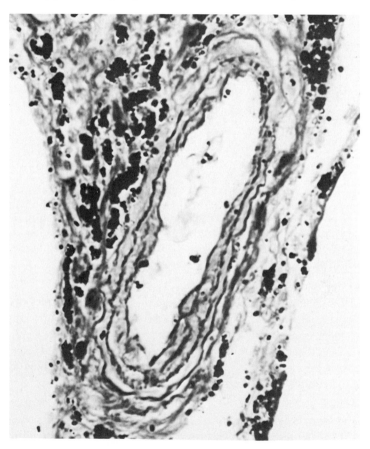

FIGURE 10 Oblique section of a small muscular pulmonary artery from a case of hematite lung. The vessel was situated on the edge of a fibrous area but was not engulfed by it. The original media of circular muscle is intact, but within the intima is a well-defined layer of longitudinal muscle. (Elastic Van Gieson, ✕ 600.)

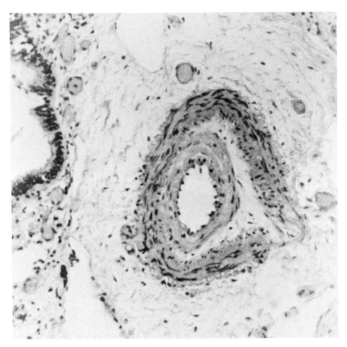

FIGURE 11   Slightly oblique section of a muscular pulmonary artery from a
woman of 54 years with scleroderma and pulmonary fibrosis. There is an eccentric lumen as a result of recanalization of a thrombus. Around the lumen a
second muscle coat has formed, although this contains fewer smooth muscle cells
than the media. (Hematoxylin and eosin, × 175.) (From Homans, John *A Textbook of Surgery*, 6th ed., 1945. Courtesy of Charles C. Thomas, Publisher,
Springfield, Illinois.)

longitudinal muscle in this type of emphysema. Liebow [61] states that he
has seen longitudinal muscle in pulmonary arteries stretcned around emphysematous bullae, an observation which we can support. The same development of intimal longitudinal muscle occurs in cases of honeycomb lung, where
the pulmonary arteries are distorted around abnormal air sacs formed by
dilatation of terminal bronchioles [62].

Hence we see that the form of pulmonary vascular disease that occurs in
primary lung disease depends more on local physical factors than on specific
diseases. Thus, any disease leading to massive pulmonary fibrosis will result in
obliterative fibrotic pulmonary vascular disease. Any condition leading to
stretching of pulmonary arteries around nodules and masses in the lung will
produce vascular disease characterized at first by intimal longitudinal muscle.
Thus, Naeye [63] reported changes in the pulmonary vasculature in

scleroderma, a condition which gives rise to interstitial fibrosis and honey-comb lung. While he regards them as characteristic of scleroderma there is certainly a case to be made that they are in fact features of interstitial pulmonary fibrosis and honeycomb lung. Two histologic features that we have noted as occurring in a striking manner in scleroderma appear to be related more to organization and recanalization of thrombus within the vascular lumen. These are, first, the development of a prominent second muscular coat composed of circularly oriented smooth muscle fibers around the lumen (Fig. 11). Second, dilated branches may arise from a sclerosed parent vessel and contain within their lumina structures (Fig. 12) which resemble super-ficially the plexiform lesions of plexogenic pulmonary arteriopathy found in association with congenital cardiac shunts and primary pulmonary hyperten-sion. They are, however, not true plexiform lesions since they lack the thin-walled peripheral vessels and the accompanying fibrinoid necrosis; they are probably an expression of organization and recanalization of thrombus.

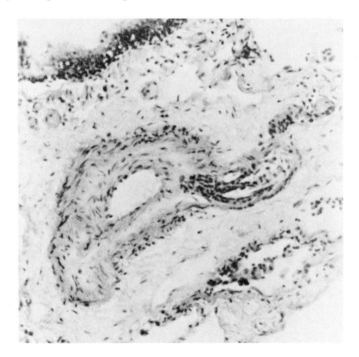

FIGURE 12 Oblique section of a muscular pulmonary artery from the same case. Around the lumen is a thin layer of muscle cells. To the right arises a branch which contains within its lumen a structure which resembles a plexiform lesion. (Hematoxylin and eosin, × 175.) (From Homans, John, *A Textbook of Surgery*, 6th ed., 1945. Courtesy of Charles C. Thomas, Publisher, Springfield, Illinois.)

C.   Vessels Beyond Fibrotic Areas

In cases of massive or interstitial fibrosis of the lung, the pulmonary blood vessels far removed from the sites of fibrosis may show histologic abnormalities.   These are not the changes generally associated with fibrosis but rather with its functional effects such as chronic hypoxemia induced by disorders of ventilation and perfusion.   Thus, in a study of honeycomb lung [62], we found it possible to compare and contrast the state of the pulmonary blood vessels in normal lung and that involved by honeycomb change since the cysts of the latter are often sharply confined to a subpleural zone in this disease. We found that intimal fibroelastosis occurred only in the arteries of those areas of lung affected by fibrosis and honeycomb change, but the development of a distinct media of circular muscle in the pulmonary arterioles was found throughout both normal and affected areas.   In addition, the medial thickness of muscular pulmonary arteries showed a greater range and a higher mean value in the frankly cystic areas.   Such findings suggest that the intimal changes are associated directly with fibrosis and honeycomb change in the surrounding lung.   In contrast, the muscularization of the pulmonary arterioles results from pulmonary hypertension brought about by the fibrosis and this hemodynamic effect is exerted throughout the entire pulmonary arterial tree.

D.   Functional Implications [33]

The functional effects of pulmonary fibrosis depend upon which part of the pulmonary vascular tree is involved, the pulmonary capillary bed or the pulmonary arteries and arterioles.   It has been appreciated for many years that a widespread increase of the thickness of the alveolocapillary membrane by the laying down of fibrous or other tissues in the interstitium of the alveolar wall will diminish the diffusing capacity for oxygen [64].   Since that time there have been many reports of a diminution in the diffusing capacity for oxygen and carbon monoxide in various forms of interstitial fibrosis.   The most obvious cause for the impaired diffusing capacity appeared to be the increased distance interposed between the alveolar gas and the capillary blood and the term "alveolar-capillary" block came into use to describe the physiological derangement.   It has since become clear that this original concept was too simplistic and requires elaboration.   Separate measurement of the diffusing capacity of the alveolocapillary membrane (DM) and the volume of blood in the pulmonary capillaries (VC) has shown that both these quantities are decreased in pulmonary fibrosis [65,66].   Hence, a diminution in the pulmonary capillary volume also contributes to the decreased diffusing capacity. When dilatation of terminal bronchioles occurs to give rise to honeycomb lung as a progression of interstitial pulmonary fibrosis, inequalities of ventilation–perfusion and abnormal anatomical shunts–develop [67,68]. As a result of these effects on the pulmonary capillaries the affected patient is breathless, especially on effort. At first there is no cyanosis at rest, but the arterial oxygen saturation falls during exercise. Finally, arterial unsaturation is present even while resting. The hyperventilation keeps the arterial PCO_2 low.

As discussed earlier in this chapter, the pulmonary arteries and arterioles in cases of fibrosis of the lung, show, after an initial phase of intimal muscularization (Fig. 10), progressive fibrotic occlusion (Figs. 8 and 9). This leads to the development of an increase in pulmonary vascular resistance, pulmonary arterial hypertension, and right ventricular hypertrophy. It is worthy of note, however, that this progression of events does not always occur. Thus, in some cases of honeycomb lung of several years duration with pronounced pulmonary vascular changes of the type described earlier there is no development of right ventricular hypertrophy [62]. This may be related to the formation of numerous thin-walled dilated vessels that may allow the blood flow to bypass the occluded terminal radicles of the pulmonary arterial tree. We have seen such vessels in histologic sections and plexus of such vessels about 50 μm in diameter have been demonstrated radiographically in cases of interstitial pulmonary fibrosis. By this means Turner-Warwick [69] showed these vascular plexi to consist of newly formed anastomotic channels connecting muscular pulmonary arteries and systemic blood vessels. Her injection studies also revealed large, isolated subpleural pulmonary-systemic anastomoses up to 1.5 mm in diameter, and she thought these had arisen from dilatation of preexisting anastomoses brought about by pulmonary hypertension. Similar pulmonary-systemic anastomoses have been demonstrated radiographically by Livingstone et al. [70]. There is also physiological evidence for intrapulmonary venoarterial shunts in lungs from cases of scleroderma showing interstitial fibrosis [71]. Two possible functions for these complex precapillary anastomoses in the lung are to allow blood to bypass occluded terminal radicles of the pulmonary arterial tree and to allow a collateral supply of blood to enter the affected honeycomb areas of lung from the systemic circulation.

IV. Granulomas: Granulomatous Pulmonary Arteritis

Some of the diseases classified as granulomas can involve the pulmonary vasculature to give rise to granulatomous pulmonary arteritis. Such diseases include tuberculosis, sarcoidosis, and the very rare pulmonary syphilis. In addition to the granulomatous arteritis, this group of diseases is characterized by progressive obliteration of pulmonary arteries and veins and an associated increase in size of the bronchial vessels with the development of bronchopulmonary

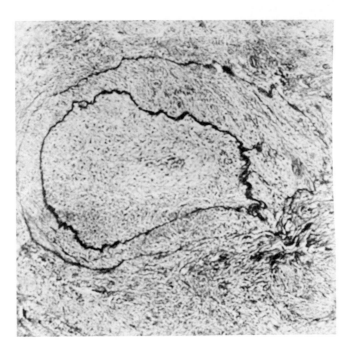

FIGURE 13   Muscular pulmonary artery in a woman aged 38 years with pulmonary tuberculosis. The artery lies within a caseous lesion and is entirely necrotic. The inner and outer elastic membranes are the only recognizable remnants. (Elastic Van Gieson, X 120.) (From Homans, John, *A Textbook of Surgery,* 6th ed., 1945. Courtesy of Charles C Thomas, Publisher, Springfield, Illinois.)

anastomoses. Elastic pulmonary arteries adjacent to areas of caseation and cavitation may show caseous necrosis of the media [72], the affected part of the arterial wall usually being in continuity with an area of caseation in the lung parenchyma. Muscular pulmonary arteries may be totally engulfed by an area of caseation, and under these circumstances there may be total caseous necrosis of the media and the adventitia. Not infrequently, only the elastic laminae remain to show the previous structure of the vessel while the lumen becomes filled with caseous matter and thrombus (Fig. 13).

When elastic pulmonary arteries show focal caseous necrosis of the media and lie near tuberculous cavities they may become eroded to form aneurysms. These are the so-called aneurysms of Rasmussen [73,74], later referred to by Calmette [75] and by Brenner [72]. Such aneurysms may rupture into the walls of tuberculous cavities leading to massive pulmonary hemorrhage [76].

Inflammatory changes in the walls of the pulmonary blood vessels are frequently severe. Sometimes a nonspecific, diffuse chronic inflammatory exudate is seen throughout a fibrosed artery, with lymphocytes predominating. Occasionally there may be a specific tuberculous arteritis with granulomas in the walls of pulmonary arteries consisting of epithelioid cells, Langhans' giant cells, and lymphocytes (Fig. 14). Sometimes tubercles have a dumbbell appearance, there being one granuloma in the adventitia and one arising from the intima and bulging into the lumen, with a connected bar of affected media [59] (Fig. 14). Thrombosis over such affected segments of the artery is common. Occasionally, isolated tuberculous vegetations may occur in the intima of large pulmonary arteries and veins [77]. In fibrotic areas in the tuberculous lung the pulmonary arteries show medial or intimal fibrosis in the various forms described earlier. The intimal fibrous tissue is usually infiltrated

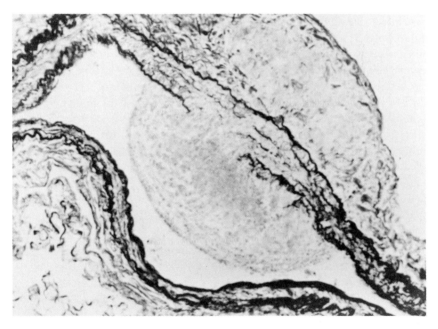

FIGURE 14   Oblique section of a muscular pulmonary artery from a man aged 38 years who died of tuberculous pericarditis and myocarditis with tuberculous lesions of the lung and spleen. One tuberculous granuloma is present in the adventitia and another arises from the intima and bulges into the lumen. They are connected by an involved segment of the underlying media which shows disruption. (Elastic Van Gieson, X 150.) (From Homans, John, *A Textbook of Surgery,* 6th ed., 1945. Courtesy of Charles C Thomas, Publisher, Springfield, Illinois.)

with lymphocytes and mononuclear cells and an occasional Langhans' giant cell. In general, pulmonary veins show similar histologic changes to those seen in the pulmonary arteries. Erosions of tuberculous lesions into pulmonary veins and venules will lead to systemic miliary tuberculosis. Often the muscular pulmonary arteries do not develop medial hypertrophy in pulmonary tuberculosis, and this is a reflection of the fact that pulmonary hypertension in this disease is often absent or moderate. Since pulmonary arterial hypertension due to tuberculosis of the lung is always acquired, the pattern of the elastic tissue of the pulmonary trunk resembles that of the normal adult pulmonary trunk [16,59].

The pathologic changes which may overtake the pulmonary blood vessels in syphilis of the lung are similar to those which we have already described as occurring in tuberculosis. Pulmonary syphilis is a very rare condition occurring at a rate of only 0.39 in 1000 necropsies. It may occur in one of the following four conditions: acute syphilitic interstitial pneumonia, diffuse interstitial fibrosis, gross scarring, and gumma formation. Pulmonary vascular syphilis is mainly a disease of the pulmonary trunk and major conducting arteries of the pulmonary circulation [72]. The histologic changes in the small pulmonary arteries in syphilis are similar to those in tuberculosis. Those vessels in close proximity to a gumma show gummatous necrosis of the media and adventitia with partial or complete occlusion of the lumen by thrombosis or fibrosis. Further away from the gummatous areas, the pulmonary arteries show nonspecific changes, such as intimal fibrosis infiltrated by lymphocytes and plasma cells, a change which has traditionally assumed the designation of "endarteritis obliterans." Those vessels so affected may show thrombosis. It should be noted that in the absence of gummas or demonstrable spirochetes there is no unequivocal evidence that these changes are due to syphilis [59]. Syphilitic periarteritis also occurs in the pulmonary vasculature.

Pulmonary arteries and veins are frequently affected by granulomatous and fibrotic lesions in sarcoidosis. Usually the granulomas lie in the vascular adventitia whereas the media and intima are less often involved. In some cases of sarcoidosis, extensive granulomatous arteritis has been described [78,79]. The media of the muscular pulmonary arteries in such granulomatous arteritis may show separation of the smooth muscle cells by a highly vacuolated, basophilic material which resembles mucin and stains metachromatically with toluidine blue [79]. The media may show focal involvement by a granulomatous arteritis, the granulomas consisting of epithelioid cells, lymphocytes, plasma cells, and giant cells.

When the granulomas are large, they project into the lumen of the vessel [59]. The intima lying over the granulomas may show severe fibrosis, and some affected vessels may contain thrombi. There is pronounced rupture and fraying of the elastic laminae, but giant cells do not appear to be closely related to the fragments of elastica as in giant cell arteritis. The various cell inclusions and mineral bodies classically associated with sarcoidosis have been found in association with the vascular granulomas. Thus, asteroid bodies, anisotropic crystals, and Schaumann's bodies may all be found. Some pulmonary vessels show severe intimal fibrosis, and a pronounced exudate of lymphocytes may surround them. Necrotizing arteritis in the pulmonary arteries has also been described in sarcoidosis of the lung.

V. Bronchopulmonary Anastomoses

A. Bronchopulmonary Anastomoses in the Normal Lung

Another potent mechanism for disturbance of the pulmonary circulation is primary lung disease, and a potential cause for the development of pulmonary vascular disease is the formation of bronchopulmonary anastomoses. Blood vessels linking the pulmonary and systemic circulations are to be found in the normal adult lung, but they are rare. Our illustrations of serial sections of them reveal that they may be considered to be branches of bronchial arteries since they have longitudinal muscle in the intima [59]. They are tortuous and of small caliber and run only a short course of less than 300 μm. Before entering the pulmonary artery the anastomotic vessel changes in structure so that it first becomes transitional in appearance between a bronchial and pulmonary artery and then assumes the structure of its pulmonary component. Such anastomoses occur in the area of distribution of bronchial arteries; namely, the hilus of the lung, the bronchial walls, and that part of the pleura supplied by the bronchial arteries. It seems unlikely that such narrow, tortuous vessels are of hemodynamic significance in the pulmonary circulation of a normal adult.

Such is not the case with the frequent straight and wide bronchopulmonary anastomoses which are to be found in the normal fetal and newborn lung. The original common pulmonary vascular plexus during development of the heart provides an excellent opportunity for the formation of different types of vascular communication during this early period of life. The structure of the neonatal bronchopulmonary anastomosis is like that of the adult except that no longitudinal muscle is found in the intima, an expected finding at a time of life when bronchial arteries are devoid of longitudinal muscle.

There appear to be two main stimuli for the production of bronchopulmonary arterial anastomoses in disease. These are a diminished pulmonary blood flow, which is of importance in cardiac disease, and the formation of new tissue within the lung, which is of greater importance in primary lung disease. Thus they occur in such congenital cardiac anomalies as Fallot's tetralogy, tricuspid atresia, and pulmonary atresia and in hematological disease such as sickle cell anemia [80]. They also occur as a result of the development of inflammatory or neoplastic tissue which occurs in diseases such as bronchiectasis, lung abscess, pulmonary tuberculosis [81], and bronchial carcinoma [82]. The formation of numerous thin-walled vessels in granulation tissue provides the same facility for the development of bronchopulmonary anastomoses as the original common pulmonary vascular plexus.

B.   Bronchopulmonary Anastomoses in Lung Disease

In bronchiectasis, bronchopulmonary anastomoses occur in relation to, and distal to, the large bronchiectatic sacs which begin in the third and fourth order of branching [83]. Before communicating with one another, the bronchial and pulmonary arteries form helices, those of the systemic vessels being tighter, wider, and more numerous. Numerous anastomoses may occur around a single bronchus and may exceed 1 mm in diameter. The bronchial artery is the same size as, or slightly smaller than, the vessel it joins. Such anastomoses may be enlargements of preexisting normal channels in the lung similar to those described above. This could explain why such connections can occur in areas remote from disease. On the other hand, the anastomoses may develop from the capillary-sized vessels of granulation tissue resulting from inflammatory changes preceding and accompanying the bronchiectasis [83]. In bronchiectasis, and in bronchial carcinoma and interstitial pulmonary fibrosis, many minute end-to-end anastomoses are to be found both subpleurally and within the lung [84].

Another quite distinct form of bronchopulmonary anastomosis arises from the vasa vasorum of the large, elastic pulmonary arteries [85]. These nutrient vessels are derived from the bronchial arteries and may pass into the lumen of the pulmonary artery to help recanalize a thrombus which is occluding it.

As well as occurring in congenital cardiac anomalies, such anastomoses have been reported in lung diseases such as chronic bronchitis and emphysema [86] and pulmonary tuberculosis [87]. They are also to be found developing as a result of widespread pulmonary vascular occlusion in sickle cell disease [80].

These bronchopulmonary anastomoses appear to have functional significance in cases of bronchiectasis and pulmonary tuberculosis. As a result of blood flow through these connections, the oxygen saturation of blood in the pulmonary arteries of lungs or lobes extensively damaged by either of these diseases may be equal to that of systemic arteries [88]. The pulmonary arterial blood pressure may be elevated as a result of these shunts, and the pressure curve obtained may be of arterial type, clearly transmitted from bronchial arteries through the bronchopulmonary anastomoses [88]. It contrasts with the pulmonary arterial wedge tracing which would be anticipated under such circumstances and which we have reported in detail elsewhere [33]. The elevation of pulmonary arterial pressure results in medial hypertrophy and intimal fibroelastosis of muscular pulmonary arteries [59]. There is, not uncommonly, thrombosis with recanalization in affected pulmonary arteries. When pulmonary hypertension becomes severe in bronchiectasis, the blood flow in the bronchopulmonary anastomoses may conceivably be reversed, leading to shunting of blood away from diseased areas into healthy lung parenchyma. The bronchial collateral flow leads to strain on the left ventricle since the output of the left ventricle exceeds that of the right by a closed circuit from the left ventricle via bronchial arteries to the left atrium. Under these circumstances, considerable left ventricular hypertrophy may develop. The extent of bronchial collateral flow can be calculated, and we have recently considered the methods employed for this at length [33].

Acknowledgments

The authors gratefully acknowledge the permission of Dr. Jesse E. Edwards, Professor C. A. Wagenvoort, and Charles C. Thomas, Springfield, Illinois, to reproduce Figures 11, 12, 13, and 14.

References

1. Bowden, D. H., V. W. Fischer, and J. P. Wyatt, Cor pulmonale in cystic fibrosis. A morphometric analysis, *Am. J. Med.,* **38**:226–232 (1965).
2. Naeye, R. L., Kyphoscoliosis and cor pulmonale. A study of the pulmonary vascular bed, *Am. J. Pathol.,* **38**:561–573 (1961).
3. Auchincloss, Jr., J. H., E. Cook, and A. D. Renzetti, Clinical and physiological aspects of a case of obesity, polycythemia and alveolar hypoventilation, *J. Clin. Invest.,* **34**:1537–1545 (1955).
4. Sieker, H. O., E. H. Estes, G. A. Kelser, and H. D. McIntosh, A cardiopulmonary syndrome associated with extreme obesity, *J. Clin. Invest.,* **34**: 916 (1955).
5. Burwell, C. S., E. D. Robin, R. D. Whaley, and A. G. Bickelmann, Extreme obesity associated with alveolar hypotension: A Pickwickian syndrome, *Am. J. Med.,* **21**:811–818 (1956).
6. Heath, D., and D. R. Williams, *Man at High Altitude.* Edinburgh, Churchill Livingstone, 1977.

7. Hicken, P., D. Heath, D. B. Brewer, and W. Whitaker, The small pulmonary arteries in emphysema, *J. Pathol. Bacteriol.*, **90**:107–114 (1965).
8. Dunnill, M. S., An assessment of the anatomical factor in cor pulmonale in emphysema, *J. Clin. Pathol.*, **14**:246–258 (1961).
9. Heath, D., Longitudinal muscle in pulmonary arteries, *J. Pathol. Bacteriol.*, **85**:407–412 (1963).
10. McLean, K. H., The significance of pulmonary vascular changes in emphysema, *Aust. Ann. Med.*, **7**:69–84 (1958).
11. Hasleton, P. S., D. Heath, and D. B. Brewer, Hypertensive pulmonary vascular disease in states of chronic hypoxia, *J. Pathol. Bacteriol.*, **95**:431–440 (1968).
12. Rotta, A., A. Cánepa, A. Hurtado, T. Velásquez, and R. Chavez, Pulmonary circulation at sea-level and at high altitudes, *J. Appl. Physiol.*, **9**:328–336 (1956).
13. Peñaloza, D., F. Sime, N. Banchero, and R. Gamboa, Pulmonary hypertension in healthy man born and living at high altitudes, *Med. Thorac,* **19**: 449–460 (1962).
14. Recavarren, S., and J. Arias-Stella, Right ventricular hypertrophy in people born and living at high altitudes, *Br. Heart J.*, **26**:806–812 (1964).
15. Arias-Stella, J., and M. Saldaña, The terminal portion of the pulmonary arterial tree in people native to high altitudes, *Circulation*, **28**:915–925 (1963).
16. Heath, D., J. W. DuShane, E. H. Wood, and J. E. Edwards, The structure of the pulmonary trunk at different ages and in cases of pulmonary hypertension and pulmonary stenosis, *J. Pathol. Bacteriol.*, **77**:443–456 (1959).
17. Saldaña, M., and J. Arias-Stella, Studies on the structure of the pulmonary trunk. I. Normal changes in the elastic configuration of the human pulmonary trunk at different ages, *Circulation*, **27**:1086–1093 (1963).
18. Saldaña, M., and J. Arias-Stella, Studies on the structure of the pulmonary trunk. II. The evolution of the elastic configuration of the pulmonary trunk in people native to high altitudes, *Circulation*, **27**:1094–1100 (1963).
19. Saldaña, M., and J. Arias-Stella, Studies on the structure of the pulmonary trunk. III. The thickness of the media of the pulmonary trunk and ascending aorta in high altitude natives, *Circulation*, **27**:1101–1104 (1963).
20. Heath, D., H. Helmholz, H. B. Burchell, J. W. DuShane, J. W. Kirklin, and J. E. Edwards, Relation between structural changes in the small pulmonary arteries and the immediate reversibility of pulmonary hypertension following closure of ventricular and atrial defect, *Circulation*, **18**:1167–1174 (1958).
21. Abraham, A. S., J. M. Kay, R. B. Cole, and A. C. Pincock, A haemodynamic and pathological study of the effect of chronic hypoxia and subsequent recovery on the heart and pulmonary vasculature of the rat, *Cardiovasc. Res.*, **5**:95–102 (1971).
22. Heath, D., C. Edwards, M. Winson, and P. Smith, Effects on the right

ventricle, pulmonary vasculature and carotid bodies of the rat of exposure to, and recovery from simulated high altitude, *Thorax*, 28:24–28 (1973).

23. Fishman, A. P., Hypoxia on the pulmonary circulation. How and where it acts, *Circ. Res.*, **38**:221–231 (1976).

24. Naeye, R. L., Pulmonary vascular changes with chronic unilateral pulmonary hypoxia, *Circ. Res.*, **17**:160–167 (1965).

25. Bergofsky, E. H., Ions and membrane permeability in the regulation of the pulmonary circulation. In the *Pulmonary Circulation and Interstitial Space*. Edited by A. P. Fishman and H. H. Hecht. University of Chicago Press, 1969, p. 289.

26. Altura, B. M., and B. W. Zweifach, Pharmacologic properties of antihistamines in relation to vascular reactivity, *Am. J. Physiol.*, **209**:550–556 (1965).

27. Haas, F., and E. H. Bergofsky, Role of the mast cell in the pulmonary pressor response to hypoxia, *J. Clin. Invest.*, **51**:3154–3162 (1972).

28. Kay, J. M., and R. F. Grover, Lung mast cells and hypoxic pulmonary hypertension. In *Progress in Respiration Research*, Vol. 9, *Pulmonary Hypertension*. Basel, Karger, 1975, pp. 157–164.

29. Kay, J. M., J. C. Waymire, and R. F. Grover, Lung mast cell hyperplasia and pulmonary histamine-forming capacity in hypoxic rats, *Am. J. Physiol.*, **226**:178–184 (1974).

30. Mungall, I. P. F., Hypoxia and lung mast cells: influence of disodium cromoglycate, *Thorax*, **31**:94–100 (1976).

31. Williams, A., D. Heath, J. M. Kay, and P. Smith, Lung mast cells in rats exposed to acute hypoxia, and chronic hypoxia with recovery, *Thorax*, **32**: 287–295 (1977).

32. Tucker, A., I. F. McMurtry, A. F. Alexander, J. T. Reeves, and R. F. Grover, Lung mast cell density and distribution in chronically hypoxic animals, *J. Appl. Physiol.*, **42**:174–178 (1977).

33. Harris, P., and D. Heath *The Human Pulmonary Circulation*, 2nd Ed. Edinburgh, Churchill Livingstone, 1977.

34. Stark, R. D., R. C. Joshi, and J. M. Bishop, Failure of an antagonist of histamine-chlorpheniramine to modify the pulmonary vascular response to hypoxia in chronic bronchitis, *Cardiovasc. Res.*, **11**:219–222 (1977).

35. Berkhov, S., Hypoxic pulmonary vasoconstriction in the rat. The necessary role of angiotensin II, *Circ. Res.*, **35**:256–261 (1974).

36. Alexander, J. M., M. D. Nyby, and K. A. Jasberg, Effect of angiotensin on hypoxic pulmonary vasoconstriction in isolated dog lung, *J. Appl. Physiol.*, **41**:84–88 (1976).

37. Zakheim, R. M., L. Mattioli, A. Molteni, K. B. Mullis, and J. Bartley, Prevention of pulmonary vascular changes of chronic alveolar hypoxia by inhibition of angiotensin I-converting enzyme in the rat, *Lab. Invest.*, **33**: 57–61 (1975).

38. Gould, A. B., and S. A. Goodman, The effect of hypoxia on the renin-angiotensinogen system, *Lab. Invest.*, **22**:443–447 (1970).

39. Molteni, A., R. N. Zakheim, K. Mullis, and L. Mattioli, Effects of chronic hypoxia on lung and serum angiotensin-I-converting enzyme activity, *Proc. Soc. Exp. Biol. Med.*, **147**:263–265 (1974).

40. Dingemans, K. P., and C. A. Wagenvoort, Ultrastructural study of contraction of pulmonary vascular smooth muscle cells, *Lab. Invest.*, **35**:205–212 (1976).

41. Smith, P., and D. Heath, Evagination of vascular smooth muscle cells during the early stages of *Crotalaria* pulmonary hypertension, *J. Pathol.*, **124**: 177–183 (1978).

42. Smith, P., and D. Heath, Ultrastructure of hypoxic hypertensive pulmonary vascular disease, *J. Pathol.*, **121**:93–100 (1977).

43. Smith, P., D. Heath, and F. Padula, Evagination of smooth muscle cells in the hypoxic pulmonary trunk, *Thorax*, **33**:31–42 (1978).

44. Fay, F. S., and C. M. Delise, Contraction of isolated smooth-muscle cells. Structural changes, *Proc. Natl. Acad. Sci. USA*, **70**:641–645 (1973).

45. Smith, P., D. Heath, and W. Mooi, Observations on some ultrastructural features of normal pulmonary blood vessels in collapsed and distended lungs, *J. Anat.*, **128**:85–96 (1978).

46. Spiro, D., R. G. Lattes, and J. Weiner, The cellular pathology of experimental hypertension. I. Hyperplastic arteriosclerosis, *Am. J. Pathol.*, **47**: 19–49 (1965).

47. Aikawa, M., and S. Koletsky, Arteriosclerosis of the mesenteric arteries of rats with renal hypertension, *Am. J. Pathol.*, **61**:293–322 (1970).

48. Buck, R. C., Intimal thickening after ligature of arteries, *Circ. Res.*, **9**:418–426 (1961).

49. Esterly, J. A., S. Glagov, and D. J. Ferguson, Morphogenesis of intimal obliterative hyperplasia of small arteries in experimental pulmonary hypertension. An ultrastructural study of the role of smooth muscle cells, *Am. J. Pathol.*, **52**:325–347 (1968).

50. Weibel, E. R., and R. A. Vidone, Fixation of the lung by formalin stream in a controlled state of air inflation, *Am. Rev. Respir. Dis.*, **84**:856–861 (1961).

51. Hicken, P., D. Heath, and D. B. Brewer, The relation between the weight of the right ventricle and the percentage of abnormal air space in the lung in emphysema, *J. Pathol. Bacteriol.*, **92**:519–528 (1966).

52. Leopold, J. G., and J. Gough, The centrilobular form of hypertrophic emphysema and its relation to chronic bronchitis, *Thorax*, **12**:219–235 (1957).

53. Dunnill, M. S., Quantitative methods in histology. In *Recent Advances in Clinical Pathology*. Edited by S. C. Dyke. London, Churchill, 1968.

54. Hicken, P., D. B. Brewer, and D. Heath, The relation between the weight of the right ventricle of the heart and the internal surface area and number of alveoli in the human lung in emphysema, *J. Pathol. Bacteriol.*, **92**:529–546 (1966).

55. Swigart, R. H., Polycythaemia and right ventricular hypertrophy, *Circ. Res.*, **17**:30–38 (1965).

56. Levine, B. E., D. B. Bigelow, R. D. Hamstra, H. J. Beckwitt, R. S. Mitchell, L. M. Nett, T. A. Stephen, and T. L. Petty, Role of long-term continuous oxygen administration in patients with chronic airway obstruction and hypoxaemia, *Ann. Intern. Med.,* **66**:639–650 (1967).

57. Stuart-Harris, C., Problems in the design and assessment in the organization of long-term oxygen therapy in chronic cor pulmonale, *International Congress on Cor Pulmonale Chronicum,* European Society for Clinical Physiology and European Society of Cardiology, Münich, March, 1976.

58. Wells, A. L., Pulmonary vascular changes in coal-worker's pneumoconiosis, *J. Pathol. Bacteriol.,* **68**:573–587 (1954).

59. Wagenvoort, C. A., D. Heath, and J. E. Edwards, *The Pathology of the Pulmonary Vasculature.* Springfield, Ill., Thomas, 1964.

60. Heath, D., W. Mooi, and P. Smith, The pulmonary vasculature in haematite lung, *Br. J. Dis. Chest,* **72**:88–94 (1977).

61. Liebow, A. A., Biochemical and structural changes in the ageing lung. In *Aging of the Lung.* Edited by L. Cander and J. H. Moyer. New York, Grune & Stratton, 1964, p. 99.

62. Heath, D., T. D. Gillund, J. M. Kay, and C. F. Hawkins, Pulmonary vascular disease in honeycomb lung, *J. Pathol. Bacteriol.,* **95**:423–430 (1968).

63. Naeye, R. L., Pulmonary vascular lesions in systemic scleroderma, *Dis. Chest,* **44**:374–379 (1963).

64. Austrian, R., J. H. McClement, A. D. Renzetti, Jr., K. W. Donald, R. L. Riley, and A. Cournand, Clinical and physiologic features of some types of pulmonary diseases with impairment of alveolar-capillary diffusion; syndrome of "alveolar-capillary block," *Am. J. Med.,* **11**:667–685 (1951).

65. McNeill, R. S., J. Rankin, and R. E. Forster, The diffusing capacity of the pulmonary membrane and the pulmonary capillary blood volume in cardio-pulmonary disease, *Clin. Sci.,* **17**:465–482 (1958).

66. Bates, D. V., C. J. Varvis, R. E. Donevan, and R. V. Christie, Variations in the pulmonary capillary blood volume and membrane diffusion component in health and disease, *J. Clin. Invest.,* **39**:1401–1412 (1960).

67. Finley, T. N., E. W. Swenson, and J. H. Comroe, Jr., The cause of arterial hypoxemia at rest in patients with alveolar-capillary block syndrome, *J. Clin. Invest.,* **41**:618–622 (1962).

68. Arndt, H., T. K. C. King, and W. A. Briscoe, Diffusing capacities and ventilation: Perfusion ratios in patients with the clinical syndrome of alveolar capillary block, *J. Clin. Invest.,* **49**:408–422 (1970).

69. Turner-Warwick, M., Precapillary systemic pulmonary anastomoses, *Thorax,* **18**:225–237 (1963).

70. Livingstone, J. L., J. G. Lewis, L. Reid, and K. E. Jefferson, Diffuse interstitial pulmonary fibrosis, *Q. J. Med. N.S.,* **33**:71–103 (1964).

71. Conner, P. K., and F. A. Bashour, Cardiopulmonary changes in scleroderma. A physiologic study, *Am. Heart J.,* **61**:494–499 (1961).

72. Brenner, O., Pathology of the vessels of the pulmonary circulation, *Arch. Intern. Med.,* **56**:211–237, 457–497, 724–752, 976–1014, 1189–1241 (1935).

73. Rasmussen, V., Om haemoptyse, navnlig den lethale, i anatomisk og klinisk henseende, *Hosp. Tidende,* **11**:33, 37, 41, 45, 49 (1868).

74. Rasmussen, V., Fortsatte iagttagelser over haemoptyse, *Hosp. Tidende,* **12**: 41, 45 (1869).

75. Calmette, A., *Tubercle Bacillus Infection and Tuberculosis in Man and Animals.* W. Soper and G. Smith, translators. Baltimore, 1923, p. 191.

76. Plessinger, V. A., and P. N. Jolly, Rasmussen's aneurysms and fatal haemorrhage in pulmonary tuberculosis, *Am. Rev. Tuberc.,* **60**:589–603 (1949).

77. Gross, P., Tuberculous vegetations of the trunk of the pulmonary artery, *Am. J. Pathol.,* **9**:17–22 (1933).

78. Bottcher, E., Disseminated sarcoidosis with a marked granulomatous arteritis, *Arch. Pathol.,* **68**:419–423 (1959).

79. Michaels, L., N. J. Brown, and M. Cory-Wright, Arterial changes in pulmonary sarcoidosis, *Arch. Pathol.,* **69**:741–749 (1960).

80. Heath, D., and I. McK. Thompson, Bronchopulmonary anastomoses in sickle-cell anaemia, *Thorax,* **24**:232–238 (1969).

81. Marchand, P., J. C. Gilroy, and V. H. Wilson, An anatomical study of the bronchial vascular system and its variations in disease, *Thorax,* **5**:207–221 (1950).

82. Cudkowicz, L., and J. B. Armstrong, The blood supply of malignant pulmonary neoplasms, *Thorax,* **8**:152–156 (1952).

83. Liebow, A. A., M. R. Hales, and G. E. Lindskog, Enlargement of the bronchial arteries and their anastomoses with the pulmonary arteries in bronchiectasis, *Am. J. Pathol.,* **25**:211–231 (1949).

84. Turner-Warwick, M., Bronchial artery patterns in lung and heart disease (Ph.D. thesis). University of London, 1961.

85. Cudkowicz, L., and J. B. Armstrong, Observations on the normal anatomy of bronchial arteries, *Thorax,* **6**:343–358 (1951).

86. Cudkowicz, L., and J. B. Armstrong, The bronchial arteries in pulmonary emphysema, *Thorax,* **8**:46–58 (1953).

87. Cudkowicz, L., The blood supply of the lung in pulmonary tuberculosis, *Thorax,* **7**:270–276 (1952).

88. Roosenburg, J. G., and H. Deenstra, Bronchial-pulmonary vascular shunts in chronic pulmonary affections, *Dis. Chest,* **26**:664–671 (1954).

7

Pulmonary Vascular Disease in Acquired Heart Disease

LEWIS DEXTER

Peter Bent Brigham Hospital
Harvard Medical School
Boston, Massachusetts

Pulmonary vascular disease associated with acquired heart disease such as mitral stenosis is almost completely reversible by surgical correction of the mitral stenosis. In contrast, pulmonary vascular disease of similar severity associated with congenital heart disease is often not reversible (see Chapter 8). The purpose of this chapter is to describe the nature, behavior, and reversibility of pulmonary vascular disease in acquired heart disease.

I. Historical Introduction

In 1936, Thompson and White [1] published a paper entitled, "Commonest cause of hypertrophy of the right ventricle—left ventricular strain and failure," and it was properly deduced that the right ventricle hypertrophied because of the high back-pressure in the lungs as a consequence of left ventricular failure. Since this was before the time of cardiac catheterization, no direct measurements of pressure were made.

Parker and Weiss [2] described histologic changes in pulmonary arteries and arterioles in mitral stenosis that were similar to those seen in systemic arterioles in patients with essential and even malignant hypertension, and which they accurately interpreted as being a manifestation of the presence of pulmonary hypertension.

The introduction of the cardiac catheter by Cournand and Ranges [3] led to the early appreciation of pulmonary hypertension in a variety of circumstances, but specifically (for the purpose of this chapter) in mitral stenosis [4-6] and in left ventricular failure from any cause [7-9].

II. Definition of Pulmonary Vascular Disease

Pulmonary vascular disease is usually defined as anatomical narrowing of the pulmonary vasculature, particularly the muscular arteries. In a broader sense it can be defined as a raised pulmonary vascular resistance, a physiological term implying an abnormal obstruction to blood flow through the lung. Such a definition includes not only anatomical narrowing of blood vessels, but also mechanical plugging (e.g., pulmonary emboli, schistosomiasis, thrombosis), reduction of pulmonary vascular volume (e.g., surgical ablation, destruction of parenchyma by disease), and vasoconstriction. In mitral stenosis and left ventricular failure, we are mainly concerned with anatomical narrowing of vessels and vasoconstriction.

Pulmonary vascular resistance (PVR) is calculated by the Poiseuille resistance equation:

$$PVR = \frac{PA_m - LA_m \times 80}{PBF}$$

where PVR = pulmonary vascular resistance (dyn sec cm^{-5}; dsc)
     PA_m = mean pressure in pulmonary artery, mmHg
     LA_m = mean pressure in left atrium, mmHg
     PBF = pulmonary blood flow (cardiac output), liters/min
     80 = specific gravity of mercury = 1.36, multiplied by gravity factor
           = 980, multiplied by 60 sec/min, divided by 1000 ml/min

Many authors prefer R units, which omits the factor 80 and is then expressed as mmHg liter^{-1} min^{-1}. This is easily obtained by dividing dsc units by 80.

There are many objections to this equation, which was derived by Poiseuille in 1842 from the use of water instead of blood, rigid tubes of finite size instead of distensible tubes of varying size down to capillaries, and steady instead of pulsatile flow. In the Poiseuille analysis, the relation of pressure to flow is a straight line. In a vascular bed, it is curvilinear. The shortcomings of this equation have been well described [10-12].

Despite these shortcomings, there is no other method of measuring resistance. When, as a result of an intervention, there are small changes in resistance, one must beware of drawing conclusions. When changes are large, one is on firmer ground [10]. The changes in mitral stenosis are so large that errors of interpretation become minimized.

III. Acquired Heart Diseases and Pulmonary Vascular Disease

Acquired heart diseases leading to pulmonary vascular disease have but one basic physiological abnormality—pulmonary venous hypertension. The list includes [5,7-10,13,14] stenosis of the pulmonary veins as they enter the left atrium, cor triatriatum (congenital, not acquired heart disease), mitral stenosis, left ventricular failure of any etiology, and others [10].

Of these, the best studied is mitral stenosis. Reasons are threefold. First, it is an operable lesion and accordingly has frequently been studied diagnostically by cardiac catheterization, i.e., physiologically. Second, biopsies of lung are readily available at the time of surgery for histologic study. Third, mitral stenosis represents a very slowly progressive narrowing of the mitral valve wherein there is ample time for compensatory mechanisms, specifically pulmonary vascular disease, to develop. Mitral regurgitation of rheumatic origin is usually combined with different degrees of mitral stenosis and runs a chronic course, with pulmonary vascular disease as a common accompaniment. Of the many causes of left ventricular failure producing pulmonary vascular disease, the next-best example is aortic stenosis. Pulmonary vascular disease in association with left ventricular failure of other etiologies is relatively uncommon, or at most mild. This is attributable to the fact that pulmonary vascular disease takes time to develop. Almost all other types of left ventricular failure are relatively acute and of short duration. The patient is acutely ill and either dies or improves. Unlike the patient with mitral stenosis, it is not common for these patients to be on the borderline of pulmonary edema for months or years.

For various reasons, most of the discussion which ensues will be concerned with pulmonary vascular disease, associated with mitral stenosis.

IV. The Normal Adult Lung

A. Physiology

Formerly, the pulmonary vasculature was considered to be a passive system which allowed the right ventricle to pump to the left ventricle whatever

TABLE 1   Pressure, Flows, and Resistances in Pulmonary and Systemic Circuit of Normal Adult Man at Rest

Circulation	Range of pressure (mmHg)		Blood flow (liters min^{-1}m^{-2})	Resistance (dyn sec cm^{-5})
	SD	Mean		
Right atrium		0–5		
Right ventricle	25–25/0–5			
Pulmonary artery	15–25/5–10	9–15		
Pulmonary capillaries		5–10		
Pulmonary veins		5–10		
Left atrium		5–10		
Left ventricle	110–130/5–10			
Aorta	110–130/70–90	85–100		
Systemic capillaries		25		
Systemic veins		5–10		
Pulmonary			3.1	
Systemic			3.1	
Pulmonary vascular				60–100
Total systemic				900–1200

amount of blood was delivered to it by way of the venous return. It does this at a low pressure. As cardiac output rises as a result of exercise, fever, or other cause, the lung seems to accept the increased blood flow without appreciable change of pressure. As we shall see, however, the vasculature has active tone and it has a vasoconstrictor capability which, compared to that in the systemic circulation, is weak.

Pulmonary Pressures and Flow

The lung is normally a high-flow, low-pressure, low-resistance organ (Table 1). Practically the entire cardiac output passes through it at pressures that are about one-sixth those of the systemic circulation. The pulmonary vascular resistance, defined as the relation of pressure divided by flow, is likewise very low compared with that of the systemic circulation. Although the lung has many functions, its main purpose is gas exchange. The pulmonary vasculature is admirably constructed for this purpose. The pulmonary capillary pressure is normally 5 to 10 mmHg [15]. According to Starling's law of edema formation, edema is produced when hydrostatic pressure exceeds oncotic pressure. Oncotic pressure is normally in the vicinity of 25 mmHg. With a normal hydrostatic pressure of only 5 mmHg, it is clear that the pulmonary parenchyma (alveoli, interstitial space) is normally kept in a relatively dehydrated state which is optimal for gas exchange.

Pulmonary Capillary Wedge Pressure

Pulmonary capillary wedge pressure has been used interchangeably with left atrial pressure in this chapter. Although its validity as a measure of left atrial pressure has been challenged, evidence indicates that the two are identical in mitral stenosis if recorded correctly. As pointed out originally [15] and re-emphasized [16], (1) the pressure in the wedge position must have a waveform that is left atrial in contour, (2) a blood sample with an oxygen saturation of 98% *must* be obtained from the wedge position, and (3) originally it was considered necessary to record pressures with both a membrane and a saline manometer and obtain equality of both pressures. This is not currently considered necessary. If (1) and (2) are observed, the pulmonary capillary wedge pressure is equal to the left atrial pressure in mitral stenosis [16,17]. If a blood sample fully saturated with oxygen cannot be obtained, any pressure so obtained must be disregarded. All pulmonary capillary wedge pressures reported here were validated as described above.

Pulmonary Vascular Tone

Although at first glance, the pulmonary vasculature appears to be passive, this is not at all the case. It is endowed with tone of the smooth muscle of the media. As Szidon and Fishman and coworkers [18,19] have emphasized, it has very little reservoir function and has a tone which is maintained by α-adrenergic mechanisms. The left side of the heart receives in diastole that amount of blood which was ejected by the right ventricle in the preceding systole [20]. This is perhaps the main way in which the two ventricles maintain absolute equality of output. Starling's law of contractility makes up for minor discrepancies of output of the two ventricles.

Pulmonary Blood Volume

The pulmonary blood volume is normally 271 ml/m^2, with a range of 204 to 314 ml/m^2, and is similar in mitral stenosis [21,22].

Pulmonary Vascular Reserve

The pulmonary vasculature has a large reserve capacity. Unilateral pneumonectomy is followed by practically full exertional capacity over a wide range, providing the opposite lung is normal. There is no appreciable change in pulmonary arterial pressure or cardiac output [23]. The normal lung tolerates unilateral obstruction of a pulmonary artery with a balloon at the end of a catheter with little change of cardiac output and with a rise of only a few millimeters of mercury of pulmonary arterial pressure (see below). In those dying of pulmonary embolism, the pulmonary arterial blood volume is regularly reduced by 65% or more [24].

Thus, there is not only an enormous pulmonary vascular reserve, but even in the face of the most severe pulmonary vascular disease, it maintains its primary function of performing adequate gas exchange. Perhaps the best evidence for this is that in those with terminal primary pulmonary hypertension, the arterial oxygen saturation is characteristically normal [25].

B. Histology

The vasculature of the normal adult lung has been described in detail by Brenner [26], Heath and Edwards [27], Harris and Heath [10], and Wagenvoort and Wagenvoort [28]. The following is a brief summary of their descriptions.

The size of the *trunk of the pulmonary artery* is about the same as that of the aorta, but its media is only about half the thickness.

The *trunk and main branches* of the pulmonary artery have elastic laminae that are interrupted and fragmented with mucopolysaccharides and collagen in the spaces between the elastic fibers. The intima is thin and consists of a single layer overlying the internal elastic membrane. The muscularis is relatively sparse.

Elastic pulmonary arteries consist of the next branches down to a diameter of approximately 1000 μm. In these vessels, the elastica is continuous and not fragmented, and the muscular elements are sparse.

Muscular pulmonary arteries have an external diameter of about 1000 down to 100 μm. They have a distinct muscular media and internal and external elastic laminae. These are the resistance vessels. The change from elastic vessels to muscular vessels is gradual. The amount of smooth muscle in the media is scanty compared with arterioles in the systemic circuit. Thus, there is a relatively wide lumen with a sparse amount of muscle. The thickness of the media is normally only about 5% of the external diameter of the vessel.

There is a change to *arterioles* when the diameter of the muscular artery is about 70 to 100 μm. They arise as a termination or as a side branch from a small muscular artery. There is no muscular layer. There is only a single elastic lamina as a continuation of the external elastic lamina, and the intima consists of a single layer of endothelial cells. With age, some intimal fibrosis occurs even in the absence of pulmonary hypertension. These arterioles terminate in a thin-walled branch, devoid of muscle, to supply a dense network of capillaries.

The network of *capillaries* in the alveolar walls assumes a roughly hexagonal shape. The capillaries are 10 to 15 μm long. This length is sufficient to ensure saturation of the red cell with oxygen over a wide range of flows. The average diameter of the capillary is 8.3 μm. This is just enough to allow red cells to pass through freely, the normal red cell having a diameter of 7 μm. Walls of the alveolar capillaries consist of endothelial cells overlying a basement membrane. On the alveolar side, an extremely thin layer of epithelium rests on a thin basement membrane. A thin, though variable space lies between the alveolar and capillary basement membranes. This space contains reticulin fibers. The thickness of the air-blood barrier is 1.6 to 1.8 μm. It has been stated that the total alveolocapillary surface area in humans is about the size of a tennis court.

Venules collect blood from capillaries and extend to a diameter of 60 to 100 μm. They consist of endothelium resting on a broad basement membrane, with occasional bundles of smooth muscle external to the basement membrane. As the venule increases in caliber, the number of smooth muscle cells increases and an elastic membrane develops between muscle and endothelium.

When the venule becomes 60 to 100 μm in diameter, it gradually assumes the character of a *vein* with progressive loss of muscle cells. The media merges with adventia and eventually consists of dense collagen interspersed with elastic fibers. The intima consists of a sheet of endothelium overlying an internal elastic lamina. There are no valves. The four pulmonary veins empty into the left atrium.

From the viewpoint of this chapter, the most striking aspect of the pulmonary vasculature is the scantiness of muscle fibers in arteries and veins.

Lymphatics are not present in the alveolocapillary space. They arise in the pleura and in the tiny connective tissue septa around pulmonary arteries and veins and in the mucosa and adventitia of bronchi. They form superficial and deep networks which anastomose in the region of the hilus and tracheobronchial lymph nodes.

A rich *supply of nerve fibers* has been demonstrated in the walls, particularly the adventitia, of the large elastic pulmonary arteries and veins and down to the muscular pulmonary arteries. None are found in arterioles and capillaries. These are both sympathetic (derived from the second to sixth thoracic ganglia and the stellate ganglia) and parasympathetic (supplied by the vagus nerve). The large pulmonary veins have a rich nerve supply which becomes scanty and disappears in the region of the venules and capillaries.

The precise function of these nerves has been difficult to ascertain in normal individuals for reasons well described by Harris and Heath [10]. The normal mean pressure in the pulmonary artery is 11 mmHg and in the left atrium, 5 mmHg; the difference is 6 mmHg. The flow is about 6 liters/min. The pulmonary vascular resistance is low (80 dyn sec cm^{-5}). A halving of resistance may lead to a diminution of the pressure gradient from 6 to 3 mmHg. The observed alterations of pressure and flow are of the same order as the errors of measurement. Thus, investigations of the role of nerves in altering vasomotor activity of the normal lung are fraught with methodological limitations and errors. Both physiological and pharmacologic evidence indicate, however, that "tone" and probably vasoconstriction are mediated by α-adrenergic stimulation [18,19]. α-Adrenergic blocking with tolazoline (Priscoline) [22,27-31] produces pulmonary vasodilatation. Parasympathetic stimulation with acetylcholine [22,32,33] produces pulmonary vasodilatation, as does β-adrenergic stimulation with isoproterenol [22,34-36]. They also produce an increase in cardiac output. All their actions are weak compared with their effect on systemic vessels, probably reflecting the small amount of muscle in the walls of the pulmonary vessels. As a result, therapy with these agents has usually, but not always [37], been disappointing.

V. Mitral Stenosis: Natural History

The natural history of mitral stenosis before the advent of cardiac surgery was well described by several authors and reviewed by Roy and Gopinath [38]. Except for the rare congenital form, the etiology of mitral stenosis is rheumatic fever. Acute rheumatic fever occurs in childhood, e.g., at age 8 years. The patient may become febrile 10 to 14 days after a β-hemolytic streptococcal infection; many joints become hot, swollen, and tender; and all layers of the heart become involved in an inflammatory process—endocardium (valvulitis), myocardium (myocarditis), and pericardium (pericarditis). The course of illness is prolonged, anywhere from months to years. It finally subsides, but may recur. It may leave no significant trace of abnormality in pericardium or myocardium. However, Bland and Jones [39] showed that 20 years later, one-third of the patients in their study had died, one-third had no heart disease, and one-third had progressive valve deterioration. In the case of mitral stenosis, the commissures of the valves become involved in a sealing-off process, the nature and course of which is not entirely clear. The orifice of the mitral valve which is normally about $4\frac{1}{2}$ cm^2 becomes narrower and narrower and finally can become as small as 0.3 cm^3, 7% of the cross-sectional area of the normal valve. The slowness of the narrowing of the mitral orifice allows time for many compensations to occur. Clinically, patients reduce their physical activities because of shortness of breath beginning at an average age of 31 years. There comes a point at which the patient is short of breath at rest because of pulmonary congestion. The orthopneic position must be assumed. This is followed by death at an average age of 48 years [40]. Chronicity is one of the hallmarks of the clinical course. The clinical manifestations have been described by Lewis et al. [41], Dexter [42], Wood [43], and Ryan [17]. This natural history gives little insight into the course of the individual patient. Some will die at an early age, and some will become octogenarians.

Relating pathophysiology to clinical symptoms individualizes the natural history and also provides an insight into the development and response to pulmonary vascular complications in these patients [5,6,41,42].

In systole, the mitral valve closes. In diastole, it opens. There is normally a pressure difference between the left atrium and left ventricle of 1 or 2 mmHg for several milliseconds in early diastole. During the remainder of diastole, there is no measurable difference. As the mitral valve narrows as a result of the rheumatic process, it is the diastolic orifice that narrows. As with many organs of the body, there is a large reserve of function. It is not until the orifice is less than half its normal size that there is a significant pressure difference across the valve at rest, and it is at about this point that patients slow down in their physical activities. The process of narrowing of the orifice continues. When the orifice approaches an area of 1.0 cm^2, the left atrial pressure at rest approaches 25 mmHg. The left ventricular diastolic pressure remains at the normal value of about 5 mmHg. The resting cardiac output has become variably reduced. The left atrial pressure of 25 mmHg has necessitated a similar rise of pressure in the lung. The pulmonary venous, pulmonary capillary, and pulmonary arterial diastolic pressures are 25 mmHg, and the pulmonary arterial systolic pressure has risen from the normal of about 18 mmHg to about 35 or 40 mmHg. At this point, the patient is dyspneic on the slightest exertion, is orthopneic, and has attacks of paroxysmal nocturnal dyspnea and of acute pulmonary edema. This is the time when hemoptysis of red blood in varying amounts may occur. The only chamber of the heart that is enlarged is the left atrium. The EKG reveals no evidence of ventricular hypertrophy. Bland and Sweet [44] described this stage of mitral stenosis as tight mitral stenosis with a normal-sized heart.

The pulmonary vascular resistance begins to rise at about this point (see below) in the majority of patients and influences all subsequent clinical manifestations [41–43]. When the pulmonary vascular resistance rises to between 400 and 800 dyn sec cm^{-5}, about half the patients become less dyspneic and instead develop the fatigue syndrome. However, the heart is enlarged due to an increase in the size of the right ventricle, the pulmonary arteries are enlarged by X-ray, and the EKG develops the pattern of right ventricular hypertrophy.

In the few in whom the pulmonary vascular resistance rises above 800 dyn sec cm^{-5}, the right ventricle fails, dyspnea recurs as the dominant symptom, and the heart and pulmonary vessels become larger by X-ray.

The various bodily changes that occur as mitral stenosis becomes progressively severe are pulmonary hypertension, at first passive and then reactive (as indicated by a rise of pulmonary vascular resistance), a reduction of flow across the mitral valve (cardiac output), lymphatic hypertrophy as pulmonary edema impends [45–47], distension of the trunk and main branches of the pulmonary artery by X-ray, and right ventricular hypertrophy and eventual failure as the pulmonary arterial pressure rises to high levels.

VI. Pulmonary Vascular Resistance

Since the emphasis of this chapter is the complication of a high pulmonary vascular resistance (PVR) in acquired heart disease, let us now consider the nature and behavior of the pulmonary vascular resistance in mitral stenosis.

A. Histologic Changes in Vessels in Pulmonary Venous Hypertension

Heath and Edwards [27] described six grades of histologic change in the pulmonary vessels of patients with pulmonary hypertension.

Grades of Histologic Change

Grade I changes consist of medial hypertrophy of muscular arteries and muscularization of the normally amuscular arterioles.

Grade II changes consist of cellular intimal proliferation in pulmonary arterioles and small muscular arteries. This proliferation may lead to vascular obliteration. There is little or no intimal change in the larger pulmonary arteries.

Grade III changes are characterized by progressive intimal fibrosis with a change from cellular to fibrous tissue. Elastosis, fragmentation of the internal elastic lamina, extension of intimal changes into the larger pulmonary arteries, and longitudinal muscle fibers in arterioles and muscular arteries may all be observed.

Grade IV changes are characterized by "dilatation" lesions and a decrease of medial thickness. Intimal thickening and elastosis are more severe than in grade III. Three types of dilatation lesions are described and include plexiform lesions, angiomatoid lesions, and vein-like branches of occluded pulmonary arteries.

Grade V change consists of numerous dilatation lesions throughout the lung and macrophages containing hemosiderin.

Grade VI lesions are characterized by fibrinoid necrosis of the media with generalized pulmonary arteritis.

Grades I through III are considered to be reversible both histologically and clinically and grades IV through VI to represent fixed irreversible lesions [10,27,28]. Grade IV to VI lesions are seen in idiopathic (primary) pulmonary hypertension and some types of congenital heart disease. In chronic pulmonary venous hypertension (mitral stenosis), pulmonary vascular changes usually extend only through grade III [10,27,28]. There are histologic changes in pulmonary capillaries and veins, but these are not the site of an increased resistance to flow, as indicated by the equality of pulmonary capillary wedge and left atrial pressures. Accordingly, they will not be discussed further.

Although there is a paucity of information regarding the fate of the histologic changes in the lungs of patients undergoing mitral surgery, what little there is suggests the return of the pulmonary vasculature to or almost to normal postoperatively [28,48].

The reasons for less severe vascular lesions in mitral stenosis than in congenital heart disease and primary pulmonary hypertension with similar pulmonary arterial pressures are speculative. However, there are obvious differences. The pressure gradient across the lung (PA-LA pressure) is about 25 mmHg less in mitral stenosis than in the other diseases with similar elevations of pulmonary arterial pressure due to the elevated left atrial pressure in mitral stenosis. In those with congenital heart disease, the left atrial pressure is usually normal. In contrast to congenital heart disease, the pulmonary blood flow is reduced in mitral stenosis, whereas it is initially high in congenital heart disease with left-to-right shunts. In primary pulmonary hypertension, cardiac output is normal or low. Chronicity is probably not a distinguishing factor. Medial hypertrophy of pulmonary arteries has been produced experimentally within 2 weeks by creating a shunt between systemic and pulmonary arteries [49,50], and more advanced lesions (plexiform) have been produced with time by the same method [50-52]. Experimental pulmonary venous hypertension in dogs has occasionally resulted in vasoconstrictive pulmonary hypertension [50] and pulmonary vascular lesions [53]. Using calves, which are known to have a highly vasoreactive pulmonary vasculature, Silove et al. [54] were able to produce not only pulmonary hypertension and an elevated PVR, but also grades I, II, and III pulmonary vascular lesions.

Regional Differences in Pulmonary Vascular Lesions

In patients with congenital heart disease, vascular lesions are uniform throughout the lung. In contrast, the bases of the lungs of patients with mitral stenosis have more vascular change than the apexes. This has been demonstrated histologically [10,28] and by measurement of regional flow [55-57].

The elastic arteries are either dilated or normal in the upper parts of the lung, but those in the lower parts are narrow. Medial hypertrophy of the muscular arteries and arterioles is much more pronounced in the basal segments than in the apexes, but intimal changes do not have a regional distribution [28]. Wagenvoort and Wagenvoort [28] suggested that the development of smooth muscle cells in the media of arteries (as well as veins) in mitral stenosis is related to the higher pressure at the bases. This is particularly the case in mitral stenosis, where patients are characteristically orthopneic in the later stages of their disorder when pulmonary hypertension supervenes. This is in contrast with most other types of pulmonary hypertension, in which orthopnea and pulmonary venous hypertension are not prominent features. The difference in hydrostatic pressure between apex and base in the upright (orthopneic) position in the average adult is 30 to 36 cmH_2O or 22 to 26 mmHg.

B.   Pulmonary Vascular Resistance in Mitral Stenosis

The following discussion is an expansion of our original studies [5,6] and is based on 100 patients with mitral stenosis without significant regurgitation or abnormality of the aortic valve (see Table A in Appendix 1). One-plus regurgitation was based on cineangiography wherein radio-opaque material was observed to regurgitate into the proximal chamber and to be totally expelled during the next systole or diastole. It was therefore considered to be hemodynamically insignificant. None of the patients had regurgitation of greater magnitude.

Relation of PVR to Size of Mitral Orifice

The relationship between the size of the orifice of the mitral valve calculated by the Gorlin equation [58] and the appearance of an increase of pulmonary vascular resistance is shown in Figure 1. The striking feature is that there is no change in pulmonary vascular resistance until the mitral valve orifice approaches 1.0 cm^2. Since there is no reason to think that there should be a direct cause-and-effect relation between the size of the mitral orifice and the appearance of an increase of PVR, the following relationships have been examined.

Pulmonary Vascular Resistance (PVR)
and Pulmonary Capillary Wedge (PCW) Pressure

The relation of PVR to PCW pressure was described by our group [5] as indicating that resistance in the lung rose when the pulmonary capillary wedge pressure approached 25 mmHg. It was postulated that arteriolar constriction possibly occurred as a reflex when pulmonary edema impended. It now appears that these postulations are not quite accurate. With greater experience, it is apparent that there is *not* an abrupt increase of pulmonary vascular resistance when the pulmonary capillary wedge pressure reaches 25 mmHg (see Fig. 2). Instead, PVR begins to rise, at least in some individuals, before this pressure is reached. Thus, the curve relating PVR to PCW is rounded instead of being at right angles. Figure 2 also indicates that this is not a uniform response. Of these patients, 5% had no increase in PVR even though their PCW was 25 mmHg or more. Only a small number (7%) had an excessive elevation of PVR (over 1000 dyn sec cm^{-5}). This is in agreement with the findings of others [17,43]. The remainder of the patients had intermediate increases of PVR.

The curves relating pulmonary vascular resistance to pressure are somewhat spurious because PCW pressure is present in both ordinate and abscissa. To avoid this and to exclude the influence of flow, the following relationships have been examined.

Pulmonary Capillary Wedge (PCW) and Pulmonary Artery Diastolic (PA$_d$) Pressures

The relation of PCW to PA$_d$ shows that as the PCW pressure rises, there is at first a corresponding rise of PA$_d$—passive pulmonary hypertension (Fig. 3).

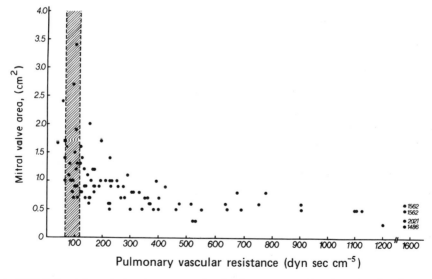

FIGURE 1 The relation between mitral valve cross-sectional area and pulmonary vascular resistance (PVR) in 100 patients with mitral stenosis. Note that pulmonary vascular resistance generally remained normal (shaded area) until the valve area approached 1.0 cm^2. It then rose to a variable extent in most cases.

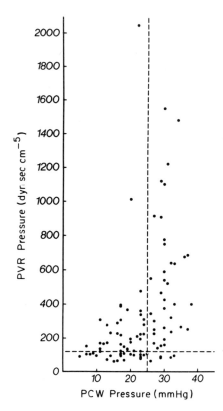

FIGURE 2 The relation between pulmonary vascular resistance (PVR) and pulmonary capillary wedge (PCW) pressure in 100 patients with mitral stenosis. Note that the pulmonary vascular resistance began to rise above normal (horizontal dotted line) before the PCW pressure approached 25 mmHg. A small number (about 7%) developed no increase in PVR despite wedge pressures of 25 mmHg, and only 8% had extreme elevations of PVR, i.e., over 1000 dsc (two had values of 1562 dsc and appear as only one dot in the figure).

The dotted line represents the normal equality of these two pressures. Divergence above the dotted line indicates that the PA_d has risen more than can be attributed to a passive rise of pulmonary artery pressure. This divergence begins in certain cases at a much lower pressure than 25 mmHg. This confirms the plot of PVR versus PCW, emphasizing that precapillary obstruction may appear before the time that pulmonary edema is impending. The divergence of pressure below the line represents the error of pressure measurement. The PA_d should never be less than PCW unless mitral regurgitation with a large V wave is present. None of these patients had significant mitral regurgitation.

The PA_d was less than the PCW mean pressure in 28 patients: by 1 mmHg in 15, by 2 mmHg in 5, by 3 mmHg in 4, by 4 mmHg in 2, and by 6 mmHg in 2. The mean difference was −2.0 ± 1.5 mmHg. The 1- and 2-mmHg differences can be considered as methodological in routine cardiac catheterizations. The 4- and 6-mmHg differences were because the measurements were not made in rapid succession. However, since these represent the findings, it seems fair to assume that deviation above the line was of the same magnitude as that below the line (2 ± 1.5 mmHg).

Pulmonary Capillary Wedge and Pulmonary Artery Mean (PA_m) Pressure

The relation of PCW to PA_m (Fig. 4) begins, in some patients, to diverge from the normal difference (6 mmHg) at about 17 mmHg. These divergences are in the same patients as shown in the plot of PCW against PA_d (Fig. 3).

Pulmonary Blood Flow

The third factor in the resistance formula is pulmonary blood flow (or cardiac output). As shown in Figure 5, the cardiac output in mitral stenosis was variable. In some, it was normal or even high. This generally occurred in patients with mild mitral stenosis without an increase of pulmonary vascular resistance. In the majority of symptomatic patients, it was reduced, as has been reported by many [4,5,10,17,59–62]. In 33% of our cases, the cardiac index at rest was 2 liters min^{-1} m^{-2} or less, a reduction of one-third or more below normal. It has been shown repeatedly that on exercise, the output does not rise in normal fashion [5,10,17,59–62].

Little emphasis has been given to the role of a reduced pulmonary blood flow on the genesis of the increase of calculated pulmonary vascular resistance in mitral stenosis. Unlike congenital heart disease with left-to-right shunts where the pulmonary blood flow is high, in mitral stenosis it is low. Figure 6

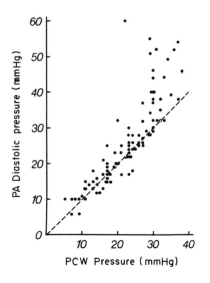

FIGURE 3 Relation between pulmonary arterial (PA) diastolic and pulmonary capillary wedge (PCW) pressure in 100 patients with mitral stenosis. Normally, these two pressures are the same, as indicated by the dashed line. The PA diastolic pressure begins to rise above the PCW pressure in some cases beginning somewhere in the vicinity of 15 mmHg. In many cases, there is no deviation from the line of equality even though the pressures were at the pulmonary edema level of 25 mmHg. See text for further discussion.

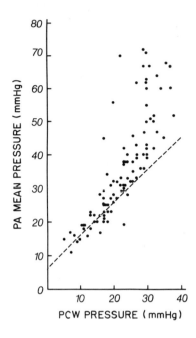

FIGURE 4 Relation between pulmonary arterial (PA) mean pressure and pulmonary capillary wedge (PCW) mean pressure in 100 patients with mitral stenosis. The dashed line represents the normal relationship between these two pressures. As in Figure 3, the PA_m pressure in some cases rose higher than the PCW pressure beginning at 15 to 20 mmHg, although a few remained on the line of equality despite pressures in excess of this. There were variably elevated PA_m pressures in excess of PCW pressure in the majority of patients whose PCW pressure exceeded 25 mmHg.

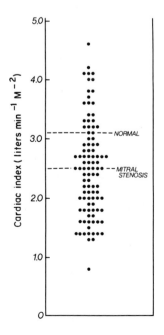

FIGURE 5 Cardiac index in 100 patients with mitral stenosis. In about a quarter of the patients, cardiac index was normal or even high. These patients generally hald mild degrees of mitral valve narrowing: 75% had cardiac indices on the low side of normal—some to extremely low values. The truly low values invariably had not only a narrow mitral valve of 1 cm^2 or less, but also an elevated pulmonary vascular resistance.

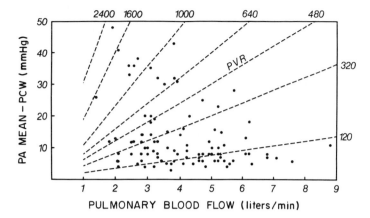

FIGURE 6 Relationships of transmural pressure (PA_m − PCW (or LA) mean pressure), pulmonary blood flow, and pulmonary vascular resistance (dotted lines) in 100 patients with mitral stenosis. An increase of pressure is associated with an increase of calculated PVR, as is a reduction of pulmonary blood flow. The influence of flow on resistance is least at low pressures and greatest at higher pressures, whereas the influence of pressure on resistance is uniformly influential in determining the calculated PVR.

is designed to show the relative roles played by pulmonary blood flow on the one hand and pressure difference across the lung (PA-LA) on the other, in relation to PVR. Although there *can* be marked reductions of cardiac output without much effect on PVR, providing ΔP is similarly reduced, a low output at elevated pressures results in impressive elevations of PVR. In studying this figure, one becomes impressed with the fact that (1) the PA-LA pressure is much less than in congenital heart disease, i.e., despite an elevation of PA pressure, the LA pressure is subtracted from it; and (2) the pulmonary blood flow (normally about 5.5 liters/min in adults) plays an important role in the calculation of pulmonary vascular resistance. Take, for example, the patient with a PA-LA of 26, and PBF of 1.4, and a PVR of 1562 in Figure 6. If the PA-LA remained at 26 and the PBF rose to 5.5, the PVR would fall to 378, just a quarter of the former value. One might say that this is playing with figures, but as we shall see, this is exactly what happens following mitral valve replacement. Hence, the role of cardiac output in the genesis of the increase of PVR must be emphasized. It must also be emphasized again that it is a mathematical relationship that exists in the resistance equation. Care must be exercised in the interpretation of this relationship. Interpretation will be postponed to Section IX.

Another approach that bears on the behavior of the pulmonary vasculature with respect to flow is that which occurs with unilateral pulmonary arterial balloon occlusion.

VII. Unilateral Pulmonary Arterial Balloon Occlusion

Carlens et al. [63] were the first to perform unilateral PA occlusion with a balloon on the end of the catheter. Brofman and colleagues [64] carried out this procedure in normal patients. Charms et al. [65] studied patients with mitral stenosis and severe pulmonary hypertension and observed a doubling of blood flow through the unoccluded lung and only small increases of pressure in the pulmonary artery. The pulmonary vascular resistance almost halved. There have been many observations of the effect of unilateral PA occlusion with a balloon in a variety of heart and pulmonary diseases with almost identical results [66–72].

Our studies, previously reported only in abstract form [73], will be included here the first time in complete detail because they illustrate the profound influence of flow on PVR even in the presence of severe compromise of the pulmonary circulation.

The studies were carried out in 36 patients, 11 with mitral stenosis, 4 with mitral regurgitation, 5 with aortic valve disease, 7 with miscellaneous disorders (patient 21, left ventricular failure, ? cause; patient 22, low cardiac output, ? cause, patient 23, chronic obstructive pulmonary disease; patients 24 and 25, primary pulmonary hypertension; patient 26, almost normal; and patient 27, constrictive pericarditis), and 9 cases of atrial septal defect (ASD). Although the latter are congenital, not acquired, heart diseases, they are included because they had very high pulmonary blood flow or high pulmonary vascular resistance.

Balloon occlusion was maintained for 10 min. Methodology and values are found in Appendix 2, Tables A and B. There was relative uniformity in the pattern of response to unilateral PA balloon occlusion without distinctive differences in the different diseases.

A. Hemodynamic Effects on Systemic Circulation

Figures 7 and 8 show the effect of unilateral pulmonary arterial occlusion on the *left side of the heart and systemic circulation*. Although there were individual variations, no statistically significant changes occurred in arterial O_2 saturation, O_2 consumption, cardiac output, pulse rate, stroke volume, arterial pressure, or LA mean pressure. In Figure 8, a momentary fall of a few millimeters of mercury of brachial arterial pressure is shown, but this was exceptional. It was not observed in other cases. In a few cases, there was a slight decrease of cardiac output which others have likewise reported [68,70], but the overall and probably fundamental response was the maintenance of a normal systemic circulation, as all other reports have demonstrated [64–72] and as are summarized in Table 2.

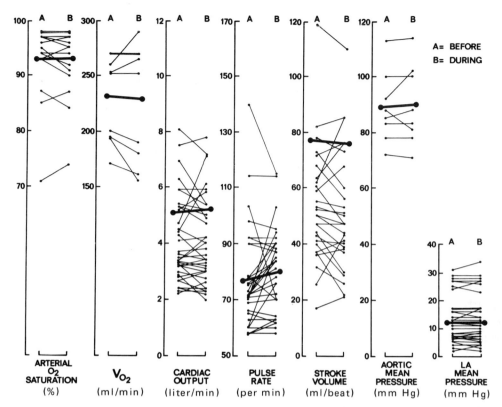

FIGURE 7 Effects of unilateral PA occlusion with a balloon on the systemic circulation. A = before, B = at the end of 10 min of occlusion. The heavy lines indicate averages. Although there were individual variations, there were no significant changes in the systemic circulation.

TABLE 2 Effect of Unilateral Pulmonary Artery Occlusion on Systemic Circulation[a]

O_2 sat (%)	V_{O_2} ml/min	CO (liters/min)	PR (per min)	SO (ml/beat)	Ao_m (mmHg)	LA_m (mmHg)
-1[b]	-1	-2	$+1$	0	$+1$	0

[a]O_2 sat = arterial O_2 saturation; V_{O_2} = O_2 consumption; CO = cardiac output; PR = pulse rate; SO = stroke output; Ao_m = arterial mean pressure; LA_m = left atrial mean pressure.
[b]All values listed are average % change.

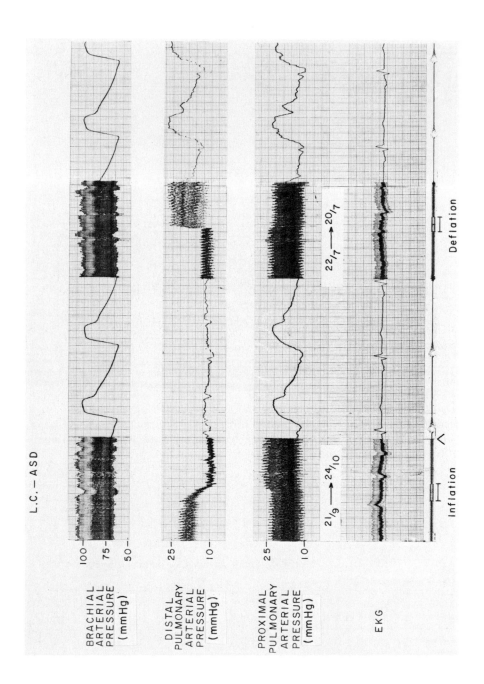

FIGURE 8 Effect of balloon inflation and deflation on pressures and EKG in patient 29 with an atrial septal defect. With inflation of the balloon, pressure in the PA distal to the balloon fell to left atrial level. This PA pressure was somewhat damped. In the PA proximal to the balloon, i.e., in the unoccluded lung, systolic pressure rose by 3 mmHg over a period of about 10 sec and gradually fell by 2 mmHg. The brachial arterial pressure, both systolic and diastolic, had a momentary drop of a few mmHg incident to inflation of the balloon. This did not occur in other cases. On deflation of the balloon, there was no detectable effect in the brachial arterial pressure, the pressure in the distal lumen rose from a left atrial to pulmonary arterial level, and systolic pressure proximal to the balloon fell slowly by 2 mmHg over a period of 10 sec. Major time lines are at 10-sec intervals.

TABLE 3   Effect of Unilateral Pulmonary Artery Occlusion on Unoccluded Lung[a]

PA-LA mean pressure (mmHg)	Blood flow (liters/min)	Mean transit time (sec)	Pulm blood volume (liters)	Pulm vascular resistance (dyn sec cm^{-5})
+24	+76	−24	+46	−33

[a]Values listed are average % change.

B.   Hemodynamic Changes in the Unoccluded Lung Alone

Hemodynamic changes in the unoccluded lung alone during unilateral PA occlusion are shown in Appendix 2, Table C. It is assumed that blood flow was equal in the two lungs before inflation and that each lung had half the pulmonary blood flow and pulmonary blood volume, the same pulmonary arterial pressure and mean transit time, and twice the PVR. These are the control values shown in the table. Results to be described are summarized in Table 3.

Pressure

Figure 8 shows a rise in PA systolic pressure on balloon inflation. The rise took between 10 and 15 sec to reach a peak and then decreased so that it was 3 mmHg above control level for the ensuing 10 min. On deflation, there was a fall of 2 mmHg of PA systolic pressure. The values are noted in Figure 8. Figure 9 shows values for each patient. For the whole group, the mean increase of PA *mean* pressure was 4.1 ± 3.9 mmHg and varied between −5 and +16 mmHg. The mean increase of PA *systolic* pressure was 9.1 ± 7.4 mmHg, with a range of 0 to 33 mmHg. The PA *diastolic* pressure varied little, except for patient 7 in whom it rose 26 mmHg during occlusion. Omitting this patient, the others had an average rise of PA diastolic pressure of 1.5 ± 2.5 mmHg, with a range of −4 to +6 mmHg. The PA *pulse* pressure during occlusion rose 7.6 ± 6.7 mmHg, with a range of −2 to +24 mmHg. The PA_m-LA_m pressure increased 3.8 ± 3.9 mmHg, with a range of −3 to 14 mmHg. This small rise of pressure represents the 24% increase noted in Table 3. As mentioned above, there was no statistical change in LA pressure during occlusion, and specifically not in mitral stenosis. *In summary,* there was only a small rise of PA and of PA-LA pressures as a result of balloon occlusion.

Flow through the unoccluded lung doubled statistically, but there were great variations. The variation in response ranged from as little as +33% (in patient 7 mentioned above with the greatest rise of PA pressure) to as much as +225% in patient 9 with aortic valve disease. Even in patients with ASD and large pulmonary blood flows before occlusion, flow increased impressively

$$Pi = \frac{PA_m + LA_m}{2}$$

This gives an estimate of the pressure acting to distend the pulmonary vascular bed. Figure 10 and Table C, Appendix 2, show the relation between PBV and Pi, i.e., the relative compliance PBV/Pi. There was a wide scatter of values before occlusion. The relative compliance of the vasculature for the unoccluded lung before balloon inflation was 5.54 ± 3.89 ml m^{-2} mmHg^{-1}, or twice this value, 11.08, if applied to both lungs. This value is slightly lower than that obtained by Milnor et al. [74], which was 14.7 ml m^{-2} mmHg^{-1}.

In every case, the relative compliance increased with occlusion, i.e., the PBV rose appreciably without a proportionate increase of pressure. Thus, they became more compliant, i.e., less "stiff" during this maneuver.

This is contrary to Yu's findings in cardiac patients undergoing exercise [22]. Values for normal showed an increase from 25.4 to 30.2 ml m^{-2} mmHg^{-1} (Table 17-1 in [22]). In patients with aortic regurgitation, there was essentially no change during exercise (24.5 and 25.0 ml m^{-2} mmHg^{-1} (Table 17-2 in [22]). For patients with aortic stenosis, mitral regurgitation and mitral

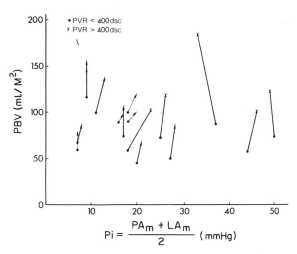

RELATIVE COMPLIANCE OF PULMONARY VASCULATURE
BEFORE AND DURING UNILATERAL PA BALLOON OCCLUSION

FIGURE 10 Relative compliance of pulmonary vasculature of the unoccluded lung alone in response to unilateral pulmonary arterial balloon occlusion. See text for discussion.

stenosis, values decreased from 22.0 to 14.0, 14.9 to 12.3, and 13.5 to 10.0, respectively (Tables 17-3 to 17-5 in [22]).

The increase in values in our patients and the decrease in values in Yu's patients with heart disease, who were not too dissimilar to our patients, is not attributable to methodology since this was similar in both studies, but rather to the type of procedure. Unilateral balloon occlusion produced a doubling of flow with little change of distending pressure. From Yu's Table III, exercise produced less of an increase in flow and greater increases in distending pressure. The LA pressures rose little in normal patients and in those with aortic regurgitation during exercise, while in those with aortic stenosis, mitral regurgitation, and mitral stenosis, there was a considerable increase in LA pressure during exercise. The difference in results appear to be attributable to the difference between balloon occlusion and exercise.

The Compliance of the Pulmonary Vasculature

In our patients undergoing unilateral PA occlusion, $\Delta PBV/\Delta Pi$ varied from 8 to 82 and averaged 29 ± 24 ml m^{-2} mmHg^{-1} (see Table D, Appendix 2). Yu's patients undergoing exercise averaged 71.5 ml m^{-2} mmHg^{-1} for normals, 34.7 for aortic regurgitation, 6.3 for aortic stenosis, 9.3 for mitral regurgitation, and 6.1 for mitral stenosis (see Yu's Table 17).

The Coefficient of Distensibility

of the pulmonary vascular bed was calculated using the equation

$$ C = \frac{1}{V} \frac{\Delta V}{\Delta P} $$

where C = coefficient of distensibility, V = pulmonary blood volume of unoccluded lung before balloon occlusion, ΔV = increase of pulmonary blood volume of unoccluded lung during balloon occlusion, and ΔP = change of distending pressure (Pi) during balloon occlusion. The coefficient of distensibility during balloon occlusion in our patients was much higher than those of Yu [22] during exercise (see Table E, Appendix 2). The average for our patients was 0.41 ± 0.37, with a range of 0.09 to 1.29. In Yu's patients, the average for normals was 0.23, for aortic regurgitation 0.12, for aortic stenosis 0.03, for mitral regurgitation 0.04, and for mitral stenosis 0.02.

There was no relation between compliance values and the level of PA pressure or PVR. In any event, the values obtained indicate how compliant the pulmonary vasculature was in these lungs, some of which had considerable elevations of pulmonary arterial pressure and pulmonary vascular resistance, and how distensible they became as a result of an increase of flow.

Comment on Unilateral Balloon Occlusion of PA

The systemic circulation was essentially unaffected by unilateral PA occlusion even though there was a high PVR in some cases or a large PBF as in some of those with ASD. Thus, even in those where the lung was compromised by extensive abnormality, it remained the true servant of the systemic circulation by remarkable adaptations to the sudden burden of its size being reduced by one-half. Unaffected on the average were the cardiac output, pulse rate, stroke output, LA pressure, arterial pressure, O_2 consumption, and arterial O_2 saturation.

The lung's adaptation was remarkable. The PA pressure increased only slightly, the PA mean by an average of only 4.1 mmHg, and the PA systolic by 9.1 mmHg. The flow was unchanged, signifying that it doubled through the unoccluded lung. It seems reasonable to conclude that the basic alteration was aimed at maintaining this flow to provide the left side of the heart with its normal quota of blood.

Changes in the lung as a result of this maneuver were (1) an increase of PBV in the unoccluded lung, presumably by distension of the vasculature or recruitment of new vessels; (2) an increase of blood flow velocity (decrease of MTT); and (3) a fall of PVR.

Compared with preocclusion, the PVR increased from a mean of 368 to 495 dyn sec cm^{-5}, an increase of 35% due to the reduction of vasculature by balloon occlusion, but in the unoccluded lung alone, the PVR fell by 34%. This fall of PVR required a widening of the pulmonary vasculature at some point, but whether by vasodilatation or recruitment of new vessels is speculative. Recruitment of new vessels seems possible but surprising in those who had considerable pulmonary hypertension and in those with very high pulmonary blood flows (ASD) in whom recruitment might have already been expected to have maximally occurred.

Widimský and associates [72] observed that in some patients with mitral stenosis, particularly in those with a very high pulmonary vascular resistance, exercise produced a much greater increase of pulmonary arterial pressure than did unilateral balloon occlusion of the pulmonary artery. The increase of flow was less during exercise than during occlusion. Furthermore, the pulmonary vascular resistance rose with exercise and fell with occlusion. The authors pointed out that with balloon occlusion, there was vasodilatation and no rise of left atrial pressure, that during exercise there was vasoconstriction and the left atrial pressure became elevated. They suggested that the fundamental difference in vasomotor response in these experiments was due to the different responses of the left atrial pressure. When it was unchanged by balloon occlusion, vasodilatation occurred. Its elevation during exercise resulted in vasoconstriction. Such vasoconstriction occurred only in those with marked elevation of pulmonary vascular resistance to begin with. These patients might be considered to have been in the group of hyperreactors.

The differences between balloon occlusion and exercise underscores the differences in physiological events. Balloon occlusion produces a doubling of blood flow without much change of pressure. Exercise is more complicated. Pressures in pulmonary artery rise, left atrial pressure rises in disease, catechols are released, and other changes occur during exercise, many or all of which can affect pulmonary vascular compliance and distensibility. Balloon occlusion produces none of these.

The differences in our values for relative compliance, compliance, and distensibility during balloon occlusion from those found by Yu [22] during exercise are probably due to these factors. For further details of interpretation, the reader is referred to several publications [10,11,22,74].

Aramendia et al. [75] were able to block the rise of PA pressure from unilateral balloon occlusion of the pulmonary artery in dogs by injecting the wall of the pulmonary artery with xylocaine in the area of balloon occlusion. Cardiac output was unaffected, indicating a doubling of flow through the unoccluded lung. The pulmonary vascular resistance through the unoccluded lung, though not calculated, must have halved. The rise of pulmonary arterial pressure was concluded to have been neurogenically mediated. However, neither the rise of pulmonary arterial pressure nor the fall of pulmonary vascular resistance could be blocked by reserpine, hexamethonium bromide, atropine, guanethidine, or vagotomy. These findings indicated that the rise of pulmonary arterial pressure was neurogenically mediated, but threw doubt on a neurogenic mechanism for the fall of pulmonary vascular resistance from unilateral pulmonary arterial occlusion.

Questions arise about the genesis of the fall of PVR. There are several possibilities. The first is that it was purely mechanical. The venous return to the right ventricle was delivered into the lung. When one lung was suddenly occluded with a balloon, the right ventricle ejected its contents into the unoccluded lung. In other words, the unoccluded lung suddenly received twice as much blood as before. Pressure rose slightly, its vascular volume increased, and vessels became distended; perhaps this is all that is necessary to explain what transpired.

This mechanical interpretation, which seems to explain all the findings, fails in one important respect. What is the regulatory mechanism? What is the signal from the systemic circulation which makes right ventricle and lung adapt in the way described to maintain the homeostasis of the systemic circulation? To my knowledge, no neurogenic, humoral, or myogenic mechanism has been clearly demonstrated and yet it seems that there almost has to be one.

It is clear, however, that an increase of pulmonary blood flow (the denominator of the resistance equation) results in an impressive reduction of pulmonary vascular resistance.

VIII. Postoperative Reduction of Pulmonary Vascular Resistance

It has been recognized for years that surgical relief of mitral stenosis results in a reduction of pulmonary vascular resistance to almost normal levels. The first studies were carried out in patients who underwent mitral valvuloplasty and commissurotomy [76-81]. It immediately became apparent that relief of the stenosis resulted in a fall of pulmonary vascular resistance, in striking contrast to the majority of patients with similar elevations of pulmonary vascular resistance in association with congenital heart disease.

With the advent of prosthetic valves, surgical relief of mitral stenosis became consistent and studies of the response of pulmonary vascular resistance to mitral valve replacement became more reliable.

Dalen and associates [82,83] monitored patients with mitral stenosis who had an average pulmonary vascular resistance of 1088 dyn sec cm^{-5} preoperatively and who underwent mitral valve replacement with a discoid mitral valve. As shown in Figure 11, the immediate results of surgery were dramatic. The left atrial pressure fell from 28 to 10 mmHg immediately. The pulmonary arterial mean pressure fell to a similar extent, from 71 to 47 mmHg. The PA-LA mean pressure difference of 39 mmHg preoperatively was unchanged on the first 3 days, postoperatively, but by the eighth day had narrowed to 29 mmHg. Thus, the immediate effect of mitral valve replacement was a disappearance of passive pulmonary hypertension and only a slight reduction of the pressure difference across the lung.

Cardiac output rose immediately to normal levels 2 days after the mitral valve obstruction had been relieved. There was a higher than normal output thereafter consistent with the normal response to surgery.

The pulmonary vascular resistance fell precipitously after surgery, almost entirely on the basis of an increase in cardiac output and only to a slight degree on the basis of a small reduction of the PA-LA gradient. The PVR at the end of 24 hr had fallen from a mean of 1234 to a mean of 737 dyn sec cm^{-5}, and at the end of 8 days to 312 dyn sec cm^{-5}. It is hard to explain these findings on a basis other than vasodilatation.

Figure 12 shows late results of mitral valve replacement reported by Zener et al. [84] and Braunwald et al. [85], plotted in such fashion that the relationships of PA-LA mean pressures, PBF, and PVR are shown by the

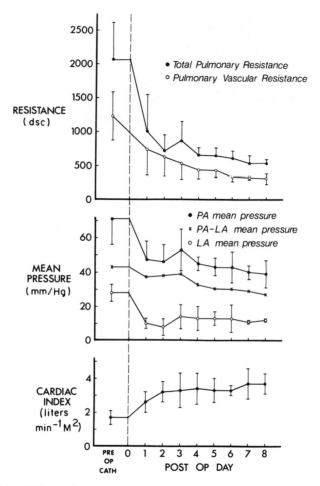

FIGURE 11   Effect of mitral valve replacement on PA-LA mean pressure, pulmonary blood flow (cardiac output), and pulmonary vascular resistance. See text for discussion.

dotted lines. There is not only a striking fall of pressure gradient in most patients, but an equally impressive increase of PBF. The result is that almost all lines slope downward and to the right, crossing to lower levels of PVR. Thus, with time, there was an adjustment of pressure and flow to the lower pulmonary vascular resistance.

Table 4 shows the preoperative and early postoperative findings in the patients reported by Dalen et al. [82,83] and the late postoperative findings by Zener et al. [84] and Braunwald et al. [85]. The late results show that the PVR had not returned entirely to normal. Their mean value was 246

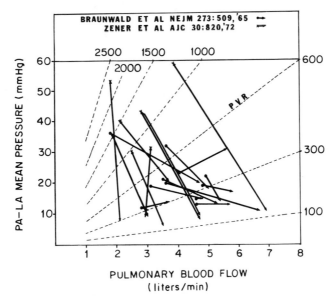

FIGURE 12   Late effects of mitral valve replacement on PA-LA mean pressure, pulmonary blood flow, and pulmonary vascular resistance. See text for discussion.

dyn sec cm^{-5}, about 3 times normal. The residual mild elevation of PVR, which by itself is clinically insignificant, may have been on the basis of residual histologic changes in the pulmonary vasculature previously described, even though there is some evidence that even these disappear after relief of mitral stenosis [28,48]. The cardiac index in the study of Braunwald et al. had become normal; in that of Zener et al., it was somewhat lower than normal. The PA-LA pressure in both studies was still about twice normal.

TABLE 4   Hemodynamic Response to Mitral Valve Replacement

Parameter	Pre-op [83]	2-10 Days Post-op [83]	7.6 Months Post-op [85]	26 Months Post-op [84]
PA mean pressure (mmHg)	71	36	27	26
LA mean pressure (mmHg)	31	10	12	13
PA-LA gradient (mmHg)	40	26	15	13
Pulmonary vascular resistance (dyn sec cm^{-5})	1088	491	243	246
Cardiac index (liters min^{-1} m^{-2})	1.7	4.0	3.0	2.6

IX. Discussion

The rise of pulmonary vascular resistance in association with mitral stenosis has led to an analysis of the numerator (PA-LA mean pressures) and of the denominator (pulmonary blood flow) of the resistance equation. PVR rises if there is a rise of the pressure at a given flow or a fall of flow at a given pressure (Fig. 6).

A. Pressure

It is clear that the first response to narrowing of the mitral valve is a rise of pressure in the left atrium with a corresponding rise of pressure in the pulmonary artery. Eventually, and starting in some individuals well before the threat of pulmonary edema, the pulmonary arterial diastolic pressure rises more than the PCW pressure, i.e., a gradient appears between PA_d and PCW (Fig. 3). Normally there is none. There are several possible causes, but all are speculative.

Intrinsic Neurogenic Reflex

There is no known intrinsic reflex vasoconstrictor pathway between pulmonary veins or capillaries and muscular pulmonary arteries which are the resistance vessels. The pulmonary arterioles and capillaries are devoid of nerve fibers. If there is a reflex in this region, it remains to be described.

Intrinsic Myogenic Reflex

In 1902, Bayliss [86] showed that the smooth muscle of systemic arteries responded to stretch, as do other types of smooth muscle. An increase of intraluminal pressure produced constriction and a decrease, relaxation (vasodilatation). Neither he nor subsequent workers have demonstrated this response in pulmonary blood vessels, but there is no reason to believe that these would not respond in a similar fashion.

Harris and Heath [10] suggested that the Bayliss myogenic reflex might occur in the lung of patients as a response to any type of pulmonary hypertension. In mitral stenosis, it would be the stimulus provided by passive pulmonary hypertension. Subsequently, there would be a vicious circle. The higher the PA pressure rose, the greater would be the vascular constriction, which in turn would produce a higher pressure.

That something of the sort may occur is suggested by the angiographic and radiologic narrowing of the pulmonary vasculature seen in patients with pulmonary hypertension. The main and lobar branches of the pulmonary artery are usually quite prominent and dilated, but beyond them they are narrow and constricted, to which the term "pruning" is sometimes applied. Whether they are narrowed because of myogenic or other type of reflex constriction is unknown.

There have been several explanations for the redistribution of blood flow from the bases to the apexes of the lung in mitral stenosis. Patients with mitral stenosis are characteristically orthopneic and therefore have higher hydrostatic pressures at the bases throughout the day and night rather than during waking hours alone. Most explanations for the diversion of blood flow from the bases to the apexes of the lung in mitral stenosis depend basically on the hydrostatic pressure difference between apex and base, the difference being 30 to 35 cmH_2O (22 to 26 mmHg).

1. Histologic narrowing of vessels are greater at the base than at the apex, presumably due to the higher basal pressures [10,28]. There is no doubt that this is at least a partial if not the complete explanation.

2. West et al. [87] attributed an increase of PVR in the basal portions of the lung to perivascular edema compressing the vessels, but Ritchie et al. [88] were unable to confirm their findings.

3. The Bayliss myogenic reflex [86] would produce greater narrowing of vessels at the base than at the apex because of the higher intraluminal pressure, but the abnormal redistribution of blood flow as shown by pulmonary angiography and perfusion scanning [55-57] is not restored to normal by recumbency, as might be anticipated if this were the explanation. Dawson [89] produced evidence that vessels at the lung base were more vasoreactive than those at the apexes and remained so irrespective of the position of the body.

Central Neurogenic Mechanisms

It has been pointed out above that sympathetic α-adrenergic stimulation increases pulmonary vascular tone and produces vasoconstriction, i.e., an increase of PVR. Parasympathetic and β-adrenergic stimulation decrease pulmonary vascular tone and produce pulmonary vasodilatation. PVR can thus be altered by appropriate adrenergic and parasympathetic agonists and antagonists [18,19,28-36]. These have been used effectively in predicting the reversibility and irreversibility of the raised PVR in mitral stenosis and other forms of pulmonary hypertension.

The most direct experimental evidence that the sympathetic nervous system is involved in the genesis of the rise of pulmonary vascular resistance as a result of pulmonary venous hypertension is that of Ferri and Rovati and their colleagues [90,91]. They reported that the abnormal rise of pulmonary arterial pressure was abolished by the sympatholytic agent, imidazoline, and the ganglionic blocking agent, hexamethonium, but not by atropine, vagotomy, or cervical sympathectomy. Norepinephrine made the pulmonary hypertension more severe. They concluded that the rise of PA pressure, out of proportion to the rise of pulmonary venous pressure, was sympathetically mediated.

The bulk of evidence, even though not completely convincing, points to α-sympathetic activity as the most important factor in producing the increase of PVR in association with pulmonary venous hypertension.

Humoral Agents

The lung produces, as well as destroys, a variety of humoral agents: prostaglandins, serotonin, histamine, and bradykinin [92–94]. Prostaglandins E_2 and $F_{2\alpha}$ are pulmonary vasoconstrictors. Serotonin is a strong pulmonary vasoconstrictor in certain species such as dog and cat, but not in humans. Bradykinin is a vasodilator. Histamine produces pulmonary venous constriction [95].

I shall not allude further to these agents. Attractive as it is to think of one or more of these substances as playing an important role in maintaining pulmonary vascular tone and raising the PVR in mitral stenosis and other forms of pulmonary venous hypertension, currently there is no evidence in support of such activity. The future may clarify their place in pulmonary vascular function.

Hypoxia

Hypoxia is a well-known pulmonary vasoconstrictor and has recently been reviewed in detail by Fishman [96]. Donald [97] and Jordan [98] suggested that uneven ventilation and alveolar hypoxia, as a result of thickened alveolar membranes, might be responsible for constriction of muscular pulmonary arteries in patients with mitral stenosis. However, Walston et al. [99] found no significant correlation between pulmonary arterial pressure and arterial oxygen saturation in mitral stenosis. Half of their patients with a mean PA pressure over 30 had an arterial oxygen saturation of 95% or higher. This does not exclude an influence of hypoxia when it exists, but makes it difficult to accept it as a primary factor in the production of the chronic pulmonary hypertension of mitral stenosis.

Acidosis

In some subjects, hydrogen ion concentration is an important stimulus to the persistence of a high pulmonary arterial pressure, particularly if there is associated hypoxia [100]. In subjects with hypoventilation, the administration of 100% oxygen may have little or no effect on elevated pulmonary arterial pressures unless the pH of blood is raised. In mitral stenosis, acidosis is uncommon. Due to chronic hyperventilation, the arterial PCO_2 is characteristically low and there is a compensated alkalosis with a normal blood pH.

Histologic Changes

The advanced changes of dilatation lesions, arteritis, and plexiform lesions seen so commonly in congenital heart disease and primary pulmonary hypertension are not found in patients with mitral stenosis. Instead, they progress only to stage 3 of the classification of Heath and Edwards [27,28]. In congenital heart disease, stage 1 to 3 lesions are considered to be reversible by surgery, and the same is true in mitral stenosis [27,28].

There are two differences in the changes in the resistance vessels in mitral stenosis from those that occur in congenital heart disease. (1) Hypertrophy of the media is much more pronounced in the arterioles of those with mitral stenosis, as might be expected because of the passive elevation of pressures in these vessels transmitted back from the left atrium. In congenital heart disease, histologic changes occur in muscular arteries which are the resistance vessels and do not extend into the arterioles. (2) Intimal lesions are much less severe in mitral stenosis, presumably due to the fact that the pressure gradient across the lung (PA-LA) is some 25 mmHg less than in those with congenital heart disease with the same PA pressure in whom the left atrial pressure is normal, and that the pulmonary blood flow tends to be low in mitral stenosis in contrast to being high in congenital heart disease.

Since the intimal lesions are thought to be on a "traumatic" basis [28,101], the combination of higher pressures and flows in congenital heart disease would produce lesions of greater severity than in those with mitral stenosis in whom the transmural pressure (PA-LA) as well as the flow are considerably less.

Concept of a Protective Mechanism

It was originally suggested [102] that the raised PVR in mitral stenosis was a protective mechanism to prevent pulmonary edema by protecting the pulmonary capillaries from a high pulmonary arterial pressure and therefore pulmonary edema. Although this is an attractive concept and widely quoted, Lucas and Dotter [61] pointed out that it did *not* protect the capillaries. On exercise, the PCW rose above the pulmonary edema threshold just as much in those with a high as in those with a normal pulmonary vascular resistance.

The way in which an increase of PVR plays a protective role is by further reducing cardiac output [10,17], which allows the orifice of the mitral valve to become progressively smaller without necessitating a further rise of left atrial and therefore pulmonary capillary pressure. At a resting left atrial pressure of about 25 mmHg (pulmonary edema level), the orifice of the mitral valve can diminish from 1.0 cm^2 to as little as 0.3 cm^2, provided that flow is reduced from about 2.7 to about 1.4 liters min^{-1} m^{-2}.

B.   Flow

Considerable emphasis is placed in this article on flow and its influence on the pulmonary vascular resistance in mitral stenosis. Little attention has been paid to it in the literature. It appears to exert an important influence on pulmonary vascular function. Flow is in the denominator of the resistance equation. At any given PA-LA mean pressure, a reduction of flow results in a higher calculated PVR, and an increase of flow results in a lower calculated PVR. Although this is a mathematical necessity, it appears to have considerable biologic significance.

Relation of PBF to PVR

Figure 6 provides an "eye-ball' evaluation of the relation of pulmonary blood flow to pulmonary vascular resistance at any given PA-LA mean pressure. One cannot escape the influence of flow on the calculation. It appears to have about as much influence on the calculation as does the elevation of pressure.

Unilateral PA Occlusion

The reason these studies were included is that they provide a striking example of the influence of flow on PVR. The elevated PA pressures were only slightly increased by unilateral PA occlusion with a balloon. Since the return flow to the left atrium and to the systemic circulation remained the same, the PA pressure remained little altered, increasing just enough to ensure a normal return to the left ventricle in order to maintain an unchanged flow to the systemic circulation. This necessitated a doubling of flow to the unoccluded lung, which was accomplished by increasing the pulmonary blood volume, by vasodilatation or recruitment of new vessels, by increasing the velocity of blood flow through the lung (more rapid mean transit time), and by a dramatic fall of pulmonary vascular resistance. The precise mechanism by which the PVR fell has never been elucidated, but from the work of

Aramendia et al. [75], it would appear to be independent of nervous regulation. Their work was done on normal dogs. Because pressures and resistances are so low in, and flows so high through the normal lung, it is frequently extremely difficult to detect the role of regulatory mechanisms. Studies should be carried out in patients with pulmonary hypertension associated with mitral stenosis and other diseases using α- and β-blocking agents to determine their influence on the pulmonary vascular response to unilateral pulmonary artery occlusion. Until experiments of this type are carried out, it is difficult to be sure that neurogenic influences have been excluded.

Another explanation is that the fall of PVR is on a purely mechanical basis. The total right ventricular stroke output, previously delivered to two lungs, was delivered to one lung as a result of unilateral PA occlusion. The slight increase in PA pressure was sufficient to produce either passive dilatation of the pulmonary vasculature or recruitment of previously nonperfused vessels. However, the studies of Aramendia et al. [75] suggest that the tone of the pulmonary vasculature was readjusted in response to the new circulatory state. The rise of PA pressure (but not the fall of PVR) was abolished by local anesthesia of the wall of the PA at the site of balloon occlusion.

Rudolph and Auld [103] perfused dog lungs and showed that by increasing the pulmonary blood flow PVR fell even when the vessels were constricted with serotonin. It seems likely, therefore, that increasing pulmonary blood flow may override vasoconstriction from drugs (serotonin) and presumably from other causes of pulmonary vasoconstriction such as those present in mitral stenosis and other diseases causing pulmonary hypertension and by sympathetic α-adrenergic stimulation.

Mitral Valve Replacement

The immediate effect of mitral valve replacement was twofold. (1) A prompt elimination of passive pulmonary hypertension. The LA pressure fell to a normal level, and with it, there was a corresponding fall of pulmonary arterial pressure. The PA-LA mean pressure difference narrowed only slightly from that which was present preoperatively. (2) With relief of the mitral stenosis, the cardiac output rose rapidly to normal levels.

The pulmonary vascular resistance fell in an almost one-to-one relation to the increase of pulmonary blood flow (cardiac output), which is similar to the pulmonary vascular response to unilateral balloon occlusion of the pulmonary artery. Over the course of 10 days, the PA-LA pressure narrowed somewhat and, in the studies of others, narrowed further over the ensuing months, but still remained about twice normal.

The PVR fell despite a reduction of the distending pressures in pulmonary arteries (PA_m) and pulmonary veins (LA_m). Rudolph and Auld [103], in perfusion experiments on dog lungs, demonstrated a reduction of PVR when these two pressures were elevated. The fall of PVR in the presence of a reduction of these two pressures indicated vasodilatation when vasoconstriction on a mechanical basis might have been anticipated.

X.   Summary

The pulmonary vascular disease associated with acquired heart disease has been discussed mainly in relation to mitral stenosis, the acquired heart disease that has been studied in greatest detail.

Pulmonary vascular disease has been defined in terms of pulmonary vascular resistance, calculated by the following formula:

$$PVR = \frac{PA\text{-}LA}{PBF} \times 80$$

where PVR = pulmonary vascular resistance (dyn sec cm^{-5}); PA = pulmonary arterial mean pressure (mmHg); LA = left atrial mean pressure (mmHg); PBF = pulmonary blood flow (liters/min); and 80 = conversion factor.

Although the calculation of PVR is fraught with difficulties of measurement and interpretation in the normal lung, where pressures are low and flow is high, it has significance and is susceptible of interpretation in the abnormal lung, where pressures are high and the flow is low.

PVR is a measure of resistance to flow through the pulmonary vasculature. Included in this resistance calculation in mitral stenosis are anatomical narrowing of pulmonary arteries and arterioles, plus arterial and arteriolar vasoconstriction.

In mitral stenosis, there is at first a passive pulmonary hypertension. As pressure rises in the left atrium in response to narrowing of the mitral valve, there is a corresponding rise of pressure in pulmonary veins, pulmonary capillaries, and pulmonary artery—passive pulmonary hypertension.

When these pressures become 18 to 20 mmHg, there is a greater rise of pressure in the pulmonary artery so that its diastolic pressure begins to exceed that in the left atrium, pulmonary veins, and pulmonary capillaries. This is referred to as reactive pulmonary hypertension.

Reactive pulmonary hypertension becomes excessive, exceeding 1000 dyn sec cm^{-5} in about 7% of patients with mitral stenosis (the hyperreactors), fails to occur in about 5% (hyporeactors), and in the remainder it becomes elevated to a variable extent.

Anatomical narrowing from muscular hypertrophy and intimal proliferation eventually occurs in pulmonary veins, arterioles, and arteries in response to the increase in pressure within their lumina.

These lesions do not progress beyond stage 3 of Heath and Edwards [27], presumably due to the lower flow rate and to the less severe transmural pressure in mitral stenosis than in congenital heart disease. In mitral stenosis, the LA pressure of approximately 25 mmHg is subtracted from the PA mean pressure to obtain the transmural pressure. In congenital heart disease and in primary pulmonary hypertension, the LA pressure is usually about 5 mmHg. In congenital heart disease, flows are characteristically high initially. In any event, hypertensive lesions in the pulmonary vasculature do not develop to a severity of stages 4, 5, and 6, which Heath and Edwards consider to be irreversible.

The precise genesis of reactive pulmonary hypertension remains unexplained. Two possibilities are the neurogenic theory, which implies an increase of vascular tone and resistance by α-adrenergic stimuli; and the myogenic reflex of Bayliss [86], who showed that vascular smooth muscle, like all smooth muscles, reacts to an increase of intraluminal pressure by constriction and to a lowering of intraluminal pressure by relaxation.

In considering the resistance formula, one has usually considered the pressure to be high because the resistance is high. In a way, this is true. The pressure is set at whatever level is necessary to overcome the resistance to flow through lung and mitral valve to ensure the left ventricle and systemic circulation with an adequate amount of blood.

However, the flow appears to be just as important in determining the resistance. Although the PA-LA mean pressure difference eventually becomes increased in mitral stenosis, coincidentally the flow becomes reduced and, with exceptions, appears to play as much a role as the elevated pressures in producing an increase in PVR.

Unilateral balloon occlusion of the pulmonary artery in mitral stenosis and other disorders produces a dramatic fall in PVR which is entirely on the basis of an increase in flow to the unoccluded lung.

Following mitral valve replacement, there is an immediate disappearance of passive pulmonary hypertension, i.e., the LA pressure falls to normal with a corresponding fall in PA pressure. The PA-LA mean pressure difference remains practically unchanged.

There is an immediate fall in PVR associated with an increase in pulmonary blood flow (cardiac output) due to relief of the mitral valve obstruction. There is, in fact, a direct relation, as in unilateral balloon occlusion between the increase in pulmonary blood flow and the fall in the PVR.

Over the course of 10 days, the PA-LA mean pressure difference decreases somewhat and continues to narrow over the succeeding weeks or months.

The final value for PVR months later reaches a level about 4 times the normal, which is physiologically but not clinically significant.

It is concluded that the pulmonary vascular responses to mitral stenosis (and other left-sided lesions which produce pulmonary venous hypertension) are (1) a modest degree of anatomical narrowing of pulmonary arterioles and muscular arteries which does not reach a degree of severity to become irreversible and self-perpetuating after relief of mitral stenosis surgically, and (2) vasoconstriction, which is centrally mediated by α-adrenergic stimulation and perhaps abetted by intrinsic myogenic vasoconstriction.

Appendix 1

Patients (100) with mitral stenosis of varying degrees of severity were studied. None had more than one-plus mitral or aortic regurgitation angiographically. One-plus regurgitation was defined as that amount which completely disappeared on the next systole or diastole when injected into the left ventricle and entered the left atrium in systole, or into the aorta just distal to the aortic valve and entered the left ventricle in diastole. Eight patients had 2+ or 3+ tricuspid regurgitation.

Patients were studied in a fasting state or else an hour or more following a light breakfast consisting of clear fluids, toast, and jam. Almost all the patients received Valium, 10 mg, before the study for relief of anxiety. Right and retrograde left heart catheterizations were performed in the usual fashion. Cardiac output was measured either by the direct Fick principle or by the indicator-dilution method using indocyanine green.

Pressures were measured using a P-23D Statham manometer connected to a multichannel recorder. Pulmonary capillary wedge pressures were measured in all cases and were validated by wave-form and an oxygen saturation of 98%. These were considered the same as left atrial pressures. Pressures were measured in pulmonary artery, left ventricle, and aorta. Flows were measured in most cases in close relation to pressures. The cross-sectional area of the mitral valve was calculated by the method of Gorlin and Gorlin [58]. The pulmonary vascular resistance was calculated as follows:

$$PVR = \frac{PA_m - LA_m}{PBF} \times 80$$

where PVR = pulmonary vascular resistance (dyn sec cm^{-5}); PA_m = pulmonary arterial mean pressure (mmHg); LA_m = left atrial (or pulmonary capillary wedge) mean pressure (mmHg); PBF = pulmonary blood flow (cardiac output) (liters/min); 80 = conversion factor to dsc units.

TABLE A Hemodynamic Values in Patients with Mitral Stenosis

Patient	Age (years)	Sex (M/F)	Body surface area (m²)	Mitral valve area (cm²)	PVR (dyn sec cm⁻⁵)	RAm	PA S	PA D	PA m	PCWm	Cardiac index (liters min⁻¹ m⁻²)	MR	AR	TR
1	20	F	1.32	1.2	106	3	50	24	32	24	4.0			
2	48	M	1.42	0.3	520	6	67	29	43	30	1.4			
3	15	F	1.18	0.9	189	—	54	32	39	30	3.2			
4	46	F	1.58	0.6	222	7	53	32	42	32	2.3			
5	55	F	1.00	0.9	229	9	50	26	33	27	2.1			
6	55	F	1.75	0.5	400	8	60	46	52	38	1.6	+		
7	50	F	1.54	0.6	372	5	72	38	50	30	2.8			
8	55	M	1.90	1.0	251	6	63	27	43	27	2.7	+		
9	62	F	1.45	0.5	300	7	62	32	39	27	2.2	+	+	
10	61	F	1.56	0.5	342	6	65	25	38	26	1.8			
11	40	F	1.56	0.7	400	4	64	32	47	33	1.8	+	+	
12	64	F	1.69	0.7	139	5	55	29	36	28	2.7		+	
13	60	F	1.45	0.5	552	11	82	28	46	26	2.0	+		
14	48	F	1.68	0.7	95	5	44	22	31	22	2.5		+	
15	46	F	1.50	1.0	84	5	43	26	35	26	3.8	+	+	
16	54	F	1.33	1.2	171	3	60	25	40	27	4.6	+	+	
17	63	F	1.47	0.5	464	7	78	34	47	29	2.1	+		++
18	43	M	2.00	1.0	233	7	82	35	50	32	3.1	+		

TABLE A (continued)

Patient	Age (years)	Sex (M/F)	Body surface area (m²)	Mitral valve area (cm²)	PVR (dyn sec cm⁻⁵)	RA_m	PA S	PA D	PA m	PCW_m	Cardiac index (liters min⁻¹ m⁻²)	MR	AR	TR
19	51	M	1.84	0.5	686	18	99	54	67	37	1.9	+		
20	26	F	1.65	0.8	674	5	108	52	68	36	2.3	+		
21	63	F	1.33	0.6	750	7	88	37	60	30	2.4	+		
22	62	F	1.95	0.6	636	7	108	44	64	33	2.0	+		
23	62	F	1.22	0.6	903	22	100	37	62	27	2.5	+		
24	58	M	1.57	0.3	1220	12	102	52	67	31	1.5	+	+	
25	51	F	1.51	0.5	1562	18	93	40	71	30	1.4		+	
26	62	F	1.83	0.8	775	25	82	44	62	30	1.8	+		+++
27	62	M	1.71	0.4	1100	16	92	46	63	30	1.4	+		
28	50	F	1.70	0.5	1126	10	104	55	67	29	1.6	+	+	
29	57	F	1.90	0.5	905	16	110	51	72	29	2.0	+	+	
30	68	F	1.55	0.9	141	4	40	17	29	23	2.2	+		+
31	32	F	1.55	1.7	64	3	37	12	20	15	4.1			
32	42	F	1.10	0.9	171	5	40	20	26	20	2.6			
33	48	F	1.37	0.6	369	2	46	23	31	19	1.9			
34	69	F	1.75	0.8	305	6	38	19	25	17	1.2	+		
35	43	F	1.59	0.7	154	2	60	28	40	29	3.6			
36	40	F	1.69	1.1	79	3	47	25	30	23	4.2			

No.	Age	Sex										Grade
37	41	F	1.72	1.4	128	2	27	18	25	17	2.9	
38	38	F	1.72	1.0	95	3	27	14	20	12	2.9	+
39	62	F	1.52	0.9	425	12	80	40	55	30	3.1	++
40	24	M	2.00	1.0	160	14	56	30	40	30	2.5	++
41	53	M	2.00	1.4	63	5	—	—	32	26	2.9	++
42	57	M	1.83	0.9	170	4	32	15	18	11	1.8	++
43	63	M	1.33	1.4	228	5	31	16	22	14	2.1	++
44	51	F	1.59	0.8	126	3	35	17	27	21	2.4	
45	68	M	1.82	0.9	110	6	30	16	21	17	1.6	+
46	22	F	1.73	0.7	353	2	85	38	60	37	3.0	
47	62	F	1.73	1.0	92	4	35	17	23	17	3.0	++
48	64	F	1.61	1.0	210	5	59	22	33	22	2.6	+
49	45	F	1.78	1.4	67	4	32	17	20	16	2.7	
50	64	F	1.66	3.4	103	5	24	10	16	8	3.7	
51	51	F	1.51	0.5	1562	18	93	40	71	30	1.4	+
52	53	F	1.53	2.0	154	4	25	10	17	7	3.4	
53	67	M	1.48	1.3	108	3	25	6	14	9	2.5	+
54	19	F	1.90	1.3	121	3	29	13	19	11	2.8	+
55	31	F	1.43	0.9	136	4	43	19	27	19	3.3	
56	60	F	1.48	0.7	280	7	58	26	38	24	2.7	+
57	70	M	2.07	1.0	89	8	42	22	29	23	2.6	+
58	56	F	1.33	0.3	2021	9	110	60	70	22	1.4	+
59	42	M	1.80	1.3	82	5	46	28	36	29	3.8	
60	60	F	1.42	1.0	393	4	75	25	45	17	4.0	

TABLE A (continued)

Patient	Age (years)	Sex (M/F)	Body surface area (m²)	Mitral valve area (cm²)	PVR (dyn sec cm⁻⁵)	RA$_m$	PA S	PA D	PA m	PCW$_m$	Cardiac index (liters min⁻¹ m⁻²)	MR	AR	TR
61	55	F	1.56	1.0	226	11	58	24	38	23	3.4	+		+
62	32	F	1.47	1.2	136	2	28	10	19	11	3.2	+	+	
63	57	F	1.55	1.0	65	3	31	12	17	14	2.4	+		
64	59	F	1.94	0.8	123	5	50	22	31	23	2.7			
65	46	F	1.49	1.9	105	7	38	20	28	20	4.1			
66	30	F	1.18	0.6	516	4	82	32	51	31	2.6			
67	75	F	1.60	0.6	475	7	71	26	42	23	2.0	+		
68	36	F	1.53	1.7	164	2	24	10	15	5	3.2			
69	60	F	1.53	0.8	312	7	65	28	40	24	2.7	+		
70	63	F	1.84	1.6	122	3	25	10	16	9	2.5	+		
71	67	F	1.43	0.9	102	0	47	22	29	23	3.3	+	+	
72	31	F	1.56	1.6	71	3	29	13	18	13	3.6			
73	?	F	1.69	0.8	171	1	33	18	22	13	2.5		+	
74	53	F	1.35	1.1	213	4	42	15	25	17	2.2	+	+	
75	64	F	2.14	1.5	100	6	50	25	32	21	4.1			
76	54	F	1.09	1.2	164	4	35	15	25	17	3.6	+		
77	52	F	1.62	0.9	276	6	34	15	23	13	1.8	+	+	
78	62	F	1.55	0.9	256	3	31	13	19	11	1.6			

No.	Age	Sex													
79	31	F	1.64	2.4	58	1	19	6	11	7	3.3	+			
80	50	F	1.56	0.9	104	4	41	23	27	21	2.8	+	+		
81	70	M	2.07	0.7	361	6	56	28	37	23	1.5	+	+		
82	47	F	1.50	1.0	98	3	35	15	20	15	2.7	+	+		
83	50	F	1.53	1.7	196	5	41	20	32	20	3.2	+	+		
84	55	F	1.52	0.8	91	5	29	11	15	10	2.9	+	+		
85	50	F	1.60	0.9	100	9	38	24	28	24	2.0	+	+	+	
86	45	M	2.11	0.8	344	9	58	30	38	23	1.7	+	+		
87	58	F	1.50	0.6	152	8	29	19	23	19	1.4				
88	51	F	1.63	0.5	1107	16	104	32	56	20	1.6	+	+		
89	55	F	1.62	0.6	229	8	32	13	22	16	1.3				
90	48	F	1.65	0.7	111	5	40	15	22	17	2.2				
91	60	F	1.47	0.5	384	4	34	20	29	17	1.7	+	+		
92	49	M	1.48	1.1	148	7	34	17	23	18	1.8	+	+		
93	59	F	1.37	0.3	534	12	79	29	42	30	1.3	+	+	+	
94	47	M	1.77	0.3	1486	25	84	49	60	34	0.8	+	+	+	+++
95	40	F	2.02	2.7	95	9	32	14	20	14	2.5				
96	59	F	1.56	0.5	640	12	72	38	52	32	1.6	+			+++
97	39	M	1.23	1.1	291	9	51	21	28	16	2.7	+			
98	55	M	1.57	1.0	194	6	45	23	31	23	2.1	+	+		
99	51	F	1.25	0.7	267	6	59	39	45	35	2.4	+	+		
100	61	F	1.60	0.5	225	5	53	18	33	24	2.0	+			

Appendix 2

Unilateral pulmonary artery balloon occlusion was performed 39 times in 36 patients: 11 patients had predominant mitral stenosis, 4 had predominant mitral regurgitation, 5 had aortic regurgitation, 7 had miscellaneous disorders, and 9 had atrial septal defect (ASD). The miscellaneous disorders consisted of idiopathic cardiomyopathy (patient 21), low cardiac output, ? cause (patient 22), chronic obstructive pulmonary disease (patient 23), primary pulmonary hypertension (patients 24, 25), "almost normal" (patient 26), and constrictive pericarditis (patient 27). The patients with ASD were included because some had very high pulmonary blood flows, others very high pulmonary vascular resistances. The procedure was explained, and each patient consented willingly to the procedure.

A triple-lumen catheter was positioned in either the right or the left pulmonary artery. Left heart catheterization was performed by either paravertebral [104] or transseptal [105] puncture of the left atrium.

After completion of diagnostic studies, simultaneous injections of T-1824 dye and ^{131}I-labeled human serum albumin (RISA) were made into the pulmonary artery and left atrium, respectively; 1- or 2-sec blood samples were obtained from the brachial artery in a wheel-type fraction collector, the timed movement of which was recorded in a multichannel electronic recorder. Injections were recorded either by a foot pedal or directly from the syringes by electrical contacts. Radioactivity of a plasma aliquot of each tube was determined in a well-type scintillation counter; T-1824 was determined in a Beckman DU spectrophotometer. Standards prepared from each injectate were analyzed in the same way. The midpoints of injections of both indicators were used as zero times for the respective dye curves. The midpoint in time after injection recorded for each tube was assigned to the concentration of the appropriate indicator in that tube. Each time-concentration curve was plotted semilogarithmically, and cardiac output and mean transit time determined as described by Hamilton et al. [106].

In every volume calculation, the average of the two simultaneous cardiac outputs was used. These two values were within 10% agreement in each case.

Calculation of pulmonary blood volume was as follows:

$$
\begin{array}{llll}
V\,(PA\text{-}BA) & = & CO \times MTT\,(PA\text{-}BA) \\
- \,V\,(LA\text{-}BA) & = & CO \times MTT\,(LA\text{-}BA) \\
\hline
V\,(PA\text{-}LA) & = & CO \times MTT\,(PA\text{-}LA) & = PBV
\end{array}
$$

where V = volume, PA = pulmonary artery, BA = brachial artery, LA = left atrium, MTT = mean transit time, and PBV = pulmonary blood volume. This volume was the true pulmonary blood volume plus some unknown portion of the left atrium with which the left atrial injection of RISA did not mix.

Pressures in pulmonary artery, left atrium, and brachial artery were measured before balloon occlusion and when these were steady, were measured throughout the 10-min period of balloon occlusion and for several minutes after the balloon had been deflated using Statham P23D pressure transducers recorded on a multichannel electronic recorder.

The balloon was inflated in either the right or left branch of the pulmonary artery. Pure carbon dioxide was used to inflate the balloon for two reasons. If the balloon should rupture, CO_2 is so soluble that it does not embolize. Second, should untoward side effects occur, its low viscosity allows the balloon to be rapidly deflated. In none of the cases here reported were any side effects encountered, but in one case (not included in the table) of Eisenmenger's complex (ventricular septal defect with systemic pressure in the PA and a right-to-left shunt), balloon inflation was quickly followed by systemic hypotension, cyanosis, and bigeminy. The balloon was immediately deflated, with prompt restoration to normal of blood pressure, color, and cardiac rhythm.

Occlusion of the PA was considered to be complete when pressure in the catheter lumen distal to the balloon fell from pulmonary arterial level to left atrial level, pressure configuration was left atrial in contour, and a blood sample with an O_2 saturation of 98% was obtained. See Figure 8 for illustration.

Arterial O_2 saturation was determined spectrophotometrically, oxygen consumption was measured as previously described [107], and pulmonary vascular resistance was calculated as described in Appendix 1, except that in this instance, the left atrial pressure was measured directly.

TABLE A Hemodynamics of Unilateral PA Balloon Occlusion[a]

	Patient	Age	Sex	BSA (m^2)	Arterial O$_2$ sat (%) A	B	O$_2$ Consumption (ml/min) A	B	Cardiac output (liters/min) A	B	Pulse rate (per min) A	B
1	G.W.	48	M	1.98	–	–	–	–	3.4	3.4	58	62
2	I.T.	44	F	1.70	–	–	–	–	3.0	2.8	60	60
3	M.A.	52	M	1.77	–	–	–	–	2.7	3.0	103	70
4	Z.N.	62	F	1.50	–	–	–	–	2.3	2.3	72	90
5	R.M.	49	M	1.71	–	–	–	–	3.6	3.4	66	64
6	G.A.	39	F	1.53	–	–	–	–	3.5	3.6	98	95
7	V.M.	46	F	1.34	94	92	–	–	2.9	2.0	78	90
8	E.F.	58	F	1.50	–	–	–	–	2.7	2.4	–	–
9	K.K.	47	M	1.66	–	–	–	–	2.4	2.2	–	–
10	A.D.	70	F	1.76	97	96	–	–	3.7	3.8	–	–
11	L.S.	52	F	1.52	–	–	–	–	2.8	3.0	70	103
12	B.S.	27	F	1.45	–	–	–	–	2.2	3.6	60	88
13	A.M.	49	F	1.62	–	–	–	–	3.2	3.0	60	60
14	A.E.	38	M	1.92	–	–	–	–	2.4	2.4	140	114
15	H.M.		M	1.76	–	–	–	–	5.2	5.8	72	76
16	F.B.	60	F	1.51	–	–	–	–	3.3	3.1	76	84
17	M.R.	32	F	1.67	87	84	–	–	4.1	4.2	60	75
18	R.J.	20	M	1.94	–	–	–	–	5.4	5.2	69	70
19	N.R.	49	M	1.93	94	94	–	–	3.4	4.0	72	86
20A	C.M.	32	M	1.72	–	–	–	–	5.3	4.7	72	78
20B	(R)	32	M	1.72	–	–	–	–	5.3	4.0	72	84
21	M.G.	63	F	2.02	–	–	–	–	4.7	7.1	73	94
22	L.V.	37	F	1.46	–	–	–	–	3.2	3.4	78	84
23	A.G.	40	M	1.54	71	74	–	–	4.5	4.0	90	90
24	F.L.	51	F	1.80	–	–	–	–	4.3	3.4	92	88
25A	C.F.	66	F	1.29	93	90	–	–	7.0	5.4	114	114
25B	(L)	66	F	1.29	93	90	–	–	–	–	–	–
26	R.S.		M		97	97	–	–	6.3	4.9	–	–
27	J.M.	58	M	1.75	–	–	–	–	3.3	3.2	63	63
28	P.H.	19	F	1.81	98	98	259	290	14.6	16.5	78	70
29	L.C.	52	M	1.60	97	95	201	190	8.1	7.2	65	62
30	G.C.	26	M	1.78	96	97	253	266	26.9	28.6	90	87
31A	J.H. (R)	22	M	2.08	98	98	279	279	6.9	6.9	58	63
31B	(L)	22	M	2.08	98	98	279	279	6.9	6.4	58	58
32	S.S.	43	F	1.58	93	95	194	154	4.4	6.1	71	72
33	K.G.	19	F	1.61	98	–	169	–	28.6	–	80	–
34	E.R.	38	F	1.41	85	87	252	252	3.2	3.3	145	–
35	P.F.	19	F	1.45	94	92	196	181	7.5	7.8	92	92
36	S.R.	43	F	1.40	95	91	172	162	3.3	2.4	75	81
				Mean	93	92	225	228	5.7	5.6	79	80
				SD	±7	±6	±43	±55	±5.7	±5.8	±21	±15

TABLE A

Stroke output (ml per beat)		PA (mmHg) A		PA (mmHg) B		LA (mmHg)		PVR (dyn sec cm^{-5})		PBV (ml)		BA (mean mmHg)	
A	B	S/D	M	S/D	M	A	B	A	B	A	B	A	B
59	68	27/11	20	31/13	20	14	14	141	114	292	214	–	–
50	47	34/21	24	40/21	25	16	17	213	314	153	118	–	–
26	43	44/22	29	48/24	33	25	23	118	266	181	156	–	–
32	26	37/16	24	56/21	33	12	12	417	730	177	184	–	–
55	53	26/13	19	40/13	24	16	16	67	188	306	173	72	71
36	38	46/35	40	79/44	56	25	27	342	644	–	–	–	–
37	22	75/33	49	100/36	59	27	26	606	1319	–	–	–	–
–	–	116/51	82	125/53	80	17	17	1924	2098	221	185	–	–
–	–	85/49	60	92/58	63	28	28	1066	1271	192	167	–	–
–	–	38/13	20	42/17	25	13	17	151	168	–	–	–	–
40	29	28/8	14	28/12	19	8	8	171	293	–	–	–	–
37	41	34/11	24	36/10	22	13	13	400	200	–	–	85	88
53	50	30/14	21	39/15	25	12	11	225	373	–	–	88	81
17	21	63/38	46	65/39	51	31	34	500	566	–	–	–	–
72	76	25/10	17	33/12	21	4	4	200	234	348	244	–	–
43	37	17/7	11	20/8	11	3	2	194	323	178	121	–	–
68	56	22/10	16	31/10	21	10	10	117	209	–	–	–	–
78	74	28/15	21	32/15	23	11	11	148	184	346	192	–	–
47	47	70/40	50	82/43	58	27	27	541	619	–	–	–	–
74	60	16/8	11	19/6	13	7	5	60	136	398	254	–	–
74	60	16/8	11	18/8	13	7	6	660	112	398	270	–	–
64	76	45/25	32	50/30	40	29	29	51	124	–	–	–	–
41	40	16/7	11	22/8	14	3	2	200	282	195	129	–	–
50	44	66/28	45	73/28	47	4	4	728	859	221	184	–	–
47	39	112/45	68	113/45	63	5	3	1171	1410	318	333	113	113
61	47	41/20	28	64/19	34	6	7	251	400	–	–	–	–
–	–	41/20	28	61/22	36	6	/	–	–	–	–	–	–
–	–	20/6	11	33/12	21	5	5	76	261	–	–	–	–
52	51	26/15	19	34/16	22	17	17	48	125	347	211	–	–
187	236	19/7	11	23/17	15	5	5	33	48	–	–	–	–
125	116	22/7	13	22/7	15	6	6	69	100	–	–	78	78
299	329	25/11	17	40/15	24	8	8	27	45	–	–	100	100
119	110	22/12	15	28/10	17	7	7	93	116	–	–	–	–
119	110	22/12	15	35/8	17	8	9	81	100	–	–	–	–
62	85	20/14	22	35/17	26	5	5	309	275	–	–	92	102
358	–	24/13	19	31/16	24	6	–	36	–	–	–	–	–
22	–	90/53	62	90/53	62	2	4	499	1405	–	–	–	–
82	85	61/19	34	78/20	38	0	0	362	389	–	–	83	83
44	30	88/43	60	95/46	68	7	8	283	1998	–	–	–	–
70	70	41 29	29	50 29	33	12	12	333	495	267	196	89	90
±54	±62	±20±14	±18	±22±15	±18	±9	±9	±391	±538	±86	±58	±13	±14

[a]Patients 1 to 11, mitral stenosis. Patients 12 to 15, mitral insufficiency. Patients 16 to 20, aortic valve disease. Patients 21 to 27, miscellaneous disorders. Patients 28 to 36, atrial septal defect.

TABLE B Hemodynamics in Unoccluded Lung Alone[a]

Patient	Pulmonary blood flow (liters/min)		Stroke output (ml per beat)		PA_m-LA_m (mean pressure mmHg)		PVR (dyn sec cm^{-5})		PBV (ml)		MTT (sec)	
	A	B	A	B	A	B	A	B	A	B	A	B
1	1.7	4.2	30	68	6	6	282	114	146	214	8.6	5.1
2	1.5	2.8	25	47	8	8	426	314	77	118	5.1	4.2
3	1.4	3.0	13	43	4	10	236	266	91	156	6.7	5.2
4	1.2	2.3	16	26	12	11	834	730	89	184	7.7	8.0
5	1.8	3.4	28	53	3	8	134	188	153	173	8.5	5.1
6	1.8	3.6	18	38	15	29	684	644	–	–	–	–
7	1.5	2.0	19	22	22	33	1202	1319	–	–	–	–
8	1.4	2.4	–	–	65	63	3848	2098	111	185	8.2	7.7
9	1.2	2.2	–	–	32	35	2132	1271	96	167	8.0	7.6
10	1.9	3.8	–	–	7	8	302	168	–	–	–	–
11	1.4	3.0	20	29	6	11	342	293	–	–	–	–
12	1.1	3.6	19	41	11	9	800	200	–	–	–	–
13	1.6	3.0	27	50	9	14	450	373	–	–	–	–
14	1.2	2.4	9	21	15	17	1000	566	–	–	–	–
15	2.6	5.8	36	76	13	17	400	234	174	244	6.7	4.2
16	1.7	3.1	22	37	8	9	388	232	89	121	5.4	3.9
17	2.1	4.2	34	56	6	11	234	209	–	–	–	–
18	2.7	5.2	39	74	10	12	296	184	173	192	6.4	3.7
19	1.7	4.0	24	47	23	31	1082	619	–	–	–	–
20A	2.7	4.7	37	60	4	8	120	136	199	254	7.5	5.4
20B	2.7	5.0	37	60	4	7	120	112	199	270	7.5	5.4

21	2.4	7.1	32	76	3	11	102	124	–	–	–	–
22	1.6	3.4	21	40	8	12	400	282	98	129	6.1	3.8
23	2.3	4.0	25	44	41	43	1456	859	111	184	4.9	4.6
24	2.2	3.4	24	39	63	60	2342	1410	159	333	7.4	9.8
25A	3.5	5.4	31	47	22	27	502	400	–	–	–	–
25B	–	–	–	–	22	29	–	–	–	–	–	–
26	3.2	4.9	–	–	6	16	152	261	–	–	–	–
27	1.7	3.2	26	51	2	5	96	125	174	211	10.5	6.6
28	7.3	16.5	94	236	6	10	66	48	–	–	–	–
29	4.2	7.2	63	116	7	9	138	100	–	–	–	–
30	13.5	28.6	150	329	9	16	54	45	–	–	–	–
31A	3.5	6.9	60	110	8	10	186	116	–	–	–	–
31B	3.5	6.4	60	110	7	8	162	100	–	–	–	–
32	2.2	6.1	31	85	17	21	618	275	–	–	–	–
33	14.3	–	179	–	13	–	72	–	–	–	–	–
34	1.6	3.3	11	–	60	58	2998	1405	–	–	–	–
35	3.8	7.8	41	85	34	38	724	389	–	–	–	–
36	1.7	2.4	22	30	52	64	2566	1988	–	–	–	–
Mean	2.9	5.1	39	70	17	21	735	492	134	196	7.2	5.5
SD	±2.9	±4.7	±36	±62	±17	±17	±901	±539	±43	±58	±1.5	±1.8

[a]Patients 1 to 11, mitral stenosis. Patients 12 to 15, mitral insufficiency. Patients 16 to 20, aortic valve disease. Patients 21 to 27, miscellaneous disorders. Patients 28 to 36, atrial septal defect.

Note: Methods are the same as those described in Appendix 2, Table A. It is assumed that each lung had the same blood flow. Therefore, before inflation, each lung received half the total pulmonary blood flow, half the stroke output of the right ventricle, and half the pulmonary blood volume. PA and LA pressures would be the same. The MTT would be the same. The pulmonary vascular resistance of each lung alone would be twice the value of the two combined.

TABLE C Relative Compliance of Pulmonary Vasculature of Unoccluded Lung Alone Before and During Unilateral Balloon Occlusion of the Pulmonary Artery[a]

Patient	Before		During		PBV/Pi	
	PBV (ml/m²)	Pi (mmHg)	PBV (ml/m²)	Pi (mmHg)	Before (ml m⁻² mmHg⁻¹)	During (ml m⁻² mmHg⁻¹)
1	74	17	108	17	4.35	6.35
2	45	20	69	21	2.25	3.29
3	51	27	88	28	1.89	3.14
4	59	18	123	23	3.28	5.35
5	89	18	101	20	4.94	5.05
8	74	50	123	49	1.48	2.51
9	58	44	101	46	1.32	2.20
15	99	11	139	13	9.00	10.69
16	59	7	80	7	8.43	11.43
18	89	16	99	17	5.56	5.82
20A	116	9	148	9	12.89	16.44
20B	116	9	157	9	12.89	17.44
22	67	7	88	8	9.57	11.00
23	72	25	119	26	2.88	4.58
24	88	37	185	33	2.38	5.61
27	99	18	121	20	5.50	6.05
Mean	78	21	116	22	5.54	7.31
SD	±22	±13	±31	±13	±3.89	±4.72

[a] $Pi = \dfrac{PA\text{-}LA}{2}$, where PA = pulmonary arterial mean pressure (mmHg), LA = left atrial mean pressure (mmHg). PBV = pulmonary blood volume of unoccluded lung. PBV/Pi = relative compliance of pulmonary vasculature.

TABLE D   Compliance of Pulmonary Vasculature

Patient	ΔV (ml/m^2)	ΔPi (mmHg)	$\dfrac{\Delta V}{\Delta Pi}$ (ml m^{-2} mmHg^{-1})
1	52	0.0	
2	29	0.5	58
3	55	6.0	9
4	60	4.5	13
5	20	2.5	8
8	40	−1.0	
9	49	1.5	33
15	40	2.0	20
16	21	−0.5	
18	10	1.0	10
20A	32	0.0	
20B	41	0.5	82
22	21	1.0	21
23	47	1.0	47
24	97	−3.5	
27	21	1.5	14
Mean	40 ± 21	1.1 ± 2.2	29 ± 24

[a] ΔV = difference of PBV before and during balloon occlusion.
ΔPi = difference of $\dfrac{PA_m - LA_m}{2}$ before and during balloon occlusion. $\dfrac{\Delta V}{\Delta Pi}$ = compliance of pulmonary vasculature.

TABLE E   **Coefficient of Distensibility of Pulmonary Vasculature**

Patient	PBV (ml m^{-2} mmHg^{-1})	ΔPBV (ml m^{-2} mmHg^{-1})	ΔPi (mmHg)	$\dfrac{1}{V}\dfrac{\Delta PBV}{\Delta Pi}$
1	74	52	0.0	
2	45	29	0.5	1.29
3	51	55	6.0	0.18
4	59	60	4.5	0.23
5	89	20	2.5	0.09
8	74	40	−1.0	
9	58	49	1.5	0.56
15	99	40	2.0	0.20
16	59	21	−0.5	
18	89	10	1.0	0.11
20A	116	32	0.0	
20B	116	41	0.5	0.71
22	67	21	1.0	0.31
23	72	47	1.0	0.65
24	82	97	−3.5	
27	99	21	1.5	0.14
			Mean	0.41
			SD	±0.37

[a]PBV = pulmonary blood volume before unilateral PA balloon occlusion. ΔPBV = increase of PBV during occlusion. ΔPi = increase of $\dfrac{PA + LA}{2}$ pressure (mmHg) during occlusion. $\dfrac{(1/V)(\Delta PBV)}{\Delta Pi}$ = coefficient of distensibility of pulmonary vasculature.

References

1. Thompson, W. P., and P. D. White, Commonest cause of hypertrophy of the right ventricle – left ventricular strain and failure, *Am. Heart J.,* 12: 641–649 (1936).
2. Parker, F., and S. Weiss, The nature and significance of the structural changes in the lungs in mitral stenosis, *Am. J. Pathol.,* 12:573–598 (1936).
3. Cournand, A., and H. A. Ranges, Catheterization of the right auricle in man, *Proc. Soc. Exp. Biol. Med.,* 46:462–466 (1941).
4. Hickam, J. B., and W. H. Cargill, Effects of exercise on cardiac output and pulmonary arterial pressure in normal persons and in patients with cardiovascular disease and pulmonary emphysema, *J. Clin. Invest.,* 27:10–23 (1948).
5. Gorlin, R., F. W. Haynes, W. T. Goodale, C. G. Sawyer, J. W. Dow, and L. Dexter, Studies of circulatory dynamics in mitral stenosis. Altered dynamics at rest, *Am. Heart J.,* 41:30–45 (1951).
6. Gorlin, R., C. G. Sawyer, F. W. Haynes, W. T. Goodale, and L. Dexter, Effects of exercise on circulatory dynamics in mitral stenosis, *Am. Heart J.,* 41:192–203 (1951).
7. Lewis, B. M., H. E. J. Houssay, F. W. Haynes, and L. Dexter, Dynamics of both right and left ventricles at rest and during exercise in patients with heart failure, *Circ. Res.,* 1:312–320 (1953).
8. Heath, D., E. V. Dox, and J. N. Harris-Hones, The clinicopathological syndrome produced by co-existing pulmonary arterial and venous hypertension, *Thorax,* 12:321–328 (1957).
9. Smith, R. C., H. B. Burchell, and J. E. Edwards, Pathology of the pulmonary vascular tree. IV. Structural changes in the pulmonary vessels in chronic left ventricular failure, *Circulation,* 10:801–808 (1954).
10. Harris, P., and D. Heath, *The Human Pulmonary Circulation: Its Form and Function in Health and Disease,* 2nd ed. Edinburgh, London, and New York, Churchill, Livingstone, 1977.
11. Burton, A. C., *Physiology and Biophysics of the Circulation,* 2nd ed. Chicago, Yearbook Medical Publishers, 1972, p. 91.
12. McDonald, D. A., *Blood Flow in Arteries.* Baltimore, Williams & Wilkins, 1974, pp. 17–30.
13. Edwards, J. E., and H. B. Burchell, Multilobal pulmonary venous obstruction with pulmonary hypertension. "Protective" arterial lesions in the involved lobes, *Arch. Intern. Med.,* 87:372–378 (1951).
14. Korn, D., R. W. DeSanctis, and S. Sell, Massive calcification of the mitral annulus. A clinicopathologic study of fourteen cases, *N. Engl. J. Med.,* 267:900–909 (1962).
15. Hellems, H., F. W. Haynes, and L. Dexter, Pulmonary "capillary" pressure in man, *J. Appl. Physiol.,* 2:24–29 (1949).
16. Rapaport, E., and L. Dexter, Pulmonary "capillary" pressure. In *Methods in Medical Research,* Vol. 2. Chicago, Yearbook Medical Publishers, 1958, pp. 85–93.

17. Ryan, T. J., Mitral valve disease. In *Clinical Cardiovascular Physiology*.
     Edited by H. J. Levine. New York, Grune & Stratton, 1976, pp. 523–561.
18. Szidon, J. P., and A. P. Fishman, Autonomic control of the pulmonary cir-
     culation. In *Symposium on the Pulmonary Circulation and Interstitial
     Space*. Edited by A. P. Fishman and H. H. Hecht. Chicago and London,
     University of Chicago Press, 1969, pp. 239–268.
19. Ingram, R. H., J. P. Szidon, R. Skalak, and A. P. Fishman, Effects of
     sympathetic nerve stimulation on the pulmonary arterial tree of the iso-
     lated lobe perfused in situ, *Circ. Res.*, **22**:801–815 (1968).
20. Franklin, D. L., R. L. Van Citters, and R. F. Rushmer, Balance between
     right and left ventricular output, *Circ. Res.*, **10**:17–26 (1962).
21. Dock, D. S., W. L. Kraus, L. B. McGuire, J. W. Hyland, F. W. Haynes, and
     L. Dexter, The pulmonary blood volume in man, *J. Clin. Invest.*, **40**:317–
     328 (1961).
22. Yu, P. N., *Pulmonary Blood Volume in Health and Disease*. Philadelphia,
     Lea & Febiger, 1969.
23. Cournand, A., R. L. Riley, A. Himmelstein, and R. Austrian, Pulmonary
     circulation and alveolar ventilation-perfusion relationships after pneumo-
     nectomy, *J. Thorac. Surg.*, **19**:80–116 (1950).
24. L. Dexter, and G. T. Smith, Quantitative studies of pulmonary embolism,
     Am. J. Med. Sci., **247**:641–648 (1964).
25. Kuida, H., G. J. Dammin, F. W. Haynes, E. Rapaport, and L. Dexter,
     Primary pulmonary hypertension, *Am. J. Med.*, **23**:166–182 (1957).
26. Brenner, O., Pathology of the vessels of the pulmonary circulation, *Arch.
     Intern. Med.*, **56**:211–237, 457–497, 724–752, 976–1014, 1189–1241
     (1935).
27. Heath, D., and J. E. Edwards, The pathology of hypertension pulmonary
     vascular disease. A description of six grades of structural changes in the
     pulmonary arteries with special reference to congenital cardiac defects,
     Circulation, **18**:533–547 (1958).
28. Wagenvoort, C. A., and N. Wagenvoort, *Pathology of Pulmonary Hyper-
     tension*. New York and London, Wiley & Sons, 1977.
29. Dresdale, D. T., M. Schultz, and R. J. Michtom, Primary pulmonary hyper-
     tension. I. Clinical and hemodynamic study, *Am. J. Med.*, **11**:686–705
     (1951).
30. Dresdale, D. T., R. T. Michtom, and M. Schultz, Recent studies in primary
     pulmonary hypertension, including pharmacodynamic observations on
     pulmonary vascular resistance, *Bull. N.Y. Acad. Med.*, **30**:195–207 (1954).
31. Vogel, J. H. K., Pulmonary hypertension: evaluation and treatment, *Hosp.
     Med.*, **13**:69–73 (1977).
32. Braun, K., G. Izak, and S. Z. Rosenberg, Pulmonary arterial pressure after
     priscoline in mitral stenosis, *Br. Heart J.*, **19**:217–221 (1957).
33. Grover, R. F., J. T. Reeves, and S. G. Blount, Jr., Tolazoline hydrochloride
     (priscoline). An effective pulmonary vasodilator, *Am. Heart J.*, **61**:5–15
     (1961).
34. Wood, P., E. M. Bester, M. K. Towers, and M. B. McIlroy, The effect of

acetyl choline on pulmonary vascular resistance and left atrial pressure in mitral stenosis, *Br. Heart J.,* 19:279–286 (1957).

35. Söderholm, B., and L. Werkö, Acetylcholine and the pulmonary circulation in mitral valvular disease, *Br. Heart J.,* 21:1–8 (1959).

36. Aviado, D. M., The pharmacology of the pulmonary circulation, *Pharmacol. Rev.,* 12:159–239 (1960).

37. Shettigar, U. R., H. N. Hultgren, M. Specter, R. Martin, and D. H. Davies, Primary pulmonary hypertension. Favorable effect of isoproterenol, *N. Engl. J. Med.,* 295:1414–1415 (1976).

38. Roy, S. B., and N. Gopinath, Mitral stenosis. Symposium on cardiac surgery (L. Werkö and L. Dexter, eds.), *Circulation,* 38(V):68–76 (1968).

39. Bland, E. F., and T. D. Jones, Rheumatic fever and rheumatic heart disease. A twenty year report of 1000 patients followed since childhood, *Circulation,* 4:836–843 (1951).

40. Olesen, K. H., The natural history of 271 patients with mitral stenosis under medical treatment, *Br. Heart J.,* 24:349–357 (1962).

41. Lewis, B. M., R. Gorlin, H. E. J. Houssay, F. W. Haynes, and L. Dexter, Clinical and physiological correlations in patients with mitral stenosis, *Am. Heart J.,* 43:2–26 (1952).

42. Dexter, L., Profiles in valvular heart disease. In *Cardiac Catheterization and Angiography.* Edited by W. Grossman. Philadelphia, Lea & Febiger, 1974, pp. 243–268.

43. Wood, P., An appreciation of mitral stenosis, *Br. Med. J.,* 1:1051–1063, 1113–1124 (1954).

44. Bland, E. F., and R. H. Sweet, A venous shunt for advanced mitral stenosis, *JAMA,* 140:1259–1265 (1949).

45. Rabin, E. R., and E. C. Mayer, Cardiopulmonary effects of pulmonary venous hypertension with special reference to pulmonary lymphatic flow, *Circ. Res.,* 8:324–335 (1960).

46. Uhley, H. N., S. E. Leeds, J. J. Sampson, and M. Friedman, Role of pulmonary lymphatics in chronic pulmonary edema, *Circ. Res.,* 11:966–970 (1962).

47. Kerley, P., Part one: Cardiovascular system. In *A Textbook of X-ray Diagnosis,* Vol. 2, 2nd ed. Edited by S. C. Shanks and P. Kerley. London, Saunders, 1951, pp. 3–190.

48. Ramirez, A., E. T. Grimes, and W. H. Abelmann, Regression of pulmonary vascular changes following mitral valvuloplasty. An anatomic and physiologic case study, *Am. J. Med.,* 45:975–982 (1968).

49. Ferguson, D. J., E. M. Berkas, and R. L. Varco, Process of healing in experimental arteriosclerosis, *Proc. Soc. Exp. Biol. Med.,* 89:492–494 (1955).

50. Geer, J. C., B. A. Glass, and H. M. Albert, The morphogenesis and reversibility of experimental hyperkinetic pulmonary vascular lesions in the dog, *Exp. Mol. Pathol.,* 4:399–415 (1965).

51. Downing, S. E., S. E. Pursel, R. A. Vidorne, H. M. Brandt, and A. A. Liebow, Studies on pulmonary hypertension with special reference to pressure-flow

relations in chronically distended and undistended lobes, *Med. Thorac.*, 19:268–282 (1962).

52. Harley, R. A., P. J. Friedman, M. Saldaña, A. A. Liebow, and C. B. Carrington, Sequential development of lesions in experimental extreme pulmonary hypertension, *Am. J. Pathol.*, 52:52a (1968).

53. Saldaña, M. E., R. A. Harley, A. A. Liebow, and C. B. Carrington, Experimental extreme pulmonary hypertension and vascular disease in relation to polycythemia, *Am. J. Pathol.*, 52:935–981 (1968).

54. Silove, E. D., W. D. Tavernor, and C. L. Berry, Reactive pulmonary arterial hypertension after pulmonary venous constriction in the calf, *Cardiovasc. Res.*, 6:36–44 (1972).

55. Dollery, C. T., and J. B. West, Regional uptake of radioactive oxygen, carbon monoxide, and carbon dioxide in the lungs of patients with mitral stenosis, *Circ. Res.*, 8:765–771 (1960).

56. West, J. B., and C. T. Dollery, Distribution of blood flow and ventilation-perfusion ratio in the lung measured with radioactive CO_2, *J. Appl. Physiol.*, 15:405–410 (1960).

57. Friedman, W. F., and E. Braunwald, Alterations in regional pulmonary blood flow in mitral valve disease studied by radioisotope scanning, *Circulation*, 34:363–376 (1966).

58. Gorlin, R., and S. G. Gorlin, Hydraulic formula for calculation of the area of the stenotic mitral valve, other cardiac valves, and central circulatory shunts, *Am. Heart J.*, 41:1–29 (1951).

59. Draper, A., R. Heimbecker, R. Daley, D. Carroll, G. Mudd, R. Wells, W. Falholt, E. C. Andrus, and R. J. Bing, Physiologic studies in mitral valvular disease, *Circulation*, 3:531–542 (1951).

60. Eliasch, H., The pulmonary circulation at rest and on effort in mitral stenosis, *Scand. J. Clin. Lab. Invest.*, 4(Suppl. IV):1–99 (1952).

61. Lucas, D. S., and C. T. Dotter, Modifications of the pulmonary circulation in mitral stenosis, *Am. J. Med.*, 12:639–649 (1952).

62. Donald, K. W., J. M. Bishop, and O. L. Wade, A study of minute to minute changes of arterio-venous oxygen content difference, oxygen uptake and cardiac output and rate of achievement of a steady state during exercise in rheumatic heart disease, *J. Clin. Invest.*, 33:1146–1167 (1954).

63. Carlens, E., H. E. Hanson, and B. Nordenström, Temporary unilateral occlusion of the pulmonary artery. A new method of determining separate lung function and of radiologic examinations, *J. Thorac. Surg.*, 22:527–536 (1951).

64. Brofman, B. L., B. L. Charms, P. M. Kohn, J. Elder, R. Newman, and M. Rizika, Unilateral pulmonary artery occlusion in man. Control studies, *J. Thorac. Surg.*, 34:206–227 (1957).

65. Charms, B. L., B. L. Brofman, and P. M. Kohn, Pulmonary resistance in acquired heart disease, *Circulation*, 20:850–855 (1959).

66. Brofman, B. L., Experimental unilateral pulmonary artery occlusion in humans, *Circ. Res.*, 2:285–286 (1954).

67. Hanson, H. E., Temporary unilateral occlusion of the pulmonary artery in man, *Acta Chir. Scand. [Suppl.]*, **187**:7–55 (1954).
68. Denolin, H., Contributions à l'étude de la circulation pulmonaire en clinique, *Acta Cardiol. Suppl.*, **10**:9–224 (1961).
69. Söderholm, B., Hemodynamics of the lesser circulation in pulmonary tuberculosis, *Scand. J. Clin. Lab. Invest. [Suppl.]*, **26**:1–111 (1957).
70. Uggla, L. G., Pulmonary hypertension in tuberculosis of the lungs. A clinical study in advanced cases examined with cardiac catheterization and temporary unilateral occlusion of the pulmonary artery, *Acta Tuberc. Scand. [Suppl.]*, **41**:7–179 (1957).
71. Sloan, H., J. D. Morris, M. Figley, and R. Lee, Temporary unilateral occlusion of the pulmonary artery in the preoperative evaluation of thoracic patients, *J. Thorac. Surg.*, **30**:591–597 (1955).
72. Widimský, J., Hurych, J., Staněk, V., and J. Kasalický, Effect of unilateral pulmonary artery occlusion on pulmonary circulation in patients with pulmonary hypertension in mitral stenosis, *Br. Heart J.*, **31**:172–177 (1969).
73. Dock, D. S., L. B. McGuire, J. W. Hyland, F. W. Haynes, and L. Dexter, The effect of unilateral pulmonary artery occlusion upon calculated pulmonary blood volume, *Fed. Proc.*, **19**:97 (1960).
74. Milnor, W. R., A. D. Jose, and C. J. McGaff, Pulmonary vascular volume, resistance and compliance in man, *Circulation*, **22**:130–137 (1960).
75. Aramendia, P., C. M. Taquini, A. Fourcade, and A. C. Taquini, Reflex vasomotor activity during unilateral occlusion of the pulmonary artery, *Am. Heart J.*, **66**:53–60 (1963).
76. Werkö, L., G. Biörck, C. Crafoord, H. Wulf, H. Krook, and H. Eliasch, Pulmonary circulatory dynamics in mitral stenosis before and after commissurotomy, *Am. Heart J.*, **45**:477–490 (1953).
77. Carlotti, J., F. Joly, J. R. Sicot, and G. Voci, Étude hémodynamique pré et post-opératoire due rétrécissement mitral, *Sem. Hop. Paris*, **29**:2079–2087 (1953).
78. Goodale, Jr., F., G. Sanchez, A. L. Friedlich, J. G. Scannell, and G. S. Myers, Correlation of pulmonary arteriolar resistance with pulmonary vascular changes in patients with mitral stenosis before and after valvulotomy, *N. Engl. J. Med.*, **252**:979–983 (1955).
79. Donald, K. W., J. M. Bishop, O. L. Wade, and P. N. Wormald, Cardiorespiratory function two years after mitral valvotomy, *Clin. Sci.*, **16**:325–350 (1957).
80. Lyons, W. S., R. G. Tompkins, J. W. Kirklin, and E. H. Wood, Early and late hemodynamic effects of mitral commissurotomy, *J. Lab. Clin. Med.*, **53**:499–516 (1959).
81. Belcher, J. R., Restenosis of the mitral valve, *Br. Heart J.*, **20**:76–82 (1958).
82. Dalen, J. E., L. Dexter, I. S. Ockene, and J. Carlson, Precapillary pulmonary hypertension: its relationship to pulmonary venous hypertension, *Trans. Am. Clin. Clin. Assoc.*, **86**:207–218 (1974).

83. Dalen, J. E., J. M. Matloff, G. L. Evans, F. G. Hoppin, Jr., P. Bhardwaj, D. E. Harken, and L. Dexter, Early reduction of pulmonary vascular resistance after mitral valve replacement, *N. Engl. J. Med.*, **277**:387–394 (1967).

84. Zener, J. C., E. W. Hancock, N. E. Shumway, and D. C. Harrison, Regression of extreme pulmonary hypertension after mitral valve surgery, *Am. J. Cardiol.*, **30**:820–826 (1972).

85. Braunwald, E., N. S. Braunwald, J. Ross, and A. G. Morrow, Effects of mitral valve replacement on the pulmonary vascular dynamics of patients with pulmonary hypertension, *N. Engl. J. Med.*, **273**:509–514 (1965).

86. Bayliss, W. M., On the local reactions of the arterial wall to changes of internal pressure, *J. Physiol. (London)*, **28**:220–231 (1902).

87. West, M. B., C. T. Dollery, and B. E. Heard, Increased vascular resistance in the lower zone of the lung caused by perivascular edema, *Lancet*, **2**: 181–183 (1964).

88. Ritchie, B. C., G. Schauberger, and N. C. Staub, Inadequacy of perivascular edema hypothesis to account for distribution of pulmonary blood flow in lung edema, *Circ. Res.*, **24**:807–814 (1969).

89. Dawson, H., Regional pulmonary blood flow in sitting and supine man during and after acute hypoxia, *J. Clin. Invest.*, **48**:301–310 (1969).

90. Ferri, F., V. Rovati, M. Panesi, R. Romanelli, and E. Righini, Su la natura riflessa della ipertensione arterioa del piccolo circola da ostacolato deflusso delle vene pulmonari, *Rass. Fisiopatol. Clin. Ter.*, **28**:608–622 (1956).

91. Rovati, V., F. Ferri, R. Romanelli, M. Panesi, and E. Righini, Influenza del sistema neuro-vegativo nella genesi della ipertensione polmonare riflessa sperimentale, *Rass. Fisiopatol. Clin. Ter.*, **28**:623–638 (1956).

92. Kadowitz, P. J., and A. L. Hyman, Influence of a prostaglandin endoperoxide analogue on the canine pulmonary vascular bed, *Circ. Res.*, **40**: 282–287 (1977).

93. Piper, P. J., Conditions of release of prostaglandins from the lung. In *Lung Metabolism*. Edited by A. F. Junod and R. De Haller. New York, Academic Press, 1975, pp. 315–321.

94. Junod, A. F., Metabolism of vasoactive agents in lung, *Am. Rev. Respir. Dis.*, **115**:51–57 (1977).

95. Gilbert, R. P., L. B. Hinshaw, H. Kuida, and M. B. Visscher, Effects of histamine, 5 hydroxytryptamine and epinephrine on pulmonary hemodynamics with particular reference to arterial and venous segment resistances, *Am. J. Physiol.*, **194**:165–170 (1958).

96. Fishman, A. P., Hypoxia on the pulmonary circulation. How and where it acts, *Circ. Res.*, **38**:221–231 (1976).

97. Donald, K. W., Pulmonary vascular resistance in mitral valvular disease. In *Pulmonary Circulation*. Edited by W. R. Adams and I. Veith. New York and London, Grune & Stratton, 1959.

98. Jordan, S. C., Development of pulmonary hypertension in mitral stenosis, *Lancet*, **2**:322–324 (1965).

99. Walston, A., R. H. Peter, J. J. Morris, Y. Kong, and V. S. Behar, Clinical implications of pulmonary hypertension in mitral stenosis, *Am. J. Cardiol.,* **32**:650–655 (1973).

100. Bergofsky, E. H., D. E. Lehr, and A. P. Fishman, The effect of changes in hydrogen ion concentration on the pulmonary circulation, *J. Clin. Invest.,* **41**:1482–1502 (1962).

101. Fry, D. L., Acute vascular endothelial changes associated with increased blood velocity gradients, *Circ. Res.,* **22**:165–197 (1968).

102. Dexter, L., R. Gorlin, B. M. Lewis, F. W. Haynes, and D. E. Harken, Physiologic evaluation of patients with mitral stenosis before and after mitral valvuloplasty, *Trans. Am. Clin. Clin. Assoc.,* **62**:170–180 (1950).

103. Rudolph, A. M., and P. A. M. Auld, Physical factors affecting normal and serotonin-constricted pulmonary vessels, *Am. J. Physiol.,* **198**:864–872 (1960).

104. Björk, V. O., G. Malmström, and L. G. Uggla, Left auricular pressure measurements in man, *Ann. Surg.,* **138**:718–725 (1953).

105. Ross, Jr., J., E. Braunwald, and A. G. Morrow, Trans-septal left heart catheterization, *Clin. Res.,* **7**:229 (1959).

106. Hamilton, W. F., J. W. Moore, J. M. Kinsman, and R. G. Spurling, Studies on the circulation. IV. Further analysis of the injection method, and of changes in hemodynamics under physiological and pathological conditions, *Am. J. Physiol.,* **99**:534–551 (1932).

107. McDonald, L., J. B. Dealy, Jr., M. Rabinowitz, and L. Dexter, Clinical, physiological and pathological findings in mitral stenosis and regurgitation, *Medicine,* **36**:237–280 (1957).

8

Congenital Heart Disease and Pulmonary Hypertension

JOSEPH K. PERLOFF

University of California, Los Angeles
School of Medicine
Los Angeles, California

I. Introduction

Pulmonary arterial pressure was measured as early as 1852, but almost a
century elapsed before cardiac catheterization permitted rapid development of
our knowledge of the pulmonary circulation [1,2]. This chapter deals with
pulmonary hypertension occurring in the setting of congenital heart disease
and focuses on the pulmonary circulation in the fetus, at birth, in the neonate,
and during subsequent growth, development, and aging. The stage is then set
for a discussion of congenital heart disease and pulmonary hypertension—its
nature, course, and management.

The mature pulmonary circulation is a low-pressure, high-flow system
that functions primarily to accomplish gas exchange between blood returning
from the systemic circulation and air ventilating the alveoli. However, the un-
expanded fetal lung serves no respiratory gas exchange function. Owing to the
thick muscular media of the fetal pulmonary arterioles, the intrinsic pulmonary vascular resistance is of the same magnitude as the systemic [3]. During
fetal life, approximately one-fourth of the systemic venous return reaches the
right ventricle, the remainder entering the left ventricle through the foramen

ovale. Approximately two-thirds of the right ventricular output is directed into the descending aorta through the ductus arteriosus, leaving only a small fraction of systemic venous return to perfuse the lung. Control of the pulmonary circulation in fetal lungs is dominated by active vasomotor influences [3]. The vascular tone of the pulmonary circulation in lambs is readily demonstrable, highly labile, and easily altered by stimulation of autonomic nerves, by pharmacologic agents, or by small changes in arterial PO_2 and PCO_2 [4]. Asphyxia in fetal lambs induced by brief occlusion of the umbilical cord causes at least a threefold increase in pulmonary vascular resistance [4]. In immature fetal lambs, this effect is mediated locally, i.e., within the lungs. In fetal lambs near term, the local reaction is augmented by a substantial contribution from adrenergic-mediated reflex pulmonary vasoconstriction [4].

It is appropriate at this juncture to examine the principle immediate and delayed circulatory alterations at birth and in the neonatal period [3,5]. The immediate changes consist of: (1) a colossal fall in pulmonary vascular resistance associated with expansion of the lungs; (2) a pronounced rise in systemic vascular resistance associated with elimination of the low-resistance placental circulation; (3) a fall in blood flow to the right atrium owing to abolition of umbilical venous return; (4) an abrupt rise—as much as 10-fold—in pulmonary blood flow, which is promptly translated into a rise in left atrial volume and pressure; (5) functional closure of the valve of the foramen ovale caused by a rise in left atrial and a fall in right atrial pressure; and (6) constriction of the ductus arteriosus at about 12 hr after birth largely in response to an increase in systemic arterial PO_2 [6]. With the first breath after birth, pulmonary vascular resistance falls dramatically not only because of mechanical expansion of the lungs and distension of intrapulmonary vessels, but also because of changes in alveolar tensions of oxygen and carbon dioxide leading to a release of hypoxic-mediated vascular tone. Pulmonary blood flow increases rapidly, pulmonary resistance soon falls below systemic, and conditions for a left-to-right shunt are established via the ductus arteriosus. During the first few days of life, the ductus can open and close intermittently. Even though pulmonary vascular resistance normally decreases 10-fold in the first few days of life, fluctuations in vasomotor tone can be sufficient to cause transient right-to-left shunting. By the first week of life, the ductus arteriosus is functionally closed, and by 6 months of age, pulmonary resistance has virtually fallen to adult levels. Several delayed changes are important and complete the picture [3]. The thick-walled fetal pulmonary arterioles are designed to meet the full force of systemic right ventricular pressure the instant the lungs expand. After this need has been met, the arterioles gradually involute. With the establishment of respiration at birth, there is a marked rise in alveolar and systemic arterial oxygen tensions to which the pulmonary arterioles are exquisitely sensitive [7], setting the stage for dilatation and anatomical involution. It is believed that regression of pulmonary arteriolar smooth muscle begins at about 2 weeks, but may take as long as 2 years to reach the fully mature state. However, experimental documentation of this regression by means of quantitative anatomy has been difficult. It is noteworthy that in children born at high altitudes, the regression either does not take place or arteriolar smooth muscle lost during the neonatal period is quickly regained [8]. For example, by 1 year of age, children born at high altitudes still have pulmonary arterial pressures comparable to normal sea-level newborns. Similarly, fragmentation of elastic fibers in the proximal pulmonary trunk, characteristic of the normal adult at sea level [9], is rarely seen at altitudes above 13,000 feet, and then only after the fifth decade of life. The larger pulmonary arteries may also play a role in determining the total drop in pressure across the lungs after birth [10]. Maturational changes may affect the neonatal disparity in size between the main and branch pulmonary arteries as well as the angulation at the origins of the right and left branches; both these factors have been held responsible for a physiological drop in pressure distal to the pulmonary trunk [10]. Still another delayed change relates to the fetal right ventricular wall, which slowly loses its relative thickness during the first year of life. Adaptive hypertrophy is an expected feature of the fetal right ventricle, which ejects at systemic pressure via the ductus arteriosus. After birth, with the stimulus of right ventricular afterload eliminated, there is a gradual reduction in thickness relative to septum and left ventricle. The thick neonatal right ventricular wall does not undergo regression; it merely does not increase its thickness as rapidly as the septum and left ventricular free wall in the growing infant [11].

In the normal human, the resting supine mean pulmonary arterial pressure at sea level ranges from 10 to 20 mmHg. Although early studies failed to disclose a relationship between age and pulmonary arterial pressure, the current consensus is that the pressure in the pulmonary artery increases by an average of 0.8 mmHg per decade. A similar tendency can be shown for the relationship between pulmonary vascular resistance and age. The magnitude of change in pulmonary resistance with exercise has also been the subject of controversy. Early observations in human subjects found large decreases in pulmonary vascular resistance and small increments in pressure during exercise [12]. These findings were interpreted as indicating either good distensibility of the vascular bed or availability of additional vascular channels which allowed the pulmonary circulation to accommodate to increases in blood flow with only small rises in pressure. As a corollary to this assumption, increments in pulmonary artery pressure occurring during exercise were considered evidence of an abnormality in the pulmonary circulation. In subsequent studies in human subjects and in dogs, only a slight tendency toward a decrease in pulmonary vascular resistance was identified. In low-pressure systems, the computation of vascular resistance is technically difficult [13]. However, by using unilateral occlusion of a pulmonary artery and by measuring the blood flow and pressure drop across one lung at rest and during exercise, it is possible to construct a pressure-flow diagram extended over a large range of pressures and flows. Pulmonary vascular resistance can be obtained from the slope of this pressure-flow relationship. When computed with this method, pulmonary vascular resistance does not change during increases in blood flow up to 4 times the basal level.

Normal pulmonary arteries in the adult are thinner and less muscular than systemic arteries of comparable size. The autonomic innervation is relatively sparse and chiefly distributed to the adventitia and outer media of large pulmonary vessels. The combination of less smooth muscle and fewer adrenergic nerve endings provides the structural basis for the comparatively modest intrinsic vasomotor activity of the adult pulmonary circulation, and for the relatively greater importance of passive effects. In keeping with the anatomical distribution of adrenergic innervation of pulmonary vessels, the effects of sympathetic nerve stimulation on the pulmonary circulation of the dog are more prominently seen in large vessels, resulting in decreases in vascular compliance but not increases in pulmonary vascular resistance. The pulmonary circulation has been shown experimentally to respond to many biologically vasoactive substances—amines, polypeptides, and prostaglandins. The functional significance and clinical implications of these responses have not yet been defined. Alveolar hypoxia is the best known pulmonary vaso-constrictive influence [7]. There is considerable variation in the response to acute hypoxia among different species. Even within the same species there appears to be a genetically determined predisposition governing the magnitude of the response. The site of action is probably not limited to precapillary vessels. Acidemia acts synergistically with hypoxia to increase pulmonary vascular resistance. Exposure to chronic alveolar hypoxia not only provokes vascular smooth muscle hypertrophy in pulmonary arterioles, but the hypertrophy regresses after cessation of the hypoxic stimulus [14]. It has been assumed that the vascular smooth muscle hypertrophy accompanying *chronic* hypoxia is the consequence of sustained pulmonary vasoconstriction in response to mechanisms analogous to the vasoconstrictor response to *acute* hypoxia [15]. The hypothesis, though plausible, has not yet been tested.

Much of current clinical reasoning about the pulmonary circulation is based on the calculation of vascular resistance (R), which relates the mean pressure drop across the lungs (PA − LA = ΔP) to cardiac output (CO) according to the expression: R = ΔP/CO. This formula is a linear hydraulic equivalent of Ohm's law and is valid for rigorous analysis only when rigid cylindrical vessels of fixed dimensions are perfused by a homogeneous fluid

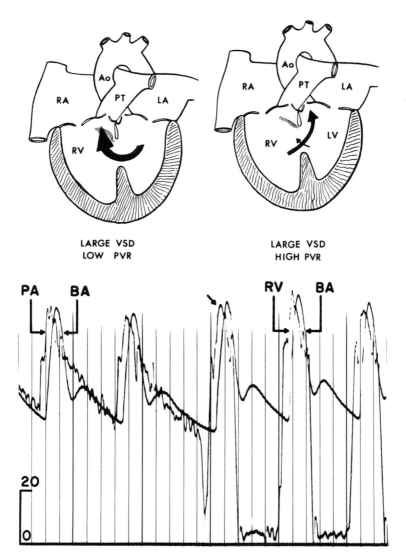

FIGURE 1 Above, schematic illustrations of large ventricular septal defect with low pulmonary vascular resistance (pure left-to-right shunt) and large ventricular septal defect with high pulmonary vascular resistance and reversed shunt (Eisenmenger's complex). The peak systolic pressures in the pulmonary trunk are identical in both. Below, tracings from an 18-year-old boy with Eisenmenger's complex. The pulmonary arterial (PA), brachial arterial (BA), and right ventricular (RV) systolic pressures are identical. (With permission, J. K. Perloff, *The Clinical Recognition of Congenital Heart Disease*, 2nd ed.)

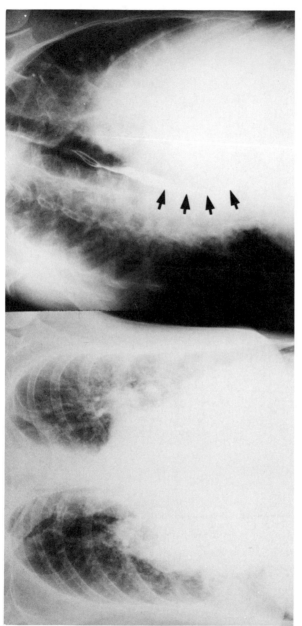

FIGURE 2 X-ray from a 60-year-old woman with an ostium secundum atrial septal defect, a 2.5:1 left-to-right shunt, and a pulmonary arterial pressure of 60/35 mmHg. Rapid clinical deterioration followed the onset of atrial fibrillation. The posteroanterior projection shows increased pulmonary vascularity with dilatation of the pulmonary trunk and both branches. The immense right atrium is seen far to the right of the vertebral column, and the dilated right ventricle occupies the cardiac apex. In addition, the right anterior oblique projection shows retrodisplacement of the esophagous due to left atrial enlargement (arrows). The patient underwent successful surgical repair of her atrial septal defect. (With permission, J. K. Perloff, *The Clinical Recognition of Congenital Heart Disease,* 2nd ed.)

flowing in a laminar stream. The law describing liquid flow through such rigid cylindric tubes was established by Poiseuille. By assuming laminar flow and constant viscosity, changes in resistance in the pulmonary circulation can be interpreted as resulting from changes in vessel geometry, principally the vessel radius.

From the above considerations, it follows that the level of mean pulmonary arterial pressure is governed primarily by an interplay among the following variables: (1) the magnitude of pulmonary blood flow; (2) the geometry, particularly the cross-sectional area and reactivity of the arteriolar bed; (3) the level of pulmonary venous pressure; and (4) the viscosity of blood. An additional variable is of major importance in congenital heart disease, namely, a free communication (or communications) between the greater and lesser circulations resulting in an obligatory rise in pulmonary arterial pressure to systemic levels [16]. A case in point is a large (nonrestrictive) ventricular septal defect. In this setting, pulmonary vascular resistance can be low, normal, or elevated (Fig. 1). Thus, pulmonary hypertension can occur with a normal pulmonary resistance, but the converse is not the case; i.e., a high pulmonary vascular resistance does not permit normal pulmonary arterial pressure unless flow is reciprocally reduced. There is an important corollary. If pulmonary arterial pressure is normal in the presence of a left-to-right shunt, an increase in flow seldom causes a serious rise in pulmonary vascular resistance, and if such a rise occurs at all, it is usually moderate in degree and late in the course of the disease (typical ostium secundum atrial septal defect; Fig. 2). If pulmonary arterial pressure is at or near systemic (as with nonrestrictive ventricular septal defect), a progressive rise in pulmonary vascular resistance to or above systemic levels occurs relatively early in the natural history if survival permits and if pulmonic stenosis does not develop [17]. Progressive structural changes in the pulmonary arterioles with reduction in cross-sectional areas of the pulmonary vascular bed constitute the important pathogenic mechanism for maintenance of pulmonary hypertension if the provoking causes are removed (abolition of the left-to-right shunt, closure of the ventricular septal defect). The most widely used pathologic classification of the pulmonary arteriolar lesions is derived from Heath and Edwards [18]. The first three grades include medial hypertrophy (which is vasoreactive and potentially reversible), cellular intimal proliferation, and fibrosis. Later, the arteriolar lesions are characterized by cellular fibrous vascular occlusion, dilatation lesions (plexiform lesions, vein-like channels, cavernous and angiomatoid lesions) in arterioles and small muscular arteries, and necrotizing arteritis. Thinning of the media may occur, and microscopic in situ thrombi are common. Considerable controversy exists concerning the mechanism and significance of the individual lesions just described. In an experimental model of pulmonary hypertension, all stages have been reproduced, and arterial necrosis

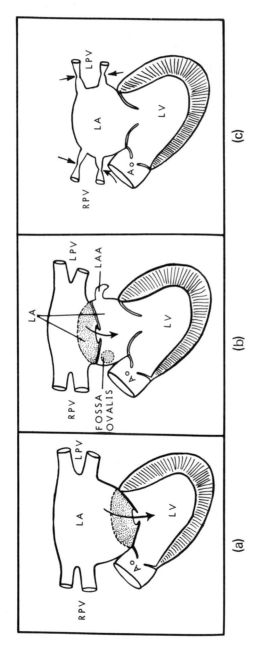

FIGURE 3 (a) Schematic illustration of the usual type of congenital mitral stenosis. The obstruction is at valvular level. (RPV, LPV = right and left pulmonary veins; LA = left atrium; LV = left ventricle; Ao = aorta). (b) Schematic illustration of the usual variety of cor triatriatum. A fibrous or fibromuscular diaphragm partitions the left atrium. The proximal compartment receives the pulmonary veins and is a high pressure zone; the distal compartment contains the fossa ovalis and left atrial appendage (LAA) and is a low-pressure zone. (c) Schematic illustration of one of the main types of pulmonary vein stenosis. The veins are narrowed near their junctions with the left atrium. (With permission, J. K. Perloff, *The Clinical Recognition of Congenital Heart Disease*, 2nd ed.)

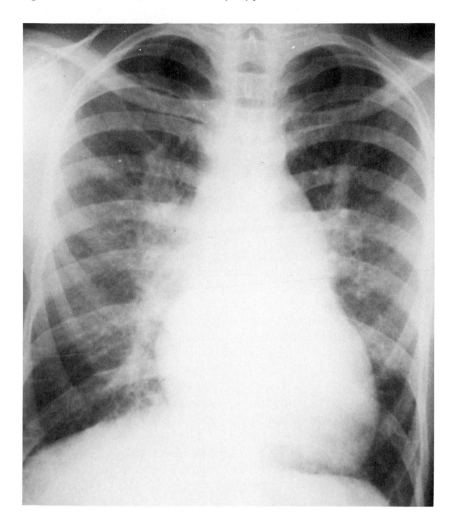

FIGURE 4 X-ray from an 18-year-old boy with cor triatriatum and a pulmonary arterial systolic pressure in excess of systemic. The lungs' fields exhibit marked pulmonary venous congestion with Kerley's lines in the right costrophrenic angle. The pulmonary trunk is conspicuously dilated. The right atrium forms a convex shadow to the right of the vertebral column, and an enlarged right ventricle occupies the apex. Note the absence of left atrial appendage. The patient underwent surgical correction. (With permission, J. K. Perloff, *The Clinical Recognition of Congenital Heart Disease,* 2nd ed.)

preceded the development of plexiform or angiomatoid lesions. The newly formed vessels were shown to originate from the bronchial circulation. Irrespective of how the increased pulmonary vascular resistance is initiated, it tends to reinforce itself (self-perpetuating) by provoking a sequence of changes that progressively increases the resistance to flow through the lungs. The degree of anatomical vascular disease forms a continuum from mild to severe. Early in the natural history, vasoconstriction contributes to the elevated arteriolar resistance, and in many instances, especially in young children, intra-pulmonary arterial infusion of acetylcholine or tolazoline results in sharp reductions in calculated resistance [19]. In the late stages, the resistance is fixed and nonvasoreactive.

Acute, mild elevations of pulmonary *venous* pressure are transmitted passively into the pulmonary arterial bed. If cardiac output remains constant, the increment in pulmonary artery pressure is somewhat less than the corresponding increment in pulmonary venous pressure because the concomitant distension of the vascular bed lowers the resistance. In clinical states characterized by chronic, severe elevations of venous pressure (for example cor triatriatum, Figs. 3b and 4) other factors come into play and may predominate. Pulmonary arterioles undergo the structural changes described above, so that pulmonary artery pressure rises to a greater extent than the increment provoked solely by the passive rise in pressure in the left atrium and pulmonary veins.

Sustained alveolar hypoventilation (defined as alveolar hypoxia coupled with a rise in alveolar and arterial PCO_2 above 45 mmHg) characterizes the pulmonary hypertension of idiopathic respiratory center depression [20]. The magnitude of pulmonary hypertension depends upon the duration and severity of chronic hypoxia [21]. In addition, *upper* airway obstruction in older children sometimes causes alveolar hypoventilation and severe pulmonary hypertension which can be mistaken for the pulmonary hypertension of congenital heart disease [22,23].

II. Pulmonary Hypertension in Specific Types of Congenital Heart Disease

A. Pulmonary Venous Behavior

Let us now turn to the causes of pulmonary hypertension *specifically* related to congenital heart disease, dealing with these causes first from a general point of view. Pulmonary hypertension may result from high pressure in the pulmonary venous bed. Venous pressure can be transmitted passively into the pulmonary arteries or can provoke pulmonary arteriolar constriction (reactive) resulting in disproportionate elevation of pulmonary arterial pressure (see

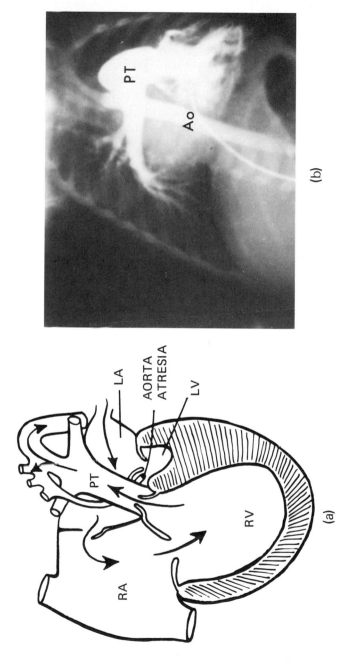

FIGURE 5 (a) Schematic illustration of the essential anatomical and circulatory derangements in aortic atresia. There is complete closure of the aortic orifice together with hypoplasia of the ascending aorta. A hypoplastic but patent mitral valve communicates with a small, blind, left ventricular cavity. Blood leaves the left atrium through an interatrial communication formed by herniation of the foramen ovale into the right atrium. The right ventricle supplies the entire pulmonary and systemic circulations; the systemic bed is reached through a ductus arteriosus which also provides retrograde flow into the ascending aorta and coronary arteries. (b) Angiocardiogram from a 48-hr-old male infant with aortic atresia. The necropsy (and angiographic) findings correspond to those in the schematic illustration. (With permission, J. K. Perloff, *The Clinical Recognition of Congenital Heart Disease*, 2nd ed.)

above). High pulmonary venous pressure secondary to congenital heart disease results from obstruction of pulmonary veins, obstruction within the left atrium proper (Figs. 3b and 4), obstruction at the mitral orifice (Figs. 3a and 5), or high left ventricular filling pressure. Congenital obstruction of pulmonary veins is caused by pulmonary vein stenosis (Fig. 3c) or by total anomalous pulmonary venous connection in which the confluence of veins gives rise to a vascular channel that is obstructed on its way to the right atrium either above or below the diaphragm (Fig. 6). Obstruction within the left atrium can take the form of cor triatriatum. Obstruction at the mitral orifice can be due to congenital mitral stenosis or mitral atresia.

High left ventricular filling pressure is perhaps the most common cause of passive elevation in pulmonary venous and pulmonary arterial pressures. Any anomaly that provokes left ventricular failure or reduces left ventricular compliance triggers this mechanism. It is important to emphasize that if left ventricular failure and high pulmonary venous pressure occur prior to involution of the fetal pulmonary arterioles (in the neonate or infant), reactive constriction of the pulmonary arterioles can result in severe pulmonary hypertension [17]. Witness the infant with coarctation of the aorta, left ventricular failure, reactive pulmonary hypertension, and pure right ventricular hypertrophy in the electrocardiogram.

B. Pulmonary Arteriolar Behavior

The behavior of the pulmonary arterioles is a key ingredient in the pulmonary hypertension of congenital heart disease. Increased pulmonary arteriolar resistance can be variable (vasoreactive) or fixed (nonvasoreactive). Once an increase in pulmonary vascular resistance is established, a vicious cycle is initiated, with progressive anatomical disease of the arterioles and in turn a progressive increase in resistance. Pulmonary vascular disease begets pulmonary vascular disease. In patients with large congenital communications between the two circulations—for example, communications at ventricular or great artery level, complete transposition of the great arteries with large ventricular septal defect, double outlet right ventricle, etc.—pulmonary hypertension occurs with pulmonary vascular resistances ranging from normal or nearly so to suprasystemic [16,19,24–26]. In addition, excessive "palliative" shunts, especially the Potts-Smith-Gibson (no longer done), occasionally Waterston, and uncommonly Blalock-Taussig anastomoses can have the same undesirable effect [27]. In infants born with large communications at either great artery, ventricular or atrial level, the inherently high neonatal pulmonary vascular resistance initially exhibits a strong tendency to fall, but subsequently displays one of four patterns [17]: (1) normal regression of the fetal pulmonary arteriole with a proportionate fall in resistance; (2) delayed

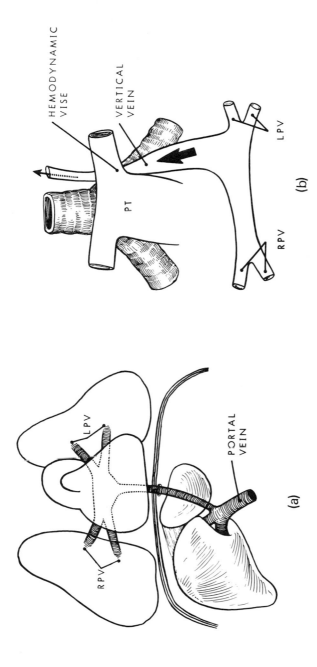

FIGURE 6 Two varieties of total anomalous venous connection with obstruction. (a) Schematic illustration showing the confluence of pulmonary veins giving rise to a vascular channel that enters the abdominal cavity through the diaphragmatic hiatus and terminates in the portal vein (RPV, LPV: right and left pulmonary veins). (b) Schematic illustration showing the anomalous vertical vein compressed in a "hemodynamic vise" as it passes upward between the pulmonary trunk (PT) and left bronchus. (With permission, J. K. Perloff, *The Clinical Recognition of Congenital Heart Disease*, 2nd ed.)

or incomplete regression; (3) recurrence of an elevated pulmonary vascular resistance after partial or complete regression (the latter two patterns provoked by the stimulus of the left-to-right shunt itself); or (4) persistence of the high pulmonary vascular resistance of the newborn [28]. In the presence of delayed or incomplete regression or occurrence of an elevated pulmonary vascular resistance after partial or incomplete regression, the pulmonary vascular disease is generally self-perpetuating and progressive unless the stimulus of the left-to-right shunt is surgically abolished while still large enough to permit, after removal, acceptable regression of pulmonary arteriolar disease. It is appropriate at this point to call attention to "persistence of the fetal circulation" (noninvolution of fetal arterioles) in full-term neonates without heart or lung disease [21,28]. There is a strong correlation between persistence of the fetal circulation and perinatal distress (intrauterine hypoxia). The same mechanism may exist (and cause hypertensive pulmonary vascular disease) in infants with certain types of congenital cardiac defects [24]. The comparative histology of the proximal pulmonary trunk and aortic root has been used to determine whether the pulmonary hypertension was present from birth [9]. Normally, after 1 year of age, the pulmonary trunk contains far fewer elastic fibers than the aorta. Identical configuration of elastic fibers in the two great arteries is evidence that pulmonary hypertension dates from birth.

C. Prearteriolar Behavior

Prearteriolar obstructive disease of the pulmonary vascular bed causes pulmonary hypertension in congenital heart disease and takes the form of stenosis of the pulmonary trunk, its bifurcation, or its primary or peripheral branches [17,29]. Stenosis of the pulmonary artery and its branches may involve varying lengths of vessel, from segmental narrowing to diffuse tubular hypoplasia. Although this congenital anomaly can be bilateral, unilateral, single, or multiple, in order to provoke pulmonary hypertension, the obstruction must be bilateral [29].

D. Alveolar Hypoventilation

Alveolar hypoventilation is, as a rule, not a concern in the pulmonary hypertension of congenital heart disease although one form of hypoventilation can be misleading in this regard. Enlarged tonsils causing chronic upper airways obstruction results in severe alveolar hypoventilation and pulmonary hypertension [22,23]. Following tonsillectomy and adenoidectomy, a dramatic reversal of pulmonary hypertension occurs in these children. However, the responsiveness to inhaled carbon dioxide remains diminished for years after surgery, implicating altered chemosensitivity in the pathogenesis.

E. Physical and Laboratory Findings in Pulmonary Hypertension

To set the stage for comment on the manifestations of pulmonary hypertension in congenital heart disease, let us first turn briefly to the purest reflections of elevations in pulmonary arterial pressure, as in primary pulmonary hypertension. Information from the natural history, physical signs, electrocardiogram, echocardiogram, chest X-ray, and fluoroscopy are pivotal. The symptomatic history of isolated pulmonary hypertension often permits a high index of suspicion based on this information alone [17]. A young patient, generally female, describes effort syncope, chest pain resembling angina, dyspnea, weakness, and fatigue, especially with exertion. Careful questioning frequently reveals additional though less dramatic cerebral symptoms, such as lightheadedness, dizziness, or faintness, all of which tend to be provoked by effort or stress, but occasionally occur spontaneously. Increasingly frequent and severe syncopal episodes herald sudden death. Chest pain resembling angina pectoris arrests attention because the patients are of an age and sex in which angina is exceptional. The advent of right ventricular failure predicts the beginning of a progressively downhill course. Hemoptysis may arise from rupture of thin-walled, fragile plexiform lesions or necrotizing arteritis. Hoarseness results from vocal cord paralysis due to compression of the left recurrent laryngeal nerve by the dilated pulmonary trunk. Neck pulsations caused by giant jugular venous A waves (powerful right atrial contraction) may be subjectively noticed, especially following effort or excitement. On physical examination, the general appearance is usually normal, but a low cardiac output may result in cold, pallid skin which may have a mild cyanotic hue due to marked peripheral extraction of oxygen. Occasionally, a reversed shunt through a patent foramen ovale causes a fall in systemic arterial oxygen saturation and true central cyanosis. The systemic arterial pulse is likely to be small and the pulse pressure narrow owing to reduced cardiac output and stroke volume. The small arterial pulse stands in contrast to the large cervical venous pulsations—giant A waves—which are important physical signs of pulmonary hypertension with intact ventricular septum and result from an increased force of right atrial contraction against a thick-walled hypertrophied right ventricle. The V wave remains relatively inconspicuous until the advent of tricuspid regurgitation, after which the jugular venous pulse exhibits two prominent crests (A and V) and two prominent troughs (X and Y). Gross tricuspid regurgitation attenuates the X descent and exaggerates the Y trough. Precordial movement and palpation are important in a number of respects.

A right ventricular impulse is uniformly present at the lower left sternal edge and in the subxiphoid area. The increased force of right atrial contraction causes presystolic distension of the right ventricle and occasionally presystolic movement of the liver. An enlarged, hypertensive right ventricle can occupy the cardiac apex so the left ventricle may not be palpable. In the second left intercostal space, three palpable events should be sought, namely, the systolic impulse of the dilated hypertensive pulmonary trunk, a palpable second sound (pulmonic component), and a pulmonic ejection sound. Nine auscultatory signs—some major, some minor—are directly related to the effects of pulmonary hypertension per se [2]. The pulmonic ejection sound is high pitched and clicking, maximal in the second left intercostal space, and often selectively decreasing with inspiration. A short, soft midsystolic murmur results from ejection into the dilated pulmonary trunk; this murmur is typically introduced by the pulmonic ejection sound. A holosystolic murmur is caused by tricuspid regurgitation as the stressed right ventricle fails. The murmur of pulmonary hypertensive tricuspid regurgitation is located at the lower left sternal edge, but can radiate to the cardiac apex especially when the apex is occupied by the right ventricle. The murmur is high pitched, may be loud enough to generate a thrill, or very soft and just at the threshold of audibility, detected only during inspiration. Inspiratory augmentation of the murmur (Rivero-Carvallo's sign) is a feature of recognized importance. The pulmonic component of the second sound is altered by pulmonary hypertension with respect to timing, intensity, and precordial location. The sound is generally not delayed, so inspiration usually finds the second sound normally or closely split. The loudness of the pulmonic component may obscure the closely preceding and softer aortic component. Auscultation at the lower left sternal edge, however, permits analysis of the transmitted but attenuated pulmonic component and may allow ready detection of splitting. The Graham Steel murmur of high-pressure pulmonary regurgitation is generally best heard in the second and third left intercostal spaces. The murmur begins with the loud pulmonic component of the second sound, is high in frequency, and is typically decrescendo. Fourth heart sounds characteristically accompanying presystolic distension of the right ventricle are best detected at the lower left sternal edge or subxiphoid area and often get selectively louder with inspiration. A third heart sound is a manifestation of right ventricular failure. With the development of tricuspid regurgitation, the third heart sound increases. Inspiration may augment the third sound in a fashion analogous to the fourth sound. Two minor auscultatory points follow. Occasionally, middiastolic or presystolic murmurs occur in isolated pulmonary hypertension, and probably represent prolonged vibrations of third and fourth heart sounds. Rarely, there is an early diastolic sound with the timing of an opening snap; the validity of this observation is in question and verification is not yet convincing.

The electrocardiogram exhibits varying degrees of pure right ventricular hypertrophy, reflecting an increase in mass due to an increase in free wall and generally in septal thickness. The P waves show right atrial abnormalities. The PR interval is normal or slightly prolonged and the QRS axis in the frontal plane varies from normal to vertical to frank right axis deviation. Right ventricular hypertrophy may be manifested by no more than an abnormal rightward shift of the frontal QRS axis. At the other end of the spectrum, right precordial leads exhibit tall monophasic R waves with ST segment depressions and marked asymmetric T-wave inversions. Deep S waves then appear in the left precordium. It is noteworthy that in the newborn infant, upright right precordial T waves are normal for 72 hr, but subsequently invert with the fall in neonatal pulmonary vascular resistance and pressure. Persistence of upright right precordial T waves beyond 72 hr usually means persistent elevation of right ventricular systolic pressure. The X-ray exhibits enlargement of the pulmonary trunk and its main branches, but the distal branches are diminished and the peripheral lung fields clear ("pruned" appearance). Signs of pulmonary venous congestion are uniformly absent. The aorta appears small in contrast to the dilated pulmonary trunk. Enlargement of the right ventricle (left anterior oblique) is more readily identified after the onset of failure and dilatation. Left ventricular enlargement does not occur, although its presence may be erroneously suggested in the left oblique or lateral view because of displacement by an enlarged right ventricle. Echocardiographic analysis (see below) prevents this error. Right atrial enlargement varies from slight to marked and is best identified in the simple posteroanterior projection. Left atrial enlargement is categorically absent and must be pointedly excluded. At fluoroscopy, increased pulsations of the pulmonary trunk and its main branches should not be mistaken for pulsations of a left-to-right shunt.

Three noninvasive or minimally invasive studies are useful: pulmonary function tests, ventilation/perfusion isotope scans, and echocardiography. I shall deal briefly only with the latter. The echocardiogram is valuable in the diagnosis of pulmonary hypertension [30,31]. Information is best considered in the following categories: the pulmonic valve echoes and the echocardiograms from right ventricle, septum, and left ventricle; and from mitral, tricuspid, and aortic valves. In the pulmonic valve echogram, the most striking feature is absence or decrease of the A wave, since even powerful right atrial contraction cannot raise right ventricular end-diastolic pressure sufficiently to reach the high pulmonary arterial diastolic pressure; thus, movement is not imparted to the pulmonic leaflets in presystole. Once the valve opens, however, it does so relatively rapidly (accelerated B-C slope). During midsystole there is notching (or fluttering) of the posterior leaflet. When right ventricular systolic time intervals are derived from fast-speed echocardiograms, the preejection period (PEP) is prolonged (increased duration of right ventricular isovolumetric contraction), while the right ventricular ejection time (RVET) is normal (provided that the chamber has not failed); accordingly, the PEP/ RVET is increased. During diastole, the slope of the pulmonic valve echo (E-F slope) is not only flat, but sometimes slightly reversed.

Now let us turn attention to echocardiographic information unrelated to the pulmonic valve. The ventricular septum may be thick (right ventricular hypertrophy), but the left ventricular posterior wall is normal, increasing the septal/posterior wall ratio. The left ventricular internal dimensions are normal to reduced, while the right ventricular dimensions are normal or increased. With the advent of right ventricular volume overload—pulmonary or tricuspid regurgitation—systolic septal motion flattens or becomes frankly anterior (i.e. paradoxic). With pulmonary regurgitation, there may be diastolic fluttering of the tricuspid valve. The anterior mitral leaflet may exhibit a diminished diastolic (E-F) slope, probably due to a decreased rate of left ventricular filling. If left ventricular stroke volume is materially reduced, the aortic leaflets drift toward each other in late systole. Cardiac catheterization identifies the presence and degree of pulmonary hypertension and elevated pulmonary vascular resistance, as well as the presence or absence of vasoreactivity of the pulmonary arterial bed.

Information from the history, physical signs, electrocardiogram, echocardiogram, and chest X-rays should bring the diagnosis into focus so that the catheterization laboratory can be used to clarify ambiguities and concentrate principally on the physiology of the pulmonary vascular bed itself. It should be understood that the physiological reserve in patients with severe pulmonary vascular obstructive disease is limited. Contrast angiography (pulmonary arteriography), by dilating systemic arterioles and increasing pulmonary venous return in the face of fixed pulmonary vascular resistance, can be lethal. Response to exercise should be avoided in the catheter laboratory; a further rise in pulmonary arterial pressure during exercise is predictable since the pulmonary vascular resistance falls little if at all in the face of increased venous return. Attention should be directed instead to simple pharmacologic interventions that shed light on vasoreactivity of the pulmonary arterioles. In vasoreactive pulmonary hypertension, for example, oxygen inhalation or intrapulmonary arterial tolazoline (priscoline) will cause a transient fall in pulmonary resistance when properly calculated by simultaneously determining pulmonary arterial pressure and flow [19].

F.   Conditions Which Mimic Pulmonary Hypertension

An important corollary to the foregoing clinical manifestations of pulmonary hypertension is represented by disorders that cause mistaken clinical impressions of elevated pressures in the pulmonary bed. A number of such disorders (some entirely innocent) are important in this regard. A decrease in anteroposterior chest dimensions, especially due to absence of thoracic kyphosis (straight back syndrome) is an example [32]. The heart is displaced forward. Proximity of the heart to the anterior chest wall results in a palpable right ventricle and pulmonary trunk, a palpable second sound at the left base, occasionally an rSr′ pattern in lead V_1, a lateral chest X-ray showing the heart against the sternum, and a posteroanterior X-ray that may show a relatively prominent main pulmonary artery. Attention to the configuration of the thoracic spine with the patient sitting bolt upright during the physical examination, and confirmed in the lateral chest X-ray avoids error. In severe cyanotic Fallot's tetralogy (or pulmonary atresia), events originating in the aortic root are exaggerated since a dilated aorta is left uncovered by the small hypoplastic pulmonary trunk. Thus, aortic ejection sounds may be present and vary with respiration, implying pulmonic origin; a short midsystolic murmur and a loud, single second sound at the "pulmonary area" superficially resemble pulmonary hypertension. An analogous situation is found with truncus arteriosus. In complete transposition of the great arteries, the right ventricle is palpable (obligatory systemic pressure) and the aortic component of the second sound is loud and palpable at the left base because the aortic root is anterior to the pulmonary trunk. In congenitally corrected (L) transposition of the great arteries, the aortic root and valve are relatively anterior, with the aortic valve taking a position ordinarily occupied by the pulmonary valve in normally oriented hearts [17]. Thus, the aortic component of the second sound may be mistaken for the loud second sound of pulmonary hypertension.

III. Consequences of Pulmonary Hypertension

The consequences of pulmonary hypertension can be considered in light of the nature, course, and management of the disorder. Pulmonary hypertension causes an increased resistance to right ventricular discharge (afterload). In general terms, there are two principle sequelae. The first is the result of increased afterload per se on the contractile performance of the right ventricle. The initial response is adaptive hypertrophy, but the ultimate response is failure of the chamber as a pump. The second consequence of pulmonary hypertension is venoarterial mixing which occurs when high pulmonary vascular resistance causes unoxygenated (venous) blood to enter the systemic circulation, producing systemic arterial hypoxemia. Physiological and morphological adaptation of the right ventricle to increased afterload is variable and depends in part upon whether the afterload begins at birth or later and whether it is chronic or acute [11]. Adaptive hypertrophy is an expected feature of the normal fetal right ventricle which ejects into the aorta at systemic pressure via the ductus arteriosus. After birth, with the afterload removed, there is a gradual reduction in the thickness of the right ventricular free wall relative to septum and left ventricle. The neonatal right ventricle does not undergo regression of hypertrophy, it merely does not increase its thickness as rapidly as the left ventricle owing to the relative differences in postnatal pulmonary and systemic vascular resistances (see above). Should the fetal right ventricle continue to eject at (but not above) systemic pressure after birth, as in Eisenmenger's complex, right ventricular thickness keeps pace with left ventricle and septum, and long-term right ventricular performance is remarkably good [11]. Witness the infrequency of right ventricular failure in this anomaly even when pulmonary resistance exceeds systemic. On the other hand, if the right ventricle undergoes adaptive hypertrophy *after* normal adult ventricular wall ratios are reached, the performance of that hypertrophied right ventricle is less adequate, as in adults with mitral stenosis in whom the right ventricle fails at pressures far below systemic [11,33]. Thus, the fetal right ventricle is "designed" to eject at systemic pressure, but the normal adult right ventricle is "designed" to function as a thin-walled, compliant, low-pressure pump. If an increase in pulmonary resistance is imposed suddenly (in situ thrombi, pulmonary embolism), the right ventricle has no time to adapt and fails acutely [34]. Conversely, chronic progressive right ventricular afterload in the adult permits adaptive hypertrophy, albeit imperfect, and right ventricular failure is delayed. Still another variable affecting the hypertensive right ventricle is the coronary arterial circulation. The right and left coronary arteries are anatomically and physiologically different vascular beds, designed to perfuse low- and high-pressure ventricles, respectively. A question therefore arises. Can an anatomical right coronary artery adequately perfuse a high-pressure right ventricle? Coronary arterial flow may prove to be a long-term limitation to stressed right ventricular performance whether the afterload begins at birth or later. This concern not only applies to the hypertensive right ventricle in preoperative congenital heart disease but also to the systemic right ventricle in complete transposition of the great arteries following a Mustard repair.

Congenital heart disease can initiate pulmonary hypertension and then in turn be variously affected by it. The following sections will highlight disorders involving the pulmonary vascular bed (venous, arteriolar, prearteriolar), the pulmonary parenchyma, and alveolar hypoventilation. Certain examples will be selected; no attempt will be made to be comprehensive.

IV. Pulmonary Venous Hypertensive Disorders

Some congenital disorders resulting in high pulmonary venous pressure and pulmonary arterial hypertension include obstruction of pulmonary veins, cor triatriatum, congenital mitral stenosis, and high left ventricular filling pressure. One of the most important differences between congenital and acquired pulmonary hypertension caused by high pulmonary venous pressure is the vasoreactivity of noninvoluted or partially involuted neonatal arterioles. In total anomalous pulmonary venous connection, the four pulmonary veins usually join a single venous channel [17]. If that venous channel is obstructed on its way to the right atrium (passage between left bronchus and pulmonary trunk, or passage through the diaphragmatic hiatus, Fig. 6), pulmonary venous pressure rises dramatically and provokes severe pulmonary hypertension by stimulating vasoconstriction of the highly reactive neonatal pulmonary arterioles [17]. Clinical signs of severe pulmonary hypertension occur without a murmur unless tricuspid regurgitation ensues. The echocardiogram shows normal left heart structures, but the X-ray reveals soft-tissue densities of pulmonary venous obstruction.

The physiological consequences of cor triatriatum or congenital mitral stenosis are analogous to rheumatic mitral stenosis in the adult, although vasoreactive pulmonary arterioles are more likely to result in pulmonary hypertension disproportionate to the pulmonary venous pressure (Fig. 4). Cor triatriatum generally occurs as an isolated defect. Echocardiography is useful in identifying a normal mitral valve in the setting of high pulmonary venous and pulmonary arterial pressures, and the obstructing membrane itself is sometimes recorded [17]. Congenital mitral stenosis generally occurs with additional anomalies, especially supravalvular stenosing ring, subaortic stenosis, and coarctation of the aorta [17]. It is important to remember that one common form of congenital mitral stenosis, the parachute mitral valve, usually produces neither an opening snap nor a loud first heart sound because of the inherent anatomical derangement of valve and chordeae and not because a large hypertensive right ventricle displaces the left ventricle from the cardiac apex. Such displacement may occur, however, and render the diastolic murmur across the stenotic mitral valve inaudible. The echocardiogram focuses the fault on the mitral valve and can sometimes identify the parachute valve itself [17].

Still another form of severe obstruction to left atrial flow with pulmonary venous and pulmonary arterial hypertension results from a hypoplastic left heart—aortic/mitral atresia (Fig. 5). The mitral valve is hypoplastic or atretic and communicates with a small, blind left ventricular cavity in which endocardial fibroelastosis is commonly found. A steep rise in left atrial pressure is invariable, with pulmonary arterial hypertension a common sequel. The right ventricle is called upon to perfuse both systemic and pulmonary circulations via the ductus arteriosus. An interatrial communication is created by herniation of the valve of the foramen ovale into the right atrium, providing the small hypertensive left atrium with its only exit. Interestingly, in this setting, the pulmonary vascular resistance is *not* invariably high. When the resistance is relatively low and when an adequate interatrial communication is present, a large volume of oxygenated blood returns to the left atrium and is available for mixing with right atrial blood; systemic arterial oxygen saturation may be relatively good, but at a price. As pulmonary vascular resistance declines, blood from the pulmonary trunk preferentially enters the lungs, while systemic flow via the ductus may fall sufficiently to produce an ashen, shock-like picture with feeble pulses [17]. On the other hand, if pulmonary resistance is high, systemic flow is maintained, but at the cost of deepening cyanosis.

A high left ventricular filling pressure in an infant typically provokes constriction of the vasoreactive pulmonary arterioles and disproportionate re-active pulmonary hypertension [17]. Coarctation of the aorta is a case in point. The incidence of heart failure with coarctation is highest during two periods in the natural history, namely, during infancy and after the third decade. In the latter period, a high left ventricular filling pressure merely results in a passive rise in pulmonary arterial pressure. The pulmonary arteriolar resistance remains normal or nearly so. However, in the infant with aortic coarctation and left ventricular failure, a high pulmonary venous pressure can provoke such reactive pulmonary hypertension that right ventricular systolic pressure exceeds an elevated left ventricular pressure [17]. Further, a high left atrial pressure may result in a left-to-right shunt via a foramen ovale, so right ventricular volume overload coexists. Clinical signs of hypertensive right ventricular failure, with pure right ventricular hypertrophy on the electrocardiogram, can be misleading. Careful palpation of the brachial and femoral arterial pulses, especially after treatment of heart failure, points the way to the correct diagnosis. Echocardiography can identify an increase in left ventricular end-diastolic dimensions (and possibly a coexisting bicuspid aortic valve), but cardiac catheterization and angiocardiography confirm the anatomical diagnosis.

V.   Arteriolar Alterations in Congenital Heart Disease

Discussion of the pulmonary arteriolar bed sets the stage for comment on certain congenital diseases associated with high pulmonary vascular resistance and pulmonary hypertension. Two general consequences are important: (1) the effect of pulmonary hypertension, per se, on the right ventricle, i.e., right ventricular hypertrophy and failure; and (2) the effect of suprasystemic pulmonary vascular resistance in producing right-to-left shunts (venoarterial mixing) with progressive hypoxemia.

Primary pulmonary hypertension (see above) serves as the touchtone for the purest expression of increased pulmonary vascular resistance and elevated pressure in the pulmonary bed. The circulatory response of subjects at high altitude is important because the picture can be analogous to if not indistinguishable from primary pulmonary hypertension. In addition, this response to high altitude occurs in patients with congenital cardiac diseases which, at sea level, would be associated with little or no pulmonary hypertension. High altitude can result in a variety of responses of the pulmonary circulation— acute pulmonary edema in unacclimatized subjects; asymptomatic, apparently acclimatized subjects, with increased pulmonary vascular resistance; compensatory increase in red cell mass without abnormally low systemic arterial oxygen saturation; and chronic mountain sickness (pulmonary hypertension, cyanosis, marked increase in red cell mass, and right ventricular failure) [8,14,35,36]. It is important in this context to underscore that persistent patency of the ductus arteriosus is 6 times as frequent in people born at high altitudes as in those born at sea level [17]. The tendency for such patients to develop pulmonary hypertension is related to birth at high altitude and not simply to the size of the ductus. In ostium secundum atrial septal defect, pulmonary hypertension is infrequent in subjects born at sea level, but an increased incidence and an earlier onset of pulmonary hypertension occur when such patients are born at high altitudes [17]. The issue can be restated in relatively simple terms. Some anomalies, such as patent ductus arteriosus, are inherently more common in subjects born at high altitudes and are complicated by pulmonary hypertension far more frequently than similar anomalies at sea level. Other malformations have little or no natural tendency to coexist with pulmonary hypertension and are not inherently more frequent at high altitudes. However, when these malformations occur in subjects born at high altitudes, pulmonary hypertension provoked by the altitude itself is likely to coexist. Even at sea level, the consequences of pulmonary hypertension related to high pulmonary vascular resistance in congenital heart disease are complex and often, although not invariably, combine the effects of right ventricular failure and the chronic progressive hypoxemia of right-to-left shunts (venoarterial mixing). The shunts can occur at atrial, ventricular, or great artery level, either with normally related great arteries (ventricular concordance) and noninverted ventricles or with such anomalies as complete transposition of the great arteries, double outlet right ventricle, congenitally corrected transposition of the great arteries (ventricular inversion), a single great artery (truncus arteriosus), or a single ventricle (absent right ventricular sinus with anatomical single left ventricle) [17]. The consequences of high pulmonary vascular resistance in these settings is variable, but as a rule predictable and physiologically rational. As a point of departure, let us take an otherwise uncomplicated large subaortic (infracristal) ventricular septal defect [17].

The natural history begins with an acyanotic newborn who exhibits neither a left-to-right shunt nor a murmur until the high neonatal pulmonary vascular resistance falls sufficiently to permit the left ventricle to eject via the ventricular septal defect into the pulmonary bed. As the pulmonary vascular resistance falls, pulmonary arterial blood flow increases, the ventricular septal defect murmur appears, left ventricular volume overload is established, and left ventricular failure ensues. Pulmonary hypertension is obligatory because of the size of the ventricular septal defect (nonrestrictive) and not because of the pulmonary vascular resistance. Even if the pulmonary resistance subsequently rises again, the right ventricular systolic pressure remains unchanged, but the left-to-right shunt reciprocally decreases, left ventricular volume overload and failure diminish, and the holosystolic ventricular septal defect murmur gets shorter and softer, fading first in late systole. When pulmonary vascular resistance exceeds systemic, the left-to-right shunt is abolished altogether and replaced by a right-to-left shunt (Fig. 1). The ventricular septal defect is then silent. Relief of left ventricular volume overload has been purchased at the price of progressive hypoxemia (Eisenmenger's complex) [19]. Cyanosis and clubbing involve upper and lower extremities. The jugular venous pulse may be normal because the right ventricular pressure cannot exceed systemic (right ventricular to aortic decompression via the large ventricular septal defect); palpation identifies right ventricular and pulmonary trunk impulses and a palpable second sound at the left base, but little or no left ventricular impulse. Auscultation detects no ventricular septal defect murmur but instead a pulmonic ejection sound (dilated hypertensive pulmonary trunk) introducing a short midsystolic murmur, a loud, single, second heart sound, and perhaps a Graham Steel murmur of high-pressure pulmonary regurgitation [2]. The X-ray no longer shows shunt vascularity or pulmonary venous congestion, the heart size may be normal or nearly so, but the pulmonary trunk remains large. The electrocardiogram exhibits right ventricular hypertrophy with variable residua of prior left ventricular volume overload. Cardiac catheterization and angiocardiography show that right ventricular systolic pressure is at but not above systemic, right ventricular filling pressure is normal or nearly so, pulmonary resistance is at or above systemic, and the shunt is entirely right-to-left.

All gradations exist between the large, acyanotic, pulmonary hypertensive, low-resistance ventricular septal defect with large left-to-right shunt and congestive heart failure at one end of the spectrum, and a large, cyanotic, pulmonary hypertensive, high pulmonary resistance ventricular septal defect with a right-to-left shunt and no congestive heart failure—but with complications of hypoxemia—at the other end of the spectrum. In the latter setting (Eisenmenger's complex), right ventricular failure is uncommon because the right ventricle can decompress into the aorta via the nonrestrictive ventricular septal defect [17]. The above commentary on ventricular septal defect underscores a point worth restating—that pulmonary hypertension occurs not only because of the high pulmonary vascular resistance but also because of the large communication between the two ventricles. The pulmonary resistance may range from relatively low to suprasystemic without a change in peak systolic pressure in the right ventricle or pulmonary trunk. As pulmonary resistance rises, the arterioles are initially vasoreactive, but ultimately the resistance becomes fixed because of irreversible anatomical changes [18] (see earlier).

Let us now examine ostium secundum atrial septal defect, contrasting this disorder with ventricular septal defect as described above. In the fetus, the direction of interatrial flow is from right to left, whether by means of a true atrial septal defect or a patent foramen ovale [3]. At birth, there may be little or no shunt in either direction, because the distensibility characteristics (compliance) of the two ventricles are the same. During the newborn period, the pulmonary vascular resistance falls and the pulmonary arterioles gradually involute; the relatively thick-walled neonatal right ventricle becomes thinner and begins to offer less resistance to filling than the left ventricle. Conditions are then appropriate for flow of left atrial blood across the defect, establishing a left-to-right shunt. Despite the logic of these assumptions, there is evidence that left-to-right interatrial shunting sometimes occurs shortly after birth [3]. The fall in neonatal pulmonary vascular resistance has been held responsible for these early shunts. It has been reasoned that a decrease in resistance to right ventricular ejection results in more complete systolic emptying of that chamber, which then preferentially fills in diastole, establishing a left-to-right shunt. Even so, consideration must be given to abnormal *left* ventricular distensibility in such infants [17]. Nevertheless, a delay in the establishment of a significant left-to-right shunt provides a partial explanation for the infrequency of pulmonary hypertension in young people with atrial septal defect. The pulmonary vascular resistance *and* pulmonary arterial pressure fall to normal *before* (or even if) a significant left-to-right shunt is established. This is in contrast to large interventricular or great artery communications, in which pulmonary vascular *resistance* may fall, but pulmonary arterial *pressure* remains high. Since the neonatal pulmonary arterial pressure typically normalizes in atrial septal defect, the pulmonary arterioles involute, a process favored by *delayed* development of the left-to-right shunting.

Once involution has occurred, an increase in pulmonary arterial flow can then be met without a rise in pulmonary arterial pressure, as in normal

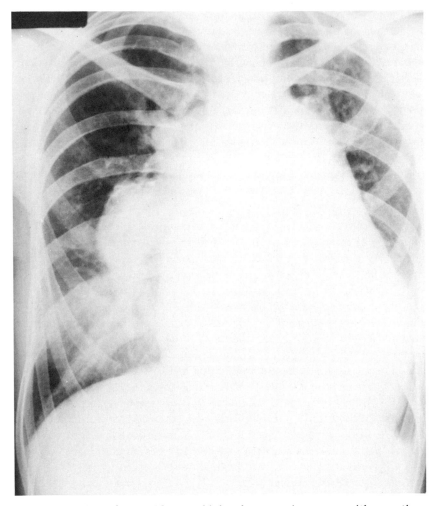

FIGURE 7   X-ray from a 28-year-old deeply cyanotic woman with an ostium secundum atrial septal defect and severe pulmonary hypertension (pulmonary vascular resistance in excess of systemic). The peripheral lung fields are clear. The pulmonary trunk is immense, and its huge right branch not only contains calcium in its upper margin, but tapers to an abrupt cutoff. The cross section of a large pulmonary arterial branch is seen just beneath the end of the right clavicle. The enlarged right ventricle occupies the cardiac apex, and its dilated outflow portion forms a relatively smooth continuity with the large pulmonary trunk above. (With permission, J. K. Perloff, *The Clinical Recognition of Congenital Heart Disease,* 2nd ed.)

individuals. Accordingly, pulmonary hypertension is not a feature of atrial septal defect in the young. An interesting exception to this rule is isolated atrial septal defect in the presence of Down's syndrome, which appears to endow the pulmonary vascular bed with a propensity for early development of high pulmonary vascular resistance [37]. When pulmonary hypertension develops in adults with atrial septal defect (Figs. 2 and 7), about 14%, the histologic alterations in the pulmonary arterioles are primarily late intimal changes. In pulmonary hypertensive ostium secundum atrial septal defect, cyanosis, when present, is symmetrical. Since the ventricular septum is intact, pulmonary arterial and right ventricular pressures can exceed systemic; a giant a wave appears in the jugular pulse (Fig. 8), and the right ventricle dilates and fails (Fig. 7). If the left-to-right shunt is entirely abolished, fixed splitting of

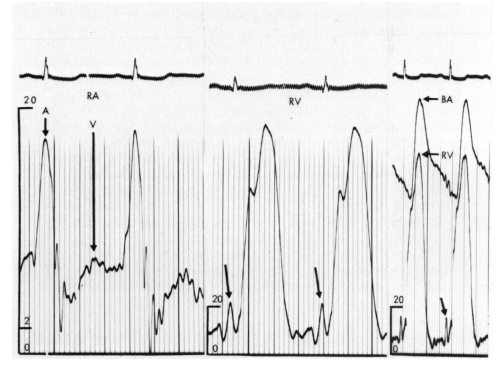

FIGURE 8 Pressure pulses from a moderately cyanotic 34-year-old man with a large ostium secundum atrial septal defect, pulmonary hypertension, and a bidirectional shunt. Giant a waves appear in the right atrium (RA) and are transmitted into the right ventricle (RV) as presystolic distension (arrows). (With permission, J. K. Perloff, *The Clinical Recognition of Congenital Heart Disease*, 2nd ed.)

the second heart sound disappears, and the echocardiogram may show normal direction of septal motion unless tricuspid regurgitation results in right ventricular volume overload [30].

And now a few comments on high pulmonary vascular resistance in some of the other congenital anomalies mentioned above: A nonrestrictive patent ductus arteriosus results in pulmonary hypertension irrespective of the level of pulmonary vascular resistance [17]. When the pulmonary resistance is above systemic, patent ductus arteriosus with reversed shunt can be identified because unoxygenated blood from the pulmonary trunk flows through the ductus into the aorta distal to the left subclavian artery so that the feet are cyanotic and the toes clubbed, whereas the hands are acyanotic and the fingers are not clubbed (differential cyanosis) (Fig. 9). This is an important clinical sign, since the continuous murmur, or indeed any ductus murmur, vanishes once the shunt is reversed; the auscultatory signs become those of pure pulmonary hypertension. The physiological consequences of an aorticopulmonary septal defect are similar to the large ductus, but differential cyanosis does not occur since the shunt is proximal to the brachiocephalic arteries. This is also the case with truncus arteriosus (Fig. 10). Double-outlet right ventricle with infracristal ventricular septal defect (subaortic), clinically resembles uncomplicated large, acyanotic pulmonary hypertensive, low-resistance ventricular septal defect, except that the electrocardiogram often (but not invariably) shows left axis deviation [17]. The echocardiogram is useful in recording an aortic wall that is not in continuity with either anterior mitral leaflet or ventricular septum. The angiocardiogram (left anterior oblique or lateral) shows that the aorta arises entirely anterior to the ventricular septum. If double-outlet right ventricle occurs with *supracristal* (subpulmonic) ventricular septal defect, there is early onset of cyanosis with an initial increase in pulmonary blood flow [17]. A relatively unique consequence of double-outlet right ventricle with supracristal ventricular septal defect occurs if a large patent ductus arteriosus coexists with suprasystemic pulmonary vascular resistance. Unoxygenated blood from the right ventricle enters the aorta, so the hands are cyanosed and the fingers clubbed, whereas oxygenated blood from the left ventricle enters the pulmonary trunk via the subpulmonic ventricular septal defect and flows through the ductus into the aorta distal to the left subclavian artery, so the feet are relatively pink and the toes not clubbed (reversed differential cyanosis) [17]. In congenitally corrected transposition of the great arteries, a large ventricular septal defect may coexist. In this malformation, the ventricles are inverted (right-to-left interchange) so the pulmonary hypertensive *venous* ventricle is an anatomical left ventricle. The electrocardiogram is helpful since V_1 may exhibit a Q wave, while V_{5-6} exhibit conspicuous absence of Q waves despite increased pulmonary blood flow and left ventricular volume overload. These initial force patterns are

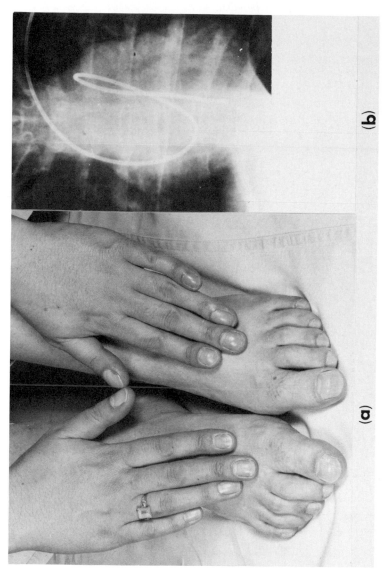

FIGURE 9 Photographs of a 20-year-old woman with patent ductus arteriosus, pulmonary hypertension, and reversed shunt. The hands are placed on the dorsum of the feet in order to compare the fingers and toes. The right hand is acyanotic and the fingers are not clubbed. The left hand exhibits mild cyanosis with clubbing (compare the thumbs). The toes are frankly cyanosed and clubbed. (b) X-ray from a 14-year-old boy with patent ductus arteriosus, pulmonary hypertension, and reversed shunt. The catheter traces the pathway of unoxygenated blood from right heart through the pulmonary trunk via the ductus into the descending aorta where the tip lies. (With permission, J. K. Perloff, *The Clinical Recognition of Congenital Heart Disease*, 2nd ed.)

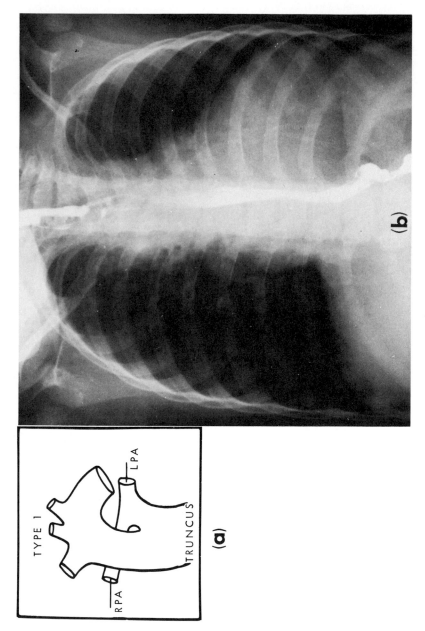

FIGURE 10 (a) Schematic illustration of truncus arteriosus type I in which a short main pulmonary artery arises directly from the truncus and gives rise to the right and left pulmonary arterial branches. Pulmonary hypertension is obligatory; pulmonary arterial systolic pressures are identical with systemic. (b) X-Ray from a 2½-year-old girl with the form of truncus arteriosus illustrated in the sketch. The slightly convex pulmonary artery segment is caused by the short, dilated main pulmonary artery as it arises from the truncus which continues as a right aortic arch. (With permission, J. K. Perloff, *The Clinical Recognition of Congenital Heart Disease*, 2nd ed.)

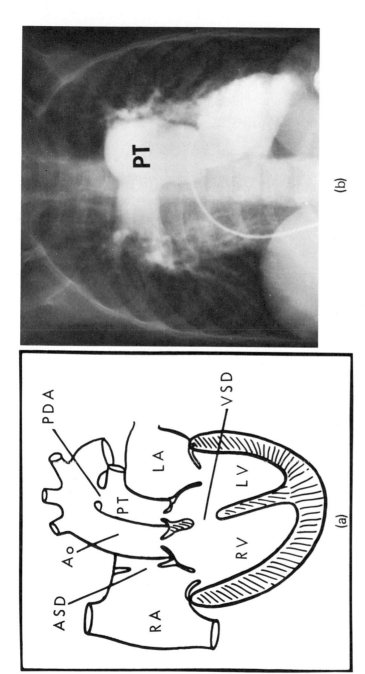

FIGURE 11 (a) Schematic illustration of complete (D) transposition of the great arteries showing the principle types of communications that join the greater and lesser circulations. A large (nonrestrictive) ventricular septal defect (VSD) and/or a large patent ductus arteriosus (PDA) result in obligatory pulmonary hypertension with identical systolic pressures in aorta (Ao) and pulmonary trunk (PT). Pulmonary hypertension can also occur with isolated atrial septal defect. (b) Angiocardiogram from a 7-year-old boy with complete transposition of the great arteries, intact ventricular septum, large atrial septal defect, and patent ductus arteriosus. The dilated transposed pulmonary trunk (PT) visualized when contrast material was injected into the left ventricle. (With permission, J. K. Perloff, *The Clinical Recognition of Congenital Heart Disease,* 2nd ed.)

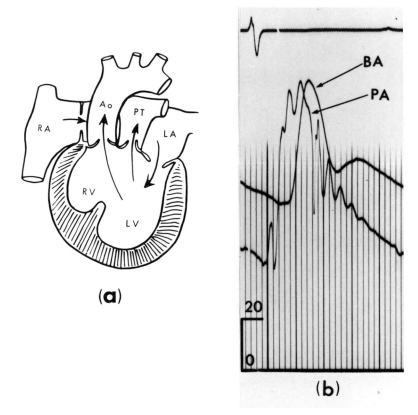

FIGURE 12   (a) Schematic illustration of tricuspid atresia with transposition of the great arteries, no pulmonic stenosis, and large ventricular septal defect. The pressure in the pulmonary trunk (PT) is necessarily systemic. The pulmonary vascular resistance determines the amount of blood entering the lungs. (b) Tracings from an 18-year-old boy (unusual longevity) with tricuspid atresia, complete transposition of the great arteries, no pulmonic stenosis, and large ventricular septal defect. The pulmonary resistance was at systemic levels. The brachial arterial (BA) and pulmonary arterial (PA) pressures were identical in systole. (With permission, J. K. Perloff, *The Clinical Recognition of Congenital Heart Disease,* 2nd ed.)

consequences of reversed (right-to-left) septal depolarization owing to inversion of the conduction system.

In the neonate with "simple" transposition of the great arteries (isolated atrial septal defect), the initial fall in pulmonary arterial pressure and pulmonary vascular resistance usually follows a normal time course. In com-

complete transposition with large ventricular septal defect, however, there is a strong tendency for the development of severe pulmonary vascular obstructive disease in the first 6 months to 1 year of life [25]. The same appears to be true for large patent ductus arteriosus with intact ventricular septum. There seems to be little doubt that early severe pulmonary vascular disease prevails in transposition with high-pressure and high-flow intercirculatory connections (Figs. 11 and 12). Nevertheless, more than an occasional infant with intact ventricular septum and closed ductus arteriosus develops advanced pulmonary vascular disease, some coming to necropsy at 3 to 11 months of age [26]. In addition, pulmonary vascular disease occurs earlier with large ventricular septal defect *and* transposition of the great arteries than with isolated ventricular septal defect of the same size [17]. Accordingly, mechanisms other than high-pressure/high-flow intercirculatory communications have been proposed to explain the particular propensity to pulmonary vascular obstruction in patients with complete transposition. Hypoxia is known to produce pulmonary arteriolar constriction, and there are two possible pathways by which hypoxemic systemic arterial blood can reach the pulmonary resistance vessels in transposition [17]. First, nutrient bronchial arteries perfuse the vasovasora of the pulmonary arteries, and second, bronchopulmonary anastomoses have been found at the precapillary level of the pulmonary vascular bed.

In addition to pulmonary hypertension (high pulmonary vascular resistance) with naturally occurring cardiac shunts, increased pulmonary resistance and pressure may result from palliative (surgical) shunts, as in Fallot's tetralogy [27]. The Potts-Smith-Gibson operation (no longer used) was the greatest offender since the communications were generally large and nonrestrictive. Pulmonary hypertension occasionally follows a Waterston shunt (ascending aorta to right pulmonary artery) but rarely follows a Blalock-Taussig anastomosis.

VI. Prearteriolar Vascular Bed in Congenital Heart Disease

Prearteriolar pulmonary vascular obstruction causing pulmonary hypertension occurs with congenital stenosis of the pulmonary artery and its branches [17,29]. The arterioles are normal since they are beyond the critical zones of pulmonary arterial narrowing. Congenital stenosis of the pulmonary artery and its branches is unique among causes of pulmonary hypertension because it elevates pulmonary systolic but not diastolic pressure, and the pulmonary valve closes at a normal (or even low) [2] pressure. Accordingly, a tell-tale increase in the pulmonic component of the second sound is not present. The chief clue is the presence of other physical signs of pulmonary hypertension, together with peripheral thoracic murmurs in right and left axillae, right anterior chest, and back [29]. The chest X-ray shows, as a rule, a nondilated pulmonary trunk, but may reveal poststenotic dilatation of the intrapulmonary branches distal to the zones of obstruction.

VII. Pulmonary Parenchymal Changes in Congenital Heart Disease

The cardiac consequences of pulmonary hypertension associated with parenchymal disease of the lung are chiefly sequelae of right ventricular failure. Coexisting hypoxemia is usually due to the parenchymal disease itself and not to pulmonary hypertension, although reversed shunt through a foramen ovale may contribute, and a decrease in alveolar PO_2 may aggravate the pulmonary hypertension. Idiopathic respiratory distress in premature infants affects the airways (distal alveolar and proximal prealveolar) and is potentially reversible. In the idiopathic respiratory distress syndrome, the combination of tachypnea, cyanosis, clinical evidence of pulmonary hypertension, and heart failure requires differential diagnosis between primary lung disease and congenital cardiac disease. In fact, the two may coexist, especially patent ductus [17]. Idiopathic respiratory distress is a feature of prematurity, and persistent patency of the ductus is much more likely in the premature infant whether idiopathic respiratory distress is present or not. Nevertheless, in the clinical management of idiopathic respiratory distress in the premature infant, it is important if not critical to identify the presence of a coexisting ductus which is likely to be large.

VIII. Hypoventilation in Congenital Heart Disease

Pulmonary hypertension (an increase in pulmonary vascular resistance) can result from alveolar hypoventilation caused by upper airways obstruction due to large tonsils in infants and young children [22]. The consequences of this form of pulmonary hypertension are right ventricular hypertrophy and failure. Hypoxia and hypercapnea are related to hypoventilation per se, although a right-to-left shunt via a patent foramen ovale may also contribute. The distinction from congenital cardiac disease is important, since removal of the offending tonsils is curative.

IX. Management of Pulmonary Hypertension in Congenital Heart Disease

The management of pulmonary hypertension, or more precisely, increased pulmonary vascular resistance in congenital heart disease, continues to be a matter of concern [11]. Let us again use ventricular septal defect as a point of departure. In infants born with large nonrestrictive ventricular septal defects, the high neonatal pulmonary vascular resistance exhibits one of four subsequent patterns described earlier: normal regression of the fetal pulmonary arterioles with a proportionate fall in resistance; delayed or incomplete regression; a rise in pulmonary vascular resistance after initial complete or partial regression; or, rarely, persistence of the high pulmonary vascular resistance of the newborn [17]. Relevant to this discussion is the patient with elevated pulmonary vascular resistance but a persistent left-to-right shunt. Selection of such patients for operation depends upon a question that is simple to pose but difficult to answer; namely, at what stage will removal of the stimulus of the left-to-right shunt still allow acceptable regression of pulmonary arteriolar disease? At what stage is the high-resistance arteriole still capable of anatomical involution? If the postoperative pulmonary vascular resistance does not adequately fall, pressure overload of the right ventricle persists and regression of hypertrophy is eclipsed. Surgical closure of large ventricular septal defects in early infancy is not followed by late development of pulmonary vascular obstructive disease, which may be the case if the defect is closed later in life [11].

In complete transposition of the great arteries (Fig. 11), the problem is more complex. In such infants with large ventricular septal defects, pulmonary vascular disease is more severe and occurs earlier than in infants with uncomplicated ventricular septal defects of the same size [24]. Accordingly, surgical intervention is appropriate in early infancy if irreversible pulmonary obstruction is to be circumvented. The Mustard operation achieves this end by redirecting venous inflows with insertion of an intraatrial pericardial partition [11]. The partition directs pulmonary venous blood across the tricuspid valve into the anatomical right ventricle, which continues to function as a systemic pump; systemic venous blood is directed across the mitral valve into the left ventricle, which still functions as the venous ventricle. A ventricular septal defect, if present, can usually be closed via the tricuspid valve without right ventriculotomy. The problem of progressive pulmonary vascular disease may be solved, but an important question remains unanswered; namely, whether an anatomical right ventricle can perform as a systemic chamber as well as an anatomical left ventricle [11]. In the patient with a large left-to-right shunt and normal pulmonary arterial pressure and resistance (as an ostium secundum atrial septal defect), adult development of elevated pulmonary arterial pressure does not preclude surgical closure of the defect [38], provided the pulmonary to systemic flow ratio is at least 2:1 (Fig. 2). Although it is not certain that the pulmonary arteriolar disease will involute after operation, there is evidence that progression is arrested. When pulmonary vascular resistance is above systemic in patients with shunts at either atrial, ventricular, or great artery level, surgical correction not only plays no useful role, but the converse is the case, since closure of the communication deprives the right ventricle of its means of decompressing into the systemic circulation. The clinical problem then becomes one of managing the compensatory rise in red cell mass so that it is optimal for tissue oxygenation but not excessive and therefore not independently hazardous [39,40].

References

1.   Cournand, A., Pulmonary circulation, *Science,* **125**:1231–1235 (1957).
2.   Perloff, J. K., Auscultatory and phonocardiographic manifestations of pulmonary hypertension, *Prog. Cardiovasc. Dis.,* **9**:303–340 (1967).
3.   Rudolph, A. B., The changes in circulation after birth. Their importance in congenital heart disease, *Circulation,* **41**:343–359 (1970).
4.   Levin, D. L., A. M. Rudolph, M. A. Heymann, and R. H. Phibbs, Morphological development of the pulmonary vascular bed in fetal lambs, *Circulation,* **53**:144–151 (1976).
5.   Dawes, G. S., Changes in the circulation at birth, *Br. Med. Bull.,* **17**:148–153 (1961).
6.   Perloff, J. K., Congenital heart diseases. In *Textbook of Medicine.* Edited by P. B. Beeson, W. McDermott, and J. B. Wyngaarden. Philadelphia, Saunders, 1979, pp. 1149–1174.
7.   Fishman, A. P., Hypoxia on the pulmonary circulation. How and where it acts, *Circ. Res.,* **38**:221–231 (1976).
8.   Arias-Stella, J., and M. Saldana, The terminal portion of the pulmonary arterial tree in people native to high altitudes, *Circulation,* **28**:915–925 (1963).
9.   Roberts, W. C., Histologic structure of the pulmonary trunk in patients with primary pulmonary hypertension, *Am. Heart J.,* **65**:230–236 (1963).
10. Danilowicz, D. A., A. M. Rudolph, J. I. E. Hoffman, and M. Heyman, Physiologic pressure differences between the main and branch pulmonary arteries in infants, *Circulation,* **45**:410–419 (1972).
11. Perloff, J. K., The pediatric congenital cardiac becomes a postoperative adult, *Circulation,* **47**:606–619 (1973).
12. Bevegard, S., A. Holmgren, and B. Jonsson, Circulatory studies in well trained athletes at rest and during heavy exercise, with special reference to stroke volume, *Acta Physiol. Scand.,* **57**:26–50 (1963).

13. Gurtner, H. P., P. Walser, and B. Fassler, Normal values for pulmonary hemodynamics at rest and during exercise, *Prog. Respir. Res.*, **9**:295–315 (1975).

14. Sime, F., D. Penaloza, and L. Ruiz, Bradycardia, increased cardiac output and reversal of pulmonary hypertension in altitude natives living at sea level, *Br. Heart J.*, **33**:647–657 (1971).

15. Szidon, J. P., and A. P. Fishman, Autonomic control of the pulmonary circulation. In *Pulmonary Circulation and Interstitial Space*. Edited by A. P. Fishman and H. H. Hecht. Chicago, University of Chicago Press, 1969.

16. McGaff, C. J., J. Ross, and E. Braunwald, The development of elevated pulmonary vascular resistance in man following increased pulmonary blood flow from systemic-pulmonary anastomoses, *Am. J. Med.*, **33**:201–212 (1962).

17. Perloff, J. K., *The Clinical Recognition of Congenital Heart Disease*, 2nd ed. Philadelphia, Saunders, 1978.

18. Heath, D., and J. E. Edwards, The pathology of hypertensive pulmonary vascular disease, *Circulation*, **18**:533–547 (1958).

19. Brammell, H. L., J. H. K. Vogel, B. Pryor, and S. G. Blount, The Eisenmenger syndrome, *Am. J. Cardiol.*, **28**:679–692 (1971).

20. Mellins, R. B., H. H. Balfour, G. M. Turino, and R. W. Winters, Failure of automatic control of ventilation (Ondine's curse). Report of an infant born with this syndrome and review of the literature, *Medicine*, **49**:487–504 (1970).

21. Siasi, B., S. J. Goldberg, G. C. Emmanouilides, S. M. Higashino, and E. Lewis, Persistent pulmonary vascular obstruction in newborn infants, *J. Pediatr.*, **78**:610–615 (1971).

22. Djalilian, M., E. B. Kern, H. A. Brown, G. W. Facer, G. B. Stickler, W. H. Weidman, and E. J. O'Connell, Hypoventilation secondary to chronic upper airway obstruction in childhood, *Mayo Clin. Proc.*, **50**:11–14 (1975).

23. Burrows, B., Arterial oxygenation and pulmonary hemodynamics in patients with chronic airway obstruction, *Am. Rev. Respir. Dis.*, **110**:64–70 (1975).

24. Bessinger, F. B., L. C. Blieden, and J. E. Edwards, Hypertensive pulmonary vascular disease associated with patent ductus arteriosus: Primary or secondary, *Circulation*, **52**:157–161 (1975).

25. Clarkson, P. M., J. M. Neutze, J. C. Wardill, and B. G. Barratt-Boyes, The pulmonary vascular bed in patients with complete transposition of the great arteries, *Circulation*, **53**:539–543 (1976).

26. Lakier, J. B., P. Stanger, M. A. Heymann, J. I. E. Hoffman, and A. M. Rudolph, Early onset of pulmonary vascular obstruction in patients with aortopulmonary transposition and intact ventricular septum, *Circulation*, **51**:875–880 (1975).

27. Hofschire, P. J., Q. C. Rosenquist, P. N. Ruckerman, J. H. Moller, and J. E. Edwards, Pulmonary vascular disease complicating the Blalock-Taussig anastomosis, *Circulation*, **56**:124–126 (1977).

28. Burnell, R. H., M. C. Joseph, and M. H. Lees, Progressive pulmonary hypertension in newborn infants, *Am. J. Dis. Child.*, 123:167–170 (1972).

29. Perloff, J. K., and E. J. Lebauer, Auscultatory and phonocardiographic manifestations of isolated stenosis of the pulmonary artery and its branches, *Br. Heart J.*, 31:314–321 (1969).

30. Feigenbaum, H., *Echocardiography*, 2nd ed. Philadelphia, Lea & Febiger, 1976.

31. Nanda, N. C., R. Gramiak, T. I. Robinson, and P. M. Shah, Echocardiographic evaluation of pulmonary hypertension, *Circulation*, 50:575–581 (1974).

32. de Leon, A. C., J. K. Perloff, H. Twigg, and M. Majd, The straight back syndrome, *Circulation*, 32:193–203 (1965).

33. Roberts, W. C., and J. K. Perloff, Mitral valvular disease, *Ann. Intern. Med.*, 77:939–975 (1972).

34. Guyton, A. C., A. W. Lindsey, and J. J. Gilluly, The limits of right ventricular compensation following acute increase in pulmonary circulatory resistance, *Circ. Res.*, 2:326–332 (1954).

35. Hultgren, H. N., and E. Lundberg, Medical problems of high altitude, *Mod. Conc. Cardiovasc. Dis.*, 31:719–724 (1962).

36. Banchero, N., F. Sime, D. Penaloza, J. Cruz, R. Gamboa, and E. Marticorena, Pulmonary pressure, cardiac output, and arterial oxygen saturation during exercise at high altitude and sea level, *Circulation*, 33:249–262 (1966).

37. Laursen, H. B., Congenital heart disease in Down's syndrome, *Br. Heart J.*, 38:32–38 (1976).

38. Gault, J. H., A. G. Morrow, W. A. Gay, and J. Ross, Atrial septal defect in patients over the age of 40 years, *Circulation*, 37:261–272 (1968).

39. Rosenthal, A., L. N. Britton, D. G. Nathan, O. S. Miettinen, and A. S. Nadas, Blood volume changes in cyanotic congenital heart disease, *Am. J. Cardiol.*, 27:162–167 (1971).

40. Rosenthal, A., D. G. Nathan, A. T. Marty, L. N. Britton, O. S. Miettinen, and A. S. Nadas, Acute hemodynamic effects of red cell volume reduction in polycythemia of cyanotic congenital heart disease, *Circulation*, 42:297–307 (1970).

9

Congenital Pulmonary Vascular Disorders

JESSE E. EDWARDS

United Hospitals, Miller Division,
St. Paul, Minnesota;
University of Minnesota,
Minneapolis, Minnesota

I.   Introduction

Anomalies involving the pulmonary vessels cover a broad field. The subject is divided here according to anatomical segments and considering the conditions peculiar to each. Thus, the basic subdivision will be according to conditions affecting the pulmonary trunk, the pulmonary arterial branches, and the pulmonary veins. The concluding section will be concerned with pulmonary arteriovenous connections.

II.   Pulmonary Trunk

Among the anomalies of the pulmonary trunk are idiopathic dilatation, obstruction of the lumen, communication with the aorta, and origin of coronary arteries from this segment of the pulmonary arterial system.

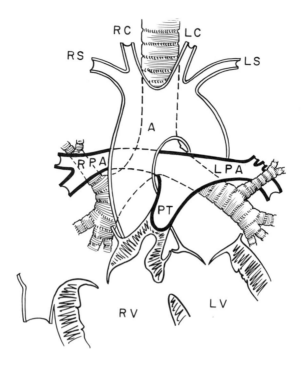

FIGURE 1   Atresia of the origin of the pulmonary trunk (PT) in tetralogy of
Fallot (pseudotruncus arteriosus). (From Edwards and McGoon [7] ; reproduced
with permission.)

A.   Idiopathic Dilatation

The pulmonary trunk may be dilated as a consequence of hemodynamic stresses
in various types of congenital cardiac disease. In contrast, idiopathic dilatation
of the pulmonary trunk is characterized by dilatation of this vessel in the absence of pulmonary stenosis, of pulmonary hypertension, and of inflammatory
disease of this vessel [1]. The condition may represent a *forme fruste* of
Marfan's syndrome [2], with histologically demonstrable cystic medial
necrosis [3].

Pulmonary valvular insufficiency has been observed in 29 and 25% of
cases reported by Brayshaw and Perloff [4] and by Ishikawa and Seki [5],
respectively. This condition may represent a complication of the dilated state
of the pulmonary trunk. Pulmonary valvular insufficiency, if present, is well
tolerated by the myocardium [6], and, in general, the prognosis is good.

B. Luminal Obstruction

Obstruction of the lumen of the pulmonary trunk may take the form of either stenosis or atresia.

Atresia and certain forms of stenosis of the pulmonary trunk characteristically are associated with an intracardiac anomalous state, usually ventricular septal defect and other features of the tetralogy of Fallot. In such an association, stenosis of the pulmonary trunk takes the form of a more-or-less uniform narrow caliber to the pulmonary trunk. Atresia may be restricted to the level of the root of the pulmonary trunk or it may involve the full length of the pulmonary trunk. When atresia is localized to the general level of the root of the pulmonary trunk, the caliber of the remainder of the vessel varies from narrower than normal to normal (Fig. 1).

When atresia involves the entire length of the vessel, the atresia may be represented by an identifiable cord-like structure, while the left and right pulmonary arteries are identifiable as confluent vessels (Fig. 2) [7]. A similar pattern of the left and right pulmonary arteries without identification of an atretic pulmonary trunk may be taken as a sign of atresia of the pulmonary trunk at an early stage in development, with loss of this vessel as an identifiable structure (Fig. 2). If the pulmonary trunk cannot be identified and the left

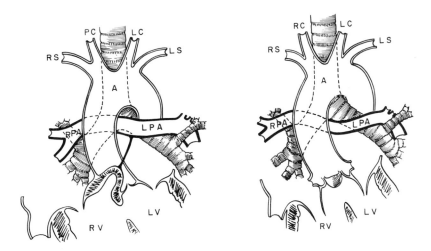

FIGURE 2 Atresia of entire length of pulmonary trunk with confluence of the left (LPA) and right (RPA) pulmonary arteries. (Left) The pulmonary trunk is identifiable. (Right) The pulmonary trunk is not identifiable. (From Edwards and McGoon [7]; reproduced with permission.)

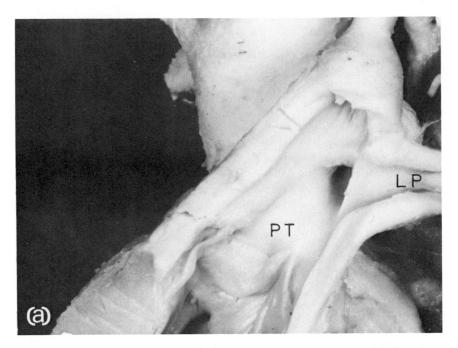

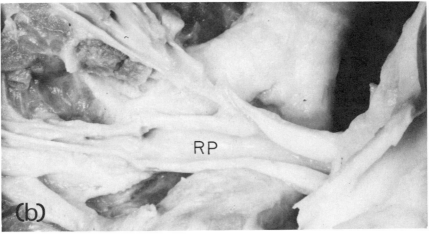

FIGURE 3   Pulmonary arterial stenosis as part of the syndrome of supravalvular aortic stenosis. (a) A pulmonary trunk (PT) shows uniformly pronounced thickening of its wall. The origin of the left pulmonary artery (LPA) is similarly involved. (b) The right pulmonary artery and its branches. The main vessel (RP) shows thickening of its wall like that observed in the left pulmonary artery and the pulmonary trunk in (a). One of the branches shows similar thickening of its wall. (From Blieden and associates [9]; reproduced with permission.)

and right pulmonary arteries are shown to exhibit "distal ductal origin" (see below), it is justifiable to consider that there is in fact true absence of the pulmonary trunk, the single arterial vessel being termed a *solitary aortic trunk* [8].

In the absence of intracardiac malformations, stenosis of the pulmonary trunk is part of the syndrome of supravalvular aortic stenosis. The change in the pulmonary trunk classically is that of uniform thickening of its media with corresponding encroachment upon the lumen. The process in the pulmonary trunk resembles that in the aorta involved by the hypoplastic type of supravalvular aortic stenosis [9]. The lesion may be associated with stenosis of peripheral pulmonary arteries (Fig. 3).

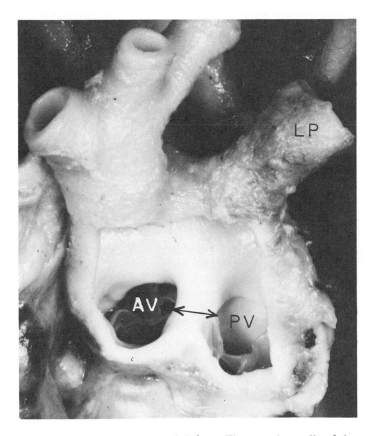

FIGURE 4 Aorticopulmonary septal defect. The anterior walls of the aorta and the pulmonary trunk have been opened to expose the aortic (AV) and pulmonary (PV) valves. The communication between the two great vessels (arrow) represents the aorticopulmonary septal defect. LP = left pulmonary artery.

C.   Communication of Pulmonary Trunk with Aorta
(Aorticopulmonary Septal Defect)

In those instances where there are both aortic and pulmonary valvular orifices
and normal branching of the pulmonary trunk, there may be a window-like
communication between the pulmonary trunk and ascending aorta (Fig. 4).
The communication, usually called aorticopulmonary septal defect or aorticopulmonary window, lies in the adjacent walls of these two vessels [10]. From
the pulmonary aspect, the defect, which is relatively large and unobstructive,
lies in close proximity to the origin of the right pulmonary artery, while from
the aortic aspect the defect lies superior to the origin of the left coronary
artery from the aorta.

This uncommon condition is not usually, and not universally, associated
with other congenital cardiovascular anomalies. In a review of 66 cases (60 from
from the literature), Neufeld and associates [11] found that patent ductus
arteriosus was the most commonly associated anomaly (12%). Less common
significant anomalies were coarctation of the aorta, anomalous origin of a pulmonary artery from the aorta, tetralogy of Fallot, and atrial septal defect.

D.   Origin of Pulmonary Arterial System
from Persistent Truncus Arteriosus

In those instances where the embryonic truncus arteriosus fails to divide into
aorta and pulmonary trunk, the condition is known as persistent truncus
arteriosus [12]. The resulting anatomical situation is a ventricular septal
defect above which arises a single arterial vessel guarded by a solitary semilunar valve. From the single arterial vessel arise the coronary arteries, aorta,
and pulmonary arterial system (Fig. 5a). The manner of origin of the pulmonary arteries is a basis for subdividing persistent truncus arteriosus into three
basic types (Fig. 5 b–d) [13]. In type I, a partial septum is present so that a
pulmonary trunk, usually of short nature, is present. From the latter, the left
and right pulmonary arteries arise. In type II, there is no pulmonary trunk,
the left and right pulmonary arteries arising independently from the posterior
aspect of the truncus arteriosus. Types I and II are the most common [14,15].
The rare type III is characterized by origin of the left and right pulmonary
arteries from the homolateral aspects of the truncus arteriosus.

Abnormalities of the truncal valve are common, of which incompetence
is a more usual consequence than stenosis [16,17]. Interruption of the aortic
arch may be associated, being observed in about 10% of cases. A right aortic
arch occurs in over 30% of cases. Origin of either the left or right pulmonary
artery may be anomalous, arising from an aortic source rather than from the
truncus or pulmonary trunk, if present.

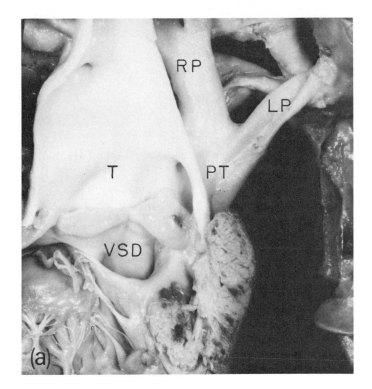

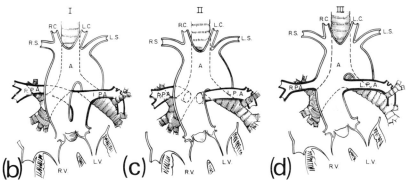

FIGURE 5 (a) Persistent truncus arteriosus. Arising above a ventricular septal defect (VSD) is a single vessel, the persistent truncus arteriosus (T). Arising from this vessel is a short pulmonary trunk (PT) and from the latter there arise the left (LP) and right (RP) pulmonary arteries. (b), (c), and (d) Variations in the manner of origin of the pulmonary arteries in persistent truncus arteriosus. (b) Type I, in which the left and right pulmonary arteries arise from a pulmonary trunk. (c) Type II. The right and left pulmonary arteries arise independently from the dorsal aspect of the truncus arteriosus. (d) Type III. The left and right pulmonary arteries arise independently from the lateral aspects of the truncus arteriosus. [(b), (c), and (d) from Edwards and McGoon [7]; reproduced with permission].

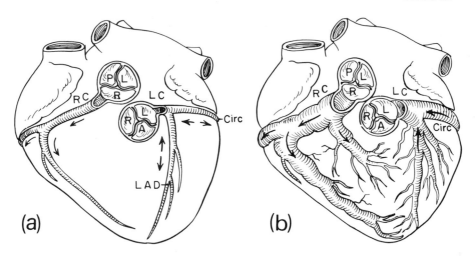

FIGURE 6   Anomalous origin of the left coronary artery (LC) from the pulmonary trunk. (a) The situation in the newborn, in whom collaterals are not well developed. The flow in the left coronary artery may be either from or toward the pulmonary trunk. (b) The situation in older children and adults, in whom a large collateral circulation is developed between the two coronary arteries. Through these collaterals, blood from the right coronary artery is carried into the left coronary arterial system for ultimate delivery to the pulmonary trunk. In (a) and (b), RC, LAD, and Circ = right, anterior descending, and left circumflex coronary arteries, respectively; P, L, and R = posterior, left, and right sinus of the aorta; A, L, and R = anterior, left, and right sinuses of the pulmonary trunk. (From Vlodaver and associates, *Coronary Arterial Variations in the Normal Heart and in Congenital Heart Disease*. Academic Press, 1975; reproduced with permission.)

E.   Anomalous Coronary Arterial Origin from Pulmonary Trunk

Uncommonly, part or all of the coronary arterial origin may be from the pulmonary trunk. While cases of both coronary arteries arising in this fashion have been described, such a situation is extremely rare. Death in the newborn period is classic [18,19]. Usually in anomalous coronary arterial origin from the pulmonary trunk, one artery arises normally from the aorta, while the other arises anomalously from the pulmonary trunk.

The more common situation is for the left coronary artery to arise anomalously [20-22], but sporadic cases have been observed in which the right coronary artery is the one involved by anomalous origin.

Origin of the left coronary artery from the pulmonary artery tends to cause death either in infancy or in childhood, but survival to adult life may occur (Fig. 6a). The longer the patient lives, the better developed is a collateral system of vessels between the normally arising right artery and the anomalously arising left coronary artery [23].

This collateral system provides a basis for an arteriovenous-like series of shunts between the two arteries terminating through the left coronary artery in the pulmonary trunk. Concomitant with this type of flow is progressive enlargement of the two coronary arteries. In the rare patient reaching adult life, the major coronary arteries may achieve diameters of about 1 cm (Fig. 6b).

Variations of origin of the left coronary artery from the pulmonary trunk are anomalous origin either of the anterior descending (Fig. 7a) or the left circumflex artery, while the other terminal branch of the left coronary artery arises independently from the aorta [24,25].

Anomalous origin of the right coronary artery from the pulmonary trunk is less common than anomalous origin of the left coronary artery (Fig. 7b). While death in infancy may occur, there is a tendency for subjects with

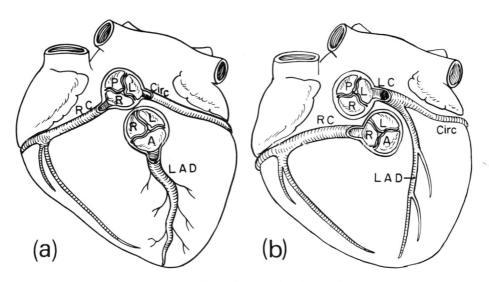

(a) (b)

FIGURE 7 (a) Anomalous origin of the anterior descending coronary artery from the pulmonary trunk, while the left circumflex artery arises from the aorta. (b) Anomalous origin of the right coronary artery from the pulmonary trunk. In (a) and (b) abbreviations are as for Figure 6. (From Vlodaver and associates. *Coronary Arterial Variations in the Normal Heart and in Congenital Heart Disease.* Academic Press, 1975; reproduced with permission.)

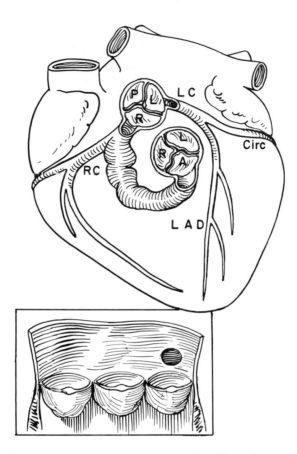

FIGURE 8 Accessory coronary artery arising from the pulmonary trunk, while the usual coronary arteries arise from the aorta. Collaterals develop in which blood from either or both coronary arteries is carried into the accessory artery for delivery to the pulmonary trunk. Insert shows accessory coronary artery arising from the pulmonary trunk. (From Vlodaver and associates. *Coronary Arterial Variations in the Normal Heart and in Congenital Heart Disease.* Academic Press, 1975; reproduced with permission.)

anomalous origin of the right artery to reach adult life without evident adverse effects [26]. There are, however, cases of premature death [27].

There are rare instances in which both coronary arteries arise from the aorta while one or several *accessory coronary arteries arise from the pulmonary trunk* (Fig. 8). The latter vessels make collateral communications with ramifications of the normally arising coronary arteries. Through such communications, arteriovenous-like shunts develop, resulting in enlargement of the accessory artery or arteries [28]. In exceptional cases, one accessory artery may achieve huge proportions, and the communicating collaterals are prominently tortuous and even aneurysmal [29].

III. Pulmonary Arterial Branches

The pulmonary arterial branches are subject to anomalous origin, stenosis, or atresia.

A. Anomalous Origin

Anomalous origin of a pulmonary arterial branch may be unilateral or bilateral. The anomalous conditions may involve origins of the pulmonary arterial branches either from the pulmonary arterial system or from the aorta or its branches.

Origin from Pulmonary Arterial System

The term, *crossed pulmonary arteries,* has been applied to that state wherein the pulmonary arteries arise either from the pulmonary trunk or from a persistent truncus arteriosus in such a way that the ostia of the two branches are malplaced. The right pulmonary artery arises to the left of and at a lower level than the origin of the left pulmonary artery. Having such origins, the pulmonary arteries cross one another as they proceed to their respective lungs (Fig. 9) [30]. The ductus arteriosus occupies a normal position, originating from the proximal segment of the left pulmonary artery. When crossed pulmonary arteries are associated with persistent truncus arteriosus, there is, in our experience, associated interruption of the aortic arch [31]. The condition of crossed pulmonary arteries, while interesting, does not itself appear to be of functional significance.

Of greater significance is the condition commonly called *vascular sling* [32,33]. This is characterized by origin of the left pulmonary artery from the right pulmonary artery, the anomalous origin being near the right pulmonary hilus and proximal to the usual branches of the right pulmonary artery. After its origin, the left pulmonary artery proceeds posteriorly in relation to the superior aspect of the origin of the right main stem bronchus. The latter may be so compressed as to be responsible for obstructive phenomena in the right lung. The left pulmonary artery then turns to the left, passing between the trachea, in front, and the esophagus, behind. Then, proceeding toward the left lung, it reaches its hilus and supplies the left lung (Fig. 10). In its course, the left pulmonary artery indents the anterior aspect of the esophagus (Fig. 11).

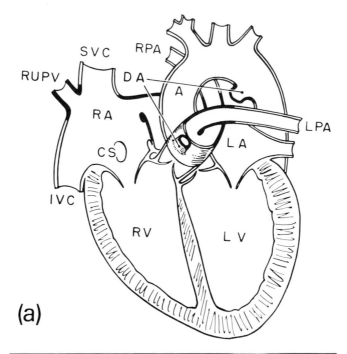

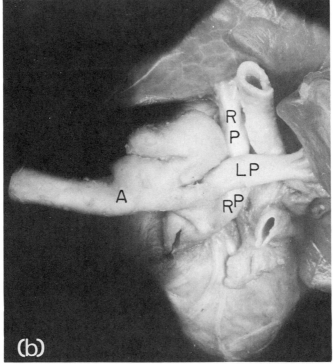

FIGURE 9

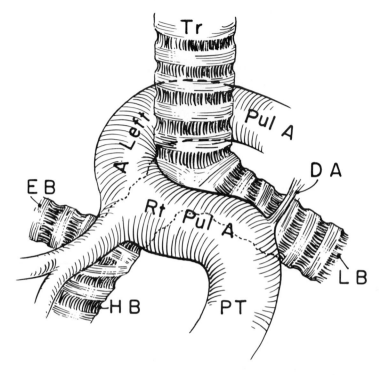

FIGURE 10 Anomalous origin of the left pulmonary artery from the right pulmonary artery (so-called vascular sling). As the left pulmonary artery proceeds toward the left, it crosses over the upper angle formed by the origin of the right main bronchus from the trachea. PT = pulmonary trunk; EB and HB = eparterial and hyparterial bronchi of right lung, respectively; LB = left main bronchus; Tr = trachea. (From Jue and associates [32]; reproduced with permission.)

Among the relatively few cases of this condition, it is inordinately common for the right bronchial tree to show the anomaly of *bronchus suis.* In this, the right upper bronchus arises from the trachea, while the trachea bifurcates into the left main stem bronchus and the right intermediate

---

FIGURE 9 (a) Diagrammatic portrayal of crossed pulmonary arteries associated with a sinus venosus atrial septal defect. LPA and RPA = left and right pulmonary arteries, respectively. (b) The aorta (A) has been retracted to the right exposing the left (LP) and right (RP) pulmonary arteries. The left pulmonary artery arises to the right of the right artery, leading to a situation in which the pulmonary arteries cross. (From Jue and associates [30]; reproduced with permission.)

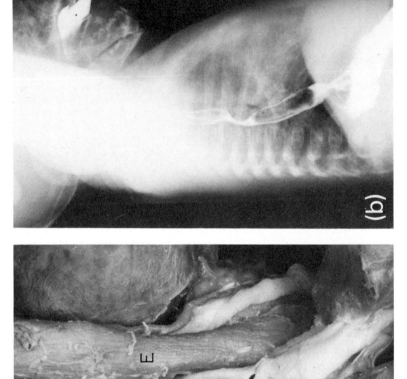

FIGURE 11 Indentation of anterior aspect of esophagus by anomalously arising left pulmonary artery. (a) The mediastinal structures viewed from the left showing the left pulmonary artery (LP) lying between the trachea (Tr) anteriorly and the esophagus (E) posteriorly. The esophagus is indented by the left pulmonary artery. (b) Lateral view of esophagram showing indentation of the anterior aspect of esophagus by anomalously arising left pulmonary artery. (From Jue and associates [32]; reproduced with permission.)

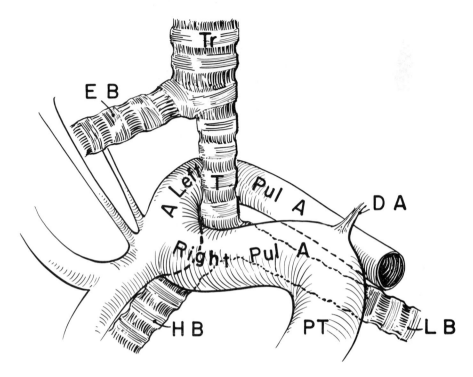

FIGURE 12   Vascular sling associated with bronchus suis. The eparterial (EB) bronchus arises independently from the trachea as the essential feature of bronchus suis. The associated anomalous origin of the left pulmonary artery from the right pulmonary artery shows the course of the left pulmonary artery to be of such nature that it passes from the right to the left in the angle formed by the hyparterial bronchus (HB) and the trachea (Tr). (From Jue and associates [32]; reproduced with permission.)

bronchus. Associated with this bronchial anomaly, the anomalous left pulmonary artery passes over the intermediate bronchus (Fig. 12).

Congenital heart disease may be associated, the most common type being the tetralogy of Fallot.

Origin from the Aorta or Its Branches

One or both pulmonary arteries may arise from the aorta or its branches, usually the innominate artery. Two forms of such anomalous origin are present. In one form, one of the pulmonary arteries arises from the ascending aorta. In the other form, termed *distal ductal origin,* one or both pulmonary arteries arise either from the aortic arch by way of the ductus arteriosus

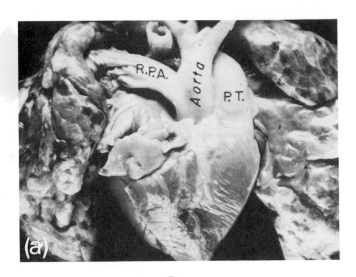

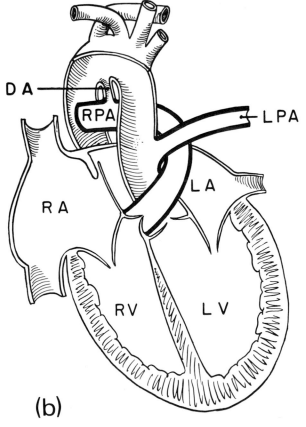

FIGURE 13

or from the base of the innominate artery. Accessory arteries to the lung from the lower thoracic or abdominal aorta occur in sequestration of the lung.

When a *pulmonary artery* displays *origin from the ascending aorta,* there is a pulmonary trunk that simply continues as the contralateral pulmonary artery (Fig. 13). It is about 4 times more common for the right pulmonary artery to arise in this fashion than the left [34]. Usually, no intracardiac anomalies are present. Origin of a pulmonary artery from the ascending aorta is to be distinguished from so-called distal ductal origin.

In *distal ductal origin of a pulmonary artery,* one or both pulmonary arteries may be involved. The stem of such origin is considered to be the dorsal segment of the corresponding sixth aortic arch, hence the term "distal ductal origin." Whether such origin is from the aortic arch or the innominate artery depends on the side in which the aortic arch is located and the pulmonary artery involved [35]. Thus, in instances of left aortic arch, the left pulmonary artery showing distal ductal origin arises from the arch (Fig. 14a) and the right pulmonary artery from the innominate (Fig. 14b). The reverse applies when the aortic arch is right-sided.

Distal ductal origin may be unilateral or bilateral. When it is unilateral, the opposite pulmonary artery arises as a continuation of the pulmonary trunk. When distal ductal origin is bilateral, there is no pulmonary trunk; the condition from the point of view of the great vessels is called *solitary aortic trunk* (Fig. 14c).

It is not uncommon that varying lengths of a pulmonary artery showing distal ductal origin are stenotic or atretic. The most common situation is for the obstruction to lie in the proximal segment and may represent postnatal closure of the ductal segment of the artery. In some cases, the artery showing distal ductal origin is atretic from its origin to the pulmonary hilus. At the latter location, a patent vessel is usually identifiable (Fig. 14d). When there is atresia of a vessel showing distal ductal origin, the contralateral vessel may also be atretic but arising from an atretic pulmonary trunk.

Apart from bronchial and other collateral arteries to the lungs in cases with pulmonary stenosis or atresia, there is the entity of *sequestration of the*

FIGURE 13   Anomalous origin of a pulmonary artery from the ascending aorta. (a) Origin of the right pulmonary artery (RPA) from the aorta. Characteristically, the vessel arises distinctly inferior to the site of origin of the innominate artery. The aortic arch was left-sided. PT = pulmonary trunk. (b) Origin of the left pulmonary artery (LPA) from the ascending aorta associated with a right aortic arch and aberrant left subclavian artery. RPA = right pulmonary artery; DA = right ductus arteriosus. [(a) from DuShane and associates, *Am. Heart J.,* **59**:782 (1960); reproduced with permission.]

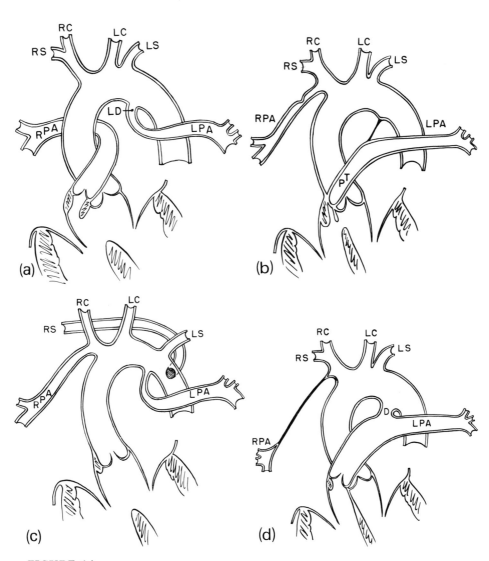

FIGURE 14

lung. In this condition, either an entire lobe or part of a lobe is not in communication with the bronchial system [36]. While the uninvolved portions of the lungs receive a normal arterial supply, the entire or principal arterial supply to the sequestered segment is by way of one or several arteries that arise from either the lower thoracic or the abdominal aorta [36,37]. While the lower lobes are more commonly involved, particularly the left, sequestration may involve the upper lobes [38].

B. Stenosis

Obstruction involving pulmonary arterial branches may take the form of local stenosis or stenoses, on the one hand, or atresia, on the other. As these may represent two separate conditions, the subject of stenosis will be considered in this section and atresia in the following.

The process of stenosis involving pulmonary arterial branches is characterized by focal obstruction or obstructions that may involve the origins of the main pulmonary arterial branches (Fig. 15) and/or one or more foci in secondary and tertiary branches (Fig. 16).

The condition is uncommon. D'Cruz and associates [39] found only 84 cases among approximately 2000 patients in whom diagnostic cardiac catheterization, angiocardiography, or both had been done. Delaney and Nadas [40], during a 7-year experience at the Children's Medical Center, Boston, found only 17 cases among subjects between the ages of 9 months and 13 years.

Relatively little has been written on the pathologic process responsible for stenosis. This appears to be focal intimal proliferation that encroaches upon the lumen and causes obstruction of involved segments. MacMahon and associates [41] additionally observed medial thickening of involved peripheral segments.

FIGURE 14   Examples of distal ductal origin of one or both pulmonary arteries. (a) Left aortic arch with distal ductal origin (LD) of left pulmonary artery (LPA) from aortic arch. RPA = right pulmonary artery. (b) Left aortic arch with distal ductal origin of the right pulmonary artery from the innominate artery. (c) Solitary aortic trunk with bilateral distal ductal origin of the pulmonary arteries associated with left aortic arch. The right subclavian artery (RS) shows aberrant origin from the aorta. (d) Distal ductal origin of the right pulmonary artery with atresia of the vessel to the pulmonary hilus. At the latter location, the right pulmonary artery is patent. D = ductus arteriosus; LPA = left pulmonary artery. (From Sotomora and Edwards [35]; reproduced with permission.)

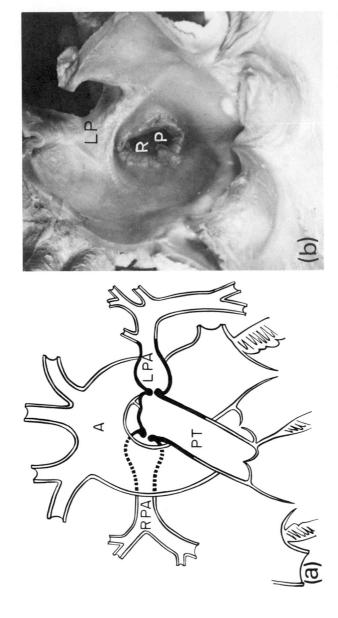

FIGURE 15   (a) Diagrammatic portrayal of localized stenosis of origin of each pulmonary artery.   (b) Interior of pulmonary trunk.   The ostium of the right pulmonary artery (RP) has not been opened, while that of the left (LP) has been opened.   There is a proliferative lesion at the ostium of each of the arteries leading to stenosis.

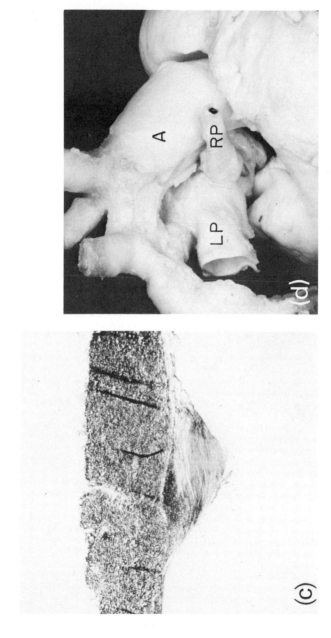

FIGURE 15 (Continued) (c) Photomicrograph of the left pulmonary arterial origin from the case shown in (b). The stenotic lesion is represented by a focus of intimal fibrous proliferation. Elastic tissue stain, ×5. (d) Aortic arch (A) and origins of the left (LP) and right (RP) pulmonary arteries from the pulmonary trunk viewed from behind. The right pulmonary artery (RP) is narrow over a long segment. LP = nonstenotic left pulmonary artery.

From angiographic studies, D'Cruz and associates classified the lesions into four types as follows: (1) localized stenosis with poststenotic dilatation, (2) segmental stenosis, (3) diffuse hypoplasia, and (4) multiple peripheral stenoses. These authors observed that among their 84 cases the stenosis was unilateral in 32 (38%) and bilateral in 52 (62%).

Pulmonary arterial stenosis may be associated with an otherwise normally developed heart, but associated cardiovascular anomalies are common, being observed in about two-thirds of cases with pulmonary arterial stenosis. Commonly associated anomalies include ventricular septal defect and pulmonary stenosis [39,40]. Less common conditions are supravalvular aortic stenosis [42], aortic coarctation, and the tetralogy of Fallot. When not associated with intracardiac anomalies, pulmonary arterial stenosis, if severe, may be confused with primary pulmonary hypertension [43]. Pulmonary arterial stenosis has been identified as a sequel of maternal rubella [44].

C.   Atresia

Atresia of a pulmonary arterial branch may be focal or diffuse. Diffuse atresia of a pulmonary artery often, but not universally, is associated with atresia of the pulmonary trunk and with the intracardiac features of the tetralogy of

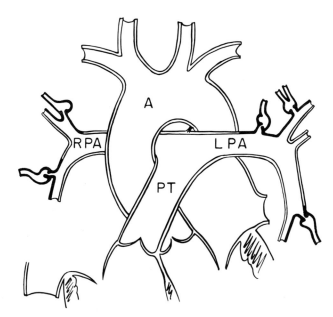

FIGURE 16   Diagrammatic portrayal of multiple sites of stenosis of peripheral pulmonary arteries.

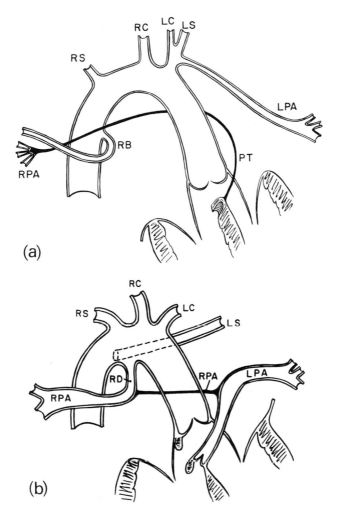

FIGURE 17 Atresia of major segments of pulmonary arterial system. (a) While the right pulmonary artery is patent at the hilus, the proximal segment of the right pulmonary artery and the entire pulmonary trunk are atretic. There is a coexistent distal ductal origin of the left pulmonary artery from the left-sided innominate artery associated with a right aortic arch. RB = bronchial artery. (b) Atresia of the proximal segment of the right pulmonary artery, while the distal segment is patent and is supplied by a right-sided ductus arteriosus (RD) arising from a right aortic arch. The left subclavian artery (LS) shows an aberrant origin from the aorta. (From Sotomora and Edwards [35]; reproduced with permission.)

of Fallot (Fig. 17). In pulmonary arteries that show "distal ductal origin," atresia may be present either in focal or diffuse nature (Fig. 14d). Regardless of the site of origin of a diffusely atretic pulmonary artery, whether from the pulmonary trunk or by distal ductal origin, there is usually patency of the vessel at the level of the pulmonary hilus [35].

IV. Pulmonary Veins

Anomalies of the pulmonary veins include isolated stenoses, anomalous connection of major veins, and combinations of the two.

A. Stenoses

Pulmonary Veno-Occlusive Disease

Pulmonary veno-occlusive disease is that condition in which there are multiple obstructive lesions in the small postcapillary veins, the venules, and small veins [45–47]. The obstructive lesions consist of fibrous thickening of the intima of involved vessels. In some vessels, fibrous septa cross the lumen, suggesting that the disease is primarily that of thrombosis (Fig. 18). If that is true, pulmonary veno-occlusive disease should be considered an acquired rather than a congenital condition. Since the majority of affected individuals are either infants or children, it is not inappropriate for this condition to be included in this chapter, with the justification that at least it needs to be included in the differential diagnosis of those congenital conditions responsible for pulmonary venous obstruction.

An interesting distinction between pulmonary veno-occlusive disease and other states causing pulmonary venous obstruction is that characteristically in the latter there is demonstrable elevation of the pulmonary arterial wedge pressure, while in the former this pressure is not elevated. This may make it difficult to differentiate clinically between pulmonary veno-occlusive disease and primary arterial pulmonary hypertension [48].

Stenosis of Individual Pulmonary Veins

Stenotic lesions may involve either anomalously terminating veins or those that join the left atrium. This section will concern itself only with the latter. Congenital stenosis may occur in one, all, or any combination of pulmonary veins. Hence, the term *stenosis of individual pulmonary veins* seems appropriately applied [49].

Characteristically, the zone of stenosis is localized to the venoatrial junction [50,51], the lesion taking the form of localized intimal fibrous proliferation

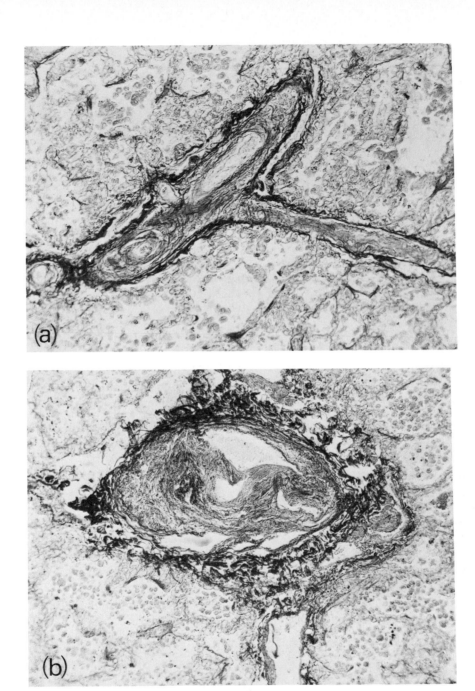

FIGURE 18   Pulmonary veno-occlusive disease. (a) A small vein and its
tributary are narrowed by intimal fibrous thickening. Elastic tissue stain; ×100.
(b) A small vein. Fibrous septa cross the lumen. Elastic tissue stain; ×100.
[From Anderson and associates: *Am. Heart J.*, **97**:233 (1979); reproduced with
permission.]

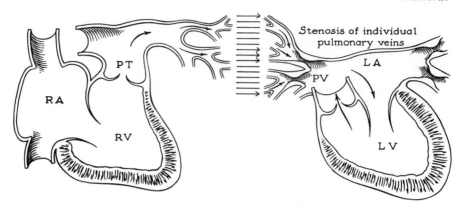

FIGURE 19   Central circulation showing stenosis of each of the pulmonary veins at their junction with the left atrium.

(Fig. 19). In severe forms, the involved veins show atresia at the junction with the left atrium. Hypoplasia of major pulmonary veins may be associated or may appear as an isolated condition of the pulmonary veins [52,53].

The process may be an isolated entity or be associated with various types of intracardiac anomalies of which atrial septal defect appears to be the most common.

B.   Anomalous Connection

When pulmonary veins fail to join the left atrium but instead terminate in a systemic vein, another pulmonary vein, or the right atrium, the term *anomalous pulmonary venous connection* applies. Synonyms include anomalous pulmonary venous drainage or anomalous pulmonary venous return. Anomalous pulmonary venous connection may take an isolated form or be associated with other cardiovascular anomalies. In the latter case the association (1) may be fortuitous, (2) may represent part of a developmental complex, or (3) the anomalous connection may represent a collateral pathway when there is significant obstruction to flow into the left ventricle.

Isolated Forms

Anomalous pulmonary venous connection as an isolated entity may be either total or partial. In the total form, no pulmonary veins join the left atrium; the pulmonary venous blood is carried either directly into the right atrium or indirectly by pulmonary venous connection to a systemic or portal vein. In the partial form, some of the pulmonary veins join the left atrium, while the

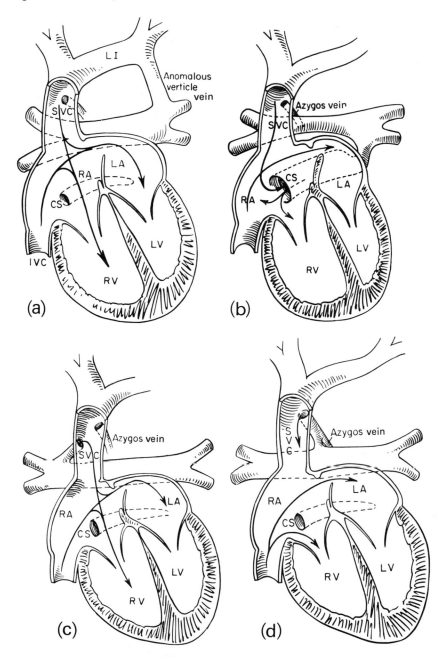

FIGURE 20 Total anomalous pulmonary venous connection. (a) To the left innominate vein (LI) through an anomalous vertical vein. (b) To the coronary sinus (CS). (c) To the superior vena cava (SVC). (d) To the azygous vein.

remainder terminate anomalously. Characteristically, in the isolated form of pulmonary venous connection, the heart is normally developed.

Total Anomalous Pulmonary Venous Connection

In total anomalous pulmonary venous connection, no pulmonary veins join the left atrium. The pulmonary venous blood is carried into the right atrium. The left atrium is supplied through an atrial septal defect. When the pulmonary veins terminate in the right atrium, they do so independently. When, as is more common, the pulmonary venous supply terminates in a systemic vein or the portal venous system, the usual veins leave the lung and then join a chamber-like confluence. The latter lies superior to the left atrium and inferior to the tracheal bifurcation. From the confluence of veins, one vessel leads to the anomalous termination into a systemic vein or an element of the portal venous system. The sites of anomalous connection may be either supradiaphragmatic or subdiaphragmatic.

Sites of supradiaphragmatic termination in order of decreasing frequency are the left innominate vein (Fig. 20), the coronary sinus, the right atrium, the superior vena cava, and the azygous vein [54,55].

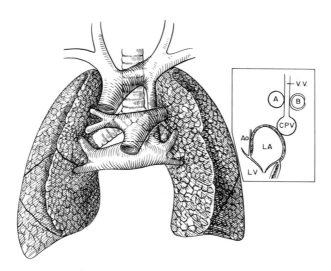

FIGURE 21   Total anomalous pulmonary venous connection to the left innominate vein, with the vertical vein ascending behind the left pulmonary artery. The insert shows the unusual course for the vertical vein (VV) as it lies between the left pulmonary artery (A) anteriorly and the left main bronchus (B) posteriorly. The arrangement creates a hemodynamic vise. (From Elliott and Edwards [56]; reproduced with permission.)

Usually, supradiaphragmatic termination is not associated with pulmonary venous obstruction, but exceptions occur. The most common of these relates to total anomalous pulmonary venous connection to the left innominate vein. More commonly, the vein that ascends from the confluence of pulmonary veins to the left innominate vein runs anteriorly to the left pulmonary hilus. Less commonly, the ascending vein runs between the left pulmonary artery, anteriorly, and the left main bronchus, posteriorly. In this position the ascending anomalous vein is compressed by what has been called a *hemodynamic vise* [56], and pulmonary venous obstruction occurs. (Fig. 21). Additionally, such a vein may be narrow and contain foci of intrinsic stenosis to compound the obstructive process [57]. A process of hemodynamic vise may also occur in anomalous connection to the superior vena cava when the vein ascending from the pulmonary venous confluence to its anomalous termination runs between the right pulmonary artery, anteriorly, and the right main bronchus, posteriorly.

When there is total anomalous connection of pulmonary veins to the coronary sinus, the latter is markedly dilated and may be confused with an accessory atrial chamber lying posteriorly to the left atrium (Fig. 20b).

Total anomalous pulmonary venous connection to the right atrium may be part of the polysplenic syndrome (see below).

When there is total anomalous pulmonary venous connection to the portal venous system, the anomalous vein leaving the confluence of pulmonary veins descends into the abdomen alongside the esophagus, accompanying this structure through the esophageal hiatus of the diaphragm. Having reached the abdominal cavity, the vein then deviates toward the right to terminate in the portal venous system (Fig. 22). In this position, veins that receive the anomalous vein include one of the following: the ductus venosus, the portal vein, or the left gastric vein.

Pulmonary venous obstruction characteristically is manifested in all cases of infradiaphragmatic connection with the portal venous system [58]. Reasons for this include the following factors: (1) high degree of resistance to flow through a long channel; (2) obstruction at the esophageal hiatus (especially during feeding); (3) a narrow state of the receiving vein, especially the ductus venosus; (4) passage of blood through the liver before reaching the right atrium; and (5) occasional occurrence of intrinsic stenosis of the anomalous vein.

A particular type of total anomalous pulmonary venous connection has been termed *atresia of the common pulmonary vein* (Fig. 23). In this condition, as in classic examples of total anomalous pulmonary venous connection, there is a chamber-like confluence of the pulmonary veins leaving the lungs. In contrast, there is no gross channel of exit from the confluence of veins [53,59-61]. Special care in dissection may reveal small veins running from

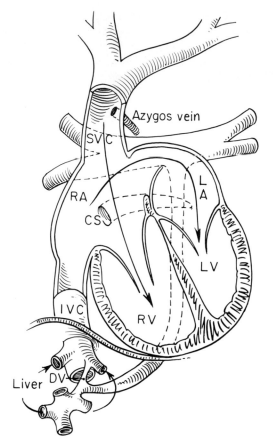

FIGURE 22   Total anomalous pulmonary venous connection to the ductus venosus (DV).

the confluence to enter the esophageal wall [59]. It is probable that the ultimate termination of pulmonary venous blood is into the somatic and visceral veins that receive the venous supply of the esophagus. High degrees of pulmonary venous obstruction are characteristic.

Partial Anomalous Pulmonary Venous Connection

Some pulmonary veins normally terminate in the left atrium, while the remaining pulmonary vein or veins terminate anomalously—*partial anomalous pulmonary venous connection.* In some circumstances, the partial anomalous pulmonary venous connection is the only anomaly; in others, it is fortuitously

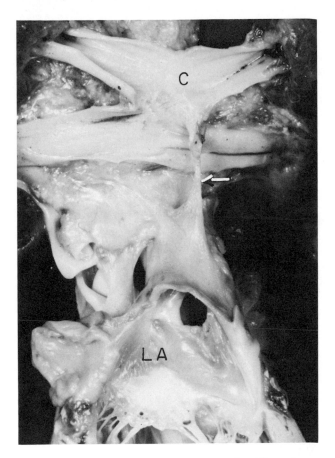

FIGURE 23 Atresia of the common pulmonary vein. The pulmonary veins join a confluence (C) from which no major vein leaves. The confluence is connected with the left atrium (LA) by an atretic strand (arrow).

associated with other anomalies; while in still others, partial anomalous pulmonary venous connection is part of a developmental complex.

Partial anomalous pulmonary venous connection, either as the sole condition or one fortuitously associated with another anomaly, most commonly involves the veins of either upper pulmonary lobe. Exceptions occur. Usually, when the left lung is involved, the left upper vein connects with the left innominate vein (Fig. 24a) [62]. When occurring on the right side, the anomalous connection is usually with the superior vena cava or the right atrium (Fig. 24b). In the latter circumstance, an intact atrial septum [63] should

distinguish the condition from one of the developmental anomalies to be
covered. Variations in detail either of solitary or multiple partial pulmonary
venous connection have been described in the comprehensive report of Blake
and associates. [55].

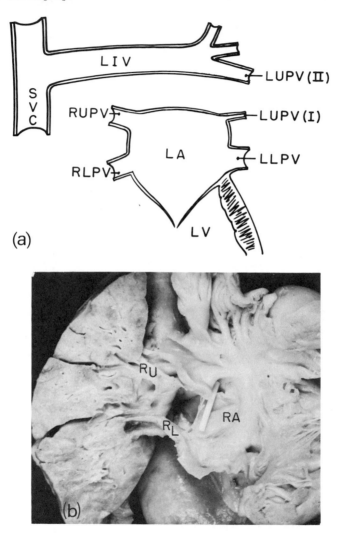

FIGURE 24 Partial anomalous pulmonary venous connection. (a) The upper
lobe of the left lung was supplied by two veins, the lower of which [LUPV (I)]
was narrow and joined the left atrium, while the upper [LUPV (II)] joined the
left innominate vein (LIV). (b) The upper and lower veins of the right lung (RU,
RL) join the right atrium (RA). Probe is in a patent foramen ovale.

Developmental Complexes Including
Anomalous Pulmonary Venous Connection

In certain developmental complexes, anomalous pulmonary venous connection forms an integral part. Such complexes are considered in the next section.

Asplenia

In the asplenic syndrome, multiple intracardiac malformations occur and total anomalous pulmonary venous connection is a common accompaniment [64]. The form of anomalous pulmonary venous connection is usually total, with ultimate termination into a systemic vein or into the portal venous system. As the coronary sinus is usually absent in the asplenic syndrome, examples of pulmonary venous connection to the coronary sinus are usually not observed.

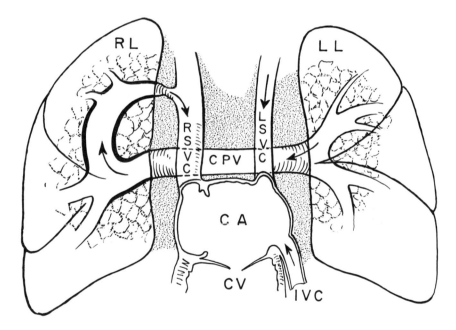

FIGURE 25 Total anomalous pulmonary venous connection in which the veins of the left lung coalesce to form a vein (CPV) that crosses the mediastinum and enters the right lung. In the latter location, this vein joins the right lower pulmonary vein. The right upper and right lower pulmonary veins are joined by a bridge within the right lung and the termination of the upper vein of the right lung is into the right of bilateral superior venae cavae. From a case of asplenia. CA and CV = common atrium and common ventricle, respectively. (From Everhart and associates [65]; reproduced with permission.)

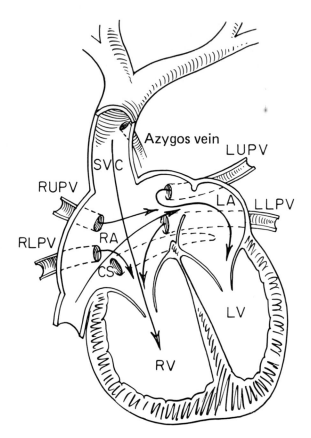

FIGURE 26   Total anomalous pulmonary venous connection to the right atrium (RA) from a case of polysplenia.

　　　Included among anomalous pulmonary venous connections associated with asplenia are situations in which one or more venous trunks cross the mediastinum to connect the veins of both lungs [65,66] before termination occurs into a systemic vein (Fig. 25). The roentgenographic shadow cast by an intrapulmonary vein may be confused with the scimitar syndrome [65] (see below).

Polysplenia

In polysplenia it is common, though not universal, that pulmonary veins join the right atrium [67]. Such termination may be total (Fig. 26) or partial. If the partial form occurs, it involves the veins of the right lung.

Sinus Venosus Atrial Septal Defect

Partial anomalous pulmonary venous connection with "sinus venosus" atrial septal defect is characterized by the presence of an atrial septal defect lying superior to the fossa ovalis and straddled by the superior vena cava (Fig. 27). The anomalous pulmonary vein or veins terminate at the general region of superior vena caval-right atrial junction. The venous supply of the upper lobe of the right lung is consistently involved, while in some cases the venous supply of the right middle and lower lobes may also participate in anomalous connection [68].

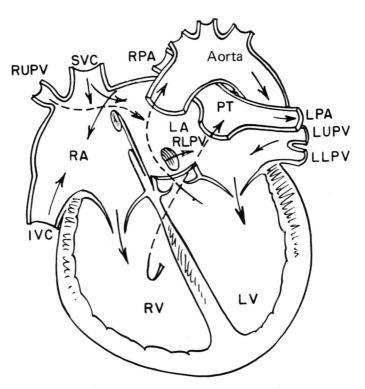

FIGURE 27   Sinus venosus type of atrial septal defect associated with anomalous termination of the right upper pulmonary vein (RUPV) to the right atrium near the superior vena caval (SVC) junction. Right lower (RLPV), left upper (LUPV) and left lower (LLPV) pulmonary veins join the left atrium (LA).

Scimitar Syndrome

Partial anomalous pulmonary venous connection to the inferior vena cava is characterized by termination of a vein from the right lung into the inferior vena cava at the general level of the diaphragm (Fig. 28). This condition may be the sole anomaly or it may be part of the *scimitar syndrome.*

The subject of the scimitar syndrome was reviewed by Kiely and associates [69]. These authors described three cases and analyzed 67 cases from the literature. The report of these authors emphasizes not only the

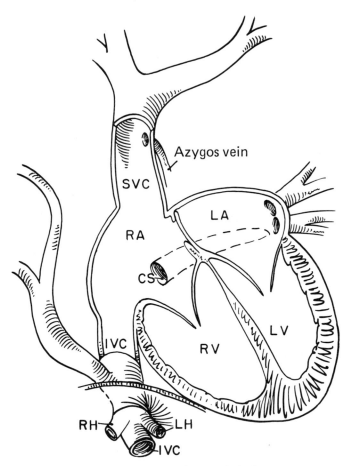

FIGURE 28   Anomalous termination of the right pulmonary venous system into the inferior vena cava (IVC). The termination may appear as an isolated phenomenon or be part of the so-called scimitar syndrome. RH and LH = right and left hepatic veins, respectively.

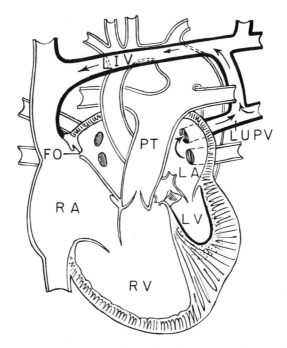

FIGURE 29 Anomalous termination of a pulmonary vein underlying an obstructive anomaly within the left side of the heart. In this instance, there is congenital aortic stenosis associated with hypoplasia of the left ventricle (LV). The foramen ovale (FO), although patent, was narrow. The main channel of egress of blood from the left atrium was by way of an anomalous connection between the left upper pulmonary vein (LUPV), on one hand, with the left innominate vein (LIV), on the other. (From Hunt and associates [74]; reproduced with permission.)

complexities of this syndrome but its variations. In summary, the scimitar syndrome may be defined as having the following characteristics: (1) anomalous connection of a right pulmonary vein with the inferior vena cava; (2) hypoplasia of the right lung; (3) dextroposition of the heart.

The right lung is small and may show deficiency of lobes. Kiely and associates observed that with about equal frequency there are one, two, or three lobes [69]. Bronchial abnormalities are common [69,70]. The anomalous venous drainage always involves the inferior lobe and may involve the entire right lung. When part of the right pulmonary venous drainage is normally to the left atrium, the upper lobe is represented by such venous drainage. Characteristically, there is but one anomalous vein, but in one of Kiely's cases there were two. These authors described two cases in which the anomalous vein joined both the inferior vena cava and, by way of a branch, the left atrium as well. Morgan and associates [71] described a case with the usual features of the scimitar syndrome in which the anomalous vein, after descending toward the inferior vena cava, turned upward to join the left atrium.

While sequestration of the lung does not occur, it is common that systemic arteries supply various parts of the right lung, most commonly its lower half. Such systemic arterial supply comes by way of arteries, usually multiple, that variously arise from the lower thoracic or upper abdominal aorta.

Cardiac anomalies may be associated with the scimitar syndrome but are uncommon. The basis for the heart's being in a dextroposition is probably related to hypoplasia of the right lung.

Association with Cardiac Anomalies

In cases with severe obstruction to the flow of pulmonary venous blood into the left side of the heart, underlying conditions include mitral atresia, aortic atresia, aortic stenosis with left ventricular hypoplasia, and cor triatriatum. In mitral and/or aortic atresia and in some cases of aortic stenosis, pulmonary venous blood flows into the right atrium through the foramen ovale. If this mechanism is inadequate, as in premature closure of the foramen ovale, a collateral venous channel may carry pulmonary venous blood into a systemic vein, usually part of the superior vena caval system (Fig. 29). Such a collateral channel, if identified by angiocardiography, may be confused with the usual channel of classic, isolated, total anomalous pulmonary venous connection.

The collateral channel usually originates in one of the major pulmonary veins, but it may begin at the left atrium, representing the so-called *levoatriocardinal vein* [72].

Details in anatomical variations in collateral channels have been reviewed in earlier publications [73-75].

V.   Pulmonary Arteriovenous Fistula

A direct connection between a pulmonary arterial branch and a pulmonary vein has variously been termed pulmonary arteriovenous fistula, pulmonary arteriovenous aneurysm, and cavernous hemangioma of the lung (Fig. 30).

The process, which tends to involve the subpleural part of the lung, may occur in any segment of either lung, but the right middle and both lower lobes seem more commonly involved [76]. Classically, the site of communication

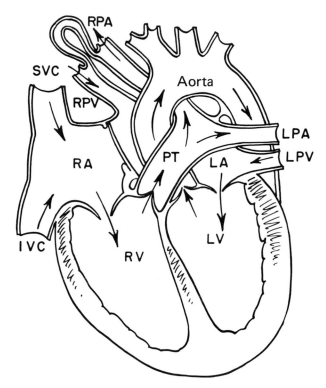

FIGURE 30 Pulmonary arteriovenous fistula involving the vascular system of the right lung. A bypassing channel exists between the right pulmonary artery (RPA) and the right pulmonary vein (RPV).

is represented by a thin-walled, aneurysm-like structure into which is fed one or more arterial branches and from which one or several veins leave [77]. Among 63 cases studied by Dines and associates [78] there were single lesions in 41 cases and multiple lesions in 22 cases. Among the latter, there were five cases with bilateral involvement.

A familial tendency has been observed, and either involved individuals or relatives may show telangiectasias of various organs as part of the Rendu-Osler-Weber syndrome [76,78,79]. Dines and associates [78] found that when the Rendu-Osler-Weber syndrome was identified, there was an increased incidence of multiplicity of pulmonary arteriovenous fistulae.

The classic functional abnormality of a pulmonary arteriovenous fistula is delivery of desaturated blood into the systemic circulation. The degree of cyanosis will depend on the volume of such delivery.

While bacterial infection of a pulmonary arteriovenous fistula has been described [80], this complication is uncommon. More common is the complication of cerebral abscess without an infection in the fistula [76]. The complication of cerebral abscess is comparable to that occurring in those forms of congenital heart disease associated with a right-to-left shunt. Rupture of the aneurysmal sac into either a bronchus or a pleural cavity has been reported [76].

A rare variant of pulmonary arteriovenous fistula was described by Lucas and associates [81]. This was characterized by absence of the parenchyma of the lower lobe of the right lung but with preservation of its vessels. The right lower pulmonary artery was joined directly to the right lower pulmonary vein. At the site of junction, an aneurysm-like structure was present.

References

1. Greene, D. G., E. deF. Baldwin, J. S. Baldwin, A. Himmelstein, C. E. Roh, and A. Cournand, Pure congenital pulmonary stenosis and idiopathic congenital dilatation of the pulmonary artery, *Am. J. Med.,* **6**:24–40 (1949).
2. Golden, R. L., and H. Lakin, The *forme fruste* in Marfan's syndrome, *N. E. J. Med.,* **260**:797–801 (1959).
3. Tung, H. L., and A. A. Liebow, Marfan's syndrome. Observations at necropsy: With special reference to medionecrosis of the great vessels, *Lab. Invest.,* **1**:382–406 (1952).
4. Brayshaw, J. R., and J. K. Perloff, Congenital pulmonary insufficiency complicating idiopathic dilatation of the pulmonary artery, *Am. J. Cardiol.,* **10**: 282–286 (1962).
5. Ishikawa, T., and I. Seki, Idiopathic dilatation of the pulmonary artery; report of a case and review of the literature, *Jpn. Heart J.,* **6**:273–283 (1965).
6. Ramsey, H. W., A. de la Torre, J. W. Linhart, L. J. Krovetz, G. L. Schiebler, and J. R. Green, Jr., Idiopathic dilatation of the pulmonary artery, *Am. J. Cardiol.,* **20**:324–330 (1967).
7. Edwards, J. E., and D. C. McGoon, Absence of anatomic origin from heart of pulmonary arterial supply, *Circulation,* **47**:393–398 (1973).
8. Manhoff, Jr., L. J., and J. S. Howe, Absence of the pulmonary artery: A new classification for pulmonary arteries of anomalous origin. Report of a case of absence of the pulmonary artery with hypertrophied bronchial arteries, *Arch. Pathol.,* **48**:155–170 (1949).
9. Blieden, L. C., R. V. Lucas, Jr., J. B. Carter, K. Miller, and J. E. Edwards, A developmental complex including supravalvular stenosis of the aorta and pulmonary trunk, *Circulation,* **49**:585–590 (1974).
10. Skall-Jensen, J., Congenital aorticopulmonary fistula. A review of the literature and report of two cases, *Acta Med. Scand.,* **160**:221–230 (1958).

11. Neufeld, H. N., R. G. Lester, P. Adams, Jr., R. C. Anderson, C. W. Lillehei, and J. E. Edwards, Aorticopulmonary septal defect, *Am. J. Cardiol.*, 9:12–25 (1962).
12. Van Mierop, L. H. S., D. F. Patterson, and W. R. Schnarr, Pathogenesis of persistent truncus arteriosus in light of observations made in a dog embryo with the anomaly, *Am. J. Cardiol.*, 41:755–762 (1978).
13. Collett, R. W., and J. E. Edwards, Persistent truncus arteriosus: Classification according to anatomical types, *Surg. Clin. N. Am.*, 29:1245–1270 (1949).
14. Bharati, S., H. A. McAllister, Jr., G. C. Rosenquist, R. A. Miller, C. J. Tatooles, and M. Lev, The surgical anatomy of truncus arteriosus communis, *J. Thorac. Cardiovasc. Surg.*, 67:501–510 (1974).
15. Calder, L., R. Van Praagh, S. Van Praagh, W. P. Sears, R. Corwin, A. Levy, J. D. Keith, and M. H. Paul, Truncus arteriosus communis. Clinical, angiocardiographic, and pathologic findings in 100 patients, *Am. Heart J.*, 92:23–38 (1976).
16. Becker, A. E., M. J. Becker, and J. E. Edwards, Pathology of the semilunar valves in persistent truncus arteriosus, *J. Thorac. Cardiovasc. Surg.*, 62:16–26 (1971).
17. Gelband, H., S. Van Meter, and W. M. Gersony, Truncal valve abnormalities in infants with persistent truncus arteriosus. A clinicopathologic study, *Circulation*, 45:397–403 (1972).
18. Roberts, W. C., Anomalous origin of both coronary arteries from the pulmonary artery, *Am. J. Cardiol.*, 10:595–600 (1962).
19. Colmers, R. A., and C. I. Siderides, Anomalous origin of both coronary arteries from pulmonary trunk. Myocardial infarction in otherwise normal heart, *Am. J. Cardiol.*, 12:263–269 (1963).
20. Cronk, E. S., J. G. Sinclair, and R. H. Rigdon, An anomalous coronary artery arising from the pulmonary artery, *Am. Heart J.*, 42:906–911 (1951).
21. Jameson, A. G., K. Ellis, and O. R. Levine, Anomalous left coronary artery arising from pulmonary artery, *Br. Heart J.*, 25:251–256 (1963).
22. Wesselhoeft, H., J. S. Fawcett, and A. L. Johnson, Anomalous origin of the left coronary artery from the pulmonary trunk. Its clinical spectrum, pathology, and pathophysiology, based on a review of 140 cases with seven further cases, *Circulation*, 38:403–425 (1968).
23. Edwards, J. E., Anomalous coronary arteries with special reference to arteriovenous-like communications, *Circulation*, 17:1001–1006 (1958).
24. Liebman, J., H. K. Hellerstein, J. L. Ankeney, and A. Tucker, The problem of the anomalous left coronary artery arising from the pulmonary artery in older children: Report of three cases, *N. Engl. J. Med.*, 269:486–494 (1963).
25. Schwartz, R. P., and F. Robicsek, An unusual anomaly of the coronary system: Origin of the anterior (descending) interventricular artery from the pulmonary trunk, *J. Pediatr.*, 78:123–126 (1971).

26. Jordan, R. A., T. J. Dry, and J. E. Edwards, Anomalous origin of the right coronary artery from the pulmonary trunk, *Mayo Clin. Proc.,* **25**: 673–678 (1950).

27. Wald, S., K. Stonecipher, B. J. Baldwin, and D. O. Nutter, Anomalous origin of the right coronary artery from the pulmonary artery, *Am. J. Cardiol.,* **27**:677–681 (1971).

28. Gobel, F. L., C. F. Anderson, H. A. Baltaxe, K. Amplatz, and Y. Wang, Shunts between the coronary and pulmonary arteries with normal origin of the coronary arteries, *Am. J. Cardiol.,* **25**:655–661 (1970).

29. Scott, D. H., Aneurysm of the coronary arteries, *Am. Heart J.,* **36**:403–421 (1948).

30. Jue, K. L., L. A. Lockman, and J. E. Edwards, Anomalous origins of pulmonary arteries from pulmonary trunk ("crossed-pulmonary arteries"). Observation in a case with 18 trisomy syndrome, *Am. Heart J.,* **71**:807–812 (1966).

31. Becker, A. E., M. J. Becker, and J. E. Edwards, Malposition of pulmonary arteries (crossed pulmonary arteries) in persistent truncus arteriosus, *Am. J. Roentgenol.,* **110**:509–514 (1970).

32. Jue, K. L., G. Raghib, K. Amplatz, P. Adams, Jr., and J. E. Edwards, Anomalous origin of the left pulmonary artery from the right pulmonary artery; report of 2 cases and review of the literature, *Am. J. Roentgenol.,* **95**:598–610 (1965).

33. Clarkson, P. M., D. G. Ritter, S. H. Rahimtoola, F. J. Hallermann, and D. C. McGoon, Aberrant left pulmonary artery, *Am. J. Dis. Child.,* **113**: 373–377 (1967).

34. Caudill, D. R., J. A. Helmsworth, G. Daoud, and S. Kaplan, Anomalous origin of left pulmonary artery from ascending aorta, *J. Thorac. Cardiovasc. Surg.,* **57**:493–506 (1969).

35. Sotomora, R. F., and J. E. Edwards, Anatomic identification of so-called absent pulmonary artery, *Circulation,* **57**:624–633 (1978).

36. Pryce, D. M., T. H. Sellors, and L. G. Blair, Intralobar sequestration of lung associated with an abnormal pulmonary artery, *Br. J. Surg.,* **35**:18–29 (1947).

37. Bruwer, A., O. T. Clagett, and J. R. McDonald, Anomalous arteries to the lung associated with congenital pulmonary abnormality, *J. Thorac. Surg.,* **19**:957–972 (1950).

38. Witten, D. M., O. T. Clagett, and L. B. Woolner, Intralobar bronchopulmonary sequestration involving the upper lobes, *J. Thorac. Cardiovasc. Surg.,* **43**:523–529 (1962).

39. D'Cruz, I. A., M. H. Agustsson, J. P. Bicoff, M. Weinberg, and R. A. Arcilla, Stenotic lesions of the pulmonary arteries. Clinical and hemodynamic findings in 84 cases, *Am. J. Cardiol.,* **13**:441–450 (1964).

40. Delaney, T. B., and A. S. Nadas, Peripheral pulmonic stenosis, *Am. J. Cardiol.,* **13**:451–461 (1964).

41. MacMahon, H. E., H. Y. Lee, and P. A. Stone, Congenital segmental

coarctation of pulmonary arteries. (An anatomic study), *Am. J. Pathol.,* **50**:15–25 (1967).

42. Beuren, A. J., C. Schulze, P. Eberle, D. Harmjanz, and J. Apitz, The syndrome of supravalvular aortic stenosis, peripheral pulmonary stenosis, mental retardation and similar facial appearance, *Am. J. Cardiol.,* **13**:471–483 (1964).

43. Snitcowsky, R., A. N. Toledo, W. Zaniolo, A. H. X. de Brito, J. A. B. Sekeff, and A. de Carvalho Azevedo, Severe pulmonary artery hypertension due to an anomaly of the pulmonary arteries, *Am. J. Cardiol.,* **13**: 542–546 (1964).

44. Esterly, J. R., and E. H. Oppenheimer, Vascular lesions in infants with congenital rubella, *Circulation,* **36**:544–554 (1967).

45. Heath, D., N. Segel, and J. Bishop, Pulmonary veno-occlusive disease, *Circulation,* **34**:242–248 (1966).

46. Liebow, A. A., K. M. Moser, and M. T. Southgate, Rapidly progressive dyspnea in a teenage boy, *JAMA,* **223**:1243–1253 (1973).

47. Wagenvoort, C. A., Pulmonary veno-occlusive disease. Entity or syndrome? *Chest,* **69**:82–86 (1976).

48. Edwards, W. D., and J. E. Edwards, Clinical primary pulmonary hypertension. Three pathologic types, *Circulation,* **56**:884–888 (1977).

49. Edwards, J. E., Congenital stenosis of pulmonary veins. Pathologic and developmental considerations, *Lab. Invest.,* **9**:46–66 (1960).

50. Reye, R. D. K., Congenital stenosis of the pulmonary veins in their extrapulmonary course, *Med. J. Aust.,* **1**:801–802 (1951).

51. Becker, A. E., M. J. Becker, and J. E. Edwards, Occlusion of pulmonary veins, "mitral" insufficiency, and ventricular septal defect. Functional resemblance to ventricular aneurysm, *Am. J. Dis. Child.,* **120**:557–559 (1970).

52. Nakib, A., J. H. Moller, V. I. Kanjuh, and J. E. Edwards, Anomalies of the pulmonary veins, *Am. J. Cardiol.,* **20**:77–90 (1967).

53. Mortensson, W., and N. R. Lundström, Congenital obstruction of the pulmonary veins at their atrial junctions. Review of the literature and a case report, *Am. Heart J.,* **87**:359–362 (1974).

54. Burroughs, J. T., and J. E. Edwards, Total anomalous pulmonary venous connection, *Am. Heart J.,* **59**:913–931 (1960).

55. Blake, H. A. R., J. Hall, and W. C. Manion, Anomalous pulmonary venous return, *Circulation,* **32**:406–414 (1965).

56. Elliott, L. P., and J. E. Edwards, The problem of pulmonary venous obstruction in total anomalous pulmonary venous connection to the left innominate vein, *Circulation,* **25**:913–915 (1962).

57. Carey, L. S., and J. E. Edwards, Severe pulmonary venous obstruction in total anomalous pulmonary venous connection to the left innominate vein. Report of a case, *Am. J. Roentgenol.,* **90**:593–598 (1963).

58. Lucas, Jr., R. V., P. Adams, Jr., R. C. Anderson, R. L. Varco, J. E. Edwards, and R. G. Lester, Total anomalous pulmonary venous connection to the

portal venous system: A cause of pulmonary venous obstruction, *Am. J. Roentgenol.,* **86**:561–575 (1961).

59.   Lucas, Jr., R. V., B. F. Woolfrey, R. C. Anderson, R. G. Lester, and J. E. Edwards, Atresia of the common pulmonary vein, *Pediatrics,* **29**:729–739 (1962).

60.   Hastreiter, A. R., M. H. Paul, M. E. Molthan, and R. A. Miller, Total anomalous pulmonary venous connection with severe pulmonary venous obstruction: A clinical entity, *Circulation,* **25**:916–928 (1962).

61.   Levine, M. A., J. H. Moller, K. Amplatz, and J. E. Edwards, Atresia of the common pulmonary vein: Case report and differential diagnosis, *Am. J. Roentgenol.,* **100**:322–327 (1967).

62.   Hickie, J. B., T. M. D. Gimlette, and A. P. C. Bacon, Anomalous pulmonary venous drainage, *Br. Heart J.,* **18**:365–377 (1956).

63.   Brody, H., Drainage of the pulmonary veins into the right side of the heart, *Arch. Pathol.,* **33**:221–240 (1942).

64.   Ruttenberg, H. D., H. N. Neufeld, R. V. Lucas, Jr., L. S. Carey, P. Adams, Jr., R. C. Anderson, and J. E. Edwards, Syndrome of congenital cardiac disease with asplenia. Distinction from other forms of congenital cyanotic cardiac disease, *Am. J. Cardiol.,* **13**:387–406 (1964).

65.   Everhart, F. J., M. E. Korns, K. Amplatz, and J. E. Edwards, Intrapulmonary segment in anomalous pulmonary venous connection. Resemblance to scimitar syndrome, *Circulation,* **35**:1163–1169 (1967).

66.   Sutherland, R. D., M. E. Korns, E. R. Pyle, and J. E. Edwards, Intrapulmonary vein contributing a segment of venous supply of contralateral lung, *Chest,* **57**:182–184 (1970).

67.   Moller, J. H., A. Nakib, R. C. Anderson, and J. E. Edwards, Congenital cardiac disease associated with polysplenia. A developmental complex of bilateral "left-sidedness," *Circulation,* **36**:789–799 (1967).

68.   Hudson, R., The normal and abnormal inter-atrial septum, *Br. Heart J.,* **17**:489–495 (1955).

69.   Kiely, B., J. Filler, S. Stone, and E. F. Doyle, Syndrome of anomalous venous drainage of the right lung to the inferior vena cava. A review of 67 reported cases and three new cases in children, *Am. J. Cardiol.,* **20**:102–116 (1967).

70.   Halasz, N. A., K. H. Halloran, and A. A. Liebow, Bronchial and arterial anomalies with drainage of the right lung into the inferior vena cava, *Circulation,* **14**:826–846 (1956).

71.   Morgan, J. R., and A. D. Forker, Syndrome of hypoplasia of the right lung and dextroposition of the heart: "Scimitar sign" with normal pulmonary venous drainage, *Circulation,* **43**:27–30 (1971).

72.   Edwards, J. E., and J. W. DuShane, Thoracic venous anomalies. I. Vascular connection of the left atrium and the left innominate vein (levoatriocardinal vein) associated with mitral atresia and premature closure of the foramen ovale. II. Pulmonary veins draining wholly into the ductus venosus, *Arch. Pathol.,* **49**:517–537 (1950).

73. Shone, J. D., and J. E. Edwards, Mitral atresia associated with pulmonary venous anomalies, *Br. Heart J.,* **26**:241–249 (1964).
74. Hunt, C. E., S. Rao, J. H. Moller, and J. E. Edwards, Anomalous pulmonary vein serving as collateral channel in aortic stenosis with hypoplastic left ventricle and endocardial fibroelastosis, *Chest,* **57**:185–189 (1970).
75. Beckman, C. B., J. H. Moller, and J. E. Edwards, Alternate pathways to pulmonary venous flow in left-sided obstructive anomalies, *Circulation,* **52**:509–516 (1975).
76. Muri, J. W., Arteriovenous aneurysm of the lung, *Am. J. Surg.,* **89**:265–271 (1955).
77. Lindskog, G. E., A. Liebow, H. Kausel, and A. Janzen, Pulmonary arteriovenous aneurysm, *Ann. Surg.,* **132**:591–606 (1950).
78. Dines, D. E., R. A. Arms, P. E. Bernatz, and M. R. Gomes, Pulmonary arteriovenous fistulas, *Mayo Clin. Proc.,* **49**:460–465 (1975).
79. Goldman, A., Arteriovenous fistula of the lung. Its hereditary and clinical aspects, *Am. Rev. Tuberc.,* **57**:266–280 (1948).
80. Maier, H. C., A. Himmelstein, R. L. Riley, and J. J. Bunin, Arteriovenous fistula of the lung, *J. Thorac. Cardiovasc. Surg.,* **17**:13–26 (1948).
81. Lucas, Jr., R. V., G. W. Lund, and J. E. Edwards, Direct communication of a pulmonary artery with the left atrium. An unusual variant of pulmonary arteriovenous fistula, *Circulation,* **29**:1409–1414 (1961).

10

Primary Pulmonary Hypertension

NORBERT VOELKEL and JOHN T. REEVES

University of Colorado Medical Center
Denver, Colorado

I. Introduction

Primary pulmonary hypertension as considered in this review is a disease of unexplained etiology within a group of disorders that affect primarily the precapillary lung vessels and lead to an increase of pressure and resistance in the pulmonary arterioles and to right heart hypertrophy and cor pulmonale. Whereas primary pulmonary hypertension has been accepted as a clinical entity [1,2], it is likely that the etiology is not homogeneous [1,3–6]. However, the disease serves as a model for the purest expression of pulmonary hypertension unmodified by coexisting cardiac or pulmonary disease [7]. The pathomorphological term "unexplained plexogenic pulmonary arteriopathy" [1] describes only one of the histologic characteristics. In this review we will use the term "primary pulmonary hypertension," acknowledging that it includes several entities (Fig. 1). Veno-occlusive disease and recurrent embolism are considered elsewhere in this volume.

Primary pulmonary hypertension can be established with certainty only if the following three criteria are met:

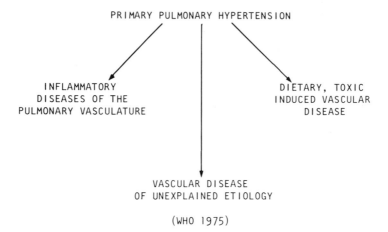

FIGURE 1

1. Demonstration of right ventricular hypertrophy in the absence of any other cardiac abnormality [4];

2. Demonstration by cardiac catheterization of an elevated pulmonary artery pressure and of a normal pulmonary wedge pressure [4];

3. Absence at autopsy of other etiologies of pulmonary hypertension; in addition, characteristic microscope findings of pulmonary arteriolar obstruction, including medial hypertrophy of the pulmonary arterioles, cellular intimal proliferation, concentric-laminar intimal fibrosis, necrotizing arteritis, and/or plexiform lesions [8].

A. History

The disease was first described by Romberg in 1891 [9] as a "sclerosis of the lung artery." Ayerza, in 1901, reported patients with heart failure and intense cyanosis (cardiacos negros). Autopsy revealed "bronchopulmonary sclerosis." The meaning of the term "Ayerza's disease" varied with each author who used it [10]. Arrillaga (1913) [11] believed that the disease was due to arteritis of the pulmonary vessels. The first systematic description of the "pathology of the vessels of the pulmonary circulation" was by Brenner in 1935 [10]. Primary pulmonary hypertension became a clinical entity after Dresdale et al. described its clinical and hemodynamic features in 1951 [2]. They considered "isolated sympathetic overactivity" as a possible etiology. Subsequently, Wood emphasized the importance of a vasoconstrictive factor in the pathogenesis of primary pulmonary hypertension [12]. In 1958, Heath and

Edwards [13] defined the structural changes in general for hypertensive pulmonary vascular disease by: (1) describing the six grades of structural changes in the pulmonary arteries, (2) demonstrating a morphological sequence of events in pulmonary hypertension, and (3) providing a structural definition of irreversibility of vascular changes. The outbreak of an epidemic of pulmonary hypertension in three European countries in 1967 [14] was attributed to the intake of aminorex, an appetite depressant amine. It became apparent that the clinical and pathologic picture of primary pulmonary hypertension could be induced by a substance taken orally. In 1970, Wagenvoort and Wagenvoort examined lung tissue from 156 pulmonary hypertensive patients from around the world, thus providing to date the largest series of autopsied patients examined in one laboratory. From their experience they provided the structural criteria for diagnosis of primary pulmonary hypertension and its separation from other forms of pulmonary hypertension, including thromboembolism [8,23].

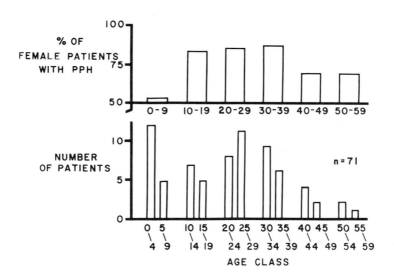

FIGURE 2 Top: Percentage of females at various ages at the time of onset of symptoms. In early childhood, males and females are affected with equal frequency, but thereafter females are affected more frequently. Bottom: Distribution of patients with primary pulmonary hypertension by age at the onset of symptoms. The largest number of patients was in the youngest age group and a second peak incidence appeared between 25 and 29 years [2,20,42,49,64,66,69, 86,87,112,120,122–125,129].

B. Frequency

Prior to the introduction of invasive catheter techniques, primary pulmonary hypertension was considered to be rare. Early reports speak of 1 case in 12,000 autopsies [15]. Now, nearly 1000 patients have been reported in the literature [8]. Using the right heart catheterization technique, its frequency was reported to be 0.17% of patients with cardiovascular disease [16], 0.25 to 1.1% in unselected right heart catheterizations [17–21], and 0.98% in autopsy series of cor pulmonale [22].

C. Sex Incidence and Age

Prior to adolescence the incidence is equal for males and females, but thereafter the incidence is predominant in females (Fig. 2). The role of femaleness in the disease is considered below. In Wagenvoort's study of autopsied patients there was a female to male ratio of 4:1, but the ratio was 0.85 for children 15 years or younger [23]. Wood [12] found a female to male ratio of 5:1. Pulmonary hypertension in patients taking aminorex had a striking (9:1) predominance of females over males [24–26]. Loogen and Both [21] reported 93 patients with primary pulmonary hypertension in which the female to male ratio was 2:1.

The distribution of ages at the time of appearance of the first symptom of primary pulmonary hypertension is shown (Fig. 2). Although all ages are represented, there is a predilection for the young, and there may be a bimodal distribution with an early peak in infancy. In Wagenvoort's 110 autopsied patients, the youngest was 4 days of age and the oldest was 69 years; the average was 23 years. Reeves and Noonan [70] reported primary pulmonary hypertension confirmed at autopsy in an 11-month-old infant in whom syncope began at age 2 months. The older mean ages (44 to 55 years) of 148 patients with pulmonary hypertension, observed in three centers in Switzerland from 1966 to 1969, probably reflected the increased incidence of pulmonary hypertension from aminorex observed in those years [31]. In the naturally occurring disease not attributed to aminorex, primary pulmonary hypertension is by and large a disease of young women (Fig. 2).

D. Familial Occurrence

Since the first documentation by Clarke et al. [32] in 1927, the familial occurrence of primary pulmonary hypertension has been well established [32–42]. Wagenvoort found in the literature reports of 63 patients from 25 families [15]. The disease has been reported in twins [43]. Massoud et al.

published the history of a family of seven children, four of whom died over a period of 7 years from primary pulmonary hypertension [44] at ages from 15 months to 20 years. In these children, the disease appeared to be congenital [45]. The possibility of a recessive trait inheritance has been suggested [46], as well as the dominant mode of inheritance [47,48]. Whatever the mode of the inheritance, the familial incidence points to the importance of some factor predisposing to primary pulmonary hypertension.

E. Natural History

Precise knowledge of the natural history is lacking because primary pulmonary hypertension is largely asymptomatic until marked vascular alterations have already developed [6,171]. Thus, the early stages of the disease are obscured. The mean survival time has been reported to be 2 to 3 years after the onset of symptoms [16]. Survival is independent of the patient's age at onset [23] and also of the pulmonary arterial pressure (Fig. 3). Patient survivals as long

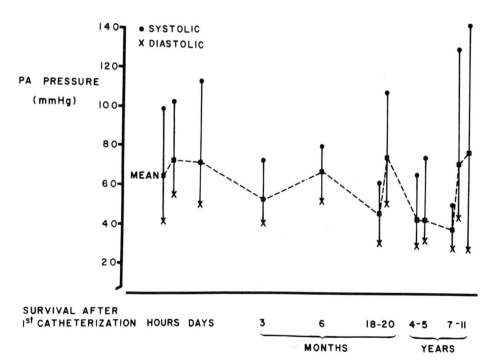

FIGURE 3   The magnitude of pulmonary hypertension at the time of initial heart catheterization is not correlated with the duration of subsequent survival [28,49,69,82,87,123–125,129].

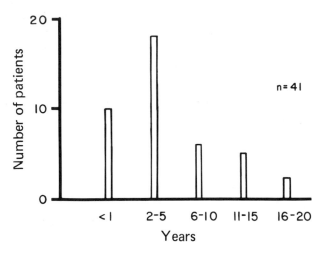

FIGURE 4   Distribution of survival times after onset of symptoms in primary
pulmonary hypertension [2,42,49,64,66,87,112,120,122,124,130].

as 19 to 29 years after onset of symptoms have been reported [23,49]. However, the distribution of survival times (Fig. 4) indicates that long survival is
unusual.

Regression of pulmonary hypertension has been reported [50]. A 10-
year-old girl with syncope had a pulmonary arterial pressure ranging from 58 to
80 mmHg at three cardiac catheterizations over a 3-year period. At age 19 years
her symptoms had disappeared. Her mean pulmonary arterial pressure had decreased to 24 mmHg, but dilatation of her pulmonary artery remained [50].
In addition, spontaneous regression of pulmonary hypertension (mean pulmonary arterial pressure falling from 71 to 17 mmHg) in a 10-year-old girl over 6
years has been observed in this institution by S. G. Blount (personal communication, 1975). Regression of pulmonary hypertension following aminorex ingestion was observed when the drug was stopped and the mean pulmonary arterial
pressure was less than 30 mmHg [51]. The rare, spontaneous regression in
primary pulmonary hypertension is important. Perhaps if the etiology can be
determined, and the cause removed early in the course of the illness, then
recovery would be possible.

II. Etiologic Factors

By definition, primary pulmonary hypertension is of unexplained etiology or
etiologies, despite considerable literature on the subject. Probably we know so
little about the etiology for several reasons.

1. The disease is uncommon, with little chance for one physician to observe the natural history and the effect of therapy on a large number of patients.

2. Symptoms tend to occur late in the course of the disease.

3. Whereas the blood pressure cuff provides a good tool for screening the population for systemic hypertension and for following the course of the disease and effects of therapy, no such tool has yet appeared for pulmonary hypertension.

4. A convincing animal model is not yet available.

The etiologic factors that have been considered, and the scanty evidence available to support each are discussed below. They include: congenital factors; familial factors; "factor associated with female maturation"; thromboembolism; autoimmune mechanism; dietary pulmonary hypertension, drugs; pulmonary hypertension in patients with hepatic dysfunction; "vasoconstricting factor."

A. Congenital Factors

The occurrence of primary pulmonary hypertension in infancy [52] raises the possibility of some congenital abnormality in the pulmonary arterial bed. Goodale and Thomas [53] considered that congenital focal aplasia or hypoplasia occurred in the media of the small pulmonary arteries. Intimal proliferation over the structural deficiencies were considered to lead to arterial stenosis and persistent hypertension. However, focal aplasia is now considered the result, and not the cause of, pulmonary hypertension of long standing. Further, the youngest infants with primary pulmonary hypertension have medial hypertrophy, not aplasia, as the striking finding [15].

Recently, the syndrome of persistence of the fetal circulation has been described, in which mean pulmonary arterial pressures over 50 mmHg persist for 60 hr after birth, during which time the infant appears to have underperfusion of the lungs [54]. The syndrome could be caused by one or more of the following: (1) failure of the pulmonary vasodilation which usually accompanies birth, (2) an insufficient number of pulmonary arterioles, (3) failure of growth of new arterioles [55], or (4) failure of regression of the fetal medial hypertrophy. Because the syndrome was only recently described, the long-term behavior of the pulmonary circulation in survivors is not known. The syndrome has features in common with primary pulmonary hypertension, and the possibility that the two disorders are related in young infants should be considered.

B.   Familial Occurrence

The familial occurrence in primary pulmonary hypertension discussed above raises the possibility that the disease or a propensity to it is inherited. The hemodynamics, clinical course, and pathologic findings in the familial cases are indistinguishable from the sporadic forms of primary pulmonary hypertension.

C.   Factors Associated with Female Maturation

Among adult patients with primary pulmonary hypertension, in patients taking aminorex [24], and in the familial occurrences [32–48], females are clearly overrepresented. Yet, the female preponderance does not appear until the age of menarche (Fig. 2). Further, the disorder was associated with pregnancy in 8 of the 56 women in the childbearing age as shown in Wagenvoort's report [23]. In eight of nine other patients, symptoms of primary pulmonary hypertension began during pregnancy, as early as the first trimester [2,42,58,69,109,117,127]. Two patients died during pregnancy. Thus, pregnancy is associated with the onset of the disease and is poorly tolerated while the disease process is active [56–58]. Yet, no specific hormone or endocrine factor has been identified in these patients. In fact, the male hormone, testosterone, apparently augments pulmonary vascular reactivity in rats at high altitude [59]. Further, normal pregnant women [60,61] have lower pulmonary arterial pressures than nonpregnant women, and pregnant dogs (unpublished results) have decreased pulmonary vascular reactivity compared to nonpregnant dogs. However, cows that have congenitally reactive pulmonary vascular beds develop pulmonary hypertension during pregnancy, whereas those with less reactive beds do not [62]. Thus it is possible that women with abnormally hyperreactive pulmonary vasculature, for example, those with primary pulmonary hypertension, may have a pulmonary pressor response to pregnancy whereas normal women do not. Hormonal influences are thus important in the pulmonary circulation, though they have been little studied as yet. However, it may be more than coincidental that both primary pulmonary hypertension and autoimmune disease occur predominantly in women.

D.   Thromboembolism

Recurrent microthromboembolism was early considered to be the etiology of primary pulmonary hypertension [27,63]. It is generally agreed that recurrent microemboli may cause irreversible pulmonary hypertension, with the obliteration of some small muscular arterioles, and intimal fibrosis leading to partial obstruction in others [6,23,168]. Indeed, there may be circumferential intimal fibrosis [23,168]. Thus, the clinical and pathologic similarities between recurrent microthromboembolism and the findings in patients with primary pulmonary hypertension provide the foundation for the controversy about whether primary pulmonary hypertension is a distinct entity or a form of recurrent thromboembolism [6,64-68].

Recurrent pulmonary microembolism, however, most often occurs over the age of 50 years [23], whereas primary pulmonary hypertension most often occurs in young women. Wagenvoort and Wagenvoort [23], on the basis of extensive studies, believe primary pulmonary hypertension and recurrent micropulmonary embolism can be differentiated on the basis of pathologic criteria: (1) careful, extensive examination in instances of microembolism may reveal bands or webs in the larger pulmonary arteries, suggesting that at some time macroembolism occurred; (2) in thromboembolic disease there is evidence of recanalization [169], i.e., webs, lattices, multiple channels, or eccentric patches of intimal fibrosis in small arteries; (3) there is less medial hypertrophy in thromboembolic disease; and (4) plexiform lesions and arterial medial fibrinoid necrosis occur in primary pulmonary hypertension but not in thromboembolic disease.

In addition, the microradiographic pattern in a patient with recurrent microembolism differs from that in patients with primary pulmonary hypertension [69]. Thus, in our view, the weight of present evidence suggests that primary pulmonary hypertension is likely not solely the result of recurrent pulmonary embolism.

E. Autoimmune Mechanism

The association of primary pulmonary hypertension with collagen diseases and Raynaud's phenomenon [70-74] suggests that the disease is part of an immunological process. Rheumatoid arthritis [75,76], polymyositis [77], scleroderma [78], dermatomyositis [79], lupus erythematosus [80-82], and Hashimoto's thyroiditis [83] have been associated with primary pulmonary hypertension. These are all diseases which, like primary pulmonary hypertension, occur primarily in women. Raynaud's syndrome has been reported in 7 to 30% of patients with primary pulmonary hypertension [8,83,84] and it precedes the appearance of symptoms of pulmonary hypertension [83]. Even a separate disorder consisting of primary pulmonary hypertension plus Raynaud's syndrome [78] has been suggested. In the familial occurrences, family members not afflicted with primary pulmonary hypertension had Raynaud's syndrome [85]. The close association with a vasoconstrictive disorder of the systemic arteries emphasizes that vasoconstriction may underlie primary pulmonary hypertension and further relates it to collagen vascular diseases which also have a high incidence of Raynaud's phenomenon.

Circulating immune complexes or local deposits of immune complexes within lung vessels have not been reported, nor has therapy with immunological suppressants been effective [86,87]. However, the link is sufficiently strong to suggest that at least some occurrences of primary pulmonary hypertension show a common etiology with autoimmune disease processes.

F.   Dietary "Primary" Pulmonary Hypertension

From 1967 to 1970 in Switzerland, Austria, and West Germany, a 20-fold increase in unexplained pulmonary hypertension was reported [88–93]. The clinical, angiographic, and histologic findings resemble the "classic" findings in primary pulmonary hypertension [95]. The epidemic followed the introduction of an appetite depressant agent aminorex (2-amino-5-phenyl-2-oxazoline, Menocil) in December 1965 and disappeared soon after the drug had been banned from the market. Approximately 2% of the patients that had taken Menocil developed pulmonary hypertension [93]. The risk of developing the disease was correlated with the dose, with up to 10% of those taking 320 or more tablets (4.4 g) developing the disease [94]. However, there was no correlation between the severity of the disease and the number of tablets the individual patient had taken [93].

The chemical structure of aminorex resembles epinephrine and amphetamine [95]. A release of catecholamines from endogenous stores by this drug [95] had been suggested, as well as a mechanism involving lung serotonin release [96,100]. Whereas it was shown that acute administration of aminorex increased the pulmonary vascular resistance in a dose-dependent fashion in anesthetized dogs [95], so far all the experimental work to demonstrate the effect of chronic application on pulmonary hemodynamics and morphology has failed to produce significant alterations [97–99]. This failure to produce chronic pulmonary hypertension with aminorex in any species investigated usually is explained by the small likelihood for pulmonary hypertension that might be even smaller in test animals. A further prerequisite is probably a high susceptibility of the pulmonary circulation to constrict when exposed to the offending agent. The aminorex episode is suggestive that a substance taken orally in humans may induce, by an as yet unknown mechanism, a fatal pulmonary hypertension which resembles primary pulmonary hypertension.

Fahlen et al. reported two patients who developed pulmonary hypertension during treatment with the antihyperglycemic biguanide phenformin. The pulmonary hypertension subsided on withdrawal of the drug and was considered to be related to lactic acidosis [101]. Thus, another oral agent has produced pulmonary hypertension, but it has not been implicated in irreversible pulmonary vascular changes.

G. Pulmonary Hypertension in Patients with Hepatic Dysfunction

Many patients with liver cirrhosis have high pulmonary blood flows and low pulmonary arterial pressures with hyporeactivity of their pulmonary vascular beds [102,103]. Clearly, however, a few patients with hepatic dysfunction develop severe pulmonary hypertension, which was thought to be caused by multiple emboli originating from the diseased liver [104]. More recent studies and review of some of the pathologic material upon which earlier studies were based have indicated the presence of concentric laminar intimal fibrosis, fibrinoid necrosis, arteritis, and plexiform lesions in the pulmonary arterial tree, thus resembling the findings in primary pulmonary hypertension [8]. Fishman [105] has reviewed certain possible mechanisms whereby liver disease could affect the lung circulation. Although the pathogenesis relating liver cirrhosis to pulmonary hypertension is not known, there are similarities of interest in their vascular arrangement [106]. Wagenvoort has reported that experimental Crotalaria-induced pulmonary hypertension is always preceded by liver injury [8].

H. The Vasoconstrictive Factor

Paul Wood (1956) proposed a "vasoconstrictive factor" in primary pulmonary hypertension, having found in some of the patients that pulmonary vasodilators acutely decreased pulmonary arterial pressure [16]. Subsequently, arguments for [39,107–110] and against [6] an increased vascular tone initiating the vascular lesions have been raised. The structural evidence for vasoconstriction began with Staemmler [111], whose studies in 1937 suggested that spasm of arterioles led to vascular muscle hypertrophy. In 1957, Short [112] found "arterial contracture" in postmortem arteriograms of patients with primary pulmonary hypertensions, and Evans et al. [52] considered the pulmonary arteries to show failure of dilatation. The recent finding that arterial hypertrophy is the dominant lesion in the lungs of infants and young children dying of primary pulmonary hypertension has led Wagenvoort to favor vasoconstriction as important in the pathogenesis [8]. Physiological evidence for the presence of vasoconstriction in primary pulmonary hypertension since the early publications of Wood [12], and Dresdale et al. [2], has largely consisted of the acute pulmonary vasodilatation in certain patients, as summarized in Section III.E. Indeed, if vasoconstriction precedes the development of intimal lesions in lung arteries, then multiple etiologies of primary pulmonary hypertension are likely (Fig. 5). Illustrations of vasomotion rising from various etiologies are given below.

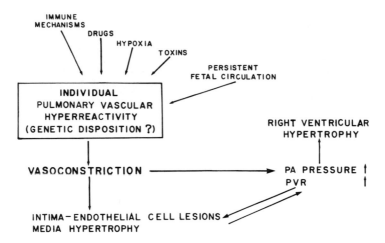

FIGURE 5 Proposed scheme for pathogenesis of primary pulmonary hypertension; i.e., any of the several stimuli may induce vasoconstriction. In susceptible individuals a vicious cycle of vasoconstriction, medial hypertrophy, and intimal damage is produced which then leads to irreversible pulmonary hypertension.

Hypoxia

The variations in individual responsiveness of the pulmonary vasculature to alveolar hypoxia of high-altitude residents [113] (Fig. 6), of patients with chronic obstructive lung disease [114], and of normal individuals [115] has been established and confirmed by angiographic studies [116]. A patient seen by S. G. Blount (personal communication, 1975) represents one end of the spectrum. A 22-year-old man developed exertional dyspnea, chest pain, and syncope within 8 months of moving from sea level to a 7000-ft resident altitude in Colorado. Cardiac catheterization revealed pulmonary hypertension (PA mean, 50 mmHg) and borderline low pulmonary flow (cardiac index, 2.9 liters). Acute administration of 100% O_2 did not lower pulmonary resistance, but Priscoline lowered the pressure and increased the pulmonary flow. The patient followed the advice to move to sea level, where symptoms disappeared and repeat catheterization within 6 months indicated that his pulmonary hypertension had abated (mean PA pressure, 20 mmHg; cardiac index, 3.4 liters min^{-1} m^{-2}). In this patient, chronic hypoxia appeared to trigger a vasoconstrictive syndrome which resembled primary pulmonary hypertension.

Persistence of the Fetal Pattern of Lung Circulation

The relatively high incidence of primary pulmonary hypertension in infants and young children as discussed above suggests that vasoconstriction continued from fetal life may contribute to the pathogenesis of the disease.

Autoimmune Disease

In one of Daoud's patients [86,103], Lupus erythematosus was present for several years before right ventricular hypertrophy by electrocardiogram and signs of pulmonary hypertension appeared. The patient then had a good vasodilator response to a continuous infusion of Isuprel (see Sec. VII), suggesting that pulmonary vasoconstriction had been present in this collagen vascular disease.

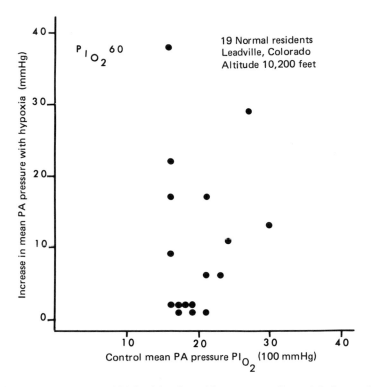

FIGURE 6 When normal high-altitude residents are made acutely hypoxic by lowering the inspired oxygen tension (PIO_2) from 100 to 60 mmHg, some individuals have virtually no increase in mean pulmonary arterial pressure (hyporeactors), while other individuals have a marked pressure increase of 15 to 40 mmHg (hyperreactors) [172].

Dietary Pulmonary Hypertension

Vasodilatation with orciprenaline and acetylcholine has been reported in pulmonary hypertensive patients with a history of aminorex intake as discussed in Section III.E.

It seems likely that a variety of pulmonary vascular constrictor influences are present in primary pulmonary hypertension. If the vasoconstriction initiates the disease process, then the vascular smooth muscle cell, as the target of the physiological and pathologic response, will be in the center of future research. Two recent observations are worth noting: (1) that mechanical stretching of the main pulmonary artery results in a rapid constriction of the peripheral pulmonary arteries [118]; and (2) that pulmonary micro-embolization with plastic microspheres evokes a vascular reflex vasodilatation in the isolated perfused lobe that was protected from embolization [119]. These observations have renewed interest in the sympathetic nerve system and its possible role in pulmonary vasoregulation. The sympathetics have been implicated in the pulmonary hypertension from aminorex [95], but the hypothesis is undocumented.

III.   Hemodynamics

A.   Pressures and Flow

Kuida et al. [120], in 1957, reported primary pulmonary hypertension in four female patients and included the hemodynamic and postmortem findings. Subsequent reports have tended to include less complete data. However, we have combined data from various published reports in which the clinical diagnosis had been verified at autopsy [120-128], providing a pattern of hemodynamic characteristics (Table 1) which are: high pulmonary arterial pressure and vascular resistance, normal pulmonary wedge pressure, and low cardiac output and index. The systemic arterial pressure was either normal or low. The findings are indistinguishable from pulmonary hypertension of other etiologies [2,21]. Only 2 of 40 patients had a systolic pulmonary arterial pressure below 50 mmHg, but 19 were above 100 mmHg. The distribution of pulmonary arterial pressure reveals relatively few patients with mean pressures below 40 or above 100 mmHg (see Fig. 20). The elevated right atrial and right ventricular diastolic pressures indicated ventricular failure. The aminorex patients represent a subgroup of patients with primary pulmonary hypertension because they have been catheterized earlier in the course of their disease and have lower pressures than most of the previously reported patients with pulmonary hypertension.

TABLE 1 Hemodynamic Measurements in Primary Pulmonary Hypertension (PPH)[a]

Measurement	Autopsy-verified cases of PPH [2,29,87,120,126]	Normal values [131]
PRA (mmHg)	10 ± 5 ($n = 21$)	4 ± 2 ($n = 30$)
PRV_{syst} (mmHg)	82 ± 28 ($n = 21$)	29 ± 6 ($n = 30$)
PAP_{syst} (mmHg)	76 ± 34 ($n = 40$)	19 ± 5 ($n = 30$)
PAP_{diast} (mmHg)	48 ± 15 ($n = 39$)	8 ± 3 ($n = 30$)
PAP_m (mmHg)	66 ± 20 ($n = 25$)	15 ± 3 ($n = 145$)[b]
P_c (mmHg)	8 ± 4.5 ($n = 21$)	8 ± 3 ($n = 30$)
CO (liters/min)	3.1 ± 0.3 ($n = 12$)	6.9 ± 1.1 ($n = 30$)
CI (liters min^{-1} m^{-2})	1.9 ± ($n = 13$)	3.7 ± 0.71 ($n = 30$)
PVR (dyn sec cm^{-5})	1280 ± 160 ($n = 8$)	150 ± 59 ($n = 30$)

[a]PRA = right atrial pressure; PRV_{syst} = right ventricular systolic pressure; PAP_{syst} = pulmonary arterial systolic pressure; PAP_{diast} = pulmonary arterial diastolic pressure; PAP_m = mean pulmonary arterial pressure; P_c = pulmonary capillary pressure; CO = cardiac output; CI = cardiac index; PVR = pulmonary vascular resistance.
[b]References 147 to 162. Systemic arterial pressure: Systolic,, 114.3 ± 15.8 ($n = 68$) [2, 4,28,29,44,46,49,50,52,56,82,87,120,126,129,142]; diastolic, 73.8 ± 13.2; mean, 84.3 + 14.0 ($n = 20$) [82,86,87,120].

B. Time Course of Pulmonary Hypertension

The survival time in primary pulmonary hypertension cannot be predicted from the measured pulmonary arterial pressures (Fig. 3). Two patients with systolic pressure above 100 mmHg survived 11 years. Results of repeated catheterization in Pedersen's autopsied patient after 10 and 11 years indicated a progressive rise in systolic pressures developed by the right heart [124]. Persistence of the pulmonary hypertension and a tendency for the cardiac output to fall was confirmed in 16 patients from the literature in whom longitudinal catheterization studies were obtained (Fig. 7). The calculated resistance rose in 12 of the 16 patients in repeat measurements 1 to 4 years after the initial measurements (Fig. 7). In four patients the resistance either

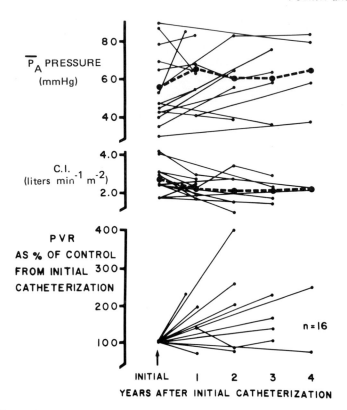

FIGURE 7 Serial hemodynamic measurements in patients with primary pulmonary hypertension. From above downward are mean pulmonary arterial pressure, cardiac index, and pulmonary vascular resistance (the latter as percentage of initial value) in 16 patients who had more than one catheterization in a 4-year period. Mean values for pressure and cardiac index are shown (-------). [20,28,82,87,125,130].

did not change or fell slightly. The measurements in two patients with documented spontaneous reversal are not shown. Both et al. [51], in their study of 14 aminorex patients, demonstrated a reversal of the pulmonary arterial pressure in six patients where the initial mean pressure did not exceed 30 mmHg. The variability of the course of the disease is impressive. Indeed, we speculate that pulmonary hypertension may arise and regress without causing symptoms and thus escape detection. At present, cardiac catheterization provides the only means for assessing pulmonary hypertension. Clearly, there is need for a noninvasive method for the monitoring of pulmonary arterial pressure in humans.

The cardiac output is low in patients with high pulmonary arterial pressures. Figure 8 shows the pressure-flow relationship in normal individuals, high-altitude residents, and patients with primary pulmonary hypertension. The primary pulmonary hypertension group has both an excessive pulmonary arterial pressure and a reduced cardiac output. Thus, measurement of pressure alone does not assess the magnitude of the pulmonary vascular derangement; both pressure and flow measurements are required. Further, cardiac output tends downward with time in primary pulmonary hypertension. Given the choice of maintaining flow at a higher pulmonary arterial pressure, or minimizing the pulmonary hypertension at the expense of pulmonary flow,

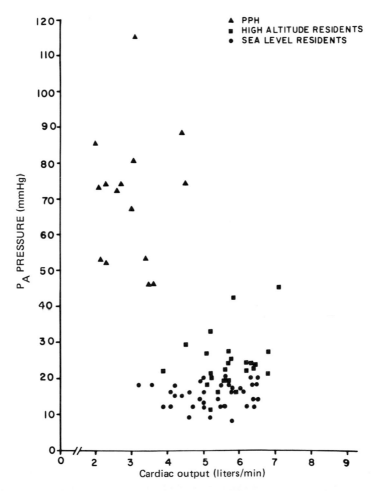

FIGURE 8 Relation of mean pulmonary arterial pressure to cardiac output at rest for normal sea-level residents [131], normal high-altitude residents [109], and patients subsequently shown by autopsy to have primary pulmonary hypertension [116–130]. The higher the pulmonary arterial pressure, the lower the cardiac output.

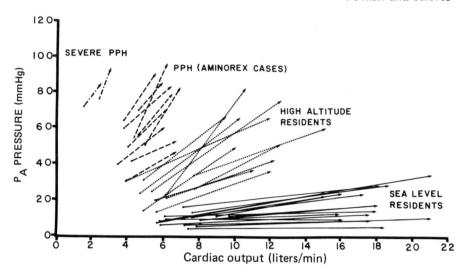

FIGURE 9   Mean pulmonary arterial pressure versus cardiac output at rest and during exercise for normal sea-level residents [131], normal high-altitude residents (– – – – –>) [113], patients with pulmonary hypertension from amino-rex (– – –>) [132], and two patients with severe primary pulmonary hyperten-sion (.-.->) [87]. The higher the resting pressure, the lower the resting flow and the smaller the increase in the flow with exercise.

the body appears to choose the latter. The data are compatible with the con-cept that the high pulmonary vascular pressure and resistance is causally related to a reduced pulmonary blood flow.

C.   Exercise

Figure 9 compares the hemodynamic data during exercise of normal indi-viduals at seal level [131], high-altitude residents [113], patients with pul-monary hypertension following aminorex intake [132], and patients with severe primary pulmonary hypertension (autopsy verified). Sea-level residents have a greater increase in flow than in pressure during exercise. High-altitude residents tend to increase pressure and flow to a nearly equal extent. Patients with pulmonary hypertension following aminorex ingestion and those with primary pulmonary hypertension tend to have large increases in pressure for a small increase in flow. The data suggest that the higher the initial pressure, the greater the increase in pressure with exercise and the smaller the increase in flow. The results support the concept that the high degree of pulmonary vascular obstruction acts to block cardiac output increase. Thus, the high resistance to flow through the lung may account both for the low flow at rest and the inadequate flow during exercise.

D. Exercise-Induced Syncope

An inadequate flow during exercise could contribute to syncope because of the inability of the heart to increase the flow to meet body demands for oxygen. In addition, exercise may trigger pulmonary vasoconstriction. Degenring [132] has shown that in patients with primary pulmonary hypertension and in aminorex-induced pulmonary hypertension, pressures and resistances in the 2 min following exercise exceeded those measured during exercise. Thus, syncope during or after exercise may be complex, reflecting one or more of the following: right ventricular failure, failure of forward flow to meet exercise demands, or pulmonary vasoconstriction [133-135].

E. Pulmonary Vascular Reactivity

In primary pulmonary hypertension, the pulmonary artery pressure may be labile so that a single value for pressure cannot be relied upon [136]. Daoud et al. [86] observed one patient in whom the mean pulmonary arterial pressure fluctuated between 40 and 70 mmHg in an apparently random fashion (Fig. 10). The pressure fluctuations were considered to reflect changing pulmonary arterial tone rather than widely fluctuating pulmonary flow. Indeed, the patient did exhibit a brisk pulmonary vasodilatation with isoproterenol.

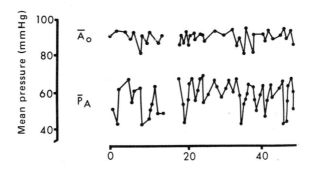

FIGURE 10   Mean pulmonary ($\overline{P}A$) and aortic ($\overline{A}o$) pressures observed for more than 40 min without intervention in a 26-year-old woman with primary pulmonary hypertension. The spontaneous fluctuations in pulmonary arterial mean pressure from 40 to 70 mmHg were not accompanied by corresponding changes in aortic pressure or (not shown) changes in heart rate. The patient subsequently showed a large fall in pressure and resistance with isoproterenol therapy for 11 days [172].

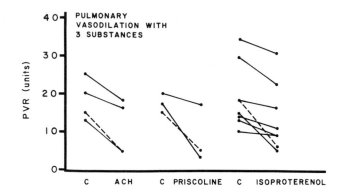

FIGURE 11 Pulmonary vascular resistance in units (mean PA pressure/cardiac index) before (c) and during infusion of pulmonary vasodilator substances [29,32,86,117,123]. Each pair of points connected by an unbroken line represents a single patient. Some patients responded well to vasodilators and others did not. The broken lines indicate the response to each of the three vasodilators in the 12-year-old boy reported by Rao et al. [29]. In this patient, acetylcholine, Priscoline, and isoproterenol were equally effective in lowering the pulmonary vascular resistance.

Pulmonary vasodilating substances such as acetylcholine, Priscoline, and β-sympathomimetics (isoproterenol, orciprenaline) have been shown to decrease pulmonary arterial pressure in primary pulmonary hypertension (Fig. 11). Other substances which have been used with variable success in an attempt to lower pulmonary arterial pressure and resistance acutely include phentolamine [20], diphenhydramine sodium, salicylate, and cortisone [86]. The evaluation of any substance requires measurement of pressure and flow. The flow may increase to such an extent that pressure may be unchanged or may even rise. If flow were not measured, the vasodilating effect of the drug would be missed. In the 12-year-old boy reported by Rao et al. [29], acetylcholine, Priscoline, and isoproterenol were equally effective in acutely lowering pulmonary pressure and resistance (Fig. 11). Among the other patients shown in Figure 11, some have a clear acute pulmonary vasodilatory response to acetylcholine, Isuprel, and Priscoline, and some do not. In the nonresponders, one must conclude that either vasoconstriction is not present, or that the agent is not an effective vasodilator.

A loss of the pulmonary vasodilating effect of acetylcholine on repeated catheterization has been attributed to a progression of irreversible intimal proliferative changes [82]. Presumably, then, pulmonary vasodilatation is possible early in the course of the disease but not late in its natural history. However, some patients with particularly high pulmonary vascular resistances demonstrated a clear fall in resistance with isoproterenol and others with more moderate resistance had a small isoproterenol effect (Fig. 11). A further confounding observation is that vasodilators may acutely lower pulmonary resistance, but quickly lose their effectiveness with repeated administration [29,86]. Rao et al. [29] abandoned Priscoline therapy in their patient when the drug became ineffective and obtained a good response to isoproterenol. Daoud has observed tachyphylaxis to isoproterenol [86]. Thus, unfortunately, it is not possible at present to predict from hemodynamic data alone which patients will respond to vasodilatation therapy or how long a favorable response might be maintained.

Acute oxygen administration has been evaluated in persons living near sea level with primary pulmonary hypertension. Oxygen caused little change in pulmonary vascular resistance (Fig. 12). Two of these patients with little or no vasodilatation with O_2 showed a brisk vasodilatation with isoproterenol. Five patients were made hypoxic by lowering their arterial oxygen tension from a mean of 76 to 46 mmHg. There was a small increase in pulmonary vascular resistance in only two of the patients (Fig. 12). The hemodynamic effect of acute administration of either oxygen or hypoxia was modest and inconsistent in these patients.

A study that tested the effect of acetylcholine infusion in nine female patients with primary pulmonary hypertension due to aminorex intake demonstrated a mean decrease of the pulmonary vascular resistance from 1074 to 767 (dyn sec cm^{-5}), mainly attributable to a vasodilatation following an increase in blood flow [137]. Similar findings were reported following administration of orciprenaline [116].

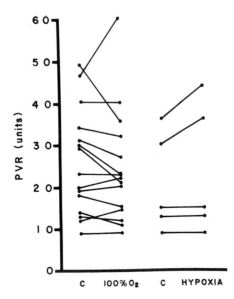

FIGURE 12   Pulmonary vascular resistance in units (mean PA pressure/ cardiac index) before (c), during 5 to 15 min of 100% oxygen breathing [20,28,56,86,87], and during alveolar hypoxia [86]. Neither oxygen breathing nor hypoxic gas mixtures had a consistent effect on pulmonary vascular resistance.

F. Right Ventricular Function

Few data dealing with the measurement of right ventricular contractility in primary pulmonary hypertension patients are available. The study of Degenring [132] demonstrated that the maximal rate of right ventricular pressure rise (dp/dt max) was 5 to 10 times the normal value. The right ventricular oxygen consumption was 5 times the normal value. With exercise, the right ventricular oxygen consumption increased further and did not fall promptly when exercise stopped. Increased myocardial norepinephrine probably contributed to the augmentation of the rate of right ventricular contraction and to the "uneconomical" increase of the myocontractility and oxygen consumption [132].

The end stage of the disease is characterized by right ventricular failure. In 50 reported fatalities [2,29,42,49,64,69,70,86,87,112,120-124, 129,130], the cause of death in 15 was severe right ventricular failure. Even in the 16 patients who died of syncope and the 16 dying of surgical or diagnostic procedures, most had signs of right ventricular failure.

G. Risks of Cardiac Catheterization and Angiography

Cardiac catheterization and angiography are particularly hazardous procedures for patients with primary pulmonary hypertension. For example, of 152 patients catheterized, 31 patients could be identified who died during cardiac catheterization or within a 36-hr period thereafter [29,64,66,69,87,112,120, 124,126-130,138-143]. The incidence may be overstated in that some patients had more than one catheterization procedure. Further, the use of the balloon-tipped, Swan-Ganz catheter may be less traumatic and therefore safer than the stiff catheters previously available. However, it is clear that catheterization and angiography carry an unusually high risk in primary pulmonary hypertension.

IV. Blood Gases, Ventilation, and Lung Function

Review of the older literature before blood gas tensions were widely employed [2,65,120] revealed an average oxygen saturation of 96.6% for 17 subjects in whom there was no shunt through the foramen ovale. The investigators concluded that, with a few exceptions [20], in primary pulmonary hypertension the arterial oxygenation was normal unless there was a right-to-left shunt through a patent foramen ovale [20]. However, the advent of blood gas tensions indicated that the values of arterial PO_2 were, in fact, low (Table 2). The decreased arterial oxygen tensions were not the result of alveolar hypoventilation, because the alveolar oxygen tensions and thus the alveolo-arterial oxygen gradients were increased (Table 2). The diffusing capacity was slightly [144,145] to strikingly [146] reduced. Herzog and Daum [146] found a normal membrane diffusion component in four patients with primary pulmonary hypertension, whereas the blood component or capillary blood volume Vc was reduced below 50% of the predicted values. Yu [147] also demonstrated a reduction in pulmonary capillary blood volume in patients with primary pulmonary hypertension.

The administration of 100% oxygen for several minutes to patients with primary pulmonary hypertension failed to increase PaO_2 to values found in normal subjects breathing oxygen [86,144,148]. These results suggest that the abnormally low PaO_2 in the air-breathing patients is not purely on the basis of a diffusion abnormality. Presumably, therefore, the mild arterial hypoxia usually observed is on the basis of ventilation-perfusion imbalance [87,146,149]. The pulmonary arterial bed in primary pulmonary hypertension is strikingly reduced due to obstructed arterioles. Although the total pulmonary flow is reduced, the flow through the patent channels may be rapid [129]. Further, capillaries draining patent arterioles are dilated [69]. The arterial PCO_2 is reduced, and several authors have reported increased frequency and volume of ventilation. Rapid flow through dilated capillary channels may be the mechanism of intrapulmonary shunting.

The effective ventilation is more than can be accounted for on the basis of the arterial hypoxemia. When the arterial CO_2 in primary pulmonary hypertension is compared to the PCO_2 in normal residents from high altitude with equivalent hypoxemia, the former have exaggerated hypocapnia (Fig. 13). Most authors have reported tachypnea. A slight decrease in dynamic compliance has been observed [88,150]. The hypocapnia could reflect a ventilatory response to low cardiac output or to intrapulmonary changes, or both. The findings are reminiscent of those in pulmonary embolism in which the hyperventilation is attributed to stimulation of intrapulmonary receptors [148,151]. Whatever the basis, it is clear that exercise dyspnea [21,56,87, 109] and increased ventilation at rest [87,144] are nearly always present in patients with primary pulmonary hypertension.

Spirometry has revealed normal vital capacities and 1-sec forced expired volumes [88]. Thus, there is no spirometric evidence of volume loss or expiratory obstruction. An increased dead space to tidal volume ratio is common [144,146] and probably reflects the loss of pulmonary arteriolar bed to ventilated lung zones.

TABLE 2 Blood Gas Measurements and Hemoglobin Concentrations from Various Sources

PaO$_2$ (mmHg)	Mean ± SE	78.5	67 ± 15	74.9 ± 15.1	63 ± 10
	No. of patients	(n = 26)	(n = 25)	(n = 13)	(n = 10)
	Source	[152]	[149]	[29,42,86,125,129]	[148]
PaCO$_2$ (mmHg)	Mean ± SE	29 ± 4	33 ± 5.6		31.0 ± 7.5
	No. of patients	(n = 26)	(n = 24)		(n = 10)
	Source	[152]	[149]		[148]
pH	Mean ± SE	7.44 ± 0.04			7.49 ± 0.11
	No. of patients	(n = 14)			(n = 10)
	Source	[29,42,86,125,144]			[148]
A-a-O$_2$ difference	Mean ± SE	49 ± 18	26.4	61	40
	No. of patients	(n = 25)	(n = 11)	(n = 2)	(n = 10)
	Source	[149]	[42,144,148]	[42,144]	[148]
Hb (mg/100 ml)	Mean ± SE	15.4 ± 2.9	16.6 ± 2		
	No. of patients	(n = 55)	(n = 21)		
	Source	[2,20,29,42,56,86,87,120]	[88]		
PaO$_2$ (mmHg) before 100% O$_2$	Mean ± SE	71.3 ± 14.6	63 ± 10		
	No. of patients	(n = 9)	(n = 10)		
	Source	[86,144]	[148]		
after 100% O$_2$	Mean ± SE	429.3 ± 89.2	453 ± 164		
	No. of patients	(n = 9)	(n = 10)		
	Source	[86,144]	[148]		

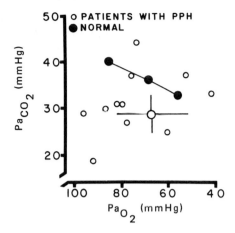

FIGURE 13 Hyperventilation in patients with primary pulmonary hypertension. Shown is P_{O_2}, P_{CO_2} diagram for arterial blood for normal residents of sea level, Denver, and Leadville, Colorado [195] (solid circles). Blood gases from 26 patients with primary pulmonary hypertension are shown as the large open circle with standard error bars [149]. The smaller open circles represent blood gas data from single patients [29,42,86,125,129,144]. Most of 37 patients with primary pulmonary hypertension fall below the normal values; i.e., they have lower P_{CO_2} values for a given P_{O_2}.

V. Pathology

A recent authoritative review of pulmonary hypertension, including primary pulmonary hypertension, has been published [8] and we will only consider: (1) the structural evidence for obstruction in the pulmonary vascular bed; (2) a brief description of lesions observed, (3) involvement of the various segments of the lung circulation, and (4) problems which remain to be solved by morphologists studying primary pulmonary hypertension.

A. Structural Evidence for Obstruction
of Lung Arteries

In the first year of life, intimal fibrosis is uncommon. Rather, the arteries show medial hypertrophy [8]. The persistence of the fetal elastic pattern in the pulmonary arterial trunk suggests that pulmonary hypertension has persisted from birth as a congenital abnormality of the pulmonary vascular bed [163,164]. Older children and adults who, through some mishap, come to autopsy relatively early in the course of their disease, show primarily medial hypertrophy [23]. Presumably, vasoconstriction in these hypertrophied

arteries largely accounts for the high pulmonary vascular resistance. In unselected autopsies of children dying with primary pulmonary hypertension, the
medial hypertrophy persists with increasing age, but is less marked (Fig. 14).
The intimal fibrosis, however, is drastically increased with age (Fig. 14).

Normally, after birth, the number of lung arteries increases rapidly with
the growth of the lung [55,165] and this increase may be retarded by vasoconstriction [54]. In the very young, failure of new vessel growth may contribute to the high resistance in primary pulmonary hypertension, although
this is conjectural at present.

In children or adults with advanced disease, severe intimal fibrosis
narrows pulmonary arterioles, producing focal obstruction. The obstruction is
compounded by the ultimate occlusion and irreversible loss of arterial segments, as evidenced by the pruned tree appearance of the postmortem pulmonary arteriograms [69,112] (see Fig. 16). Quantitative estimates from
microradiography indicate a profound loss of vessels, with but a small fraction
of the pulmonary arterioles remaining (Fig. 15). A visual impression of the
barren microvasculature is shown in Figure 16. Dilated capillaries bypass obstructed arterial segments to provide collateral flow (Fig. 16). Thus, vessel
loss may be even more severe than the measurements indicate. From the
above considerations it is clear that vasoconstriction and hypertrophy of
vessels, progressive intimal sclerosis, failure of growth of new vessels, and obliteration of existing vessels in various combinations account for the raised
pulmonary resistance in primary pulmonary hypertension.

B.   Descriptions of the Lesions Observed

Apart from the medial hypertrophy, two pathologic processes (which may be
related) have been described. Most common is the intimal fibrosis which

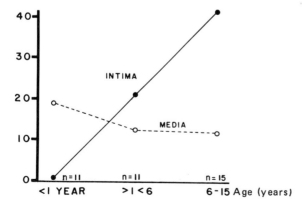

FIGURE 14   Relation of
age to relative thickness of
the media (.−.) or the intima (o−−o) expressed as
percentage of vessel dia-
meter in autopsied patients
with primary pulmonary
hypertension [23]. Medial
hypertrophy was greatest
in infants, but intimal
fibrosis was more apparent
in the older children.

apparently is laid down layer by layer on the luminal surface to provide a concentric onionskin appearance to the thickened intima of the transected vessel (Fig. 17). The second process is perivascular inflammation (pulmonary arteritis), which is followed by necrosis of the vascular wall. Wagenvoort et al. [165] proposed that it is the necrosis which precedes the formation of the plexiform lesion (see Chapter 1). The plexiform lesion has come to be one of the hallmarks of primary pulmonary hypertension because it is found in more than 70% of those with the disease, and it occurs only in two other pulmonary hypertensive disorders, i.e., those associated with congenital shunts and hepatic dysfunction [23]. Stuard et al. reported a patient with 300,000 plexiform lesions in the right lung [166]. Vogt and Rüttner in their report on seven patients with primary pulmonary hypertension found a correlation between the degree of the histologic lesions and the mean pulmonary arterial pressure and indicated that plexiform lesions were found in patients where the mean pulmonary arterial pressure was above 58 mmHg [22]. The number of plexiform lesions also increases with increasing pulmonary hypertension in patients with shunts from congenital heart disease [23]. Both the concentric intimal fibrosis and the arteritis lead to hyalinization of the wall of the pulmonary arteriole. In all these vascular lesions, fibrin deposition, platelet thrombi, recanalization, and cellular reorganization occur.

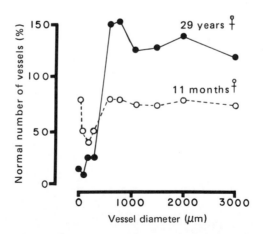

FIGURE 15 Relation of vessel size to the number of vessels predicted for a 29-year-old female (·) and an 11-month-old infant (o) dying of primary pulmonary hypertension [25]. In both patients there was a marked decrease in vessel numbers, relative to controls, for vessels below 600-μm diameter. The maximum decrease was in vessels of approximately 300 μm in diameter.

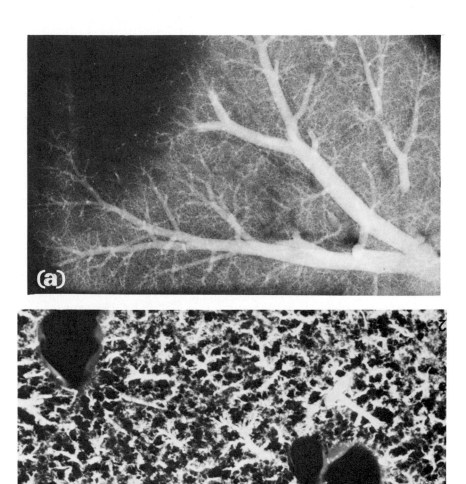

FIGURE 16a and b

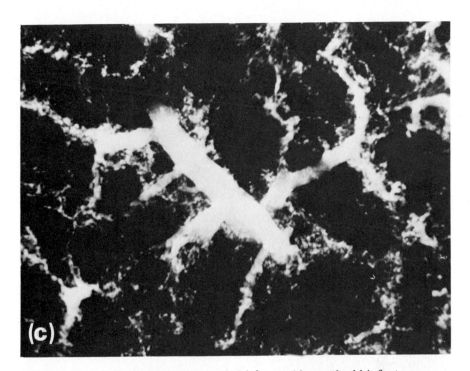

FIGURE 16   Radiographs (a) through (c) from a 10-month-old infant considered to have normal lungs [25] : (a) 1-cm thick lung slide (×2). The pulmonary arterial tree has been injected with barium sulfate and appears radio-opaque (white). Note normal vascular pattern and background haze. (b) A microradiograph (×7.5) of a 50-μm thick lung section from the lung shown in (a) above. Note the good filling of the microcirculation by the radio-opaque injection medium. (c) A microradiograph (×100) of a 50-μm thick section from the lung shown in (a). Note the details of the arterioles and the normal pattern of the lung capillaries.

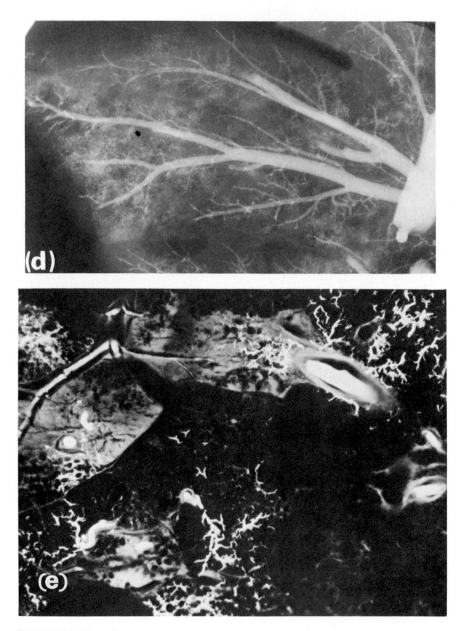

FIGURE 16d and e

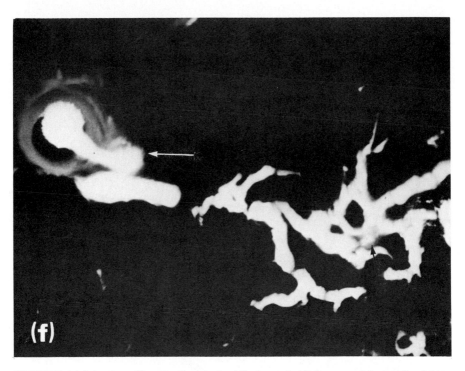

FIGURE 16 (continued)   Radiographs (d) through (f) from an 11-month-old infant dying of primary pulmonary hypertension [25]: (d) 1-cm thick lung slice (×2). Note the sparse filling of the microcirculation as evidenced by the poor background haze. (d) A microradiograph (×8.7) of a 50-μm thick section from the lung shown in (d). Note the narrowed arteries, the patchy filling of the microcirculation, and the rather large areas devoid of contrast. (f) Shown is an enlargement (×60) of the vessels in the lower midsection of (e) above. The white arrow indicates an area shown histologically to be an occluded arteriole. The opaque circle at the black arrow appeared to be dilated capillary segments. Histologic examination of this area confirmed that these were dilated capillaries.

C.   Involvement of the Various Segments of the Lung Circulation

The main pulmonary artery may become dilated, and the walls show arteriosclerosis, aneurysm, or rupture as a result of prolonged severe pulmonary hypertension [8]. The right and left pulmonary arteries and the lobar branches are usually dilated. However, the segmental arteries and the smaller muscular arteries often show a surprising lack of dilation and, in fact, are often narrowed (Fig. 16), suggesting that they may be actively involved in the

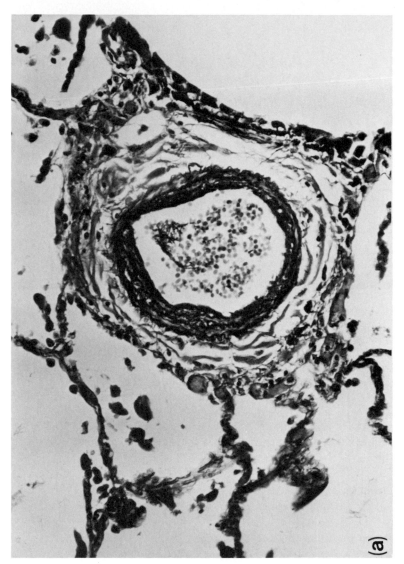

(a)

FIGURE 17a   Photomicrograph of a pulmonary arteriole approximately 250 μm in diameter from a patient with no evidence of pulmonary hypertension or pulmonary vascular disease (Vierhof-van Gieson).

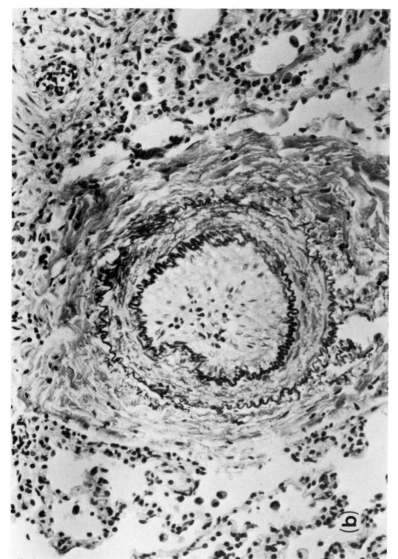

FIGURE 17b Photomicrograph of a pulmonary arteriole approximately 250 μm in diameter from a patient dying of primary pulmonary hypertension. Muscular hypertrophy can be seen between the internal and external elastic lamina. Intimal hyperplasia has nearly occluded the lumen (Vierhof-van Gieson). (Courtesy of Dr. Antony Martinez.)

vasoconstrictive process. The arteries most severely involved appear to be those less than 600 to 1000 μm in diameter. Such vessels are too small to be visualized by the usual postmortem angiograms and their loss is recognized as a loss of the background haze [164,167]. Analysis of microradiographs suggested that a large proportion of vessels less than 600 μm failed to fill with the radio-opaque injectate in the patients but not in the controls [69]. The maximum impact of the disease appeared to be on vessels approximately 200 to 300 μm in diameter. Reid has proposed that the maximum vessel loss occurs in vessels approximately 40 μm in diameter [128]. Clearly, primary pulmonary hypertension has preference for the small pulmonary arterioles, although even the muscular arteries may be involved.

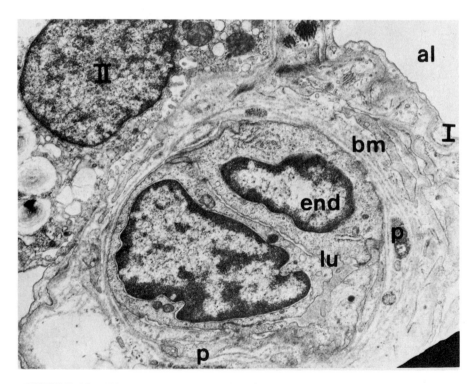

FIGURE 18   Electron micrograph of an alveolar capillary (approximately 7.0 μm in diameter) from a patient with primary pulmonary hypertension. The capillary lumen (lu) is seen as a cleft lined by plump endothelial cells (end). Concentric layers of basement membrane (bm) and pericyte processes (p) give rise to an onionskin appearance around the capillary. Types I (I) and II (II) pneumocytes, alveolus (al) (X 10,500). (Courtesy of Dr. Barbara Meyrick.)

The pulmonary hypertension and focal arterial obstruction may have a profound effect on the pulmonary capillary bed. Normally, the pulmonary capillaries (unlike the systemic capillaries) are located quite near an arterial vessel (Fig. 16). When the arterial pressure rises to a very high level the high pressure may be transmitted to the first portion of the capillary bed. The proximal capillary bed, if it remains patent, reacts to the hypertension by becoming profoundly dilated [69], as has already been shown in Eisenmenger's syndrome [168,169]. The dilated capillaries bulge into the alveolar lumen [168].

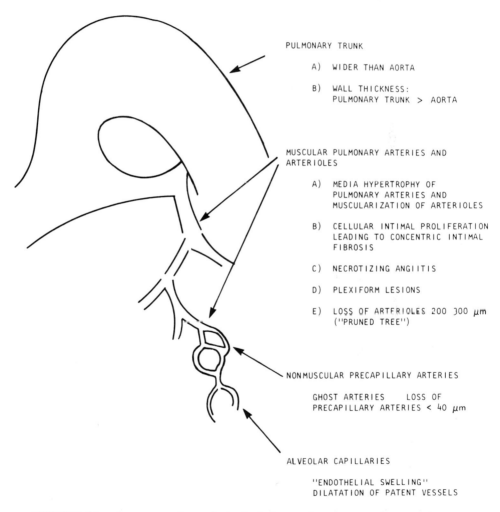

PULMONARY TRUNK

    A)   WIDER THAN AORTA

    B)   WALL THICKNESS:
        PULMONARY TRUNK > AORTA

MUSCULAR PULMONARY ARTERIES AND ARTERIOLES

    A)   MEDIA HYPERTROPHY OF
        PULMONARY ARTERIES AND
        MUSCULARIZATION OF ARTERIOLES

    B)   CELLULAR INTIMAL PROLIFERATION
        LEADING TO CONCENTRIC INTIMAL
        FIBROSIS

    C)   NECROTIZING ANGIITIS

    D)   PLEXIFORM LESIONS

    E)   LOSS OF ARTERIOLES 200 300 μm
        ("PRUNED TREE")

NONMUSCULAR PRECAPILLARY ARTERIES

GHOST ARTERIES   LOSS OF
PRECAPILLARY ARTERIES < 40 μm

ALVEOLAR CAPILLARIES

"ENDOTHELIAL SWELLING"
DILATATION OF PATENT VESSELS

FIGURE 19   Summary of morphological changes in primary pulmonary hypertension at various levels in the pulmonary vascular tree.

These dilated, tortuous vessels may contribute to the structure of the plexi-form lesion. The capillaries are also damaged by the high pressure, flow, or by released substances, resulting in endothelial swelling and even total oc-clusion (Fig. 18). Thus, in one form or another, the pulmonary circulation from the main pulmonary artery to the capillaries is involved in the disease process (Fig. 19). The veins are largely exempted [170].

D. Problems Remaining

Little electron microscopy has been reported in primary pulmonary hyper-tension [171] (Fig. 18). We thus remain largely ignorant of the details of the changes in the intimal and smooth muscle cells. That is, if vasoconstriction is the initial event, what abnormality in the contractile machinery is present? If the process originates in the intima, what are the ultrastructural changes early in the disease? In addition, we found no published reports bringing the methodology of immunopathology to bear on the disease. Yet, such investiga-tion is indicated in view of the prominence of arteritis in the pathogenesis and the close link between primary pulmonary hypertension and immune complex diseases of the collagen vascular type. Quantitative morphology, which has yielded important information thus far, needs additional stress, for example, in the area of numbers of vessels and their sizes in primary pulmonary hyper-tension. The role of the platelet and fibrin deposition, and the pathophys-iology of intimal sclerosis and its relation to medial hypertrophy, need to be clarified. Are platelet and fibrin deposition primary or secondary in the disease process? Why do some patients have a highly reactive pulmonary circulation while others with similar elevations of pressure and resistance have an unreactive vascular bed? In view of the mystery which surrounds the disease and the difficulty in obtaining lung tissue in early stages of the disease, an animal model is needed. These are but a few of the questions and prob-lems surrounding this rare but highly fatal disease.

VI. Diagnosis

One problem in primary pulmonary hypertension is the large individual varia-tion in the stage of the disease process when the first symptoms appear [6,172]. The large range of pulmonary arterial pressures at the initial cathe-terization (Fig. 20) testifies to the fact that the mean pressure may range between 30 and 122 mmHg. Thus, in many patients, the first symptoms appear at a stage when the disease is far advanced and the process is likely to be irreversible.

A. Symptoms

The symptoms described by the patients are listed (Table 3). Dyspnea on exertion is present in almost all patients and seems to be the earliest symptom (Fig. 19). Orthopnea is seen, but not consistently, and the complaint is not prominent [121]. It is unlikely that dyspnea is related to mechanical lung function, which shows little derangement. The dyspnea is not caused by hypoxemia because it occurs when hypoxemia is absent and because it is not relieved by breathing pure oxygen [148]. Dyspnea may be related to the low cardiac output because both dyspnea and low output are present in nearly all patients. During exertion, both the limitation of the cardiac output and the increase in dyspnea are most profound, and we have seen two patients in whom relief of pulmonary hypertension and increase in output relieved dyspnea. Dyspnea also could be related to stimulation of intrapulmonary receptors affected in some way by the vascular disease (see Section IV).

Anginal-type chest pain is a common finding and it occurs in other forms of pulmonary hypertension [173], precipitated in most cases by exertion. Like dyspnea, it may occur at relatively low pulmonary arterial pressures (Fig. 21). No arteriosclerotic changes have been described in the coronary arteries. The relationship of angina to myocardial ischemia is

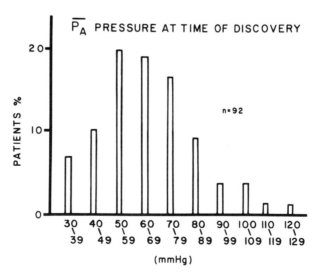

FIGURE 20   Distribution of mean pulmonary arterial pressure at the time of initial heart catheterization in 92 patients considered to have primary pulmonary hypertension [2,20,23,28,29,42,49,50,52,56,62,86,87,120,122–126,129, 130,196].

TABLE 3   Symptoms of PPH

Symptom	Harms and Voss [149]	Yu [109]	Compiled data from other authors [13,120,121,126]
Dyspnea on exertion	100% (*n* = 42)	98% (*n* = 55)	85% (*n* = 48)
Syncope	20%	55%	21%
Fatigue	—	38%	80%
Anginal-type chest pain	54%	42%	48%
Hemoptysis	7%	13%	15%
Cyanosis	—	45%	36%
Nonproductive cough	—	18%	23%
Hoarseness	—	6%	8%

uncertain, but a decreased coronary blood flow relative to the hypertrophied right ventricle has been suggested [134].

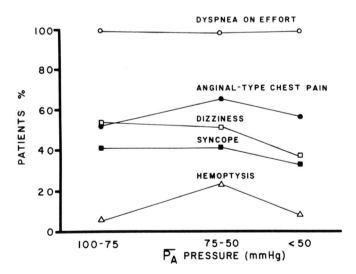

FIGURE 21   Relationship of frequency of symptoms in spontaneous primary pulmonary hypertension and pulmonary hypertension following aminorex ingestion, to level of pulmonary arterial pressure as measured at heart catheterization: 100–75 mmHg: (*n* = 13); 75–50 mmHg: (*n* = 40) <50 mmHg (*n* = 32) [21].

Syncopal attacks or dizziness usually occur with or following exertion. Loogen and Both [21] found in a retrospective study of 85 patients that syncope was uncommon at pulmonary arterial mean pressures below 40 mmHg, and tended to increase slightly in frequency with rising pressure (Fig. 19). Howarth and Lowe [134], and Dresdale et al. [2] suggested as the mechanism for syncope, acute right heart failure with a decrease of cardiac output leading to coronary [2] and cerebral [21] underperfusion. Perhaps reflex mechanisms, sensing stretch in the pulmonary artery, act to further increase pulmonary resistance [118] or depress systemic pressure [162].

Hemoptysis is evidence of advanced disease. It seems likely to us that in primary pulmonary hypertension and in patients with pulmonary hypertension from congenital heart disease, the bleeding results from rupture of the dilated capillaries which bulge into the alveoli under high pressure [168,169,191]. Yuceoglu et al. reported [123] a patient with primary pulmonary hypertension and hemoptysis who had a fatal lung hemorrhage after being placed on anticoagulants.

Cyanosis has several contributing factors. With pulmonary hypertension and right heart failure, a patent foramen ovale will permit a right-to-left shunt. Oxygen saturations in six such patients averaged 88% [56,125]. A few patients with a closed foramen ovale have such a reduced arterial PO_2 that the saturation is lowered [144]. However, peripheral cyanosis may occur in the absence of a shunt and with normal arterial saturation because the low cardiac output and the high hemoglobin concentration result in a relatively high concentration of desaturated hemoglobin in the capillaries.

Hoarseness from pressure on the recurrent laryngeal nerve caused by a dilated main pulmonary artery has been reported [123,174,175]. The concurrence of purpura and ecchymoses due to intravascular hemolysis and thrombocytopenia is rare and has been described in three patients [166,176].

B. Clinical Signs

The clinical recognition of primary pulmonary hypertension has recently been summarized [172]. In brief, the signs reflect severe pulmonary hypertension. Inspection reveals a prominent jugular venous a wave, and, in right heart failure, an elevated venous pressure [21,68,88,109]. Cyanosis has been discussed above. Palpation reveals small pulses and cold extremities consistent with a low cardiac output, and a sternal heave of right ventricular hypertrophy [21,109]. Auscultation reveals an accentuated pulmonary closure sound reflecting the high diastolic pulmonary arterial pressure, and a systolic ejection click probably caused by sudden tensing of the distended pulmonary artery [5,21]. A right ventricular third and/or fourth heart sound reflect increased resistance to right ventricular filling. A systolic murmur of tricuspid insufficiency and a diastolic murmur of pulmonary insufficiency are late findings. The phonocardiogram confirms clinical auscultation.

The electrocardiogram characteristically shows right heart hypertrophy by the usual criteria [177,178] (Fig. 22). Normal electrocardiograms are seen in fewer than 10% of the patients and these have lesser degrees of pulmonary hypertension [22]. Vectorcardiography is a relatively sensitive tool in the detection of right heart hypertrophy [179,180]. The QRS vector in the frontal plane shifts to the right (90-150°) in correlation with increasing

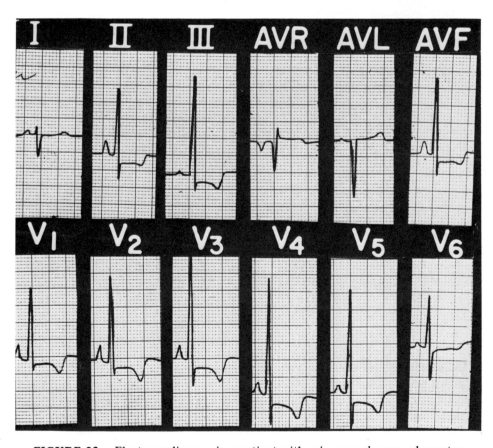

FIGURE 22   Electrocardiogram in a patient with primary pulmonary hypertension. The mean QRS axis was +120 degrees. The tall, peaked P waves indicate right atrial enlargement. The tall R waves in leads V_1-V_3 and deep S wave in V_6 and the associated T-wave changes indicate right ventricular hypertrophy. (Tracing compliments of Dr. J. Ray Pryor.)

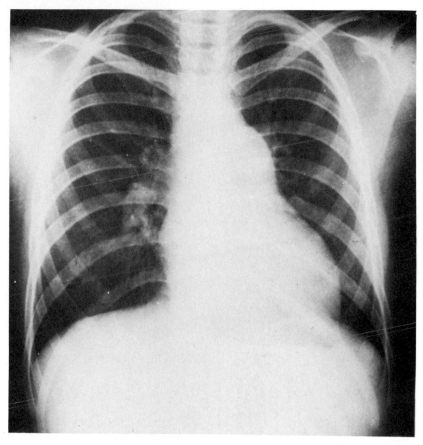

FIGURE 23   Chest roentgenogram in an 11-year-old girl with primary pulmonary hypertension showing prominence of main pulmonary artery and paucity
of vascular marking in peripheral lung fields. (Courtesy of Dr. S. Gilbert Blount.)

pulmonary arterial pressure [3,21]. P pulmonale may or may not be present
[21,172].   Atrioventricular or right bundle branch block are uncommon
findings.

The chest roentgenogram (Fig. 23) shows a prominent pulmonary
arterial trunk reflecting dilation from long-standing pulmonary hypertension
although there is not a good relation between pulmonary arterial dilation and
the measured pressure and resistance [43,181]. Occasionally there is an
abrupt decrease in the caliber of the more peripheral arterial segments, reflecting vasoconstriction [182]. The vasculature in the peripheral lung fields may
appear normal or decreased. The electrocardiogram is a more reliable indication

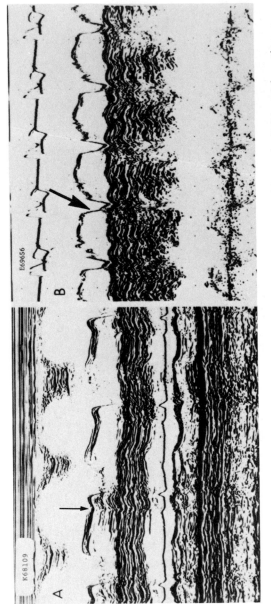

FIGURE 24 (a) Echocardiogram of the pulmonary valve in a normal subject. A slight atrial motion, a wave (arrow), in the pulmonary valve motion is seen following the P wave in the electrocardiogram. (b) Echocardiogram of the pulmonary valve in a patient with pulmonary hypertension. The a wave is absent. The velocity of opening of the pulmonary valve (at arrow) is slightly greater than in the normal subject. (Courtesy of Dr. Michael Johnson.)

of right ventricular hypertrophy than the chest film. If right ventricular failure is present, the heart may be enlarged. The lung scan may be normal even in severe pulmonary hypertension [183], although the scan in conjunction with pulmonary vasodilating drugs has been used to distinguish reactive from fixed pulmonary hypertension [184,185].

The echocardiogram (Fig. 24) reflects only pulmonary hypertension [186], but its ultimate value will be judged by the confidence with which it will allow an estimate of the pulmonary arterial pressure. Several findings indicate the presence of pulmonary hypertension but are not sensitive as to the actual magnitude of the pressure:

1. The loss of, or diminution of, the a wave in the pulmonary valve motion indicates the diastolic pressure in the pulmonary artery is above that generated by atrial systole.

2. The decreased E-F slope of the pulmonary valve probably reflects diastolic motion of the pulmonary artery itself which is altered in pulmonary hypertension [187].

3. The early closure of the pulmonary valve leaflet may reflect the decreased ejection period when pressure is high [187].

4. Increased diameter of the right ventricular chamber indicates the dilatation present.

In children, an index relating the ratio of the right ventricular preejection period to right ventricular ejection time has provided a rough estimate of pulmonary arterial pressure [188]. It remains to be seen how this may be refined and how well it may apply to adults.

Primary pulmonary hypertension is diagnosed by excluding known causes of pulmonary hypertension, particularly mitral stenosis, congenital cardiac shunts with pulmonary hypertension, recurrent pulmonary emboli, anomalies of the pulmonary veins, pulmonary parenchymal disease, and hepatic dysfunction [172]. In planning diagnostic tests one should recall that pulmonary angiography and cardiac catheterization, and particularly lung biopsy, are fraught with hazard for the patient with primary pulmonary hypertension.

VII. Therapy

A large variety of drugs and procedures have been employed in the long-term therapy of primary pulmonary hypertension with almost uniform failure (Table 4). The exceptions are intravenous isoproterenol therapy (0.5 to

TABLE 4   Effects of Therapy

Therapy and source	Administration	No. of patients	Maximum duration of Rx	Estimate of benefits	Recatheterization in at least one patient	Complications of Rx
Steroids [86,87,110,125]	oral	5	2 yr	0	+	Diabetes
Immuran [86]	oral	1	2 yr	0	+	—
Reserpine [87,110,125,192]	oral	5	3 yr	0	+	—
Anticoagulants [20,87,123,191]	oral	30	3 yr	0	+	Fatal hemoptysis
Fibrinolysis [194]	IV	3	1–3 days	0	+	Cerebral hemorrhage
Sympathectomy surgical [125]		1	—	0	+	—
Monamine [125] oxidase inhibitor	oral	2	4 wks	0	+	—
Antiserotonin [110]	oral	1	6 mo	0	+	—
Priscoline [29,87]	oral	4	3 yr	0	+	—
[29]	IV	1	2 days	0	+	—
Nitroglycerine [192]	oral	4	4 mo	3/4-0 1/4-+	+	—
Isosorbide [193] dinitrate	oral	1	4 mo	0	+	—
Isoproterenol [86,190]	oral	3	2 yr	1/3-0 2/3-+	+	—
[29,86, Blount, unpublished results]	IV	4	2–11 days	2/5-0 3/5-+	+	Catheterization failure
Banthine [87]	oral	1		0	+	
O$_2$ (Reeves, 1975, unpublished results)	nasal	1	2 yr	0	+	—
Banding of pulmonary artery [20]	surgery	4	1½ yr	0	+	Cyanosis
Descent to lower altitude (Blount, 1975, unpublished results)		1	6 mo	+	+	—

1.0 gm/min) given as a constant infusion in three of five patients and nitroglycerine in one of four patients. These apparent successes listed in the table are misleading, however, for several reasons. (1) Only therapy carried out for several days has been shown. Patients with no change or an increase in resistance with acute isoproterenol therapy did not receive chronic administration on the likelihood that it would not be beneficial. (2) Patients who were treated for several days unsuccessfully with isoproterenol are known to the authors, but have not been reported. Thus, results presented overstate the effectiveness of long-term vasodilator therapy. Indeed, successful therapy with vasodilators may be the exception rather than the rule. However, the fact that any success is possible is remarkable given the history of this disease.

A problem with all the vasodilators is that a given agent may lower resistance acutely but, with repeated administration, the vasodilating effect disappears [190]. Thus, such therapy may be regarded as symptomatic because it does not reverse the pathologic process. Further research is essential in order that the etiology of the disease be discovered. Once the mechanism is known, perhaps it can be arrested or reversed. The instances of spontaneous reversal provide hope that early recognition and therapy could lead to recovery. Thus, the ultimate hope is for a discovery of the basic mechanisms which now are unknown.

VIII. Recent Development

This is the largest clinical study known to us, to date, with 137 cases of primary pulmonary hypertension (PPH). Watanabe, S., and T. Ogata, Clinical and experimental study upon primary pulmonary hypertension, *Jpn. Circ. J.,* **40**:603–610 (1976).

References

1. *World Health Organization: Primary Pulmonary Hypertension.* Report on a WHO Meeting. Edited by S. Hatano and T. Strasser. Geneva, Publisher, 1975.
2. Dresdale, D. T., M. Schultz, and R. J. Michtom, Primary pulmonary hypertension. I. Clinical and haemodynamic study, *Am. J. Med.,* **11**:686 (1951).
3. Trell, E., and C. Lindström, Primary and thromboembolic pulmonary hypertension. Clinical and pathoanatomic observations, *Acta Med. Scand. [Suppl.],* **534**:1–30 (1972).
4. McGuire, J., R. C. Scott, R. A. Helm, S. Kaplan, E. A. Gall, and J. P. Biehl, Is there an entity primary pulmonary hypertension? *Arch. Intern. Med.,* **99**:917 (1957).

5. Wade, G., and J. Ball, Unexplained pulmonary hypertension, *Q. J. Med.*, **26**:83 (1957).
6. Blount, S. G., Primary pulmonary hypertension, *Mod. Conc. Cardiovasc. Dis.*, **36**(12):67–72 (1967).
7. Perloff, J. K., and J. P. Szidon, Pulmonary hypertension: etiologies, recognition, consequences. In *Clinical Cardiology*. Edited by J. T. Willerson, and C. A. Sanders. San Francisco, Grune and Stratton, Inc., 1977.
8. Wagenvoort, C. A. and N. Wagenvoort, *Pathology of Pulmonary Hypertension*. New York, John Willey and Sons, 1977.
9. Romberg, E., Ueber Sklerose der Lungenarterien, *Dtsch. Arch. Klin. Med.*, **48**:197 (1891).
10. Brenner, O., Pathology of the vessels of the pulmonary circulation, *Arch. Intern. Med.*, **56**:211,457,724,976,1189 (1935).
11. Arrillaga, F. C., Sclérose de l'artére pulmonaire secondaire à certains états pulmonaires chroniques, *Arch. Mal. Coeur*, **6**:518 (1913). Sclérose de l'artére pulmonaire, *Bull. Mem. Soc. Med. Hop. Paris*, **48**:292 (1924).
12. Wood, P., Pulmonary hypertension with special reference to the vasoconstrictive factor, *Br. Heart J.*, **21**:557 (1959).
13. Heath, D., and J. E. Edwards, The pathology of hypertensive pulmonary vascular disease: A description of six grades of structural changes in the pulmonary arteries with special references to congenital cardiac septal defects, *Circulation*, **18**:533 (1958).
14. Gurtner, H. P., M. Gertsch, C. Salzman, M. Scherrer, P. Stucki, and F. Wyss, Häufen sich die primär vasculären Formen des chronischen cor pulmonale? *Schweiz. Med. Wochenschr.*, **98**:1579, 1695 (1968).
15. MacCallum, W. G., Obliterative pulmonary arteriosclerosis, *Bull. Johns Hopkins Hosp.*, **49**:37 (1931).
16. Wood, P., *Diseases of the Heart and Circulation*. Philadelphia, J. Lippincott Co., 1956, p. 839.
17. Bärlocher, P., F. Schaub, and A. Bühlmann, Über die sogennante primäre pulmonale Hypertonie, *Schweiz. Med. Wochenschr.*, **88**:869 (1958).
18. Schwingshackl, H., A. Amor, and F. Dienstl, "Primäre" pulmonale Hypertonie bei sieben jüngeren Frauen., *Dtsch. Med. Wochenschr.*, **94**:639 (1969).
19. Voss, H., and H. Harms, Epidemiology and clinical aspects of primary vascular pulmonary hypertension. A report on 42 cases, *Z. Kreislaufforsch.*, **59**(10):887–891 (1970).
20. Störstein, O., L. Efskind, C. Müller, R. Rokseth, and S. Sander, Primary pulmonary hypertension with emphasis on its etiology and treatment, *Acta Med. Scand.*, **179**(2):197–212 (1966).
21. Loogen, F., and A. Both, Primary pulmonary hypertension, *Z. Kardiol.*, **65**(1):1–14 (1976).
22. Vogt, P., and J. R. Rüttner, Das cor pulmonale aus pathologisch-anatomischer Sicht, *Schweiz. Med. Wochenschr.*, **107**:549 (1977).
23. Wagenvoort, C. A., and N. Wagenvoort, Primary pulmonary hypertension. A pathologic study of the lung vessels in 156 clinically diagnosed cases, *Circulation*, **42**:1163 (1970).

24. Wirz, R., and U. Arbenz, Primär vaskuläre pulmonale Hypertonie in der Schweiz 1965–1970, *Schweiz. Med. Wochenschr.*, **100**:2147 (1970).
25. Gertsch, M., Die Häufigkeit der primär vasculären pulmonalen Hypertonie am Inselspital Bern, *Z. Kreislaufforsch.*, **59**:884 (1970).
26. von Smekal, P., K. Standfuss, and G. Rau, Increase of primary vascular pulmonary hypertension in connection with the intake of appetite depressants? Questions of respiratory regulation, *Z. Kreislaufforsch.*, **59**: (10):892–897 (1970).
27. Berthrong, M., and T. H. Cochran, Pathological findings in 9 children with "primary" pulmonary hypertension, *Bull. Johns Hopkins Hosp.*, **97**:69 (1955).
28. Farrar, J. F., R. D. Reye, and D. Stuckey, Primary pulmonary hypertension in childhood, *Br. Heart J.*, **23**:605 (1961).
29. Rao, S. B. N., J. H. Moller, and J. E. Edwards, Primary pulmonary hypertension in a child. Response to pharmacologic agents, *Circulation*, **40**(4): 583–587 (1969).
30. Burnell, R. H., M. C. Joseph, and M. H. Lees, Progressive pulmonary hypertension in newborn infants, *Am. J. Dis. Child.*, **123**:167 (1972).
31. Rivier, J. L., Hypertension artérielle pulmonaire primitive, *Schweiz. Med. Wochenschr.*, **100**:143 (1970).
32. Clarke, R. C., C. F. Coombs, G. Hadfield, and A. T. Todd, On certain abnormalities, congenital and acquired of the pulmonary artery, *Q. J. Med.*, **21**:51 (1927).
33. Van Epps, E., Primary pulmonary hypertension in brothers, *Am. J. Roentgenol.*, **78**:471 (1957).
34. Coleman, P. N., A. W. Edmunds, and F. Tregillus, Primary pulmonary hypertension in three sibs, *Br. Heatt J.*, **21**:81 (1959).
35. Fleming, H., Primary pulmonary hypertension in eight patients including mother and her daughter, *Aust. Ann. Med.*, **9**:10 (1960).
36. Van Bogaert, A., J. Wanters, R. Tosetti, and H. O'Heer, Hypertension pulmonaire primitive familiale, *Arch. Mal Coeur*, **54**:1185 (1961).
37. Boiteau, G. M., and A. J. Libanoff, Primary pulmonary hypertension: familial incidence, *Angiology*, **14**:260 (1963).
38. Parry, W. R., and D. Verel, Familial primary pulmonary hypertension, *Br. Heart J.*, **28**:193 (1966).
39. Sedziwy, L., and J. Kalczynski, Primary pulmonary hypertension in three brothers, *Acta Med. Pol.*, **7**:401 (1966).
40. Kingdon, H. S., L. S. Cohen, W. C. Roberts, and E. Braunwald, Familial occurrence of primary pulmonary hypertension, *Arch. Intern. Med.*, **118**: 422 (1966).
41. Rogge, J. D., M. E. Mishkin, and P. D. Genovese, The familial occurrence of primary pulmonary hypertension, *Ann. Intern. Med.*, **65**:672 (1966).
42. Delaye, J., R. Loire, J. Brune, C. Dalloz, J. P. Delahaye, and A. Gonin, Hereditary primary pulmonary arterial hypertension. History of 2 families and review of the literature, *Coeur Med. Interne*, **8**(1):31–45 (1969).

43. Czarnecki, S. W., and H. M. Rosenbaum, The occurrence of primary pulmonary hypertension in twins with a review of etiological considerations, *Am. Heart J.,* **75**:240 (1968).
44. Massoud, H., W. Puckett, and S. H. Auerbach, Primary pulmonary hypertension: A study of the disease in four young siblings, *J. Tenn. Med. Assoc.,* **63**(4):299–305 (1970).
45. Thilenius, O. G., A. S. Nadas, and H. Jockin, Primary pulmonary vascular obstruction in children, *Pediatrics,* **36**:75 (1965).
46. Hood, W. B., H. Spencer, R. W. Lass, and R. Daley, Primary pulmonary hypertension: familial occurrence, *Br. Heart J.,* **30**:336 (1968).
47. Melmon, K. L., Familial pulmonary hypertension, *N. Engl. J. Med.,* **269**: 770 (1963).
48. Thompson, P., and C. McRae, Familial pulmonary hypertension. Evidence of antosomal dominant inheritance, *Br. Heart J.,* **32**:758 (1970).
49. Charters, A. D., and W. C. Baker, Primary pulmonary hypertension of unusually long duration, *Br. Heart J.,* **32**(1):130–133 (1970).
50. Bourdillon, P. D., and C. M. Oakley, Regression of primary pulmonary hypertension, *Br. Heart J.,* **38**:264 (1976).
51. Both, A., F. Loogen, and W. Maurer, Follow-up studies on patients with primary vascular pulmonary hypertension taking anorectics, *Verh. Dtsch. Ges. Inn. Med.,* **77**:445–448 (1971).
52. Evans, W., D. S. Short, and D. E. Bedford, Solitary pulmonary hypertension, *Br. Heart J.,* **19**:93 (1957).
53. Goodale, Jr., F., and W. A. Thomas, Primary pulmonary arterial disease, observations with special reference to medial thickening of small arteries and arterioles, *Arch. Pathol.,* **58**:568 (1954).
54. Siassi, B., S. J. Goldberg, G. C. Emmanouilides, S. M. Higashino, and E. Lewis, Persistent pulmonary vascular obstruction in newborn infants, *J. Pediatr.,* **78**:610 (1971).
55. Reeves, J. T., and J. E. Leathers, Postnatal development of pulmonary and bronchial arterial circulations in the calf and the effects of chronic hypoxia, *Anat. Rec.,* **157**:641–656 (1967).
56. Shepherd, J. T., J. E. Edwards, H. B. Burchell, H. J. C. Swan, and F. H. Wood, Clinical, physiological and pathological consideration in patients with idiopathic pulmonary hypertension, *Br. Heart J.,* **19**:701 (1957).
57. Ichinose, S., O. Takeoka, T. Matsuura, T. Kiriyama, N. Endo, M. Ochiai, Y. Hishimoto, and I. Niki, Primary pulmonary hypertension: a case report with discussion on its pathogenesis, *Jpn. Circ. J.,* **32**:773 (1968).
58. Demas, N. W., Maternal death due to primary pulmonary hypertension, *Trans. Pac. Coast Obstet. Gynecol. Soc.,* **40**:64–67 (1972).
59. Moore, L., I. F. McMurtry, and J. T. Reeves, Effects of sex hormones on cardiovascular and hematologic responses to chronic hypoxia in rats, *Proc. Soc. Exp. Biol. Med.,* **158**:658–662 (1978).
60. Werkö, L., Pregnancy and heart disease, *Acta Obstet. Gynecol. Scand.,* **33**: 162 (1954).

61. Weir, K. E., I. F. McMurtry, A. Tucker, J. T. Reeves, and R. F. Grover, Prostaglandin synthetase inhibitors do not decrease hypoxic pulmonary vasoconstriction, *J. Appl. Physiol.,* 41:714–718 (1976).

62. Moore, L., J. T. Reeves, D. H. Will, and R. F. Grover, Pregnancy-induced pulmonary hypertension in cows susceptible to high mountain disease, *J. Appl. Physiol.,* 46:184–188 (1979).

63. Owen, W. R., W. A. Thomas, B. Castleman, and E. F. Bland, Unrecognized emboli to the lungs with subsequent cor pulmonale, *N. Engl. J. Med.,* 249: 919 (1953).

64. Rosenberg, S. A., A study of the etiological basis of primary pulmonary hypertension, *Am. Heart J.,* 68:484 (1964).

65. Ohlsen, E. G. J., Thrombo-embolic pulmonary hypertension: an experimental study, *J. Pathol.,* 106:4 (1972).

66. Kuzman, W. J., Primary pulmonary hypertension, *Med. Times,* 98(3):151–162 (1970).

67. Trell, E., Primary and chronic thromboembolic pulmonary hypertension. Nosologic spectrum, *Angiology,* 23(9):558–574 (1972).

68. Fowler, N. O., B. Black-Schaffer, R. C. Scott, and M. Gueron, Idiopathic and thromboembolic pulmonary hypertension, *Am. J. Med.,* 40:331 (1966).

69. Reeves, J. T., and J. A. Noonan, Microarteriographic studies of primary pulmonary hypertension. A quantitative approach in two patients, *Arch. Pathol.,* 95(1):50–55 (1973).

70. Winters, W. L., R. R. Joseph, and M. Learner, Primary pulmonary hypertension and Raynaud's phenomenon, *Arch. Intern. Med.,* 114:821 (1964).

71. Colonna, D., J. P. Maurst, C. Leiva, and A. Semper, Hypertension artérielle pulmonaire primitive et syndrome de Raynaud, *Coeur Med. Interne,* 3:469 (1964).

72. Gisand, G., H. Latour, P. Puech, and J. Roujon, Rapport d'un cas d'hypertension pulmonaire anociée à un syndrome de Raynaud, *Arch. Mal Coeur,* 50:154 (1957).

73. Smith, W. M., and I. G. Kroop, Raynaud: disease in primary pulmonary hypertension, *JAMA,* 165:1245 (1957).

74. Celonä, G. C., G. H. Friedell, and J. C. Sommers, Raynaud's disease and primary pulmonary hypertension, *Circulation,* 22:1055 (1960).

75. Onodera, S., and J. R. Hill, Pulmonary hypertension. Report of a case in association with rheumatoid arthritis, *Ohio Med. J.,* 61:141 (1965).

76. Gardner, D. L., J. J. Onthie, J. Macleod, and W. S. Allan, Pulmonary hypertension in rheumatoid arthritis. Report of a case with intimal sclerosis of the pulmonary and digital arteries, *Scot. Med. J.,* 2:183 (1957).

77. Pace, W. R., J. L. Decker, and C. J. Martin, Polymyositis: Report of two cases with pulmonary function studies suggestive of progressive systematic sclerosis, *Am. J. Med. Sci.,* 245:322 (1963).

78. Trell, E., and C. Lindström, Pulmonary hypertension in systemic sclerosis, *Ann. Rheum. Dis.,* 30:390 (1971).

79. Caldwell, I. W., and J. D. Aitchison, Pulmonary hypertension in derma-
     tomyositis, *Br. Heart J.*, **18**:273 (1956).
80. Slama, R., A. Crevelier, P. Coumel, and S. Snanoudj, Hypertension
     arteriélle pulmonaire primitive et lupus érythemateux disséminé, *Presse
     Med.*, **75**:961 (1967).
81. Wohl, M., Case records of the Massachusetts General Hospital, *N. Engl. J.
     Med.*, **288**:204 (1973).
82. Samet, P., and W. H. Bernstein, Loss of reactivity of the pulmonary
     vascular bed in primary pulmonary hypertension, *Am. Heart J.*, **66**:107
     (1963).
83. Rawson, A. J., and H. M. Woske, A study of etiologic factors in so called
     primary pulmonary hypertension, *Arch. Intern. Med.*, **105**:81 (1960).
84. Wallcott, G., H. B. Burchell, and A. L. Brown, Jr., Primary pulmonary
     hypertension, *Am. J. Med.*, **49**:70 (1970).
85. Seldin, D. W., M. Ziff, A. G. DeGraff, B. D. Fallis, and R. R. Burns,
     Raynaud's phenomenon associated with pulmonary hypertension, *Texas
     J. Med.*, **58**:654 (1962).
86. Daoud, F. S., D. B. Kelly, and J. T. Reeves, Isoproterenol as a potential
     pulmonary vasodilator in primary pulmonary hypertension, *Am. J.
     Cardiol.*, **42**:817–822 (1978).
87. Sleeper, J. C., E. S. Orgain, and H. D. McIntosh, Primary pulmonary hy-
     pertension. Review of clinical features and pathologic physiology with a
     report of pulmonary haemodynamics derived from repeated catheteriza-
     tion, *Circulation*, **26**:1358 (1962).
88. Gahl, K., H. Fabel, E. Greiser, D. Harmjanz, H. Ostertag, and H. S. Stender,
     Primary vascular pulmonary hypertension. Report on 21 patients, *Z.
     Kreislaufforsch.*, **59**(10):868–883 (1970).
89. Rivier, J. L., M. Jaeger, P. Desbaillets, and C. Reymond, Primary and
     anorexigenic pulmonary arterial hypertension, *Arch. Mal Coeur*, **64**(4):
     607 (1971).
90. Steim, H., K. Deibert, G. W. Lohr, and H. Reindell, Primary pulmonary
     hypertension—contribution on occurrence and etiology, *Verh. Dtsch. Ges.
     Inn. Med.*, **75**:439–443 (1969).
91. Kaindl, F., Primary pulmonary hypertension, *Wien Z. Inn. Med.*, **50**(10):
     451–453 (1969).
92. Loogen, F., and W. Kübler, Primary pulmonary hypertension, *Z. Kreis-
     laufforsch.*, **59**(10):865–867 (1970).
93. Gurtner, H. P., *Schweiz. Med. Wochenschr.*, **100**:2158 (1970).
94. Greiser, E., Epidemiologische Untersuchungen zum Zusammenhang
     zwischen Appetitzüglereinnahme und primär vasculären Hypertonie,
     Internist, **14**:437 (1973).
95. Kraupp, O., Studies on the etiology of primary pulmonary hypertension
     in animal experiments, *Wien Z. Inn. Med.*, **50**(10):493–496 (1969).
96. Lüllmann, H., M. R. Parwaresch, M. Sattler, K. U. Seiler, and A. Sieg-
     friedt, The effects of anorectic agents on the pulmonary pressure and

morphology of rat lungs after chronic administration, *Arzneimittelforsch.*, 22:2096 (1972).

97. Byrne-Quinn, E., and R. F. Grover, Aminorex (Menocil) and amphetamine: acute and chronic effects on pulmonary and systemic hemodynamics in the calf, *Thorax*, 27:127 (1972).

98. Kay, J. M., P. Smith, and D. Heath, Aminorex and the pulmonary circulation, *Thorax*, 26:262–270 (1971).

99. Kay, J. M., Crotalaria pulmonary hypertension, *Prog. Respir. Res.*, 5: 30 (1970).

100. Mielke, H., K. U. Seiler, U. Stumpf, and O. Wassermann, Influence of Aminorex (Menocil) on pulmonary pressure and on the content of biogenic amines in the lungs of rats, *Naunyn Schmiedeberg's Arch. Pharmacol.*, 274(s):R79 (1972).

101. Fahlen, M., H. Bergman, G. Helder, L. Ryden, I. Wallentin, and L. Zettergren, Phenformin and pulmonary hypertension, *Br. Heart J.*, 35: 824 (1973).

102. Massumi, R. A., J. C. Rios, and H. E. Ticktin, Hemodynamic abnormalities and venous admixture in portal cirrhosis, *Am. J. Med. Sci.*, 25:275 (1965).

103. Daoud, F. S., J. T. Reeves, and J. W. Schaefer, Failure of hypoxic pulmonary vasoconstriction in patients with liver cirrhosis, *J. Clin. Invest.*, 51: 1076–1080 (1972).

104. Naeye, R. L., "Primary" pulmonary hypertension with coexisting portal hypertension. A retrospective study of 6 cases, *Circulation*, 22:376 (1960).

105. Fishman, A. P., Dietary pulmonary hypertension, *Circ. Res.*, 35:657–660 (1974).

106. Reeves, J. T., J. E. Leathers, and C. Boatright, Microradiography of the rabbit's hepatic microcirculation. The similarity of the hepatic portan and pulmonary arterial circulations, *Anat. Rec.*, 154:103–120 (1966).

107. Fowler, N. O., R. N. Westcott, V. D. Hanenstein, R. G. Scott, and J. McGuire, Observations on autonomic participation in pulmonary arteriolar resistance in man, *J. Clin. Invest.*, 29:1387 (1950).

108. Dresdale, D. T., R. F. Michtom, and M. Schultz, Recent studies in primary pulmonary hypertension including pharmacodynamic observations on pulmonary vascular resistance, *Bull. N.Y. Acad. Med.*, 30:195 (1954).

109. Yu, P. N., Primary pulmonary hypertension: Report of 6 cases and review of literature, *Ann. Intern. Med.*, 49:1138 (1958).

110. Farrar, J. F., Idiopathic pulmonary hypertension, *Am. Heart J.*, 66:128 (1963).

111. Staemmler, M., Die Thromboendarteritis obliterans der Lungenartenrien, *Klin. Wochenschr.*, 16:1669 (1937).

112. Short, D. S., The arterial bed of the lung in pulmonary hypertension, *Lancet*, 2:12–16 (1957).

113. Vogel, J. H. K., W. F. Weaver, R. L. Rose, S. G. Blount, and R. F. Grover, Pulmonary hypertension on exertion in normal man living at 10,150 feet (Leadville, Colorado), *Med. Thorac.*, 19:461 (1962).

114. Lindsay, D. A., and J. Read, Pulmonary vascular responsiveness in the prognosis of chronic obstructive lung disease, *Am. Rev. Respir. Dis.,* **105**: 242 (1972).

115. Read, J., and J. Lee, Regional pulmonary vasoconstriction as an individual factor in the genesis of cor pulmonale, *Am. Rev. Respir. Dis.,* **96**:1181 (1967).

116. Bolt, W., Pathologische Physiologie des Cor pulmonale, *Verh. Dtsch. Ges. Kreislaufforsch.,* **000**:196 (1955).

117. Degenring, F. H., Primary vascular form of pulmonary hypertension. A comprehensive comparison with a new therapeutic and resistance-computing technic, *Arch. Kreislaufforsch.,* **67**(3):277–301 (1972).

118. Juratsch, C. E., G. C. Emmanouilides, D. Thibeault, B. Baylen, J. A. Jengo, M. M. Laks, and J. M. Criley, Main pulmonary artery distention: Potential mechanism for sustained pulmonary hypertension in the new-born, *Circulation,* **56**(Suppl. III):73 (1977).

119. Kealy, G. P., and M. J. Brody, Studies on the mechanism of pulmonary vascular responses to miliary pulmonary embolism, *Circ. Res.,* **41**:807 (1977).

120. Kuida, H., G. Dammin, F. Haynes, E. Rapaport, and L. Dexter, Primary pulmonary hypertension, *Am. J. Med.,* **23**:166 (1957).

121. Chapman, D. W., J. P. Abbott, and J. Latsor, Primary pulmonary hypertension: Review of literature and results of cardiac catheterization in 10 patients, *Circulation,* **15**:35 (1957).

122. Stucki, P., K. Bürki, and U. Baumgärtner, Über primäre pulmonale Hypertonie, *Schweiz. Med. Wochenschr.,* **93**:1823 (1963).

123. Yuceoglu, Y. Z., D. T. Dresdale, Q. J. Valensi, R. M. Narvas, and N. T. Gottlieb, Primary pulmonary hypertension with hoarseness and massive (fatal) hemoptysis. Review of the literature and report of a case, *Vasc. Dis.,* **4**:290 (1967).

124. Pedersen, L., Primary pulmonary hypertension. One case observed during twelve years, *Dan. Med. Bull.,* **14**(3):59–61 (1967).

125. Plass, R., K. H. Gunther, B. Bothig, and W. Munster, Clinical features and hemodynamics of primary pulmonary hypertension, *Dtsch. Gesundheitsw.,* **23**(1):16–22 (1968).

126. Deshmukh, M. M., S. G. Kinare, and K. K. Datey, Primary pulmonary hypertension (clinical, haemodynamic and pathological study), *J. Assoc. Physicians India,* **17**(11):661–666 (1969).

127. Jornod, J., Q. de Barros, P. R. Moret, and R. P. Baumann, Comparative study of pulmonary, gasometric and hemodynamic function in 6 cases of primary pulmonary hypertension; anatomic-pathologic examination of 3 cases, *Schweiz. Med. Wochenschr.,* **100**(50):2160–2163 (1970).

128. Reid, L., G. Anderson, and G. Simon, Comparison of primary and thromboembolic pulmonary hypertension, *Thorax,* **27**(2):263–264 (1972).

129. Snider, G. L. (Moderator), Primary pulmonary hypertension: A fatality during pulmonary angiography. Clinical conference from Boston University School of Medicine, *Chest,* **64**(5):628–635 (1973).

130. Hendrix, G. H., Familial primary pulmonary hypertension, *South. Med. J.*, **67**(8):981–983 (1974).

131. Gurtner, H. P., P. Walser, and B. Fassler, Normal values for pulmonary hemodynamics at rest and during exercise in man, *Prog. Respir. Res.*, **9**: 295 (1975).

132. Degenring, F. H., Pulmonary circulation and contractility of the right ventricular myocardium in primary pulmonary hypertonia. Studies during rest and exercise tests, *Arch. Kreislaufforsch.*, **65**(3):71–82 (1971).

133. Brill, I. C., and J. J. Krygier, Primary pulmonary vascular sclerosis, *Arch. Intern. Med.*, **68**:560 (1941).

134. Howarth, S. and J. B. Lowe, Mechanism of effort syncope in primary pulmonary hypertension and cyanotic congenital heart disease, *Br. Heart J.*, **15**:47 (1953).

135. Dressler, W., Effort syncope as an early manifestation of primary pulmonary hypertension, *Am. J. Med. Sci.*, **223**:131 (1952).

136. Fishman, A. P., Dynamics of the pulmonary circulation. In *Handbook of Physiology, Circulation,* **2**:1724 (1963).

137. Arbenz, U., P. Wirz, M. Schonbeck, A. Gadient, and F. Mahler, Effect of acetylcholine infusions on the hemodynamics of primary vascular pulmonary hypertension, *Verh. Dtsch. Ges. Inn. Med.*, **77**:1318–1321 (1971).

138. Samet, P., W. H. Bernstein, and J. Widrich, Intracardiac infusion of acetylcholine in primary pulmonary hypertension, *Am. Heart J.*, **60**: 433 (1960).

139. Marshall, R. J., H. F. Helmholz, and J. T. Shepherd, Effect of acetylcholine on pulmonary vascular resistance in a patient with idiopathic pulmonary hypertension, *Circulation*, **20**:391 (1959).

140. Calnini, P., G. G. Gensini, and M. S. Hoffman, Primary pulmonary hypertension with death during right heart catheterization. A case report and a survey of reported fatalities, *Am. J. Cardiol.*, **4**:519 (1959).

141. Ghose, J. C., S. Sarkar, and D. P. Basu, Primary pulmonary hypertension— clinical and hemodynamic features, *Am. Heart J.*, **24**:328 (1972).

142. Kleiger, R. E., M. Boxer, R. E. Ingham, and D. G. Harrison, Pulmonary hypertension in patients using oral contraceptives. A report of six cases, *Chest,* **69**:143 (1976).

143. Nanavaty, J. M., and S. A. Trivedi, Primary pulmonary hypertension; clinical and hemodynamic study of three cases, *J. Assoc. Physicians India,* **13**:661 (1965).

144. Goff, A. M. and E. A. Gaensler, Primary (idiopathic) pulmonary hypertension, *Med. Thorac.*, **22**(5):530–545 (1965).

145. Goff, A. M., and E. A. Gaensler, Respiratory pathophysiology in chronic progressive pulmonary vascular disease, *Indian J. Med. Sci.*, **497**:213 (1967).

146. Herzog, H. and S. Daum, Lung function in primary obstructive pulmonary hypertension, *Prog. Respir. Res.*, **5**:400 (1970).

147.   Yu, P. N., *Pulmonary Blood Volume in Health and Disease.* Philadelphia, Lea and Febinger, 1969.
148.   Obrecht, H. G., M. Scherrer, and H. P. Gurtner, Der Gasaustausch in der Lunge bei der primär vasculären Form des chronischen Cor pulmonale, *Schweiz. Med. Wochenschr.,* **98**:1999–2007 (1968).
149.   Harms, H. and H. Voss, Blood gas analysis in primary vascular pulmonary hypertension, *Z. Kreislaufforsch.,* **59**(10):897–901 (1970).
150.   McIlroy, M. B., and G. H. Apthorp, Pulmonary function in pulmonary hypertension, *Br. Heart J.,* **20**:397 (1958).
151.   Guz, A., Regulation of respiration in man, *Ann. Rev. Physiol.,* **37**:303–323 (1975).
152.   Kummer, F., Primary pulmonary hypertension. Lung function tests, *Wien Z. Inn. Med.,* **50**(10):484–486 (1969).
153.   Brotmacher, L., and P. Fleming, Cardiac output and vascular pressures in 10 normal children and adolescents, *Guy Hosp. Rep.,* **106**:268 (1957).
154.   Dexter, L., et al., Studies of the pulmonary circulation in man at rest, normal variations and the inter-relations between increased blood flow, elevated pulmonary arterial pressure and high pulmonary "capillary" pressures, *J. Clin. Invest.,* **29**:602 (1950).
155.   Donald, K. W., et al., The effect of exercise on the cardiac output and circulatory dynamics of normal subjects, *Clin. Sci.,* **14**:37 (1955).
156.   Doyle, J. T., J. S. Wilson, and J. V. Warren, The pulmonary vascular responses to short term hypoxia in human subjects, *Circulation,* **5**:263 (1952).
157.   Fishman, A. P., H. W. Fritts, and A. Cournand, Effects of acute hypoxia and exercise on the pulmonary circulation, *Circulation,* **22**:204 (1960).
158.   Granath, A., and T. Strandell, Relationships between cardiac output, stroke volume, and intracardiac pressures at rest and during exercise in supine position, and some anthropometric data in healthy old men, *Acta Med. Scand.,* **176**:447 (1964).
159.   Hickam, J. B., and W. H. Cargill, Effect of exercise on cardiac output and pulmonary arterial pressure in normal persons and in patients with cardiovascular disease and pulmonary emphysema, *J. Clin. Invest.,* **27**:10 (1948).
160.   Holmgren, A., B. Jonsson, and T. Sjostrand, Circulatory data in normal subjects at rest and during exercise in recumbent position, with special reference to the stroke volume at different work intensities, *Acta Physiol. Scand.,* **49**:343 (1960).
161.   Hultgren, H. N., J. Kelly, and H. Miller, Pulmonary circulation in acclimatized man at high altitude, *J. Appl. Physiol.,* **20**:223 (1965).
162.   Kjellberg, S. R., et al., *Diagnosis of Congenital Heart Disease.* Chicago, Yearbook Medical Publishers, 1955.
163.   Heath, D., and J. E. Edwards, Configuration of elastic tissue of pulmonary trunk in idiopathic pulmonary hypertension, *Circulation,* **21**:59 (1960).

164. Reid, L., Morphology of pulmonary circulation in health and disease, *Kongr. Ber. Wiss. Tag. Norddtsch Ges. Lungen Bronchialhk.,* **14**:333 (1975).

165. Wagenvoort, C. A., D. Heath, and J. E. Edwards, The pathology of the pulmonary vasculature. In *Pathology.* Edited by A. A. Editor. Springfield, Ill., Charles C. Thomas, 1964.

166. Stuard, I. D., R. S. Heusinkveld, and A. J. Moss, Microangiopathic hemolytic anemia and thrombocytopenia in primary pulmonary hypertension, *N. Engl. J. Med.,* **287**(17):869–870 (1972).

167. Anderson, G., L. Reid, and G. Simon, The radiographic appearances in primary and in thrombo-embolic pulmonary hypertension, *Clin. Radiol.,* **24**(1):113–120 (1973).

168. Harris, P., and D. Heath, *The Human Pulmonary Circulation,* 2nd ed. Edinburgh, Churchill Livingston, 1977.

169. Reeves, J. T., D. Tweedale, J. Noonon, J. E. Leathers, and M. B. Quigley, Correlation of microradiographic and histologic findings in the pulmonary vascular bed. Technique and applications in pulmonary hypertension, *Circulation,* **34**:971–983 (1966).

170. Wagenvoort, C. A. and N. Wagenvoort, A classification of "primary pulmonary hypertension," *Prog. Respir. Res.,* **5**:17 (1970b).

171. Meyrick, B., S. W. Clarke, C. Symons, D. J. Woodgate, and L. Reid, Primary pulmonary hypertension: A case report including electronmicroscopic study, *Br. J. Dis. Chest,* **68**(1):11–20 (1974).

172. Blount, S. G., and R. F. Grover, Pulmonary hypertension. In *The Heart,* 4th ed. Edited by A. Hurst and B. Logue. New York, McGraw-Hill, Inc., 1978, pp. 1456–1472.

173. Viar, W. N., and T. R. Harrison, Chest pain in association with pulmonary hypertension, *Circulation,* **5**:1 (1952).

174. Soothill, J. V., A case of primary pulmonary hypertension with paralyzed left vocal cord, *Guy Hosp. Rep.,* **100**:121 (1951).

175. Brinton, W. D., Primary pulmonary hypertension, *Br. Heart J.,* **12**:305 (1950).

176. Wang, Y., A. H. From, and W. Krivit, Disseminated pulmonary arterial thrombosis associated with thrombocytopenia: Occurrence in identical twins, *Circulation,* **31**(2):215 (1965).

177. Scott, R. C., S. Kaplan, N. O. Fowler, R. A. Helm, R. N. Westcott, I. C. Walker, and W. J. Stiles, The electrocardiographic pattern of right ventricular hypertrophy in chronic cor pulmonale, *Circulation,* **11**:927 (1955).

178. Fowler, R. S., and J. D. Keith, The electrocardiogram in pulmonary stenosis. A reappraisal, *Can. Med. Assoc. J.,* **98**:433 (1968).

179. Fischer, T., Über den frühdiagnostischen Wert der Vektorkardiographischen Zeichen des chronischen Cor pulmonale, *Z. Kreislaufforsch.,* **59**:236 (1970).

180. Halter, J., T. Moccetti, K. Gattiker, and P. Lichtlen, Die Bedeutung der Vektorcardiographie für die Diagnose des chronischen Cor pulmonale, *Verh. Dtsch. Ges. Kreislaufforsch.,* **38**:130 (1972).

181. Wettengel, R., H. Reichelt, H. Stender, E. Greiser, and H. Fabel, Vergleich hämodynamischer und röntgenologischer Parameter bei Kranken mit chronischem Cor pulmonale, *Pneumonology,* **149**:127–131 (1973).
182. Gahl, K., E. Greiser, and H. S. Stender, Radiological findings in primary vascular hypertension, *Fortschr. Geb. Roentgenstr. Nuklearmed.,* **116**(5): 589–599 (1972).
183. Luther, M., and H. Czempiel, Lung scanning in primary vascular chronic cor pulmonale, *Z. Kreislaufforsch.,* **59**(12):1061–1073 (1970).
184. Koppenhagen, K., H. Ernst, H. Paeprer, H. W. Liebenschutz, and H. Meinhold, Perfusion scintigraphy of the lung in primary vascular pulmonary hypertension, *Fortschr. Geb. Roentgenstr. Nuklearmed.,* **115**(1): 27–34 (1971).
185. Sill, V., N. Völkel, K. Scherer, D. Nowak, and R. Montz, Experimental model for pharmaco-perfusion lung scanning, *Pneumonology,* **150**:13–17 (1974).
186. Goodman, D. J., D. C. Harrison, and R. L. Popp, Echocardiographic features of primary pulmonary hypertension, *Am. J. Cardiol.,* **33**(3):438–443 (1974).
187. Weyman, A. E., Echocardiographic patterns of pulmonic valve motion with pulmonary hypertension, *Circulation,* **50**:905 (1974).
188. Hirschfeld, S., R. Mayer, D. C. Schwartz, J. Korthagen, and S. Kaplan, The echocardiographic assessment of pulmonary artery pressure and pulmonary vascular resistance, *Circulation,* **52**:642–650 (1975).
189. Daoud, F. S., and J. T. Reeves, Temporary relief of primary pulmonary hypertension with isoproterenol, *Circulation,* **46**(2):143 (1972).
190. Baughman, R., and S. R. Inkley, Letter to the editor, *N. Engl. J. Med.,* **296**:631 (1976).
191. Burkart, F., Primäre vasculäre pulmonale Hypertonie (Tagungsberichte), *Z. Kreislaufforsch.,* **59**:92 (1970).
192. Degenring, F. H., Die therapeutische Beeinflussung der primär vaskulären Form des chronischen Cor pulmonale und der weiterbestehenden pulmonalen Hypertonie nach Kommissurotomie der Mitralstenose, *Z. Kreislaufforsch.,* **59**:912–923 (1970).
193. Both, A., Therapy of primary pulmonary hypertension, *Z. Kreislaufforsch.,* **59**(10):909–911 (1970).
194. Fischer, M., H. Mösslacher, and J. Slany, Thrombolytische Therapie bei primär vaskulären pulmonaler Hypertension, *Med. Welt,* **8**:229–231 (1971).
195. Weil, J. V., G. Jamieson, D. W. Brown, R. F. Grover, O. J. Balchum, and J. F. Murray, The red cell mass-arterial oxygen relationship in normal man, *J. Clin. Invest.,* **47**:1627–1634 (1968).
196. Kleinerman, L., G. Roseteanu, and G. H. Bunghez, Primary pulmonary arterial hypertension, *Romanian Med. Rev.,* **20**:17–25 (1966).
197. Watanabe, S., and T. Ogata, Clinical and experimental study upon primary pulmonary hypertension, *Jpn. Circ. J.,* **40**:603–610 (1976).

11

Neoplasia of the Pulmonary Vascular Bed

WILLIAM M. THURLBECK

University of Manitoba and Health Sciences Center
Winnipeg, Manitoba, Canada

I. Introduction

True neoplasms of the pulmonary vessels—arteries, veins, and lymphatics—are extremely uncommon, and a computer-assisted search of the literature for the 10 years ending in 1976 produced only a handful of papers. Further, there is some question whether the best known vascular lung tumors—sclerosing hemangioma and hemangiopericytoma of the lung—should be included as examples of vascular neoplasms. The former may not necessarily be a true neoplasm and, if so, there is some question whether it is endothelial and thus vascular in origin. Hemangiopericytomas, while clearly vascular neoplasms, are not easy to diagnose with certainty, and it may be that several of the tumors in the literature diagnosed as hemangiopericytomas are other tumors. The neoplasm which most commonly involves the pulmonary vascular bed often is not thought of as being a vascular tumor, namely, lymphangitic carcinoma. This is not only a tumor involving the lymphatics of the lung, but also likely involves the pulmonary arteries in the first instance.

Supported by Negotiated Development Grant #DG-152 of the Medical Research Council.

Besides reviewing neoplasms of the pulmonary vascular bed, this chapter will also review very briefly lesions that may be confused with neoplasms, or have been thought by some to be neoplasms of the vascular system in the past, although contemporary reviews may not regard them as neoplasms.

II. Benign Neoplasms and Malformations of the Lung

A. Sclerosing Hemangiomas of the Lung [1]

Currently, the general view is that the lesions in the soft tissues previously referred to as sclerosing hemangiomas are in reality derived from histiocytes and should be regarded as variants of fibrous histiocytomas [2]. However, the term sclerosing hemangioma is still generally used in the lung.

Sclerosing hemangiomas characteristically have a papillary appearance (Fig. 1). On superficial histologic examination, this may lead to confusion with bronchiolar-alveolar carcinoma. The distinction is important since

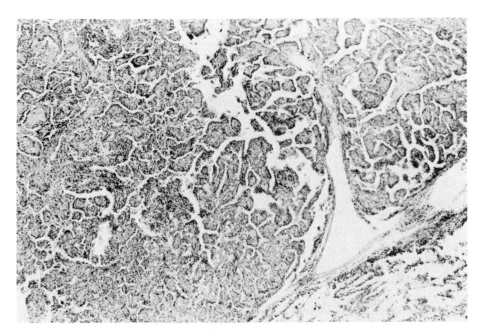

FIGURE 1   Sclerosing hemangioma of the lung. It is well demarcated from the surrounding lung and is distinctly papillary in appearance (H&E, ×60).

sclerosing hemangiomas are benign lesions. The distinction is usually easy since sclerosing hemangiomas reveal their true nature by showing areas of dense sclerosis with obliterated capillaries (Fig. 2). They also have distinct margins and do not use alveoli as a framework on which the tumor cells grow, as is the case of bronchiolar-alveolar carcinoma. Ossification of the densely sclerotic tissue may occur. Sheets of cells, apparently endothelial in origin, may be present (Fig. 3). Areas of old hemorrhage result in many hemosiderin-laden macrophages and may also be the source of foam cells which may be prominent and give the tumor a yellow color. This feature has also led to the appellation of "histiocytoma" for this tumor. Sclerosing hemangiomas are single in 85% of instances and may involve any lobe of the lung, although the right middle lobe is involved disproportionately frequently for its small size [3]. About half of the cases occur in the age range of 40 to 60 years and only about one-sixth of the cases have been found in man.

There is by no means complete agreement about the nature of origin of these tumors. The general view is that they are neoplastic in nature, but experts have argued, on the basis of light microscopy, whether they are endothelial [1] or epithelial [4] in origin. Recent electron microscopic studies have not been helpful, since one study purported to show an endothelial

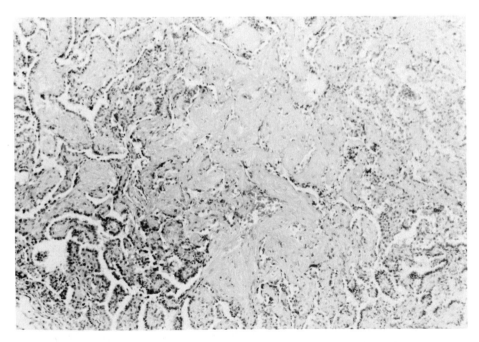

FIGURE 2   Areas of dense sclerosis are present in the lesion (H&E, ×96).

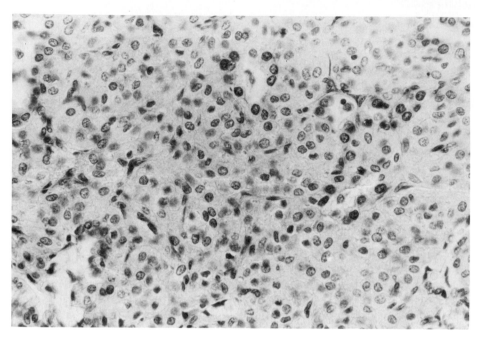

FIGURE 3   In areas, sheets of cells are seen, presumably endothelial in origin (H&E, ×380).

origin [5] but another report gave apparently convincing evidence that the great majority of the cells present in the lesions were epithelial [6].

B.   Lymphangioma [7]

A single example of a lymphangioma of the lung has been recorded. The lesion presented as a solitary 3.3 × 2.5 cm mass in the right upper lobe, close to the pleura, in a 66-year-old woman. The lesion was grayish white and focally hemorrhagic and the cut surface was smooth and slightly viscous. Histologically it was multicystic, containing fluid. The intervening stroma of tissue consisted of immature spindle- or stellate-shaped cells, and the overall appearance was that of a lymphangioma in other organs. The majority of lymphangiomas in other parts of the body appear to be malformations and occur in young subjects, but some may be true neoplasms. In this instance, the occurrence in an elderly person suggests it may be a true neoplasm rather than a malformation.

C.   Pulmonary Lymphangiomyomatosis

The lesion described above is quite different from the interesting condition of pulmonary lymphangiomyomatosis, which is likely nonneoplastic and represents a bizarre proliferation of smooth muscle cells primarily in lymphatic vessels of the lung. The condition is reasonably common, and Corrin et al., in a comprehensive review in 1975, found 34 cases in the literature in addition to their own 23 cases [8]. The clinical syndrome is characteristic—it is confined to women who are, with only occasional exceptions [9], in the child-bearing age. The chief complaint is most commonly dyspnea, which is progressive, starting generally between 25 and 34 years of age, and death occurs within 10 years of the onset of symptoms. Spontaneous pneumothorax, chylothorax, and hemoptysis are frequent complications and may occasionally be presenting complaints. Proliferation of smooth muscle in abdominal lymph nodes may produce a large mass which on occasion has been the presenting complaint. Both obstructive and restrictive patterns of pulmonary function abnormality have been reported, but a recent publication has indicated that airflow obstruction is the most characteristic pattern, with

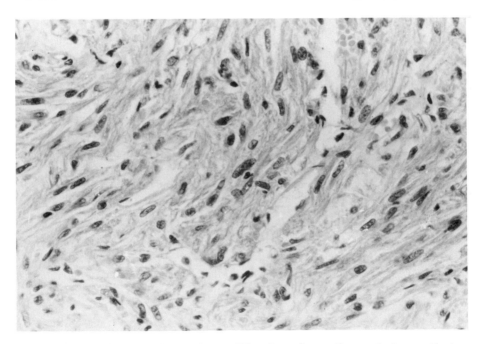

FIGURE 4   Bizarre and irregular proliferation of smooth muscle in a patient with lymphangiomyomatosis (H&E, ×380).

relative preservation of lung volume [10]. (Indeed, reported lung volumes derived from helium dilution are likely spuriously low, and the frequent presence of chylothorax and pneumothorax also complicates the problem of lung volume measurements.)

The lung lesions are characteristic. There is extensive, irrational proliferation of smooth muscle cells (Fig. 4). Special stains, staining with antibodies to smooth muscle [11], and electron microscopy [12] have indicated that the tumor cells are derived from smooth muscle. The proliferation of smooth muscle appears to be mainly from the walls of lymphatic channels leading to lymphatic obstruction. Serial section studies have suggested the muscle was solely derived from lymphatics [12], and this has been given additional credence by the smooth muscle proliferation in the lymph nodes and lymphatic channels in other parts of the body. (It is obstruction to the latter that may result in chylothorax or chylous ascites.) However, Corrin et al. [8], Carrington et al. [10], and ourselves [13] noted that there appeared to be smooth muscle proliferation of venous, arterial, and bronchiolar smooth muscle. Corrin et al. [8] considered that proliferation of venous smooth muscle led to venous obstruction which was responsible for the hemoptysis which commonly occurred in these patients and for the hemosiderosis frequently found in their lungs. Most characteristically, the lung contains many large cystic spaces (Fig. 5). These are not dilated bronchioles, as in fibrosing alveolitis, but are emphysematous spaces, often containing smooth muscle in their walls (Fig. 6). The pathogenesis of these spaces is uncertain, but it has been suggested that they are due to bronchiolar air trapping caused by proliferation of smooth muscle in the walls of the airways [12]. Identical lung and lymph node lesions are seen in tuberous sclerosis, and patients with lymphangiomyomatosis may have the renal malformations seen in tuberous sclerosis. However, the exact relationship between the two conditions is uncertain.

D.   Hemangiomas and Arteriovenous Fistula

The term hemangioma is a misnomer and the lesions referred to as "benign hemangiomas" of the lung appear to be congenital or acquired malformations, the latter usually associated with cirrhosis of the liver. The congenital lesions are usually referred to as arteriovenous fistulas that are sometimes classified into cavernous hemangiomas or capillary telangiectasia [4]. This is in some aspects confusing since these terms may suggest a neoplastic process. Although only 45 cases had been reported up to 1949 [14], arteriovenous fistulas are not uncommon and the Mayo Clinic encountered 63 examples in 20 years. The average age of presentation was 41 years, with the range of 4 to 70 years [15].

About two-thirds of the patients are women and about one-third of the lesions are multiple, but often the other lesions only become apparent after resection of an apparently solitary lesion. The blood supply is usually the pulmonary artery and the drainage into the pulmonary vein, but occasionally the blood supply is from a systemic artery (3 of 63 instances in the Mayo Clinic series) and the drainage into the vena cava. About 60% of patients have the Rendu-Osler-Weber syndrome (hereditary hemorrhagic telangiectasia), and 3 to 6% of patients with hereditary hemorrhagic telangiectasia have detectable pulmonary involvement [16,17]; presenting symptoms including hemoptysis, asymptomatic pulmonary masses, and sometimes extensive

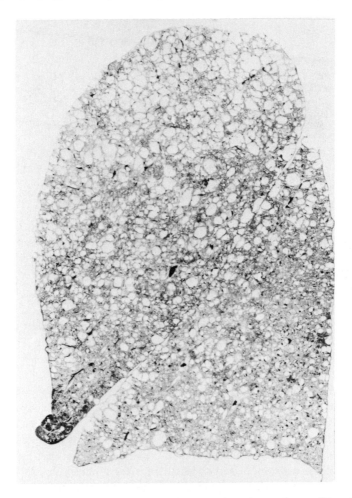

FIGURE 5 A paper-mounted, whole-lung section shows the multicystic character of the lung.

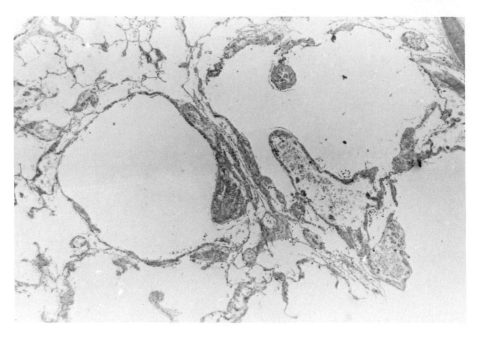

FIGURE 6   Alveolated tissue with focal areas of proliferated smooth muscle form the walls of the cystic space (H&E, ×24).

arteriovenous shunting with cyanosis. Rare complications or presenting complaints include rupture into the pleural cavities and cerebral abscess either due to septic thromboemboli from the angioma or by passage through the aneurysm of infected emboli.

About 70% of arteriovenous fistulas occur in the lower lobes close to the pleura [18]. The gross appearance is quite variable. At one extreme, there may be just one large sac; at the other, the lesion may consist of small dilated vessels, or telangiectases [19]. More usually, there is an intertwined mass of vessels of differing size interposed between supplying artery and draining vein. Random histologic sections do not disclose the true nature of the lesion and may resemble hemangiomas seen elsewhere. As opposed to systemic arteriovenous fistulas, thickening of the walls of veins and intimal proliferation are not striking because of the low pressure in the lesser circulation. Dissection and casts have shown the supplying artery and draining vein; the former may be quite small. Arteriovenous fistulas likely arise from a malformation of the capillary bed in which there is focal persistence of the fetal arteriovenous anastomoses. Since the resistance to flow is low in these regions, blood preferentially flows through them. This results in increasing dilatation of the vascular spaces, finally resulting in obvious arteriovenous fistulas.

E.   Acquired Arteriovenous Fistulas or Hemangiomas

Interest in the pulmonary vasculature in liver disease has been brought about by the association of cyanosis with cirrhosis and other chronic liver diseases. A variety of abnormalities in the pulmonary vasculature has been described. Rydell and Hoffbauer [20], using plastic casts, found a number of direct arteriovenous connections both at the hilus and at the periphery of the lung. Others have shown consistent dilatation of the small pulmonary arteries of the lung in cirrhosis and the presence of spider nevi on the pleura in about one-half of the cases. One patient had many small arteriovenous shunts throughout the lung [21]. However, the correlation between the extent of the malformation and the degree of arterial unsaturation is poor, so that the arteriovenous fistulas do not appear to account for the cyanosis which is seen in some patients with cirrhosis.

F.   Multiple Chemodectomas of the Lung

Brief mention should be made of these interesting lesions since they are so intimately connected with small pulmonary veins. They have been reviewed in detail elsewhere [3]. It is uncertain whether they are neoplasms and it is also unlikely that they are derived from blood vessels although their histogenesis is uncertain. These lesions have been found in 0.25 to 0.5% of random necropsies, although, when careful search is made, they have been found in 3 to 4% of autopsies. Of all cases reported, 84% have been in females, and there is an increased frequency in patients with chronic heart or lung disease, such as pulmonary thromboembolism, bronchitis and emphysema, mitral stenosis, and chronic heart failure. Generally, they are an incidental finding on microscopic examination of the lung, but occasionally they are recognized as 0.5- to 2-mm yellowish white nodules scattered through the lung. They resemble chemodectomas very closely using the light microscope, and this has raised the possibility that chemoreceptor tissue normally exists in the lungs and that these are tumors arising from this tissue. Recent electron microscopic studies have shown that these lesions bear no resemblance to chemoreceptor tissue, but instead, surprisingly, resemble meningiomas. The interpretation of these findings is uncertain. The exact origin of the arachnoidal cell has been ascribed to both mesoderm and neuroectoderm, so that these lesions may arise from cells that have aberrantly followed nerves out of the central nervous system during development. Others have suggested that they may be of mesothelial origin. Their close association with pulmonary venules and their association with pulmonary vascular disorders at least raise the possibility that they may originate in small veins.

III. Malignant Neoplasms of the Pulmonary Vascular System

A.   Hemangiopericytomas

These are among the more difficult tumors for pathologists to diagnose with certainty and often there will be conflict between expert histopathologists concerning the diagnosis in a particular case. All too often it is a diagnosis applied to an unusual tumor that does not fit into any commonly recognized pattern. Pericytes, the cells that lie around capillaries and are thought to be contractile, are thought to be the cells of origin [22]. The details of the presence and position of pericytes in the lung are still not available, and the relationship between the cells recently described in the alveolar wall and thought to be contractile by Kapanci et al. [23] and pericytes is also not completely clear. Hemangiopericytomas were first described by Stout and Murray in 1942 [22], and they have been described in most tissues. The histologic appearance is of sheets and clusters of spindle and elongated cells, sometimes of organoid appearance, in close relationship to vascular channels, which are frequently collapsed (Figs. 7 and 8). A stain for reticulin demarcates the endothelium of the vessel from the tumor cells, and the tumor cells are surrounded individually by reticulin. In 1974, 24 cases of hemangiopericytoma of the lung were reported [24], and at least three further cases have been reported since then [25,26]. Hemangiopericytomas of the lung occur predominantly in patients over the age of 40 and are slightly more common in women than men. Mortality was higher in men (50%) than in women (32%), and large tumors had a worse prognosis than small [24]. Although some experts doubt that it is possible to predict which hemangiopericytomas will behave in a malignant fashion, McMaster et al. [27] emphasized the importance of grading hemangiopericytomas into benign, borderline, and malignant in tumors throughout the body, and these criteria may be applied usefully to the lung as well. Liebow has indicated that, in his experience, hemangiopericytomas of the lung were relatively benign, whereas those of the chest wall occurred at an average age of about 30 years, mostly in women, and behaved in a much more malignant fashion. In a review of hemangiopericytomas, Backwinkel and Diddams [28] grouped hemangiopericytomas of the lung and mediastinum together and found that their recurrence rate (45.3%) was about that of all hemangiopericytomas (52.2%). However, the recurrence rate of hemangiopericytomas of lung and chest wall in the first year (36.3%) was the highest of any site. The diagram and text in the paper by McMaster et al. [27] support Liebow's observation that hemangiopericytomas of the chest wall frequently appear to be malignant on histologic grounds and often lead to the death of the patient.

B. Connective Tissue Tumors of the Pulmonary Arteries

At least 24 of these tumors have been reported [29], compared to only 18 sclerosing hemangiomas. This is perhaps because the latter are undramatic and familiar to most pathologists and are thus not reported, whereas the former have a much more spectacular clinical presentation. Although the clinical features have also been fairly uniform, as yet only two cases have been diagnosed during life and then on the basis of a surgical biopsy [29].

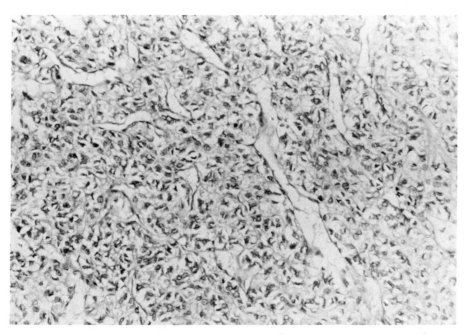

FIGURE 7 Hemangiopericytoma. Tumor cells are arranged in sheets and cords and separated from each other by tortuous capillaries, some of which are patent and others collapsed (H&E, ×240).

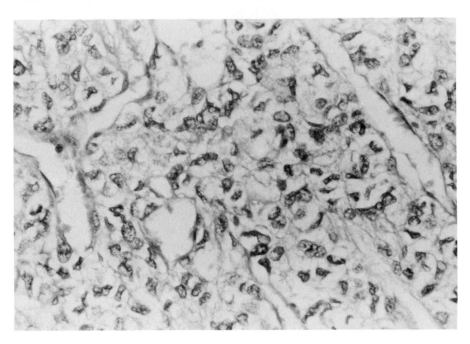

FIGURE 8   A higher-power view shows the capillaries containing red cells and the cords of tumor cells (H&E, X380).

Neoplasms of large systemic arteries and veins and the heart are well recognized, and similar tumors originate in the pulmonary trunk or the pulmonary arteries. One case has been described originating in a pulmonary arteriovenous fistula [30]. The tumors originate in the wall of the vessels and characteristically grow in the lumen and occlude the vessel to a greater or lesser extent. They may grow through the wall and involve surrounding tissues. Thrombosis of the pulmonary artery and embolization to the lung are common. Diverse histopathologic terms have been applied to these tumors. This is to be expected since malignant connective tissues are often quite varied in appearance, at times mixed, and the type of connective tissue made by them is not always characteristic. Thus, leiomyosarcomas [29–31], sarcomas [32, 33], fibrosarcomas [34], fibromyxosarcomas [35], mesenchymomas [36], chondrosarcomas [37], and osteosarcomas [38] have been described. The usual clinical presentation is of unexplained progressive right heart failure which is intractable to therapy. Other symptoms have also been noted, syncope being present in several cases [35,36,38]. Thrombocytopenia and coagulation problems have been described in two cases [32,35] and may be more common, with proper clinical search, because an extensive mass of intravascular tumor is present in many cases and this is likely to produce the complication of disseminated intravascular coagulation. One case has closely mimicked a pheochromocytoma with presenting complaints of palpitation, sweating, and hypertension [34]. One patient presented with a large pericardial effusion [29]. The majority of cases have been diagnosed at postmortem, and the clinical course has been short.

C. Hemangiosarcoma and Hemangioendotheliomas of the Lung

Spencer [4] is rightly skeptical about the occurrence of primary malignant tumors of endothelial origin in the lung. Close scrutiny of the recorded cases [39–46] suggests that only three of them may truly be hemangiosarcomas of the lung. The pathologic description of the case reported by Tralka and Katz [46] is not convincing in itself, but the clinical features of a rapid increase in size of superficial masses, together with a large pulmonary mass and a rapid course, suggests a malignant tumor, likely of vascular origin, perhaps complicating a patient with the Rendu-Osler-Weber syndrome. A very similar case was reported by Hall in 1935 [41], and a case record of the Massachusetts General Hospital [44] is also convincing (although there was some question at the time whether this really was a hemangiosarcoma, and, in retrospect, a hemangiopericytoma could be included in the differential diagnosis). The three patients were 40 to 68 years old and presented primarily with respiratory symptoms, including hemoptysis, chest pain, and dyspnea. Large hemothoraces occurred in two patients, and extensive visceral involvement (by metastases or hemangiomas as part of the Rendu-Osler-Weber syndrome) occurred in two of them.

Some cases were clearly incorrectly diagnosed. One was not documented as a hemangiosarcoma [39]. Another was a patient with pulmonary hypertension producing extensive pulmonary arterial and arteriolar plexiform lesions interpreted by the authors as being intravascular neoplasma [42], and another was probably a minute chemodectoma [42]. The other four cases were obscure, and one may have been a case of Rendu-Osler-Weber syndrome with a very large pulmonary arteriovenous fistula [40]. One case [45] appeared to be a hemangiosarcoma but involved both bowel and lung and it is not clear which was primary. A further problem is that some arteriovenous fistulas may be very cellular and apparently atypical. This histologic pattern, together with the appearance of multiple lesions in several organs in patients with the Rendu-Osler-Weber syndrome, may mimic a malignant neoplasin, and one such case has been reported [47].

D. Solitary Chemodectoma of the Lung [48]

These tumors are briefly mentioned because of the previous allusion to multiple chemodectoma-like tumors. The histogenesis of these tumors is unknown, but, histologically, they closely resemble chemodectomas found in the more usual sites such as carotid body, glomus jugulare, retroperitoneum, and elsewhere. These tumors should be regarded as malignant, although only about 5% of them metastasize [15].

IV. Metastatic Tumors to the Pulmonary Vasculature

A. Lymphangitic Carcinoma

Every chest physician is familiar with the dramatic syndrome of lymphangitic cancer of the lung. About half of the patients are dead within 3 months of diagnosis; almost 90%, within 6 months [49]. The outlook is not invariably pessimistic, however, as one report indicated that 4 of 31 patients lived more than 2 years [50]. There is also a recent case report of complete clearing of the chest roentgenogram in a patient with biopsy-proven lymphangitic carcinoma, and the chest film remained normal for 18 months [51]. Thus, with modern chemotherapy, the prognosis may not be so dismal. There is extensive involvement of pleural and deep lymphatics in lymphangitic carcinoma of the lung. Pleural effusions are commonly seen, and on gross inspection there is a linear pattern of gray-white tumor filling and extending through the lymphatics. The cut surface of the lung shows a predominant linear pattern of tumor within the lung which involves the lobular septa in which the distal and perivenous lymphatics are to be found (Figs. 9 and 10). Similarly, linear tumor is found in the lymphatics of the bronchovascular sheath (Fig. 10). Most commonly, the tumor lies in columns or sheets 2 to 3 mm thick and nodules of various size are encountered along the course of the lymphatics. In perhaps 20 to 25% of cases, the lymphatics may be grossly normal at necropsy but histologic examination shows involvement of the lymphatics [52].

Most commonly, lymphangitic cancer is a complication of adenocarcinomas, with the primary sites being in the stomach, pancreas, breast, prostate, ovary, colon, and endometrium. However, cancers other than adenocarcinoma may cause lymphangitic carcinoma and cases with primary tumors in the bladder and esophagus have been described [52]. It has been stated that carcinoma of the cervix never produces lymphangitic carcinoma, but at least six cases have been reported [52-54]. The frequency of the primary tumor will depend on the community under study and the time that the study was done. Older reports emphasized carcinoma of the stomach, but at the present time perhaps nearly half of the cases in North America are due to carcinoma of the breast. Lymphangitic carcinoma is a fairly frequent complication of cancer of the breast and has been described in 24% of such patients [52]. In Japan, where carcinoma of the stomach is still frequent, one might anticipate that it is still a common cause of lymphangitic cancer.

The present view is that lymphangitic cancer is caused in the first instance by embolization to the branches of the pulmonary artery with subsequent invasion of the arterial wall. Extension into the adjacent lymphatics then occurs, with subsequent centripetal spread of the tumor. Evidence for this view is the great frequency with which tumor emboli can be found in the

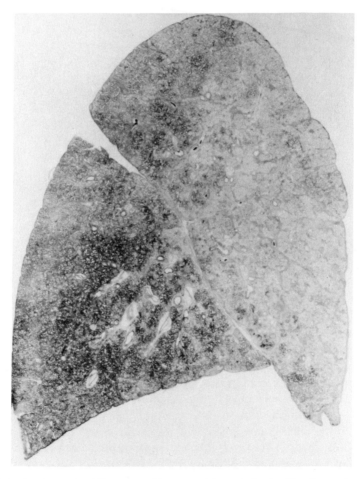

FIGURE 9 Increased linear markings are apparent in the lingular and upper lobes of this paper-mounted, whole-lung section.

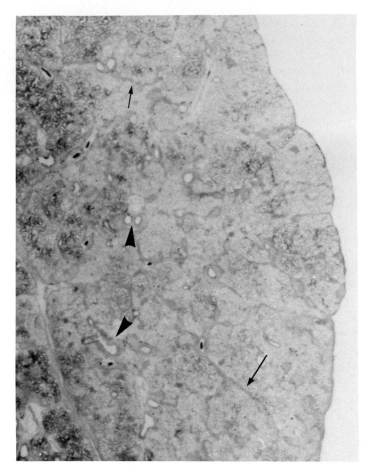

FIGURE 10   Tumor is seen in lymphatics and lobular septa (arrows) and in the bronchovascular sheath (arrowheads). Some tumor nodules are also apparent.

pulmonary arteries—in 20 of 23 cases in one series [52], including all the cases with the mildest involvement of the lung. In addition, extensive vascular obliteration is present in many cases, together with evidence of cor pulmonale. It is also true that there is usually evidence of systemic hematogenous spread of tumor to other organs in most patients with lymphangitic carcinoma. Involvement of the hilar lymph nodes, with retrograde spread of tumor, was once a popular theory. However, it is now apparent that the hilar nodes are often free of tumor; this may be true of as many as half of the cases, even on histologic examination of the lymph nodes [52].

The extensive lymphangitic anastomoses between the lymph nodes and lymph channels of the upper abdomen and the lymphatics of the lower lobes of the lung has suggested that this may be the route of spread in some instances, certainly carcinoma of the stomach and pancreas. The older literature stressed the importance of invasion of the thoracic duct by tumor, which could then lead to extensive intravascular tumor embolization. However, in the majority of reported instances, the thoracic duct is free of tumor.

There is good correlation between the appearance of the chest roentgenogram and the gross findings at necropsy [52]. The chest film is normal in about one-third of cases, but in these patients the tumor is either difficult or impossible to see grossly at necropsy. As tumor becomes more obvious grossly, so does the radiological abnormality. A nodular pattern on the chest film indicates severe involvement of the lung anatomically. The pattern seen radiologically is not just tumor in lymphatics, it is tumor in and around the lymphatics.

B. Metastases to the Lung of Malignant Vascular Tumors

Tumors of endothelial and perithelial origin may metastasize to the lung. This usually presents no diagnostic problem clinically since the primary vascular tumor generally has been identified previously. However, in some instances this may not be so and then debate may ensue whether the lesion is primary in the lung. Indeed, doubt has been expressed [4] whether the reported malignant hemangiomas of the lung were primary or secondary [40,41,45].

C. Kaposi's Sarcoma

It has been suggested that Kaposi's sarcoma may have the pericyte as the cell of origin [55]. Although primarily a dermatologic condition outside Africa, involvement of internal organs occurs in 10 to 20% of cases. Lung involvement is relatively uncommon and is usually not diagnosed during life. The lung involvement is usually in the form of multiple nodules throughout both lungs, but occasionally there may be massive involvement of an entire lung [56].

References

1. Liebow, A. A., and D. S. Hubbell, Sclerosing hemangioma (histiocytoma, xanthoma of the lung), *Cancer*, **9**:53–75 (1956).

2. Stout, A. P., and R. Lattes, Armed Forces Institute of Pathology Fascicle, *Pathology of Soft Tissue.* Washington, D.C., Armed Forces Institute of Pathology, 1966.

3. Thurlbeck, W. M., The lung–Structure, function and disease. In *International Academy of Pathology Monograph.* Edited by W. M. Thurlbeck and M. R. Abell. Baltimore, William & Wilkins, 1978, Chap. 16.

4. Spencer, H., *Pathology of the Lung (Excluding Pulmonary Tuberculosis),* 3rd ed. Oxford, New York, Toronto, Sydney, Paris, Frankfurt, Pergamon, Philadelphia, Toronto, Saunders, 1977.

5. Haas, J. E., E. J. Yunis, and R. S. Totten, Ultrastructure of a sclerosing hemangioma of the lung, *Cancer,* **30**:512–518 (1972).

6. Hill, G. S., and J. C. Eggleston, Electron microscopic study of so-called "pulmonary sclerosing hemangioma." Report of a case suggesting epithelial origin, *Cancer,* **30**:1092–1106 (1972).

7. Wada, A., R. Tateishi, T. Terazawa, M. Matsuba, and S. Hattosi, Case report: Lymphangioma of lung, *Arch. Pathol.,* **98**:211–213 (1974).

8. Corrin, B., A. A. Liebow, and P. J. Friedman, Pulmonary lymphangiomyomatosis. A Review, *Am. J. Pathol.,* **79**:348–382 (1975).

9. Joliat, G., H. Stalder, and Y. Kapanci, Lymphangiomyomatosis: A clinico-anatomical entity, *Cancer,* **31**:455–461 (1973).

10. Carrington, C. B., D. W. Cargell, E. A. Gaensler, A. Marks, R. A. Redding, J. T. Schaaf, and A. Tomasian, Lymphangiomyomatosis. Physiologic pathologic radiologic correlations, *Am. Rev. Respir. Dis.,* **116**:977–996 (1977).

11. Steffelaar, J. W., D. A. Nijkamp, and C. Hilvering, Pulmonary lymphangiomyomatosis. Demonstration of smooth muscle antigens by immunofluorescence technique, *Scand. J. Respir. Dis.,* **58**:103–109 (1977).

12. Vazquez, J. J., L. F. Fernandez-Cuervo, and B. Fidalgo, Lymphangiomyomatosis: Morphogenetic study and ultrastructural confirmation of the histogenesis of the lung lesion, *Cancer,* **35**:2321–2328 (1976).

13. Vadas, G., J. A. P. Paré, and W. M. Thurlbeck, Pulmonary and lymph node myomatosis: Review of the literature and report of a case, *Can. Med. Assoc. J.,* **96**:420–424 (1967).

14. Yater, W. M., J. Finnegan, and H. M. Griffin, Pulmonary arteriovenous fistula (varix); Review of the literature and report of 2 cases, *JAMA,* **141**:581–589 (1949).

15. Dines, D. E., R. A. Arms, P. E. Bernatz, and M. R. Gomes, Pulmonary arteriovenous fistulas, *Mayo Clin. Proc.,* **49**:460–465 (1974).

16. Sluiter-Eringa, H., N. G. M. Orie, and H. J. Sluiter, Pulmonary arteriovenous fistula. Diagnosis and prognosis of non-complainant patients, *Am. Rev. Respir. Dis.,* **100**:177–188 (1969).

17. Hodgson, C. H., and R. L. Kaye, Pulmonary arteriovenous fistula and hereditary hemorrhagic telangiectasia: A review and report of 35 cases of fistula, *Dis. Chest,* **43**:449–455 (1963).

18. Bosher, L. H., D. A. Blake, and B. R. Byrd, An analysis of the pathologic

anatomy of pulmonary arteriovenous aneurysms with particular reference to the applicability of local excision, *Surgery,* **45**:91–104 (1959).

19. Cooley, D. A., and D. G. McNamara, Pulmonary telangiectasia. Report of a case proved by pulmonary biopsy, *J. Thorac. Surg.,* **27**:614–622 (1953).

20. Rydell, R., and F. W. Hoffbauer, Multiple pulmonary arteriovenous fistulas in juvenile cirrhosis, *Am. J. Med.,* **21**:450–460 (1956).

21. Berthelot, P., J. G. Walker, S. Sherlock, and L. Reid, Arterial changes in the lungs in cirrhosis of the liver—lung spider nevi, *N. Engl. J. Med.,* **274**: 291–298 (1966).

22. Stout, A. P., and M. P. Murray, A vascular tumor featuring Zimmermann's pericytes, *Ann. Surg.,* **116**:26–33 (1942).

23. Kapanci, Y., P. M. Costabella, and G. Gabbiani, Location and function of contractile interstitial cells of the lungs. In *Lung Cells in Disease,* Proceedings of a Brook Lodge Conference, Augusta, Michigan, April 21 to 23, 1976. Edited by A. Bouhuys. Amsterdam, New York, Oxford, North-Holland, 1976, pp. 69–84.

24. Meade, J. B., F. Whitwell, B. J. Bickford, and J. K. B. Waddington, Primary hemangiopericytoma of the lung, *Thorax,* **29**:1–15 (1974).

25. Krishnan, M., C. Panicker, and W. M. C. Thomas, Malignant pulmonary hemangiopericytoma, *Aust. N.Z. J. Surg.,* **45**:157–159 (1975).

26. De Wet Lubbe, J. J., P. M. Barnard, and J. J. Van der Walt, Primary malignant hemangiopericytoma of the lung, *S. Afr. Med. J.,* **47**:2121–2122 (1973).

27. McMaster, M. J., E. H. Soule, and J. C. Ivins, Hemangiopericytoma: A clinicopathologic study and long-term followup of 60 patients, *Cancer,* **36**: 2232–2244 (1975).

28. Backwinkel, K. D., and J. A. Diddams, Hemangiopericytoma: Report of a case and comprehensive review of the literature, *Cancer,* **25**:896–901 (1970).

29. Thijs, L. G., J. A. Kroon, and T. M. Van Leeuwen, Leiomyosarcoma of the pulmonary trunk associated with pericardial effusion, *Thorax,* **29**:490–494 (1974).

30. Wang, N. S., T. A. Seemayer, M. N. Ahmed, and J. Morin, Pulmonary leiomyosarcoma associated with an arteriovenous fistula, *Arch. Pathol.,* **98**:100–105 (1974).

31. Kevorkian, J., and D. P. Cento, Leiomyosarcoma of large arteries and veins, *Surgery,* **73**:390–400 (1973).

32. Wackers, F. J. T., J. B. Van der Schoot, and J. F. Hampe, Sarcoma of the pulmonary trunk associated with hemorrhagic tendency. A case report and review of the literature, *Cancer,* **23**:339–351 (1969).

33. Jacques, J. E., and R. Barclay, The solid sarcomatous pulmonary artery, *Br. J. Dis. Chest,* **54**:217–220 (1960).

34. Wolf, P. L., R. C. Dickenman, and J. D. Langston, Fibrosarcoma of the pulmonary artery, masquerading as a pheochromocytoma, *Am. J. Clin. Pathol.,* **34**:146–154 (1960).

35. Green, J. R., L. E. Crevasse, and D. R. Shanklin, Fibromyxosarcoma of the pulmonary artery associated with syncope, intractable heart failure, polycythemia and thrombocytopenia, *Am. J. Cardiol.,* **13**:547–552 (1964).

36. Hagström, L., Malignant mesenchymoma in pulmonary artery and right ventricle. Report of a case with unusual location and histological picture, *Pathol. Microbiol. Scand.,* **51**:87–94 (1960).

37. Lowell, L. M., and J. E. Tuhy, Primary chondrosarcoma of the lung, *J. Thorac. Surg.,* **18**:476–483 (1949).

38. McConnell, T. H., Bony and cartilaginous tumors of the heart and great vessels. Report of an osteosarcoma of the pulmonary artery, *Cancer,* **25**: 611–617 (1970).

39. Baumann, E. P., and F. A. Bainbridge, Proceedings of the Pathological Society of London, *Lancet,* **1**:520 (1903).

40. Wollstein, M., Malignant hemangioma of the lung with multiple visceral foci, *Arch. Pathol.,* **12**:562–571 (1931).

41. Hall, E. M., A malignant hemangioma of the lung with multiple metastases, *Am. J. Pathol.,* **11**:343–352 (1935).

42. Plaut, A., Hemangioendothelioma of the lung. Report of two cases, *Arch. Pathol.,* **29**:517–529 (1940).

43. Barani, J. C., Un caso de angiosarcoma pulmonar, *Hoja Tisiol.,* **11**:245 (1951).

44. Case Records of the Massachusetts General Hospital, Case #40191, *N. Engl. J. Med.,* **250**:837–843 (1954).

45. Press, P., Hemangioendotheliosarcoma in the lung, *Pneumon. Coeur,* **14**: 932 (1958).

46. Tralka, G. A., and S. Katz, Hemangioendothelioma of the lung, *Am. Rev. Respir. Dis.,* **87**:107–115 (1963).

47. Powell, V., Pulmonary telangiectasis, *Thorax,* **13**:321–326 (1958).

48. Goodman, M. L., and E. G. Laforet, Solitary primary chemodectomas of the lung, *Chest,* **61**:48–50 (1972).

49. Yang, S. P., and C. C. Lin, Lymphangitic carcinomatosis of the lungs. The clinical significance of its roentgenologic classification, *Chest,* **62**:179–187 (1972).

50. Goldsmith, H. S., H. D. Bailey, and E. L. Callahan, Pulmonary lymphangitic metastases from breast carcinoma, *Arch. Surg.,* **94**:483–488 (1967).

51. Schimmel, D. H., P. J. Julien, and G. Gamsu, Resolution of pulmonary lymphangitic carcinoma of the breast, *Chest,* **69**:106–108 (1976).

52. Janower, M. L., and J. B. Blennerhassett, Lymphangitic spread of metastatic cancer to the lung. A radiologic-pathologic classification, *Radiology,* **101**:267–273 (1971).

53. Gilberg, K., and H. Rakowski, Pulmonary lymphangitic spread of cancer of the cervix, *N. Engl. J. Med.,* **289**:921 (1973).

54. Buchsbaum, H. J., Lymphangitic carcinomatosis secondary to carcinoma of the cervix, *Obstet. Gynecol.,* **36**:850–860 (1970).

55. Hashimoto, K., and W. F. Lever, Kaposi's sarcoma: Histochemical and electron microscopic studies, *J. Invest. Dermatol.,* **43**:539–549 (1964).
56. Dantzig, P. I., D. Richardson, S. Rayhanzadeh, J. Mauro, and R. Shoss, Thoracic involvement of non-African Kaposi's sarcoma, *Chest,* **66**:522–525 (1974).

AUTHOR INDEX

Numbers in brackets are reference numbers and indicate that an author's work is referred to although his name is not cited in the text. Italic numbers give the page on which the complete reference is listed.

A

Abad, J. M., 307[77], *334*

Abbott, C. J., 264[96], 265[96], *276*

Abbott, J. P., 586[121], 589[121], 594[121], 609[121], 610[121], *624*

Abdel-Fattah, M. M., 158[124], 159 [124], *225*, 323[127], *337*

Abelanet, R., 128[93], *223*

Abelmann, W. H., 121[55], 158, 200 [205], 201[205], 211[239], *221, 225, 229, 231*, 437[48], 457 [48], *483*

Abou-Zeina, A., 323[127], *337*

Abraham, A. S., 392[21], *422*

Abu-Nassar, H. J., 161[136], *225*

Adams, F. H., 291[41], 292[41], 321[41], 324[41], 328[41], *332*

Adams, P., Jr., 26[39], *99*, 122[62], *222*, 532[11], 537[32], 539– 541[32], 555[58], 559[64], *567, 568, 569, 570*

Adamson, J., 306[66], *333*

Adelstein, S. J., 352[26], *382*

Adhikari, P. K., 122[72], *222*

Adkins, P. C., 86[195], *108*

Agarwal, J. B., 324[137], *337*

Agustsson, M. H., 44[106], *103*, 545 [39], 548[39], *568*

Ahmed, M. N., 640[30], *647*

Ahmed, S. S., 308[85], *334*

Aikawa, M., 397[47], *424*

Aitchison, J. D., 581[79], *622*

Alazraki, N. P., 311[95], *335*

Albert, H. M., 89[203], *108*, 437 [50], *483*

Albrechtsen, O. K., 375[88], *385*

Alderson, P. O., 361[42], 364[42], *382*

Alexander, A. F., 394[32], *423*

Alexander, J. K., 161[136], *225*, 324[134], *337*

Alexander, J. M., 394[36], *423*

Alfenito, J. C., 306[67], *333*

Allan, W. S., 581[76], *621*

Allanby, K. D., 120[35], *220*

Alley, R. D., 62[149], *105*, 168 [152], 208[152], *226*

Alpert, J. S., 211[236], *231*, 309 [92], 329[158], *235, 339*

Altura, B. M., 250[53], *274*, 393 [26], *423*

651

SUBJECT INDEX

A